Essentials of Veterinary Immunology and Immunopathology

Ramswaroop Singh Chauhan •
Yashpal Singh Malik • M. Saminathan •
Bhupendra Nath Tripathi

Essentials of Veterinary Immunology and Immunopathology

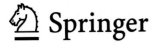

Ramswaroop Singh Chauhan
College of Veterinary & Animal Sciences
Govind Ballabh Pant University of
Agriculture & Technology
Pantnagar, Uttarakhand, India

Yashpal Singh Malik
College of Animal Biotechnology
Guru Angad Dev Veterinary and Animal
Sciences University
Ludhiana, Punjab, India

M. Saminathan
Centre for Animal Disease Research
and Diagnosis
ICAR-Indian Veterinary
Research Institute
Bareilly, Uttar Pradesh, India

Bhupendra Nath Tripathi
Sher-e-Kashmir University of Agriculture &
Technology of Jammu
Jammu, J & K, India

ISBN 978-981-99-2717-3 ISBN 978-981-99-2718-0 (eBook)
https://doi.org/10.1007/978-981-99-2718-0

© The Editor(s) (if applicable) and The Author(s), under exclusive license to Springer Nature Singapore Pte Ltd. 2024
This work is subject to copyright. All rights are solely and exclusively licensed by the Publisher, whether the whole or part of the material is concerned, specifically the rights of translation, reprinting, reuse of illustrations, recitation, broadcasting, reproduction on microfilms or in any other physical way, and transmission or information storage and retrieval, electronic adaptation, computer software, or by similar or dissimilar methodology now known or hereafter developed.
The use of general descriptive names, registered names, trademarks, service marks, etc. in this publication does not imply, even in the absence of a specific statement, that such names are exempt from the relevant protective laws and regulations and therefore free for general use.
The publisher, the authors, and the editors are safe to assume that the advice and information in this book are believed to be true and accurate at the date of publication. Neither the publisher nor the authors or the editors give a warranty, expressed or implied, with respect to the material contained herein or for any errors or omissions that may have been made. The publisher remains neutral with regard to jurisdictional claims in published maps and institutional affiliations.

This Springer imprint is published by the registered company Springer Nature Singapore Pte Ltd.
The registered company address is: 152 Beach Road, #21-01/04 Gateway East, Singapore 189721, Singapore

Foreword

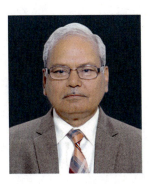

It is an esteemed privilege for me to write the foreword for the publication titled "Essentials of Veterinary Immunology and Immunopathology," authored by Prof RS Chauhan, Dr YPS Malik, Dr M. Saminathan, and Dr BN Tripathi. The field of immunopathology stands witness to rapid and remarkable advancements, underscoring the imperative of staying abreast with contemporary developments to harness them for fundamental and applied research within one's respective domains.Immunopathology has undergone substantial evolution over the past few decades, driven by ground breaking technological innovations and extensive investigative pursuits. This branch of science is poised for further expansion, as immunopathologists delve into the intricate dynamics of disease response in humans and animals, the aberrations within the immune system, and the genesis and potential remediation of immunopathological maladies. Our comprehension of immunopathology continues to evolve, elucidating how the body's immune mechanisms operate during safeguarding against infections and bodily systems implicated in immunopathogenic disorders.

The book covers pivotal subjects, including fundamental immunological concepts, biomarkers pertinent to immunopathology in veterinary medicine, hyper-reactive responses, autoimmune phenomena, immune insufficiencies, modulation of immune processes, immunopathological manifestations across diverse animal ailments, immunopathological disorders affecting different animal species, techniques in immunopathological analysis, and pivotal molecular biology techniques integral to veterinary diagnostics. To add specifically, the inclusion of detailed insights into immunological strategies employed to tackle the challenges posed by the COVID-19 pandemic enhances the relevance of the publication in the context of recent global health events. This rich repository of knowledge is meticulously crafted to cater comprehensively to the needs of students, academics, scientists, researchers, diagnostic practitioners, field veterinarians, medical professionals, and healthcare experts.

I convey my heartfelt appreciation to the authors for their stellar contributions, as their endeavour aptly consolidates the scattered knowledge pertaining to immunopathology into a coherent narrative. I am confident that this publication will emerge as a valuable resource of pertinent information for scholars, educators, and students alike. I wish to compliment the efforts made by the editors in this regard.

Uttar Pradesh Pandit Deen Dayal Upadhyaya G. K. Singh
Pashu Chikitsa Vigyan Vishwavidyalaya Evam
Go-Anusandhan Sansthan
Mathura, Uttar Pradesh, India

Contents

1	**Basic Concepts in Immunology**		1
	1.1	Natural or Paraspecific Immunity	2
	1.2	Acquired or Specific Immunity	3
	1.3	Humoral Immunity	3
		1.3.1 Immunoglobulin G (IgG)	4
		1.3.2 Immunoglobulin M (IgM)	6
		1.3.3 Immunoglobulin A (IgA)	6
		1.3.4 Immunoglobulin E (IgE)	6
		1.3.5 Immunoglobulin D (IgD)	7
	1.4	Cell-Mediated Immunity	7
	1.5	Immune Response	8
	1.6	Cells of the Immune System	9
		1.6.1 Lymphoid Channel	9
		1.6.2 Myeloid Channel	11
	1.7	Cytokines	20
		1.7.1 Interferons	20
		1.7.2 Interleukins	21
		1.7.3 Tumor Necrosis Factor (Cytotoxins)	25
		1.7.4 Colony-Stimulating Factor	26
		1.7.5 Migration Inhibitory Factor	26
	Further Reading		30
2	**Biomarkers of Immunopathology in Veterinary Medicine**		31
	2.1	Introduction	32
	2.2	Specific Cells of the Innate Immune System	33
		2.2.1 Neutrophils	33
		2.2.2 Monocytes	36
		2.2.3 Lymphocytes	37
	2.3	Receptors for Microbial Ligands	38
		2.3.1 Transmembrane PRRs	39
		2.3.2 Cytosolic PRRs	39
	2.4	Inflammatory Mediators	39
		2.4.1 Cytokines	40

		2.4.2	Interleukins	41
		2.4.3	Chemokines	41
	2.5	Anti-microbial Molecules		42
		2.5.1	Complement	42
		2.5.2	Lysozyme	42
		2.5.3	Anti-microbial Peptides	43
		2.5.4	Cathelicidins	43
		2.5.5	Defensins	43
		2.5.6	Collectins	44
	2.6	Conclusion		44
	References			45
3	**Hypersensitivity**			**49**
	3.1	Hypersensitivity		50
	3.2	Type I Hypersensitivity		52
		3.2.1	Components of Type I Hypersensitivity	52
		3.2.2	Mediators of Type I Hypersensitivity Reaction	57
		3.2.3	Clinical Manifestations	58
		3.2.4	Detection of Type I Hypersensitivity	63
	3.3	Type II Hypersensitivity		64
		3.3.1	Mechanism of Type II Hypersensitivity	65
		3.3.2	Type II Hypersensitivity to Drugs	72
		3.3.3	Type II Hypersensitivity in Infectious Diseases	72
	3.4	Type III Hypersensitivity		72
		3.4.1	Serum Sickness	74
		3.4.2	Autoimmune Complex Disease	76
		3.4.3	Arthus Reaction	76
		3.4.4	Diseases Associated with Immune Complexes	76
		3.4.5	Pathogenesis	77
		3.4.6	Clinical Findings	78
		3.4.7	Lesions	78
	3.5	Type IV Hypersensitivity		81
		3.5.1	The Tuberculin Reaction	81
		3.5.2	Johnin Reaction	85
		3.5.3	Other Intracellular Pathogens Showing DTH	85
		3.5.4	Allergic Contact Dermatitis	86
		3.5.5	Detection of Type IV Hypersensitivity	86
	Further Reading			87
4	**Autoimmunity**			**89**
	4.1	General Concept		90
	4.2	Mechanism of Induction		91
		4.2.1	Physiological Autoimmunity	91
		4.2.2	Pathological Autoimmunity	91
		4.2.3	Mechanisms of Tissue Injury	95

	4.3	Autoimmune Diseases	96
		4.3.1 Systemic Autoimmune Diseases	96
		4.3.2 Autoimmune Ocular Disease	117
	References		117
		Further Reading	118
5	**Immunodeficiency**		121
	5.1	Immunodeficiency	122
		5.1.1 Congenital Immunodeficiency	122
		5.1.2 Acquired Immunodeficiency	126
	5.2	Diagnosis of Immunodeficiency	138
	Further Reading		139
6	**Immunomodulation**		143
	6.1	Immunomodulation	144
	6.2	Need of Immunomodulation	144
	6.3	Physiological Products	146
		6.3.1 Neuroendocrine Hormones	146
	6.4	Neuropeptides	147
	6.5	Growth Hormone and Prolactin	149
	6.6	Opioid Peptides	149
	6.7	Thymic Products	150
	6.8	Cytokines	151
	6.9	Microbial Products	151
		6.9.1 *P. acnes* (Corynebacterium Parvum)	151
	6.10	Lentinan	155
	6.11	Probiotics	155
	6.12	Chemical Compounds	156
		6.12.1 Levamisole	157
		6.12.2 Thiabendazole	158
		6.12.3 Imuthiol	158
		6.12.4 Isoprinosine	158
		6.12.5 Indomethacin	158
		6.12.6 Ascorbic Acid Derivatives	159
		6.12.7 Dihydroheptaprenol	159
	6.13	Adjuvants	159
	6.14	Herbal Products	161
	6.15	Vitamins	165
	6.16	Cow Therapy	166
	References		167
7	**Immunopathology of Pneumonia in Animals**		169
	7.1	Introduction	170
	7.2	Ruminants	173
	7.3	Mycoplasmal Diseases	181
	7.4	Peste des Petits Ruminants (PPR)	182

	7.5	Chlamydiosis	183
	7.6	Parainfluenza-3	183
	7.7	Equines	183
	7.8	Swine	183
	7.9	Porcine Reproductive and Respiratory Syndrome (PRRS)	184
	7.10	Swine Influenza	184
	7.11	Other Diseases	185
	7.12	Small Animals	185
	7.13	Immunity to Pneumonia	186
	7.14	Innate Immunity	188
	7.15	Adaptive Immunity	192
		7.15.1 Humoral Immunity	192
	7.16	Cell-Mediated Immunity	193
	7.17	Immunodeficiency in Animals	197
		7.17.1 Congenital Immunodeficiency	197
		7.17.2 Acquired Immunodeficiency	198
	7.18	Immunomodulation	198
	7.19	Evasion Strategies of Microbes	199
	7.20	Evasion from Innate Immune Responses	199
		7.20.1 Interference with the Physical Barrier	199
		7.20.2 Interference with Phagocytosis by Predisposing Factors and Pathogens	199
		7.20.3 Effects of Predisposing Factors and Pathogens on the Production of Innate Defense Molecules	200
		7.20.4 Effects on Receptors on the Surface of Airway Epithelial Cells and Cell Signal Transduction	201
		7.20.5 Interference with Intracellular Killing	202
		7.20.6 Interference with IFN System	202
	7.21	Evasion of Adaptive Immune Response	203
		7.21.1 Infection of Leukocytes and Suppression of Proliferation	203
		7.21.2 Suppression of Proliferation of Leukocytes	203
		7.21.3 Infection of Cells of the Immune System	203
		7.21.4 Induction of Humoral and Cellular Immune Tolerance	203
		7.21.5 Inhibition of Antibody Activity	204
		7.21.6 Interference with Cytotoxic T-Lymphocyte Response	204
	7.22	Conclusion	204
	References		205
8	**Immunopathology of the Liver in Animals**		**217**
	8.1	Introduction	218
	8.2	Anatomy of the Liver	218
	8.3	Histology of the Liver	218

	8.4	The Bile Duct System and Gallbladder	219
	8.5	Cells of the Liver	219
	8.6	Blood Supply and Bile Flow	220
	8.7	Immunopathology of the Liver	220
	8.8	Types and Patterns of Cell Death in the Liver	222
	8.9	Necrosis	222
	8.10	Apoptosis	225
	8.11	Autoimmune Hepatitis (AIH)	226
	8.12	Key Inflammatory Pathways in the Development of AIH	226
	8.13	Immunopathology of Infectious Diseases Affecting the Liver	227
		8.13.1 Infectious Canine Hepatitis	227
	8.14	Wesselsbron Disease	230
	8.15	Rift Valley Fever	231
	8.16	Lymphoid Leukosis in Poultry	232
	8.17	Marek's Disease in Poultry	234
	8.18	Leptospirosis	236
	8.19	*Fusobacterium necrophorum*	238
	8.20	Trematodes	240
	8.21	*Cysticercus fasciolaris*	244
	8.22	*Lantana camara* toxicity	244
	8.23	Conclusion	246
	References	247
9	**Immunopathology of Diarrhea in Animals**	253
	9.1	Introduction	254
	9.2	Etiology	255
	9.3	Classification of Diarrhea	258
		9.3.1 Acute Diarrhea	259
		9.3.2 Persistent Diarrhea (PD)	259
		9.3.3 Chronic Diarrhea	259
		9.3.4 Small Bowel Diarrhea	259
		9.3.5 Large Bowel Diarrhea	260
		9.3.6 Osmotic Diarrhea	261
		9.3.7 Secretory Diarrhea	261
		9.3.8 Exudative Diarrhea	261
	9.4	Pathogenesis of Diarrhea	262
		9.4.1 Bacterial Pathogens of Diarrhea	262
	9.5	*Escherichia coli*	262
	9.6	Enteropathogenic *E. coli* (EPEC)	263
	9.7	Enterotoxigenic *E. coli* (ETEC)	263
	9.8	Enterohemorrhagic *E. coli* (EHEC)	263
	9.9	Enteroadherent or Enteroaggregative *E. coli* (EAEC)	264
	9.10	Enteroinvasive *E. coli* (EIEC)	264
		9.10.1 *Shigella*	264
		9.10.2 *Salmonella*	265

		9.10.3	*Clostridium*	266
	9.11	Viral Pathogens of Diarrhea		267
		9.11.1	Rotavirus	267
		9.11.2	Bovine Viral Diarrhea (BVD)	268
		9.11.3	Coronavirus	269
		9.11.4	Norovirus	269
	9.12	Diarrhea due to Intestinal Parasites		270
		9.12.1	Giardia	270
		9.12.2	*Cryptosporidium*	271
		9.12.3	Trichuris	271
		9.12.4	Strongyloides	271
		9.12.5	Traveler's Diarrhea (TD)	271
	9.13	Chemical Mediators Influencing the Intestinal Motility		272
		9.13.1	Serotonin	272
		9.13.2	Prostaglandins	272
		9.13.3	Claudin	273
		9.13.4	Nutrition and Diarrhea	274
	9.14	Immunity		276
	9.15	Diagnosis		277
		9.15.1	Prevention and Prophylaxis	279
		9.15.2	Public Health	280
	9.16	Conclusion		281
	References			282
10	**Immunopathology of Reproductive Disorders of Animals**			**293**
	10.1	Introduction		293
	10.2	Uterine Function		295
	10.3	Innate Immune Defense of the Uterus		296
	10.4	Adaptive Immune Defense of the Uterus		298
		10.4.1	Humoral Immunity	298
		10.4.2	Cell-Mediated Immunity	298
	10.5	Anatomical and Physiological Barriers Against Uterine Infections		299
	10.6	Prevalence of Uterine Infections		299
	10.7	Risk Factors Associated with Uterine Infections		299
	10.8	Abortion		300
	10.9	Etiology of Abortion		300
	10.10	Immunopathology of Abortions		301
	10.11	Brucellosis		310
	10.12	Mycotic Abortion in Cattle and Sheep		313
	10.13	Listeriosis		314
	10.14	Trichomoniasis		316
	10.15	Neosporosis		320
	10.16	Campylobacteriosis		321
	10.17	Leptospirosis		324

		10.18	Bluetongue Virus	327
		10.19	Infectious Bovine Rhinotracheitis	330
		10.20	Bovine Herpesvirus 4 Infection	333
		10.21	Epizootic/Enzootic Abortions	334
		10.22	Toxoplasmosis	337
		10.23	Bovine Viral Diarrhea	341
		10.24	Equine Viral Arteritis	344
		10.25	Conclusion	348
		References		349
11	**Immunopathology of Mastitis**			373
	11.1	Introduction		373
	11.2	Mastitis-Causing Pathogens		374
		11.2.1	Bacteria	374
		11.2.2	Viruses	377
	11.3	Immune Responses		383
	11.4	Host-Pathogen Interactions		384
	11.5	Mammary Immunology		385
	11.6	Physical and Chemical Barriers of the Teat		385
	11.7	Endogenous Defenses		386
	11.8	Lactoferrin		386
	11.9	Complement		387
	11.10	Cytokines		387
	11.11	Eicosanoids		388
	11.12	Immunoglobulins		389
	11.13	Pattern Recognition Receptors (PRRs)		389
	11.14	Inflammation		391
	11.15	Mammary Vascular Endothelium		391
	11.16	Localized Cellular Components of Inflammation		392
		11.16.1	Epithelial Cells	392
		11.16.2	Somatic Cells	393
	11.17	Immunopathogenesis		394
	11.18	Conclusion		397
	References			398
12	**Immunopathological Disorders of Kidneys**			405
	12.1	Introduction		405
	12.2	Glomerulonephritis		406
	12.3	Type I Membranoproliferative Glomerulonephritis		406
	12.4	Type II Membranoproliferative Glomerulonephritis		409
	12.5	Type III Membranoproliferative Glomerulonephritis		410
	12.6	Crescentic Glomerulonephritis		410
	12.7	IgA Nephropathy		411
	12.8	Postinfection Glomerulonephritis		412
	12.9	Conclusion		413

	References	414
13	**Immunopathological Disorders of Joints**	**417**
13.1	Introduction	417
13.2	Normal Cartilage, Joint Capsule, and Synovium	420
13.3	Synovium Function	421
13.4	Rheumatoid Arthritis	422
13.5	Immunopathological Mechanisms of Rheumatoid Arthritis	422
13.6	Immune-Mediated Inflammation in Rheumatoid Arthritis	423
13.7	Role of Interleukin-7 in Immunopathology of Rheumatoid Arthritis	425
13.8	Immune Target Therapy and Ongoing Immune-Modulated Therapy in Rheumatoid Arthritis	425
13.9	Psoriatic Arthritis	426
13.10	Caprine Arthritis Encephalitis Virus-Induced Arthritis	427
13.11	Temporomandibular Joint Destruction (TMJD)	427
13.12	Spondyloarthritis (SpA)	428
13.13	Ankylosing Spondylitis	429
13.14	Summary	430
	References	430
14	**Immunopathology of Skin Ailments**	**435**
14.1	Introduction	435
14.2	Cellular Components of the Skin	437
	14.2.1 Keratinocytes	437
	14.2.2 Melanocytes	438
	14.2.3 Langerhans Cell	438
	14.2.4 Macrophage	441
	14.2.5 Mast Cells	441
14.3	Mechanism Regulating Immune-Mediated Skin Injury	441
14.4	Allergic Contact Dermatitis	442
14.5	Pemphigus Foliaceus	443
14.6	Vitiligo	443
14.7	Canine Atopic Dermatitis (CAD)	446
14.8	Flea Allergy Dermatitis (FAD)	446
14.9	Chediak-Higashi Syndrome	447
14.10	Discoid Lupus Erythematosus (DLE)	448
14.11	Conclusion	448
	References	449
15	**Immunological Interventions for the Management of Coronavirus Disease 2019 (COVID-19)**	**453**
15.1	Introduction	454
15.2	Etiology	455
15.3	Transmission of COVID-19	455
15.4	Predisposing Factors	456

	15.5	Clinical Manifestations	457
		15.5.1 Pathology	457
		15.5.2 Clinical Pathology	458
		15.5.3 Diagnosis	459
	15.6	Immunological Interventions for the Management of COVID-19	460
	15.7	Immunological Interventions	460
		15.7.1 Convalescent Plasma Therapy	460
		15.7.2 Antagonists of Interleukin 6 Receptor (IL-6R) and IL-6	461
		15.7.3 Blockade of the IL-1 Pathway	461
		15.7.4 Inhibition of Janus Kinases (JAK)	461
		15.7.5 Recombinant Soluble ACE2	462
		15.7.6 Inhibition of Granulocyte Macrophage Colony-Stimulating Factor Receptor (GM-CSF-R)	462
		15.7.7 Stem Cell Therapy	463
		15.7.8 Corticosteroids	463
		15.7.9 Remdesivir	463
		15.7.10 Chloroquine Phosphate and Hydroxychloroquine	464
		15.7.11 Ivermectin	464
		15.7.12 Umifenovir (Arbidol)	465
		15.7.13 Low Molecular Weight Heparin (LMWH)	465
		15.7.14 Nonsteroidal Anti-inflammatory Drugs (NSAIDs)	465
		15.7.15 Anticancer Drugs	465
		15.7.16 Other Antiviral Compounds	466
		15.7.17 CRISPR-Based Tools	466
	15.8	Vaccines Against COVID-19	466
	15.9	Plant-Based Vaccines to Combat COVID-19	473
	15.10	Control Strategies	474
	15.11	Role of Artificial Intelligence in Controlling COVID-19 Spread	475
	15.12	One Health Approach to Counter Future Pandemics of SARS-CoV-2	475
	15.13	Conclusion	476
		References	476
16	**Immunopathology of Parasitic Diseases of Animals**		**483**
	16.1	Introduction	483
	16.2	Innate Immunity Against Parasites	484
	16.3	Parasites Recognition	484
	16.4	Adaptive Immunity to Parasites	485
	16.5	Protozoa Induced Adaptive Immunity	485
	16.6	Helminths Induced Adaptive Immunity	486
	16.7	Evasion of Immune Responses by Parasites	487
	16.8	Trichomoniasis	488

16.9	Neosporosis	489
16.10	Toxoplasmosis	491
16.11	Fasciolosis	493
16.12	*Spirocerca lupi*	495
16.13	*Cysticercus fasciolaris*	497
16.14	Diarrheal Parasites	499
16.15	Conclusion	499
	References	500

17 Immunopathological Disorders of Cattle and Buffalo 505

17.1	Introduction	506
17.2	Immunodeficiency	507
17.3	Primary Immunodeficiency	507
17.4	Chediak-Higashi Syndrome	507
17.5	Bovine Leukocyte Adhesion Deficiency	508
17.6	Transient Hypogammaglobulinemia	508
17.7	Acquired Immunodeficiency	508
17.8	Bovine Viral Diarrhea Virus	509
17.9	Bovine Immunodeficiency Virus Infection	510
17.10	Bovine Herpes Virus Infection	511
17.11	Hypersensitivity Reactions	511
17.12	Type I Hypersensitivity	513
17.13	Allergic Rhinitis	513
17.14	Acute Systemic Anaphylaxis	513
17.15	Milk Allergy	514
17.16	Insect Bite Allergy	514
17.17	Type II Hypersensitivity	514
17.18	Hemolytic Disease of Newborn Calf	515
17.19	Type III Hypersensitivity	515
17.20	Serum Sickness	516
17.21	Arthus Reaction	517
17.22	Immune Complex-Mediated Glomerulonephritis	517
17.23	Type IV Hypersensitivity	517
17.24	Tuberculin Reaction	518
17.25	Johnin Reaction	519
17.26	Allergic Contact Dermatitis	520
17.27	Autoimmunity	520
17.28	Vitiligo	521
17.29	Conclusion	521
	References	521

18 Immunopathological Disorders in Sheep, Goat, Wild Animals, and Laboratory Animals 525

18.1	Introduction	526

18.2	Hypersensitivity Reactions in Sheep, Goat, Wild Animals, and Laboratory Animals	527
18.3	Type I Hypersensitivity	527
18.4	Acute Systemic Anaphylaxis	527
18.5	Allergic Rhinitis	528
18.6	Type II Hypersensitivity	528
18.7	Blood Groups	529
	18.7.1 Sheep	529
	18.7.2 Goat	529
18.8	Blood Transfusion Reaction	529
18.9	Hemolytic Diseases	530
18.10	Type III Hypersensitivity	530
18.11	Sheep	530
18.12	Rabbit	531
18.13	Type IV Hypersensitivity	531
18.14	Immunodeficiency in Sheep, Goat, Wild Animals, and Laboratory Animals	533
18.15	Primary Immunodeficiency/Congenital Immunodeficiency	533
18.16	Severe Combined Immunodeficiency Disease (SCID)	533
18.17	Transient Hypogammaglobulinemia in Lamb	534
18.18	Secondary Immunodeficiency/Acquired Immunodeficiency	534
18.19	Bluetongue Disease	534
18.20	Border Disease	535
18.21	Jaagsiekte Disease	535
18.22	Feline Leukemia Virus	536
18.23	Mouse Mammary Tumor Virus	536
18.24	Feline Immunodeficiency Virus	536
	18.24.1 Simian Immunodeficiency Virus Infection	536
	18.24.2 Murine Leukemia Virus	537
18.25	Autoimmunity	537
18.26	Pemphigus Foliaceus	537
18.27	Autoimmune Hemolytic Anemia (AIHA)	537
18.28	Orf-Induced Autoimmunity	538
18.29	Johne's Disease	538
18.30	Autoimmune Disease in a Polar Bear	538
18.31	Conclusion	538
	References	539
19	**Immunopathological Disorders in Swine and Equine**	**543**
19.1	Introduction	544
19.2	Hypersensitivity	544
19.3	Type I Hypersensitivity	544
19.4	Pathogenesis of Type I Hypersensitivity	545
19.5	Clinical Manifestation of Type I Hypersensitivity	546
	19.5.1 Diagnosis	548

19.6	Type II Hypersensitivity and Its Pathogenesis		548
19.7	Clinical Manifestation of Type II Hypersensitivity Reaction		548
	19.7.1	Diagnosis	550
19.8	Type III Hypersensitivity and Its Pathogenesis		550
	19.8.1	Clinical Manifestation of Type III Hypersensitivity Reaction	550
	19.8.2	Diagnosis	551
19.9	Type IV Hypersensitivity and Its Pathogenesis		551
	19.9.1	Clinical Manifestation of Type IV Hypersensitivity Reaction	552
	19.9.2	Diagnosis	552
19.10	Immunodeficiency Diseases		552
19.11	Primary Immunodeficiency Diseases		553
	19.11.1	Secondary Immunodeficiency Diseases	554
19.12	Autoimmune Disorders		555
19.13	Clinical Manifestation of the Autoimmune Disorders		555
19.14	Conclusion		558
References			558

20 Immunopathological Disorders of Pet Animals 563

20.1	Introduction		563
20.2	Immunopathology		564
20.3	Types of Hypersensitivity		564
20.4	Disease Related to Type 1 Hypersensitivity		564
	20.4.1	Anaphylactic Shock	564
	20.4.2	Urticaria and Angioedema	565
	20.4.3	Canine Atopic Dermatitis	565
	20.4.4	Flea Allergy Dermatitis (Flea Bite Hypersensitivity)	565
20.5	Type 2 Hypersensitivity		566
20.6	Disease Related to Type 2 Hypersensitivity		566
	20.6.1	Incompatible Blood Transfusion	566
20.7	Type 3 Hypersensitivity		566
20.8	Disease Related to Type 3 Hypersensitivity		568
	20.8.1	Serum Sickness	568
	20.8.2	Arthus Reaction	568
	20.8.3	Glomerulonephritis	568
	20.8.4	Type 4 Hypersensitivity	568
20.9	Disease Related to Type 4 Hypersensitivity		569
	20.9.1	Allergic Contact Dermatitis	569
20.10	Autoimmune Diseases		570
20.11	Autoimmune Diseases of the Pet Animals		570
	20.11.1	Systemic Lupus Erythematosus	570
	20.11.2	Rheumatoid Arthritis	570
	20.11.3	Autoimmune Thyroiditis	571

		20.11.4	Myasthenia Gravis	571
	20.12	Immunodeficiency		571
	20.13	Disorder Related to Primary Immunodeficiency		572
		20.13.1	Severe Combined Immunodeficiency Syndrome (SCID)	572
		20.13.2	Lethal Acrodermatitis	572
		20.13.3	Chediak-Higashi Syndrome	572
	20.14	Disorder Related to Secondary Immunodeficiency		572
		20.14.1	Canine Parvovirus Infection	572
		20.14.2	Canine Distemper	573
		20.14.3	Drug Therapy Defects	573
	References			573
21	**Techniques in Immunopathology**			**577**
	21.1	Collection of Blood and Serum		578
	21.2	Leucocyte Count		579
		21.2.1	Total Leucocyte Count (TLC)	579
		21.2.2	Differential Leucocyte Count (DLC)	580
		21.2.3	Absolute Lymphocyte Count (ALC)	580
		21.2.4	Absolute Neutrophil Count (ANC)	581
	21.3	Collection of Lymphoid Cells		583
		21.3.1	Blood	583
		21.3.2	Prescapular Lymph Node	584
		21.3.3	Mesenteric Lymph Nodes	584
		21.3.4	Mucosa-Associated Lymphoid Tissue (MALT)	584
		21.3.5	Respiratory-Associated Lymphoid Tissue (RALT)	585
		21.3.6	Spleen	586
	21.4	Lymphocyte Blastogenesis Assay		586
	21.5	Macrophage Function Test		587
		21.5.1	Nitroblue Tetrazolium Test	587
		21.5.2	Bactericidal Activity	588
	21.6	Delayed-Type Hypersensitivity (DTH) Reaction		588
		21.6.1	Allergens	589
		21.6.2	Tuberculin Test	589
		21.6.3	Johnin Test	589
		21.6.4	Mallein Test	590
		21.6.5	DNCB-/DNFB-Induced DTH Reaction	590
	21.7	Gamma Globulins in Serum		592
	21.8	Measurement of Antibody Titer		594
		21.8.1	Enzyme-Linked Immunosorbent Assay (ELISA)	594
	21.9	Dot Immunobinding Assay (DIA)		597
	21.10	Agglutination Test		599
	21.11	Immunofluorescence Techniques		599
		21.11.1	Direct Method	600
		21.11.2	Indirect Method	600

	21.12	Immunoperoxidase Techniques (IPT)................	600
		21.12.1 Antigen Detection........................	602
		21.12.2 Enumeration of T and B Cells..............	605
	21.13	Peroxidase Antiperoxidase (PAP) Techniques...........	607
	21.14	Avidin-Biotin Complex Techniques..................	609
		21.14.1 Enzyme-Labeled Avidin-Biotin Method........	610
		21.14.2 Bridged Avidin-Biotin Method..............	610
		21.14.3 Avidin-Biotin Complex Method.............	610
	21.15	Detection of Immune Complex.....................	611
		21.15.1 Kidneys.............................	611
		21.15.2 Serum..............................	615
	21.16	Microscopic Evaluation of Lymphoid Organs...........	615
		21.16.1 Processing of Tissues....................	615
		21.16.2 Staining.............................	618
	21.17	Evaluation of Xenobiotics........................	619
		21.17.1 Humoral Immune Response................	619
		21.17.2 Cell-Mediated Immune Response............	620
	References..		621
22	**Molecular Biology Techniques of Pivotal Importance in Veterinary Diagnostics**.................................		**623**
	22.1	Polymerase Chain Reaction (PCR)..................	624
		22.1.1 Principle.............................	624
		22.1.2 Ingredients...........................	624
		22.1.3 Primers..............................	625
	22.2	Taq DNA Polymerase...........................	625
		22.2.1 Three Stages in PCR.....................	625
		22.2.2 Applications of PCR.....................	626
	22.3	Microarray...................................	627
		22.3.1 Principle.............................	627
		22.3.2 Types of Microarrays....................	627
		22.3.3 DNA Microarray.......................	628
		22.3.4 Applications of Microarrays................	628
	22.4	Lateral Flow (Immuno) Assay......................	628
		22.4.1 Principle.............................	628
		22.4.2 Parts of LFA Device.....................	628
		22.4.3 Material of the Sample Pad................	630
		22.4.4 Optimization..........................	631
		22.4.5 Diagnostic Applications...................	631
		22.4.6 Advantages of LFA.....................	631
	22.5	Complement Fixation Test........................	631
		22.5.1 Principle.............................	632
		22.5.2 Procedure............................	632
		22.5.3 Interpretation of Results..................	632
		22.5.4 Detection of Antigen.....................	633

	22.5.5	Quantitative Testing	633
	22.5.6	Applications of CFT	633
22.6	High-Performance Liquid Chromatography (HPLC)		634
	22.6.1	Principle	634
	22.6.2	Types of HPLC	634
	22.6.3	Procedure	635
	22.6.4	Applications of HPLC	636
22.7	Confocal Microscopy		636
	22.7.1	Principle	636
	22.7.2	Applications of Confocal Microscope	637
	22.7.3	Advantages of Confocal Microscopy	638
	22.7.4	Cons of Confocal Microscope	638
22.8	Fluorescence-Activated Cell Sorting (FACS)		638
	22.8.1	Principle	638
	22.8.2	Mechanism of FACS	639
	22.8.3	Procedure	639
	22.8.4	Quantifying the FACS Data	640
	22.8.5	Clinical Applications	642
22.9	CRISPR/Cas9 Technology		642
	22.9.1	CRISPR as the Genome-Editing Technology	642
	22.9.2	Different CRISPR Systems and Their Uses in Genome Editing	643
	22.9.3	Utilizing CRISPR-Cas9 Beyond Genome Editing	644
22.10	Conclusion		644
References			645

About the Authors

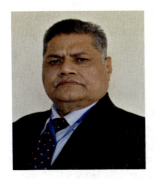

Ramswaroop Singh Chauhan born on September 10, 1958 and did Bachelors with Honors, Master and Doctoral Degrees in veterinary sciences with specialization in Veterinary Pathology from G.B. Pant University of Agriculture & Technology, Pantnagar. He served in various capacities as National Fellow, and Joint Director (CADRAD), ICAR-IVRI, Izatnagar, Director and Vice-Chancellor (Acting), ICAR-IVRI and Campus Director, IBT, Patwadangar. He has written 101 books including 35 manuals and 1 monograph. He has contributed 99 chapters in different books and published 231 research and 59 review papers. He also popularized science among the common man by publishing 346 semi-technical articles including 19 pamphlets. He is life member of several prestigious scientific bodies and has been in several executive committee. He has been awarded with several prizes, medals, and honors including Best Young Scientist Award (1992), IAAVR Award (1996), National Fellow Award (1999), Fellow NAVS (2000), Fellow SIIP (2001), K.S. Nair Memorial Award (1999), Vigyan Bharti Award (2000), Dr. C.-M. Singh Trust Award (2002), Dr. Rajendra Prasad Award (2002), Shri Ramlal Agrawal National Award (2000), Best Paper Award SIIP (2003), Best Paper Award IAVA (2001, 2002 and 2003), Best Teacher Award (2004) by GBPUAT, Fellow IAVP (2006), Gopal Gaurav (2007), Bharat Excellence Award (2007), Diplomat ICVP (2008), Intas-ISVE Best Veterinary Scientist Award (2008), Best Academician Award (2012), Moropant Pingle Go Sewa National Award (2015), Outstanding Scientist Award (2019), Research Excellence Award (2020), and Indo Asian-Claude

Bourgelat Distinguished Innovative Scientist Award-2020 in Animal Immunopathology. He has been inducted in many national and international scientific/advisory committees and boards including Member, WHO/IPCS Committee on Environmental Health Criteria; Member, Hindi Advisory Committee, Govt. of India; Chairman, IAVP/VCI Committee on revision of Veterinary Pathology Courses; Member, Central Management Committee, AIIMS; Chairman, Cow Therapy Research Group, etc. His pioneer work includes immunopathology due to pesticides, heavy metals, mycotoxins, and nanoparticles. He has supervised as Principal Investigator in more than 25 research projects funded by GBPUAT, DST, ICAR, UPCAR, Industry, DADF, ICAR-IVRI, Govt. of Uttarakhand, etc.

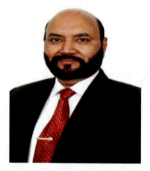

Yashpal Singh Malik is currently the Dean of the College of Animal Biotechnology, Guru Angad Dev Veterinary, and Animal Sciences University (GADVASU) Ludhiana, India. He is a recipient of the prestigious "ICAR-National Fellow" at the ICAR-Indian Veterinary Research Institute. His areas of expertise are rotaviral diseases, viral disease epidemiology, microbial biodiversity, host–virus interactions, and pathogen diagnostics. He has pursued advanced studies in molecular virology at the University of Minnesota, USA; University of Ottawa, Ontario, Canada; and Wuhan Institute of Virology, Wuhan, China. He is the recipient of several prestigious national, state and academy awards and honors, including the ICAR-Jawaharlal Nehru Award. He has authored 7 books, 62 book chapters, and over 225 research and review articles. He has been associated with societies of international repute, like, the Managing Committee Member of the World Society for Virology (USA). He has been serving as Secretary General of Indian Virological Society. Being a member in "One Health group in Federation of Asian Veterinary Association" (FAVA) for 2021–2025, he is the Indian flag bearer on the international forum. He is the Editor-in-Chief of the Journal of Immunology Immunopathology and has also edited special issues of the Springer journal Virus Disease, Bentham's The Open Virology Journal, and the Journal of Current Drug Metabolism. He has been awarded a prestigious Fellowship by the National Academy of Veterinary Sciences (India), National Academy of Dairy Sciences (India), National Academy of Biological Sciences, and Academy of Microbiological Sciences.

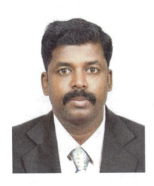

M. Saminathan (Veterinary Pathology) obtained his B.V.Sc. and A.H. (2010) degree from Madras Veterinary College, TANUVAS, Tamil Nadu, and M.V.Sc. (2013) and Ph.D. (2018) degrees from the ICAR-Indian Veterinary Research Institute, Izatnagar, India. He joined Agricultural Research Service (ARS) in 2015 and currently, working as Scientist (SS) in Centre for Animal Disease Research and Diagnosis (CADRAD), ICAR-IVRI, Bareilly, Uttar Pradesh, India. He possesses research, disease investigation, and undergraduate and postgraduate teaching experiences in veterinary pathology. His research areas of interest are mammary cancer in rat and dog, especially triple-negative mammary cancer, immunopathogenesis of bluetongue virus and rabies. He has used immunological assays like immunohistochemistry, fluorescent antibody test, fluorescence-activated cell sorting, ELISA, etc. during research. He has published around 245 publications (60 research articles, 32 review articles, 80 abstracts, and 7 lead papers in International and National Conference/Symposium, 52 GenBank submissions, 9 books and book chapters, 9 technical/popular articles, etc.). He has been awarded Dr C.M. Singh Award, IAVP-Prof. S. Ramachandran Memorial Award, IAVP-Dr Ram Raksha Kiran Shukla Award, IAVP-Dr C.M. Singh Memorial Award for best research article, IAVP-Dr Balwant Singh Memorial Young Scientist Award, IAVP-Dr Patri Rama Rao Memorial Award, IAVP-Dr B.S. Rajya Memorial Award, Scifax Young Scientist Award, and Certificate of Outstanding Reviewer by International journals. He has been actively serving as Editor, Editorial Board Member, and Reviewer in 14 International (journals like Small Ruminant Research, Biomedicine & Pharmacotherapy, Results in Applied Mathematics, Journal of Advanced Research and Microbiological Research, BMC Veterinary Research, Frontiers in Cellular and Infection Microbiology, Irish Veterinary Journal) and various National journals. He has been serving as Joint Secretary of Indian Association of Veterinary Pathologists (IAVP). His h-index is 25 and i10-index is 45 with 2440 citations.

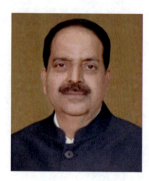

Bhupendra Nath Tripathi An FRCPath, obtained his B.V.Sc. and A.H. degree from CSA University of Agriculture & Technology, Kanpur, India, and his M.V.Sc. (1987) and Ph.D. (1990) degrees from the ICAR-Indian Veterinary Research Institute, Izatnagar, India. Currently, he is serving as Vice-Chancellor of Shr-e-Kashmir University of Agriculture & Technology Jammu. He joined Agricultural Scientist Services in 1991 and served IVRI in the capacities of Scientist, Senior Scientist, and Principal Scientist before moving in 2009 to CSWRI, Avikanagar, Rajasthan, as Head, Animal Health Division, in 2012 to Baghpat as Director of National Institute for Animal Health (NIAH), Govt of India, in 2014 to Hisar as Director of ICAR-National Research Centre on Equines & Project Coordinator, National Centre for Veterinary Type Cultures (NCVTC) and in 2020 as Deputy Director General (Animal Science), New Delhi. He was a Postdoctoral Fellow at the Institute of Animal Health, Compton, UK, and the Moredun Research Institute, Edinburgh with International Wellcome Trust Fellowship (London), UK.

His area of interest is infectious diseases with focus on understanding mechanisms by which microbial pathogens cause disease, including molecular virology to in vivo pathogenesis. He has made pioneering contributions on immuno-pathobiology, diagnosis, and vaccine development for various infectious diseases of animals. He has been granted two patent and published 7 new patents. He has published more than 175 original research papers in peer reviewed national and international journals, 20 review articles, 20 book chapters, five books, five manuals, and edited three conference proceedings.

He is a diplomat of Indian College of Veterinary Pathologists and has served as Chief Editor of Indian Journal of Veterinary Pathology. He is currently holding the Chair of the President of Indian Association of Veterinary Pathology (IAVP). He is the recipient of several awards, honors, fellowship of professional societies and academies, reviewer of high impact international journals, and has visited several countries for academic, research purposes and as a member of Indian delegation of international organizations (OIE, FAO, WHO, BIMSTEC).

Basic Concepts in Immunology

Key Points

1. Antigen is a foreign substance, which is able to stimulate the production of antibodies in the body.
2. Antibodies are protein in nature, which are specific to antigens and produced as a result of antigenic stimulation.
3. The combination of chemical, humoral, and cellular processes in the body provides immunity, which is the body's resistance against extraneous etiological factors of disease.
4. Innate immunity includes anatomical, physiological, phagocytic, and inflammatory barriers that keep out microbes.
5. Innate immunity offers quick initial protection, and adaptive immunity offers lasting effective immunity.
6. Acquired immunity is classified into humoral and cell-mediated immunity. Antibodies are the main components of humoral mechanism. T- and B-lymphocytes and macrophages are the main components of cell-mediated immunity.
7. Antibody-mediated immunity is called humoral immunity and present in body fluids, mainly in the blood.
8. Examples of cell-mediated immune response are graft rejection and graft-versus-host disease.
9. Cytokines are chemical mediators and hormonelike glycoproteins with a molecular weight of 8–25 kDa and composed of a single chain. Cytokines are known to regulate certain important biological functions.Immunity is the resistance of the body against extraneous etiological factors of disease, which is afforded by the interaction of chemical, humoral, and cellular reactions in the body. This is an integral part of the body without which one cannot think of life. During the process of evolution, nature has provided this defense mechanism in the body of all living creatures, particularly of higher animals and humans that protects them

from physical, chemical, and biological insults. It can be classified as natural or paraspecific and acquired or specific immunity.

1.1 Natural or Paraspecific Immunity

Some animal species are resistant to particular disease conditions due to presence of natural resistance against them, e.g., horses, pigs, and cats are resistant to canine distemper virus, dogs are resistant to feline panleukopenia virus, and chickens are resistant to anthrax. Even within the species, there is a natural resistance that protects some individuals while others are susceptible, e.g., Indian desi cattle zebu (*Bos indicus*) is quite resistant to piroplasmosis in comparison to *Bos taurus*. Besides, there are a number of mechanisms or barriers in the body provided by nature, which protect the host against the invading microorganisms (Table 1.1). These are as follows:

- *The skin* and *mucous membrane* prevent organisms from gaining entrance in the body.
- *Mucus* prevents from infections by trapping and keeping them away.
- *Saliva, gastric juice*, and *intestinal enzymes* kill bacteria.

Table 1.1 Summary of natural or non-specific or para-specific host defenses

Type of barrier	Mechanism of action
Anatomical barriers	
Skin	• Acts as a mechanical barrier and retards the entry of microbes • Acidic environment (pH 3–5) and retards the growth of microbes
Mucous membranes	• Normal flora competes with microbes for attachment sites and nutrients • Mucus entraps the foreign microorganisms • Cilia propel the microorganisms out of the body
Physiological barriers	
Temperature	• Normal body temperature inhibits the growth of some pathogens • Fever response inhibits the growth of some pathogens
Low pH	• Acidity of stomach contents kills most of the ingested microorganisms
Chemical mediators	• Lysozyme cleaves the bacterial cell wall • Interferon induces antiviral state in uninfected cells • The complement lyses the microorganisms or facilitates phagocytosis • Toll-like receptors recognize the microbial molecules, signal cell to secrete immunostimulatory cytokines • Collectins disrupt the cell wall of pathogen
Phagocytic/endocytic barriers	• Various cells internalize (endocytose) and break down the foreign macromolecules • Specialized cells (blood monocytes, neutrophils, tissue macrophages) internalize (phagocytose), kill, and digest the whole microorganisms
Inflammatory barriers	• Tissue damage and infection induces the leakage of vascular fluid, containing serum proteins with antibacterial activity and influx of phagocytic cells into the affected area

- *Tears, nasal* and *gastrointestinal tract secretions* are bactericidal due to presence of lysozymes.
- *Phagocytic cells*, such as neutrophils, kill bacteria through phagocytosis.
- *Macrophages* kill organisms through phagocytosis.
- *Natural antibodies* act as opsonins and help in phagocytosis.
- *Interferons* have antimicrobial properties. They are host and species specific and arrest the viral replication.
- *Interleukins, cytotoxins*, and *growth factors* stimulate the immune reactions and inflammation.
- *Natural killer cells* kill the targets coated with IgG.

1.2 Acquired or Specific Immunity

Acquired immunity develops in the body as a result of prior stimulation with antigens. It is specific to a particular antigen against which it was developed. It can be restimulated on second or subsequent exposure with antigen, and thus, it has memory for a particular antigen. It differs from natural immunity in respect to prior stimulation, specificity, and memory (Table 1.2). It can be classified as humoral and cell-mediated immunity.

1.3 Humoral Immunity

The antibody-mediated immunity is called humoral immunity and is present in the fluids of the body, mainly in the blood. The antibodies are present in the serum of the blood, which protect the body from diseases. It is specific to a particular antigen. Antibodies are formed in the blood as a result of exposure to the foreign substances including bacteria, viruses, parasites, and other substances.

Antigen is a foreign substance, which is able to stimulate the production of antibodies in the body. They may be of high molecular weight (MW) protein, polysaccharides, and nucleic acids. Simple chemicals of low MW are not able to induce immunity. However, they may be conjugated with large MW molecules, such as proteins, to become antigenic and induce antibody production. Such substances are termed as *haptens*.

Antibodies are protein in nature and are produced as a result of antigenic stimulation. Antibodies are specific to antigens. Most of the microorganisms have several antigenic determinants known as *epitopes*, and antibodies are produced against each antigenic determinant specifically. The antibody response to antigen can be enhanced if the antigen is released slowly in the body. There are several substances, like oils, waxes, alum, and aluminum hydroxide, which may be added with antigen so that it is released slowly in the body to increase the antibody production. Such substances are known as *adjuvants*. Antibodies are also known as *immunoglobulins* as they are part of globulins. They are glycoprotein in nature and are of five types: IgG, IgA, IgM, IgD, and IgE (Table 1.3; Fig. 1.1).

Table 1.2 Difference between innate and adaptive immunity

Characteristics	Innate immunity	Adaptive immunity
Initiation	Always "on"	Turned on by antigens
Cells involved	Macrophages, dendritic cells, neutrophils, natural killer cells	T- and B-lymphocytes
Cellular and chemical barriers	Skin, mucosal epithelia, and antimicrobial molecules	Lymphocytes in epithelia and antibodies secreted at epithelial surfaces
Blood proteins	Complement and others	Antibodies
Evolutionary history	Ancient	Recent
Onset	Rapid (minutes to hours)	Slow (days to weeks)
Specificity	Limited and fixed for molecules shared by groups of related microbes and molecules produced by damaged host cells	Highly diverse for microbial and nonmicrobial antigens; improves during the course of immune response
Diversity	Limited; germ line encoded	Very large; receptors are produced by somatic recombination of gene segments
Potency	May be overwhelmed	Rarely overwhelmed
Memory	None	Significant memory
Non-reactivity to self	Yes	Yes
Response to repeat injection	Identical to primary response	Much more rapid than primary response
Effectiveness	Does not improve	Improves with exposure

Table 1.3 Difference between major immunoglobulin classes in domestic mammals

Property	Immunoglobulin class				
	IgM	IgG	IgA	IgE	IgD
Molecular weight (Da)	900,000	180,000	360,000	200,000	180,000
Subunits	5	1	2	1	1
Electrophoretic mobility	β	γ	β-γ	β-γ	γ
Heavy chain	M	γ	α	ε	δ
Synthesis	Spleen and lymph nodes	Spleen and lymph nodes	Intestinal and respiratory tracts	Intestinal and respiratory tracts	Spleen and lymph nodes

1.3.1 Immunoglobulin G (IgG)

It is the main antibody found in high concentration (75%) in the serum with a MW of 150 kilodaltons (kDa). It is produced by plasma cells in the spleen, lymph nodes, and bone marrow. It has two identical light chains and two gamma heavy chains. The

1.3 Humoral Immunity

Fig. 1.1 Diagram showing (**a**) structure of antibody with its different parts, (**b**) Immunoglobulin G (IgG), (**c**) Immunoglobulin M (IgM), (**d**) Immunoglobulin A (IgA), and (**e**) Immunoglobulin E (IgE)

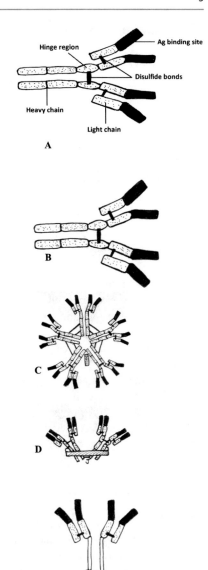

light chains may be of kappa or lambda type. IgG is the smallest immunoglobulin, which may pass through the blood vessels with increased permeability. It has the capacity to quickly bind with foreign substances leading to opsonization. Its binding with antigen may also activate the complement (Fig. 1.1b).

1.3.2 Immunoglobulin M (IgM)

This constitutes about 7% of the total serum immunoglobulins. It is also produced by plasma cells in the spleen, lymph nodes, and bone marrow. It is a pentamer consisting of five molecules of conventional immunoglobulin with MW of 900 kDa. These five molecules are linked through disulfide bonds in a circular form. A cysteine-rich polypeptide of 15 kDa binds two of the units to complete the circle and is known as "J" chain. It is produced in the body during the primary immune response. It is considered to be more active than IgG for complement activation, neutralization of antigen, opsonization, and agglutination. IgM molecules are confined to the blood and have little or no effect in tissue fluids, body secretions, and acute inflammation (Fig. 1.1c).

1.3.3 Immunoglobulin A (IgA)

It is secreted as a dimer (MW 300 kDa) by plasma cells present in the body surfaces like intestinal, respiratory, and urinary systems, mammary gland, and the skin. Its concentration is very little in the blood. IgA produced in the body surfaces is either through epithelial cells or diffused in the bloodstream. IgA is transported through intestinal epithelial cells having a receptor of 71 kDa, which binds with the secretary component covalently to form a secretary IgA. This secretary component protects IgA in the intestinal tract from digestion. It cannot activate the complement and cannot perform the opsonization. IgA can neutralize the antigen and agglutinate the particulate antigen. IgA prevents adherence of foreign particles/antigen on the body surfaces, and it can also act inside the cells. It is about 16% of the total immunoglobulins present in the serum (Fig. 1.1d).

1.3.4 Immunoglobulin E (IgE)

It is also present on the body surfaces and produced by plasma cells located in the connective tissue and mucosa beneath the body surfaces. It is in very low concentration in the serum. It can bind on receptors of mast cells and basophils. When any antigen binds to these molecules, it causes degranulation of mast cells leading to release of chemical mediators to cause acute inflammation. It mediates hypersensitivity type I reaction and is responsible to provide resistance against invading parasitic worms. It has the shortest half-life (2–3 days) and thus is unstable and can be readily destroyed by mild heat treatment. It is only 0.01% of the total immunoglobulin in the serum with a MW of 190 kDa (Fig. 1.1e).

1.3.5 Immunoglobulin D (IgD)

The IgD is absent in most domestic animals. However, it is present in very minute amount in the plasma of dogs, non-human primates, and rats. The IgD can be detected in the plasma. In the serum, it is normally lysed by proteases during clotting. It is only 0.2% of the total immunoglobulin content in the blood with MW of 160 kDa.

On the basis of their functions, antibodies may be of various types:

Antitoxins have the property to bind with toxins and neutralize them.

Agglutinins are those antibodies which can agglutinate RBCs and/or particulate material such as bacterial cells.

Precipitins can precipitate proteins by acting with antigens and inhibit their dissemination and chemical activity.

Lysins can lyse cells or bacteria through the complement.

Opsonins have the property to bind with foreign particles non-specifically leading to opsonization, making the foreign material palatable to phagocytic cells.

Complement-fixing antibodies bind with antigens and fix the complement for its lysis.

Neutralizing antibodies are those which specifically neutralize or destroy the target antigens; merely binding with antigen can't be considered as neutralizing antibodies.

1.4 Cell-Mediated Immunity

Cell-mediated immunity is a form of immune response mediated by T-lymphocytes and macrophages. The examples of cell-mediated immune response are graft rejection and graft-versus-host reactions. If a piece of the skin is surgically removed from one animal and grafted on to another animal of the same species, it usually survives for only a few days and is then destroyed by the recipient. This process of graft rejection is the manifestation of cell-mediated immunity and characterized by infiltration of mononuclear cells at the site of graft. In the process, the foreign cells are rapidly recognized and eliminated. Even cells with minor structural abnormalities are recognized as foreign by the immune system and eliminated, although they are apparently healthy. Such abnormal cells include aged cells, virus-infected cells, and tumor cells. On the skin grafting from one animal to another initially appears to be healthy, and the blood vessels will soon develop between the graft and its host. But after 1 week, these new blood vessels start to degenerate to cut the blood supply to the graft, resulting in the death of graft, and it sheds off. This slow rejection occurs in the first graft, but when a second graft is made from the same donor and placed on the same host again, it survives only for 1–2 days and is rejected promptly. This rapid rejection is known as secondary immune response or second set of reaction. The graft rejection is similar to antibody formation in terms of specificity and is mediated by T-lymphocytes found in the spleen, lymph nodes, and peripheral blood.

1.5 Immune Response

When the antigen enters the animal's body, it is trapped, processed, and eliminated by several cells, including macrophages, dendritic cells, and B cells. There are two types of antigens in the body, i.e., exogenous and endogenous. The exogenous or extracellular antigens are present freely in the circulation and are readily available for antigen-processing cells.

The endogenous or intracellular antigens are not free and are always inside the cells such as viruses. But when these viruses synthesize new viral proteins using biosynthetic process of the host cells, these proteins also act as antigen and are termed as endogenous or intracellular antigens.

The processing of antigen by macrophages is comparatively less efficient as most of the antigen is destroyed by the lysosomal proteases. An alternate pathway of antigen processing involves antigen uptake by a specialized population of mononuclear cells known as *dendritic cells* located throughout the body especially in lymphoid organs. Such dendritic cells have many long filamentous cytoplasmic processes called dendrites and lobulated nuclei with clear cytoplasm containing characteristic granules (Fig. 1.2).

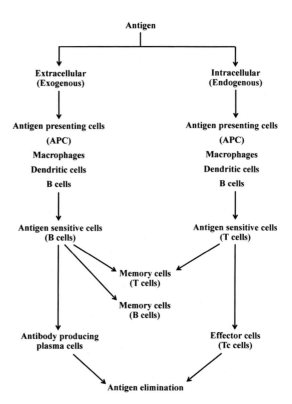

Fig. 1.2 Antigen processing in the body

Antigen-presenting cells process the exogenous antigen and convert into fragments to bind with MHC class II molecules. Such processed antigens along with MHC class II molecules and cytokines, such as IL-1, are presented to antigen-recognizing cells (T-helper cells). Macrophages also regulate the dose of antigen to prevent inappropriate development of tolerance and provide a small dose of antigen to T-helper cells. However, if the antigen is presented to T-cells without MHC class II molecule, the T-cells are turned off, resulting into tolerance. On an average, an antigen-presenting cell possesses about 2×10^5 MHC class II molecules. A T-cell requires activation by 200–300 peptide-MHC class II molecules to trigger an immune response. Thus, it is estimated that an antigen-presenting cell may present several epitopes simultaneously to T-helper cells. A counterpart of T-helper cells known as suppressor T-cells (Ts-cell) also exists, which suppress the immune response. The virus-encoded proteins and endogenous antigens are handled in a different manner from those of exogenous antigens. Such antigens are bound to MHC class Ia molecules and transported to the cell surface. Antigen-MHC class Ia molecule complex triggers a lymphocyte response, i.e., cytotoxic T-cells (Tc-cells). These cytotoxic T-cells recognize and destroy virus-infected cells. However, there is some cross-priming leading to cell-mediated immune response by exogenous antigens and humoral immune response by endogenous antigens. Some lymphocytes also function as memory cells to initiate secondary immune response (Fig. 1.3).

On the antigen exposure, there is a latent period of about 4 to 6 days, and only after that serum antibodies are detectable. The peak of antibody titer is estimated about 2 weeks after exposure to antigen and then declines after about 3 weeks. During the primary immune response, majority of the antibodies are of IgM type, whereas in the secondary immune response, they are always predominated by IgG.

1.6 Cells of the Immune System

There are many cells that participate in the immune functions of the body. These cells are present in different organs and tissues and in the blood, making a complex system. All the cells of the immune system arise from pluripotential stem cells through the two main channels:

1.6.1 Lymphoid Channel

Lymphocytes differentiate through the lymphoid channel and are of two types: T-lymphocyte and B-lymphocyte. Both the cells are equipped with surface receptors of antigens. T-lymphocytes develop from their precursors in the thymus, while B-lymphocytes differentiate from the bursa of Fabricius in birds. In mammals, B-lymphocytes differentiate in the fetal liver and in adults in the bone marrow. They acquire surface receptors for specificity. These sites of lymphocyte differentiation are known as central or primary lymphoid organs.

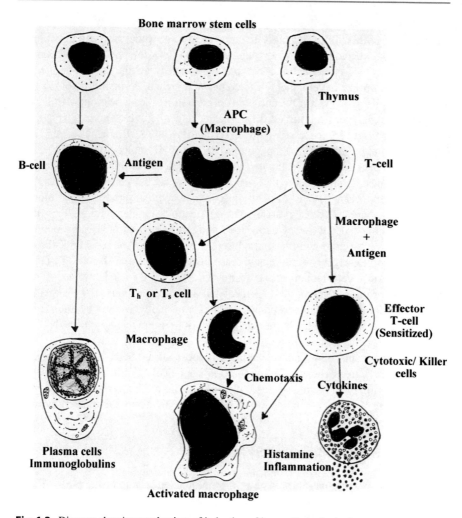

Fig. 1.3 Diagram showing mechanism of induction of immunity in the body

A third population of lymphocytes, which do not express any antigen receptors, are called natural killer cells (NK cells). They are derived from the bone marrow and can be identified functionally from T- or B-lymphocytes by their ability to lyse certain tumor cells without prior sensitization. Structurally, these are large granular lymphocytes.

1.6.2 Myeloid Channel

Monocytes (macrophages in tissue location) and granulocytes, such as neutrophils, basophils, and eosinophils, develop through myeloid channel. Besides, antigen-presenting cells, platelets, and mast cells also develop through myeloid channel.

Other cells include mainly endothelial cells, which express certain molecules for recognition of lymphocytes and their distribution in the tissue spaces. A brief description of each cell type participating in the immunological and immunopathological reactions of the body is given as under:

1.6.2.1 Lymphoid Cells

Lymphoid cells are produced in the primary or central lymphoid organs like the thymus and bone marrow. However, for their maturation, these cells migrate through the secondary lymphoid organs like the spleen, lymph nodes, tonsils, mucosa-associated lymphoid tissue, etc. In an adult person, lymphoid tissue comprises 2% of the total body weight. In blood circulation, lymphoid cells are 20–50% of the total white blood cells (Table 1.4). The lymphoid cells may survive for many years and in some cases for the whole life of an individual (Fig. 1.4).

In a blood smear, one can observe two types of lymphoid cells based on their morphological characteristics: small lymphocytes and large lymphocytes. The majority of the smaller lymphocytes are either helper or cytotoxic T-lymphocytes with a high nuclear-cytoplasm (N:C) ratio. These cells contain a cytoplasmic structure known as "Gall bodies," which are made up of lysosomes with lipid droplet. They have a well-developed Golgi apparatus. The larger lymphocytes have smaller N:C ratio and show dendritic morphology. Such cells include B-cells and NK cells, which contain large azurophilic granules.

There are a large number of molecules on the cell surface of lymphocytes, which can be used to distinguish the type of cells. These are known as **markers**. These markers are identified by a set of specific monoclonal antibodies. The lymphoid cells are classified on the basis of the presence of cluster of differentiation (CD) molecules, which is termed as CD system of classification. The CD system refers to groups or clusters of monoclonal antibodies, each binding specifically to particular cell markers. The CD system depends on the computer analysis of

Table 1.4 Peripheral blood lymphocyte populations in mammals as percentage of the total population

Species	T-cells	CD4+ T-cells	CD8+ T-cells	CD4/CD8 ratio	B-cells
Bovine	45–53	8–31	10–30	1.53	16–21
Sheep	56–64	8–22	4–22	1.55	11–50
Horse	38–66	56	20–37	4.75	17–38
Pig	45–57	23–43	17–39	1.4	13–38
Dog	46–72	27–33	17–18	1.7	7–30
Cat	31–89	19–49	6–39	1.9	6–50
Human	70–75	43–48	22–24	1.9–2.4	10–15

Fig. 1.4 (a) Photomicrograph of lymphocyte, (b) diagram of T-lymphocyte, and (c) B-lymphocyte showing different receptors

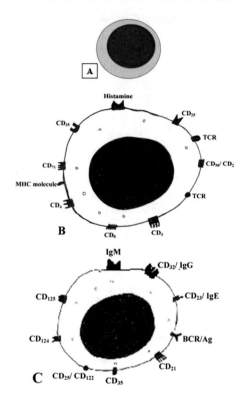

monoclonal antibodies produced in mice against human leukocyte antigens. A number is used to indicate each cell marker molecule recognized by a group of monoclonal antibodies.

Some molecules are characteristics of a particular lineage of cells. These are termed as lineage markers. The molecules for identification of cells developed during maturation stage of the cells are called maturation marker. Some markers appear only after activation of the cell by the stimulus and are known as activation markers.

E. g.	Lineage marker	CD3 present exclusively on T-cells
	Maturation marker	CD1 found on cells of the thymus during development of cells and absent on peripheral blood T-lymphocytes
	Activation marker	IL-2 and CD25 appeared only after stimulation of T-cells by antigens

As mentioned earlier, lymphoid cells comprise two types of lineages, i.e., T- and B-cells, which act specifically in response to antigens. However, there are certain cells like NK cells which do not require antigen stimulation and act on their own. Brief descriptions of all these cells along with their markers are as follows:

T-Lymphocytes

T-lymphocytes are those lymphocytes which bind to sheep red blood cells (SRBC) through CD2 molecule, while B-lymphocytes cannot perform this function. Definitive T-cell marker for T-cell lineage is the T-cell antigen receptor (TCR). The TCR is of two types: TCR1 and TCR2. TCR1 is composed of two gamma and delta polypeptides, while TCR2 has alpha and beta heterodimer of two disulfide linked polypeptides. Both the receptors are associated with a set of five polypeptides, the CD3 complex, to give the T-cell receptor complex (TCR-CD3 complex). Thus, T-cells express either TCR1 or TCR2. In the peripheral blood of human, 85–95% T-lymphoid cells have TCR2, while 15% have TCR1 (Fig. 1.4b).

The TCR2-positive T-cells can be further identified as per the following two categories:

1. Cells that carry CD4 marker and help or induce immune responses are known as T-helper (T_h) cells.
2. Cells that carry CD8 marker and perform the cytotoxicity function are known as cytotoxic T-cells (T_c cells).

The CD4 molecule recognizes its specific antigen in association with MHC class II, while CD8 recognizes antigen in association with MHC class I molecules. TCR1 cells do not express either CD4 or CD8 marker, although some of them are CD8 positive. CD4 cells are further divided into two groups:

1. Cells which influence the response of T-cells and B-cells and perform as helper function. These are also CD29+ and overlap with CD45 antigen.
2. Cells which induce suppressor or cytotoxic functions of CD8-positive cells. This also expresses CD45 molecule. T-helper cell populations are of two types: T_h-1 and T_h-2. T_h-1 is associated with helper functions to mediate cytotoxicity and local inflammation and to combat with intracellular organisms. These cells secrete interleukin-2 (IL-2) and gamma interferon. T_h-2 cells stimulate B-cell proliferation to produce antibodies, which protect the body against free-living organisms.

The CD8-positive cells also have two subpopulations: subset 1 and 2. Subset 1 expresses CD28 molecule and produces IL-2, while subset 2 responds to IL-2 and expresses CD11 and CD18 molecules. These cells have large granular lymphocyte (LGL) morphology, and the granules present in the cells perform cytotoxic functions of T-cells.

The TCR1-positive cells with CD3 molecule are found mainly in the mucosal epithelium. Though their small number is present in the peripheral blood, the majority of intraepithelial lymphocytes are TCR1 positive. These cells protect the mucosal surfaces in the body.

There are other markers, a few of which are present on all the T-cells, that include pan-T-cell markers—CD2, CD3, CD5, and CD7 molecules, and CD7 molecule present on all NK cells.

B-Lymphocytes

B-cells comprise only 5–15% of the total peripheral blood lymphocytes. These cells are defined by the presence of immunoglobulins on mature cells. In human, majority of B-lymphocytes are present in the blood, which expresses two immunoglobulins, i.e., IgM and IgD. The minority of cells also express IgG, IgA, and IgE. The B-cells of IgA phenotype are found in large numbers in mucosal surfaces. Majority of B-cells carry MHC class II antigen, i.e., CD35 and CD21 (dendritic cell markers). A marker of T-cell, the CD5 molecule, has also been found on some B-cells. It identifies the subsets of B-cells predisposed for autoantibody production and are named as B2 cells. Such cells are found predominantly in the peritoneal cavity of mouse. The conventional cells of antibody production are B2 cells (Table 1.5 and Fig. 1.4c). Plasma cells are the modified B-lymphocytes meant for antibody production. Plasma cells have smooth spherical or elliptical shape with abundant cytoplasm and eccentrically placed cartwheel-shaped nucleus. The cytoplasm stains slightly basophilic and gives a magenta shade of purplish red. In the cytoplasm, there is a distinct hyaline homogenous mass called Russell body, which lies on the cisternae of the endoplasmic reticulum. This is the accumulated immunoglobulins produced by these cells (Fig. 1.5).

Natural Killer Cells

Natural killer (NK) cells are present in the peripheral blood and comprise about 10–15% of the total peripheral blood lymphocytes. These are defined as the lymphocytes which do not have any conventional surface antigen receptors, i.e.,

Table 1.5 Differentiating features between T- and B-lymphocytes

Property	B-lymphocytes	T-lymphocytes
Development	Bone marrow, bursa of Fabricius, and Peyer's patches	Thymus
Distribution	Cortex of the lymph node and splenic follicles	Paracortex of the lymph node and periarteriolar sheath of the spleen
Circulation	No	Yes
Important surface antigen receptors	B-cell receptor (BCR)-immunoglobulin	T-cell receptor (TCR)-protein heterodimer and associated with CD2, CD3, CD4, or CD8
Mitogens	Pokeweed and lipopolysaccharide	Phytohemagglutinin, concanavalin A, Bacille Calmette-Guerin (BCG) vaccine, and pokeweed
Antigens recognized	Free foreign proteins	Processed foreign proteins in MHC antigens
Tolerance induction	Difficult	Easy
Progeny cells	Plasma cells and memory cells	Effector T-cells and memory T-cells
Secreted products	Immunoglobulins	Cytokines

1.6 Cells of the Immune System

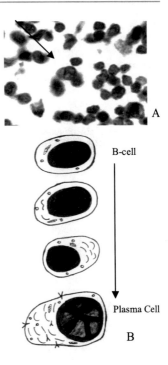

Fig. 1.5 (**a**) Photomicrograph of plasma cell. (**b**) Diagrammatic presentation of development of plasma cell from B-lymphocytes

TCR or immunoglobulin. The surface antigens present on NK cells also share with T-cells or monocytes. The molecules present on the NK cell are as follows:

1. **CD16 molecule:** It is present on NK cells and is also expressed by neutrophils, macrophages, and some T-cells.
2. **CD56 molecule:** If the CD3 molecule is absent and cells are positive for CD16 or CD56, they are definitely NK cells in man.
3. Resting NK cells also express alpha chain of IL-2 receptor. Thus, stimuli to IL-2 also activate NK cells. Alpha chain of IL-2 is also present on TCR1-, TCR2-, and CD8-positive cells. With NK cells all these are known as "lymphocyte-activated killer cells" (LAK cells), which kill fresh tumor cells.

NK cells may kill tumor cells, virus-containing cells, and the targets coated by IgG, i.e., antibody-dependent cell cytotoxicity. These cells may also release gamma interferon, cytokine IL-1, and GM-CSF. All T-, B-, and NK cells, granulocytes, and macrophages possess leukocyte functional antigen 1 (LFA-1), which is responsible for cell adhesions and intercellular communication.

1.6.2.2 Mononuclear Phagocytes

The mononuclear phagocytes develop from bone marrow stem cells, which may survive for years in the body. Mononuclear phagocytes comprise mainly two types of cells including professional phagocytes and antigen-presenting cells (APC). The

Fig. 1.6 (a) Photomicrograph of macrophage/monocyte, (b) diagram of macrophage showing different receptors, and (c) diagram showing different stages and types of phagocytic cells: 1. stem cell, 2. promonocyte, 3. monocyte, 4. microglia in the brain, 5. histiocyte in connective tissue, 6. Kupffer cell in the liver, 7. alveolar macrophages, and 8. osteoclasts in the bone

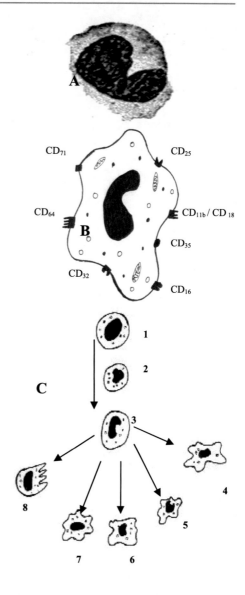

stem cells in the bone marrow differentiate as promonocytes and monocytes in the blood and migrate in the tissues as macrophages. The professional phagocytic cells destroy the particulate material, and APC present the processed antigens to lymphocytes. In man, the size of macrophages is about 10–18 μm and is larger than lymphocytes. In the blood, monocytes have horseshoe-shaped nucleus and contain faint azurophilic granules. These cells have well-developed Golgi apparatus and many intracytoplasmic lysosomes, which contain peroxidases and hydrolases for intracellular killing of microorganisms (Fig. 1.6).

1.6 Cells of the Immune System

Fig. 1.7 Diagram showing phagocytosis. (**a**). Opsonization and chemotaxis, (**b**–**c**). engulfment, and (**d**, **e**) digestion

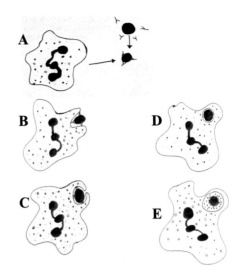

Macrophages have a tendency to adhere on the glass or plastic surface. These cells are able to phagocytose the microorganisms and tumor cells through specialized receptors (Fig. 1.7). The receptors may bind with certain carbohydrates present on the cell wall of the organisms or IgG or complement. In mice and man, monocytes have mannosyl fucosyl receptor (MFR), which binds to the surface of bacteria. These cells also bear CD14 receptor for lipopolysaccharide (LPS)-binding protein normally present in the serum and may coat on Gram-negative bacteria. Macrophages have receptors for Fc portion of IgG and is termed as CD64, which is responsible for opsonization, extracellular killing, and phagocytosis. On some mononuclear cells, particularly antigen-presenting cells (APC), receptors for the complement (CR_1 and CR_3), cytokines (IL-4, IFN, and migration inhibitory factor), and class II MHC are also present.

Antigen-Presenting Cells

Antigen-presenting cells are a heterogenous population of monocytes. These are found to be associated with immunostimulation, induction of T_h cell activity, and communication with other leukocytes. Some endothelial and epithelial cells under certain circumstances may also acquire properties of the APC when stimulated by cytokines. These cells do not have MHC II molecules and are induced to express them to act as APC.

The antigen-presenting cells are found in the skin, lymphocytes, spleen, and thymus. They migrate through the lymphatics and present antigen to T_h cells. They are rich in MHC IIa molecules.

Follicular dendritic cells are found in the secondary follicles in the lymph nodes and spleen. They present antigen to B-cells and lack in class II MHC but have complement receptor CD35 for interaction with immune complex. In the thymic medulla, such cells are rich in MCH class II and delete T-cells, which react with self-antigens, through negative selection. Somatic cells, which do not have MHC class II, may also get stimulated through cytokines (TNF, IFN) for presenting the antigen.

1.6.2.3 Polymorphonuclear Granulocytes

Polymorphonuclear granulocytes are produced in the bone marrow and are short lived only for 2–3 days. In the peripheral blood of man, these cells are 60–70% of the total leukocyte count. They may also migrate to extravascular sites in the tissues through diapedesis. These cells are not specific to antigens and non-specifically perform the phagocytosis. The deficiency of these cells may lead to increased susceptibility to infections. Mature cells have multilobed nucleus and granules. Granulocytes are neutrophils, eosinophils, and basophils.

1.6.2.4 Neutrophils

Neutrophils constitute 90% of the total circulating polymorphs and are of 10–20 µm in diameter. They are attracted by certain chemotactic factors like proteins of bacteria, C_3a, C_5a, fibrinolysin, and kinins. The stimuli of chemotaxis are responsible for their migration and diapedesis (Fig. 1.8). These cells have two types of granules:

1. **Primary granules:** Azurophilic granules are present in lysosomes containing acid hydrolases, myeloperoxidases, and muramidases.
2. **Specific or secondary granules:** They contain lactoferrin and lysozymes.

The granules are released through receptors by immune complexes.

1.6.2.5 Eosinophils

Eosinophils comprise 2–5% of the total leukocyte count in the blood. They are responsible for killing of large targets, which cannot be phagocytosed such as

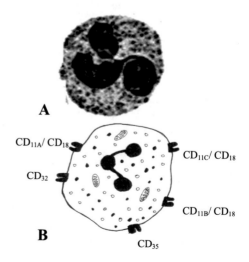

Fig. 1.8. (a) Photomicrograph of polymorphonuclear cell. (b) Diagram of polymorphonuclear cell showing different receptors

1.6 Cells of the Immune System

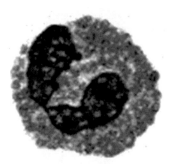

Fig. 1.9 Photomicrograph of eosinophil

Table 1.6 Comparison of two major types of mast cells

Features	Mucosal mast cells	Connective tissue mast cells
Structure	Few and variable-sized granules	Many uniform granules
Size	9 to 10 μm diameter	19 to 20 μm diameter
Proteoglycan	Chondroitin sulfate	Heparin
Histamine	1.3 pg/cell	15 pg/cell
Life span	Less than 40 days	More than 6 months
Location	Intestinal wall and lungs	Peritoneal cavity and skin
Production enhanced by IL-3	+	–

parasites. Eosinophils may also act as phagocytic cells to kill organisms, but this is not their primary function. The eosinophil contains membrane-bound granules with crystalloid core and a bilobed nucleus. The cells degranulate through fusion of granules and plasma membrane outside cell on large targets to destroy them. Eosinophils are also attracted by certain chemotactic factors like products of T-cells, mast cells, basophils, and parasites. They also bind with parasites coated with IgG or IgE. The granules in cells have major basic protein, which releases histaminase and arylsulfatase and reduces leukocyte migration to the site (Fig. 1.9).

1.6.2.6 Basophils and Mast Cells

In the blood these are less than 0.2% of the total leukocytes and have deep violet blue-colored granules. When basophils are present in the tissues, they are known as mast cells. They are also of two types (Table 1.6):

1. **Mucosal mast cells (MMC):** These cells are dependent on T-cells for proliferation. They are present in the mucosal surfaces of the body.
2. **Connective tissue mast cell (CTMC):** They are present in the connective tissue.

Basophilic granules present in these cells are rich in heparin, SRS-A, and ECF-A, which are released on degranulation. When allergens come in contact, it cross-links with IgE bound on the surface of mast cells and stimulate the cells to degranulate and release histamine, which plays an active role in allergy and against parasites (Fig. 1.10).

Fig. 1.10 Photomicrograph of basophil

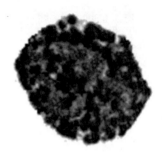

1.6.2.7 Platelets

Platelets are derived from megakaryocyte of the bone marrow, which contains granules. It helps in the clotting of the blood and is involved in inflammation and immunity. They also express MHC class I molecules and receptors for IgG-Fc portion and have low affinity to IgE. When the endothelial surface gets damaged, platelets adhere and aggregate on damaged endothelium and release substances to increase permeability, attract leukocytes, and activate the complement.

1.7 Cytokines

Cytokines are hormonelike glycoproteins in nature with a MW of 8–25 kDa and composed of a single chain. Cytokines are referred to as any chemical mediator, which acts as a signal between cells irrespective of their types. They are known to regulate certain important biological functions such as cell growth, cell activation, immunity, inflammation, tissue repair, fibrosis, morphogenesis, and chemotaxis. Cytokines are produced by cells, usually lymphocytes (**lymphokines**), monocytes (**monokines**), and others as a result of stimulation through injury. Cytokines are considered to be functional proteins and are grouped together based on their homologous amino acid sequences. The various types of cytokines are as follows:

1. Interferons (IFN)
2. Interleukins (IL)
3. Tumor necrosis factors (TNF)
4. Colony-stimulating factors (CSF)
5. Migration inhibitory factors (MIF)

1.7.1 Interferons

Interferons were first identified as antiviral agents in the year 1957. They are also found to be potent immune regulators and growth factors. Interferons are further classified as alpha, beta, gamma, omega, and tau interferon. Interferon-α is produced by leukocytes (lymphocytes, monocytes, macrophages) in response to viral infection and has 20 subtypes. Interferon-β is produced by fibroblasts as a result of virus or its

1.7 Cytokines

Table 1.7 Source and action of interferons

Interferons	Source	Action
Interferon-alpha (IFN-α)	Lymphocytes, monocytes, macrophages	Inhibits virus growth, activates macrophages
Interferon-beta (IFN-β)	Fibroblasts	Inhibits virus growth, activates macrophages
Interferon-gamma (IFN-γ)	Th-1 cells, cytotoxic T-cells, NK cells, macrophages	Stimulates T-cells, enhances NK cell activity, activates macrophages and phagocytosis, promotes antibody-dependent and cell-mediated cytotoxicity
Interferon-omega (IFN-ω)	Lymphocytes, monocytes, trophoblasts	Inhibits virus growth, activates macrophages
Interferon-tau (IFN-τ)	Trophoblasts	Inhibits virus growth, immunity to fetus through the placenta

nucleic acid, while interferon-γ is a single protein produced by T-lymphocytes in response to simulation of immunity. Alpha and beta interferons are useful in the control of cancer as these have inhibitory properties for cell growth. The curative use in renal cell carcinomas has been reported. Gamma interferon is produced by T-lymphocytes, macrophages, and natural killer cells. It activates antigen-presenting cells and regulate the functions of astrocytes, microglia, endothelial cells, and thymocytes. The excessive production of gamma interferon may play an important role in autoimmunity. Omega interferon is produced by lymphocytes, monocytes, and trophoblasts and activates macrophages and checks the viral growth in cells. Interferon-tau (IFN-τ) is produced by trophoblasts, which checks the viral growth and provides immunity to fetus through the placenta (Table 1.7).

1.7.2 Interleukins

There are at least 18 types of interleukins reported in the literature. These are the molecules produced by leukocytes and also act on leukocytes. Some of them are also produced by other cells than leukocytes. However, their targets are T- and B-lymphocytes, fibroblasts, and endothelium. The various subtypes of interleukins from interleukin-1 to interleukin-18 are described (Table 1.8).

1.7.2.1 Interleukin-1 (IL-1)

It is also known as endogenous pyrogen, lymphocyte-activating factor, or catabolin. The IL-1 is produced by B-lymphocytes, endothelial cells, fibroblasts, and macrophages. It stimulates T- and B-cell functions. By increasing the production of prostaglandins and collagenase, it induces inflammation. It acts on the brain to increase the body temperature (fever), and in the liver it may produce certain proteins

Table 1.8 Source and action of interleukins

Type of interleukin	Size in MW (kDa)	Source	Target/action
Interleukin-1 (IL-1α, IL-1β, and IL-1RA)	17	Macrophages, Langerhans cells, T-cells, B-cells, vascular endothelium, fibroblasts, keratinocytes	T-cells, B-cells, neutrophils, eosinophils, dendritic cells, fibroblasts, endothelial cells, hepatocytes, macrophages
Interleukin-2 (IL-2)	15	T-helper-1 cells (Th-1)	T-cells, B-cells, NK cells
Interleukin-3 (IL-3)	25	Activated T-cells, Th-1 cells, Th-2 cells, eosinophils, mast cells	Stimulates growth and maturation of bone marrow stem cells, eosinophilia, neutrophilia, monocytosis, increases phagocytosis, promotes immunoglobulin secretion by B-cells
Interleukin-4 (IL-4)	20	Activated Th-2 cells	B-cells, T-cells, macrophages, endothelial cells, fibroblasts, mast cells, IgE production in allergy, downregulates IL-1, IL-6, and TNF-α
Interleukin-5 (IL-5)	18	Th-2 cells, mast cells, eosinophils	Eosinophils, increases T-cell cytotoxicity
Interleukin-6 (IL-6)	26	Macrophages, T-cells, B-cells, bone marrow stromal cells, vascular endothelial cells, fibroblasts, keratinocytes, mesangial cells	T-cells, B-cells, hepatocytes, bone marrow stromal cells, stimulates acute-phase protein synthesis, acts as pyrogen
Interleukin-7 (IL-7)	25	Bone marrow, spleen cells, thymic stromal cells	Thymocytes, T-cells, B-cells, monocytes, lymphoid stem cells, generates cytotoxic T-cells
Interleukin-8 (IL-8)	8	Macrophages	T-cells, neutrophils
Interleukin-9 (IL-9)	39	Th-2 cells	Growth of Th-cells, stimulates B-cells, thymocytes, mast cells
Interleukin-10 (IL-10)	19	Th cells, B-cells, macrophages, keratinocytes, Th-2 cells	Th-1 cells, NK cells, stimulates B-cells, thymocytes, mast cells
Interleukin-11 (IL-11)	24	Bone marrow stromal cells, fibroblasts	Growth of B-cells, megakaryocyte colony formation, promotes the production of acute-phase proteins
Interleukin-12 (IL-12)	75	Activated macrophages	Th-1 cell activity, T-cell proliferation and cytotoxicity, NK cell proliferation and cytotoxicity, suppresses IgE production, enhances B-cell immunoglobulin production

(continued)

Table 1.8 (continued)

Type of interleukin	Size in MW (kDa)	Source	Target/action
Interleukin-13 (IL-13)	10	Th-2 cells	B-cells, macrophages, neutrophils, inhibits macrophage activity, stimulates B-cell proliferation, stimulates neutrophils
Interleukin-14 (IL-14)	53	T-cells, malignant B-cells	Enhances B-cell proliferation, inhibits immunoglobulin secretion
Interleukin-15 (IL-15)	15	Activated macrophages, epithelial cells, fibroblasts	T-cells, NK cells, proliferation of both cytotoxic and helper T-cells, generates LAK cells
Interleukin-16 (IL-16)	13	T-cells (CD8 cells)	T-cells, CD4 cells, chemotactic for lymphocytes
Interleukin-17 (IL-17)	17	CD4 cells	Promotes the production of IL-6, IL-8
Interleukin-18 (IL-18)	–	Monocytes Epithelial cells	Activates NK cells, enhances IFN-γ, IL-2, GM-CSF
Interleukin-23 (IL-23)	19/40	Macrophages, dendritic cells	T-lymphocytes (increase IL-17)
Interleukin-27 (IL-27)	28/13	Macrophages, dendritic cells	Th-1 lymphocytes (inhibition and/or differentiation), NK lymphocytes (increase IFN-γ)
Chemokines	8–12	Macrophages, endothelia, fibroblasts, epithelia	Increased migration of phagocytes, B-lymphocytes, and T-lymphocytes, and increased wound repair
Lymphotoxin	21–24	T-lymphocytes	Increased development of B- and T-lymphocytes and increased migration and activation of neutrophils

in response to injury. All the cells of the body have receptors of IL-1 and respond to it.

1.7.2.2 Interleukin-2 (IL-2)

Interleukin-2 is produced by T-lymphocytes comprising CD4+ and CD8+ and large granular lymphocytes. Earlier it was known as T-cell growth factor. Interleukin-2 acts upon all the T-lymphocytes to induce their activity and growth. It also induces the growth and differentiation of large granular lymphocytes and B-cells. The macrophages and oligodendrocytes are also activated by the action of IL-2. It is being used in renal cancer therapy as it activates T-cells, which produce cytotoxic anticancer effects.

1.7.2.3 Interleukin-3 (IL-3)
Earlier IL-3 was known as multispecific hemoprotein as it stimulates erythrocytes, granulocytes, macrophages, and lymphocytes. It is produced by activated T-cells, eosinophils, and mast cells.

1.7.2.4 Interleukin-4 (IL-4)
Interleukin-4, previously known as B-cell-activating factor, acts on B-cells and induces their activation and differentiation for production of IgG1 and IgE. On T-cells, IL-4 acts as growth and activating factor. It induces MHC class II expression with macrophages and inhibits cytokine (IL-1, IL-6, and TNF-α) production and their downregulation. Excess IL-4 plays an important role in anaphylaxis as a result of increased IgE production. It is produced by activated T_h-2 cells.

1.7.2.5 Interleukin-5 (IL-5)
Interleukin-5 is produced by T_h-2 cells, mast cells, and eosinophils and acts on eosinophils and promotes growth and differentiation of B-cells. In parasitic diseases, it is responsible for eosinophilia.

1.7.2.6 Interleukin-6 (IL-6)
Previously, it was known as B-cell differentiating factor. IL-6 is produced by T-lymphocytes, macrophages, B-lymphocytes, fibroblasts, and endothelial cells. It acts on B-cells and induces their differentiation into plasma cells. IL-6 stimulates production of acute-phase proteins in the liver. It is an important growth factor for multiple myeloma and also acts as pyrogen.

1.7.2.7 Interleukin-7 (IL-7)
Earlier it was known as pre-B-cell growth factor. It is produced by the bone marrow and thymic stroma. IL-7 acts on thymocytes for T-cell growth and their activation. It is also known to act as macrophage-activating factor.

1.7.2.8 Interleukin-8 (IL-8)
Interleukin-8 has 15 subtypes below the MW of 8 kDa. All these subtypes of IL-8 are produced by macrophages and endothelial cells. These are involved in migration of cells in the inflammatory process. It acts as chemotactic agent for neutrophils and T-lymphocytes.

1.7.2.9 Interleukin-10 (IL-10)
Interleukin-10 is produced by T_h cells, B-cells, and macrophages and acts on T_h cells and NK cells. It stimulates B-cell proliferation.

1.7.2.10 Interleukin-11 (IL-11)
Interleukin-11 is produced by bone marrow stromal cells and fibroblasts. It acts on B-cells for their growth and promotes production of the acute-phase proteins.

1.7.2.11 Interleukin-12 (IL-12)
Interleukin-12 is a heterodimeric cytokine produced by phagocytic cells, B-cells, and antigen-presenting cells in response to bacteria, bacterial products, and intracellular pathogens. It has clinical potential as therapeutic agent in the control of infectious diseases and cancer. It plays a central role in linking the innate and adaptive immune response. It favors the development of T-helper cells and activate them for cell-mediated immunity against pathogens.

1.7.2.12 Interleukin-13 (IL-13)
It is produced by T-helper cells and acts on B-cells, macrophages, and neutrophils. IL-13 inhibits macrophage activity and stimulates B-cell proliferation and neutrophil activity.

1.7.2.13 Interleukin-14 (IL-14)
It is produced by T-lymphocytes and malignant B-cells. It enhances B-cell proliferation and inhibits immunoglobulin secretion.

1.7.2.14 Interleukin-15 (IL-15)
Interleukin-15 is produced by epithelial cells, fibroblasts, and macrophages and acts on T-cells for their proliferation and generation of LAK cells.

1.7.2.15 Interleukin-16 (IL-16)
It is produced by CD8 cells and acts as chemotactic agent for lymphocytes and acts on CD4 cells.

1.7.2.16 Interleukin-17 (IL-17)
Interleukin-17 is produced by T-helper cells and promotes production of interleukin-6 and interleukin-8 from macrophages, T- and B-cells, and endothelial cells.

1.7.2.17 Interleukin-18 (IL-18)
Interleukin-18 is produced by monocytes and epithelial cells and acts on NK cells. It enhances the activity of gamma interferon, interleukin-2, and GM-CSF. It also has anti-tumor and anti-microbial action.

1.7.3 Tumor Necrosis Factor (Cytotoxins)

The tumor necrosis factor has direct cytotoxic effect on neoplastic cells. It is produced by macrophages and T-cells and is associated with apoptosis. It induces fever and other acute-phase inflammatory responses. It stimulates the synthesis of certain lymphokines and activates endothelial cells and macrophages. Tumor necrosis factor-alpha is produced by macrophages, T- and B-cells, and fibroblasts. It activates macrophages and enhances immunity and inflammatory reaction. Tumor necrosis factor-beta is produced by T-helper cells, which activates cytotoxic T-cells, neutrophils, macrophages, and B-lymphocytes.

1.7.4 Colony-Stimulating Factor

1.7.4.1 Macrophage Colony-Stimulating Factor
It is produced by monocytes, endothelial cells of blood capillaries, and fibroblasts. It acts on monocyte precursor cells for their proliferation.

1.7.4.2 Granulocyte Colony-Stimulating Factor
It is produced by macrophages, endothelial cells, and fibroblasts. It acts on stem cells of granulocytes and stimulates them for their proliferation and differentiation.

1.7.4.3 Granulocyte-Monocyte Colony-Stimulating Factor
It is produced by T-lymphocytes, macrophages, endothelial cells, and fibroblasts. It stimulates the granulocyte and macrophage precursors for their proliferation. It induces phagocytosis, superoxide production, and antibody-dependent cellular cytotoxicity (ADCC) by neutrophils.

1.7.5 Migration Inhibitory Factor

Migration inhibitory factor (MIF) is produced by T-cells and acts on macrophages. It inhibits the migration of macrophages, and thus, macrophages remain present at the site of injury.

1.7.5.1 Mechanism of Action
Cytokines are effective in very low concentration even at a dose of 10^{-12} gm/ml. They bind with high-affinity receptors on the cell surface, which transmit the cytokine signals to the nucleus. Cytokines regulate the intensity and duration of the immune response by stimulation or inhibition of the activity of various cells. Binding of a given cytokine to responsive target cells stimulates expression of cytokine receptors, which in turn affect other target cells. Thus, cytokines secreted by a single lymphocyte following antigen-specific activation can influence the activity of various cells involved in the immunity.

The cytokine actions are non-specific. However, there is some specificity regulated by cytokine receptors present on various cells. The cytokine receptors are expressed on a cell only after that cell has interacted with antigen. Thus, the non-specific activity of cytokines is limited to antigen-primed lymphocytes (Table 1.9).

The cytokines do not operate individually in vivo. A mixture of cytokines can exert an effect, which is not seen with any of the cytokines used alone. There can be both synergistic and antagonistic effects. There are some inhibitors of cytokines in vivo, *which* might operate in three different ways:

1. Cytokine-like mediators, which bind to the cytokine receptors.
2. Extracellular domains of the cytokine receptors that have been shed by the cell.
3. One cytokine can switch off the response to another.

Table 1.9 A summary of the major mediators of inflammation

Inflammatory mediator	Primary source	Inflammatory action
Cytokines and chemokines		
IL-1β, IL-6, and TNF-α	Macrophages	Leukocyte and endothelial activation; systemic reactions
CXCL8 (IL-8)	Leukocytes	Leukocyte activation and chemotaxis
Plasma proteins		
C3a	Complement activation	Mast cell degranulation; smooth muscle contraction
C5a	Complement activation	Leukocyte chemotaxis; mast cell degranulation; smooth muscle contraction; vascular permeability
Bradykinin	Kinin-kallikrein system	Vasodilation; vascular permeability; pain
Vasoactive amines		
Histamine	Mast cell degranulation	Vascular permeability; smooth muscle contraction
Serotonin (5-hydroxytryptamine)	Mast cell degranulation	Vascular permeability; smooth muscle contraction
Eicosanoids		
Leukotriene B4	Leukocytes	Leukocyte activation and chemotaxis; vascular permeability
Leukotrienes B4, D4, and E4	Leukocytes (particularly mast cells)	Smooth muscle contraction; vascular permeability
Prostaglandin E2	Leukocytes (particularly mast cells)	Vasodilation; vascular permeability; pain

The cytokine receptor antagonists include IgG adherent monocyte product of a protein (18 kDa), which binds with IL-1 receptor present on the cell surface, and thus, the action of IL-1 is inhibited due to lack of receptor. Other inhibitors of cytokine actions bind with cytokine itself. These are the soluble serum inhibitors of cytokines derived from extracellular domain of the receptors by enzymatic cleavage.

Many cytokines are being studied for their therapeutic and prophylactic potential. The use of interleukins in domestic animals for increased antibody production, increased cellular cytotoxic responses, and altered cell trafficking has been reported. The administration of cytokines in cattle and pigs provide effective protection against diseases without any clinical defects. The natural cytotoxic cell responses are increased, and the number of immunocytes was found increased in the mammary gland due to use of cytokine therapy.

The cytokines are rapidly inactivated or cleared from the body. This may limit the duration of cytokine immunotherapy. Thus, the timing of cytokine administration is critical; the careful timing may be helpful in the control of infectious diseases. There is a fear that repeated or prolonged use of cytokines may increase the risk of inducing antibodies against them. The excessive release or administration of cytokines can lead to shock syndrome: hemorrhagic necrosis, the Shwartzman reaction, and necrosis. Shock syndrome occurs when certain bacterial products, like lipopolysaccharides (LPS), are released during septicemic stage. It leads to fever, circulatory collapse, diffuse intravascular coagulation, and hemorrhagic necrosis. Schwartzman reaction is observed when Gram-negative organisms are injected into the skin of rabbits, and after 24 h another intravenous injection of the same organism is given. The reaction consists of hemorrhagic necrosis that occurs at the prepared site of the skin. These reactions are mediated by cytokines particularly interleukin-1 and tumor necrosis factor.

1.7.5.2 Historical Milestones

2650 BC	India	Foundation of immunology was laid when variolation against smallpox was performed by inoculating live organisms from disease pustules. It protected the host from smallpox
300–500 BC	Charak	Developed 1st immunomodulator "Chyawan Prash to increase Jeevani Shakti"
600 AD	Acharya Madhava	Diagnosis of diseases
1794–1823	Edward Jenner	Father of Immunology, prevented smallpox though cowpox virus
1877	Paul Erlich	Recognition of mast cells
1879	Louis Pasteur	Attenuation of bacteria *Pasteurella multocida* for vaccine
1884	Elie Metchnikoff	Phagocytosis of bacteria by mammalian neutrophils
1885	Louis Pasteur	Rabies vaccination development
1890	Von Behring	Protective effects of antibody, Tetanus culture filtrate as vaccine
	Rod Porter and Gerry Edelman	Structure of immunoglobulin
1891	Robert Koch	Delayed-type hypersensitivity
1894	Paul Ehrlich	Side chain theory of antibody production
1901	Karl Landsteiner	A, B, and O blood groupings
1901	Emil Adolf von Behring	Nobel prize for the discovery of serum antibody
1901–1908	Carl Jensen and Leo Loeb	Transplantable tumors
1902	Ricket and Portier	Anaphylaxis
1903	Sir Almroth Wright	Described opsonins
1905	Robert Koch	Nobel prize for immune response in tuberculosis
1906	Clemens von Pirquet	Coined the word allergy
1908	Ilya Ilyich Mechnikov and Paul Ehrlich	Nobel prize for phagocytosis and antitoxins
1913	Charles Richet	Nobel prize for anaphylaxis

(continued)

1.7 Cytokines

(continued)

1919	Jules Bordet	Nobel prize for complement
1941	Albert Coons	Immunofluorescence technique
1942	Jules Freund and Katherine McDermott	Adjuvants
1944	Medawar	Immunological basis of graft rejection
1949	Macfarlane Burnet and Frank Fenner	Immunological tolerance hypothesis
1950	Richard Gershon and K Kondo	Discovery of suppressor T cells
1952	Ogden and Bruton	Discovery of agammaglobulinemia (antibody immunodeficiency)
1953	Morton Simonsen and WJ Dempster	Graft-versus-host reaction
1953	James Riley and Geoffrey West	Discovery of histamine in mast cells
1955–1959	Niels Jerne, David Talmage, and Macfarlane Burnet	Clonal selection
1956	Rose and Witebsky'e	Thyroid autoantibodies/autoimmunity
1957	Ernest Witebsky and coworkers	Induction of autoimmunity in animals
1957	Alick Isaacs and Jean Lindemann	Discovery of interferon (cytokine)
1960	Sir Frank Macfarlane Burnet and Peter Brian Medawar	Nobel prize for immunological tolerance
1961	Jaeques Miller	Immunological junction of thymus
1967	Kimishige Ishizaka and coworkers	Identification of IgE as the reaginic antibody
1970	WHO	Eradication of smallpox

Cells of immune system |
1972	Gerald M. Edelman and Rodney R. Porter	Nobel prize for antibody structure
1974	Rolf Zinkernagel and Peter Doherty	MHC restriction
1975	Kohler and Milstein	Monoclonal antibodies used in genetic analysis
1977	Rosalyn Sussman Yalow	Nobel prize for development of radioimmunoassay
1980	Baruj Benacerraf, Jean Dausset, and George D. Snell	Nobel prize for the discovery of the major histocompatibility complex
1984	Niels K. Jerne, Georges J.F. Kohler, and César Milstein	Nobel prize for production of monoclonal antibodies
1987	Susumu Tonegawa	Nobel prize for mechanism of antibody diversity
1990	Joseph E. Murray and E. Donnall Thomas	Nobel prize for transplantation
1990	NIH team	Gene therapy for SCID using cultured T cells
1993	NIH team	Treatment of SCID using genetically altered umbilical cord cells
1996	Peter C. Doherty and Rolf M. Zinkernagel	Nobel prize for major histocompatibility complex restriction
2011	Ralph M. Steinman	Nobel prize for role of the dendritic cell in adaptive immunity

(continued)

(continued)		
2011	Bruce A. Beutler and Jules A. Hoffman	Nobel prize for activation of innate immunity
2011	B. Hoffmann, M. Beer, T. Mettenleiter	Discovery of Schmallenberg virus
2011	Carl H. June	First successful use of CAR T cells expressing the 4-1BB costimulatory signaling domain for the treatment of CD19+ malignancies
2012	A.M. Zaki, R. Fouchier, W.I. Lipkin	Discovery of MERS coronavirus
2016	Yoshinori Ohsumi	Nobel Prize for his discoveries of mechanisms for autophagy
2018	Tasuku Honjo and James Allison	Nobel prize for their discovery of cancer therapy by inhibition of negative immune regulation
2020	Harvey J. Alter, Michael Houghton, and Charles M. Rice	Nobel Prize for the discovery of hepatitis C virus
2023	Katalin Karikó and Drew Weissman	Discovery of nucleoside base modifications that enabled the development of effective mRNA vaccines against COVID-19

Further Reading

Chauhan RS (1998) An introduction to immunopathology. G.B. Pant University, Pantnagar

Chauhan RS (2002) Illustrated veterinary pathology. IBDC, Lucknow

Chauhan RS, Singh GK (2001) Cytokines and immunity. In: Singh GK, Chauhan RS (eds) Advances in veterinary anatomy, pp 164–175

Higgins DA (1981) Markers for T- and B-lymphocytes and their application to animals. Veter Bull 51:925–963

Maliszewski C, Gallis B, Baker PE (1990) The molecular biology of large animal cytokines. Adv Vet Sci Comp Med 35:181–313

Poster P (1979) Structural and functional characteristics of immunoglobulins of the common domestic species. Adv Vet Sci Comp Med 23:1–21

Singh GK, Chauhan RS (2001) Immunocytology: an anatomical perspective. In: Singh GK, Chauhan RS (eds) Advances in veterinary anatomy, pp 79–91

Thomas ML (1989) The leukocyte common antigen family. Annu Rev. Immunol 7:339–369

Tizard IR (1996) Veterinary immunology: an introduction, 5th edn. W.B. Saunders Co., Singapore

Biomarkers of Immunopathology in Veterinary Medicine

Key Points

1. Biomarkers are biological molecules or characteristics, which can be distinctively and consistently assessed as an indication of normal physiological, pathobiological, or pharmacodynamic processes.
2. Specific cells of innate immune system, receptors for microbial ligands, antimicrobial molecules, and inflammatory mediators are the potential biomarkers of immunopathology.
3. Pathogen-associated molecular patterns (PAMPs) are unique molecules and exogenous signals from microbial invaders.
4. Damage-associated molecular patterns (DAMPs) are endogenous signals consist of molecules released from the dead or damaged cells.
5. Pattern-recognition receptors (PRRs) are present on sentinel cells, which are located throughout the body and recognize the DAMPs and PAMPs.
6. Most prevalent PRRs are TLRs and RLRs like RIG-I, MDA-5, and NOD-like receptors.
7. The first PRRs to be discovered were the TLRs.
8. IgG2 antibodies are produced in response to polysaccharide antigens, whereas the IgG1 subclass primarily reacts to protein antigens.
9. Interleukins are a type of cytokines produced by leukocytes and a variety of different body cells.
10. Chemokines are broad class of small secreted proteins that signal through G protein-coupled heptahelical chemokine receptors on cell surfaces and induce cell migration.
11. Antimicrobial peptides (AMPs) are essential components of the innate immune system in humans, animals, and plants, and they serve as the first line of defense against foreign invaders like bacteria, fungi, and viruses.
12. Collectins are soluble mammalian collagen-containing C-type lectins that serve diverse functions in the innate immune system and represent an important group of PRRs.

© The Author(s), under exclusive license to Springer Nature Singapore Pte Ltd. 2024
R. S. Chauhan et al., *Essentials of Veterinary Immunology and Immunopathology*, https://doi.org/10.1007/978-981-99-2718-0_2

13. Biomarkers are commonly used in biological research, illness diagnosis, monitoring, and treatment prognostication in veterinary medicine.Biomarkers are the biological molecules or characteristics they can be distinctively and consistently assessed as an indication of normal physiological, pathobiological, or pharmacodynamic processes. Specific cells of the innate immune system, receptors for microbial ligands, antimicrobial molecules, and inflammatory mediators are the potential biomarkers of immunopathology, which are frequently employed for biological research, disease diagnosis, and monitoring as well as therapeutic prognostication in veterinary medicine (Linde et al. 2008; Llibre and Duffy 2018).

2.1 Introduction

Biomarkers are the biological molecules or characteristics they can be distinctively and consistently assessed as an indication of normal physiological, pathobiological, or pharmacodynamic processes. Specific cells of the innate immune system, receptors for microbial ligands, antimicrobial molecules, and inflammatory mediators are the potential biomarkers of immunopathology, which are frequently employed for biological research, disease diagnosis, and monitoring as well as therapeutic prognostication in veterinary medicine (Linde et al. 2008; Llibre and Duffy 2018). Specific biomarkers should be measurable with little or no variability, should have a sizeable signal-to-noise ratio, and change promptly and reliably in response to changes in the condition, disease, or its therapy. The use of clinical biomarkers has the advantages of being simpler and less expensive to measure than final clinical end-points.

Biomarkers can be used as prognostic indicators in disease screening, diagnosis, characterization, monitoring, and treatment in veterinary medicine. Immunological biomarkers are cytokines (IL-1β, IL-6, IL-12p70, IFN-γ, TNF-α, adiponectin, and leptin), chemokines (IL-8, MIP-1α or CCL3, MIP-1β or CCL4, and RANTES or CCL5), soluble forms of cell receptors (soluble CD14 (sCD14), sCD25 or IL-2Rα, sCD40L, sCD120b or sTNF-RII, sCD126 or sIL-6R, sCD130 or sgp130, and sCD163), and immune activation markers (T- and B-lymphocyte phenotype) can serve as surrogate markers for cellular activation and play an important role in the function of the immune system. Complex interactions between the immune cells of the innate and adaptive immune systems are modified by the release of a variety of cell mediators that trigger inflammatory responses, which help to eliminate and destroy foreign antigens.

The cytokines are small signalling molecules that orchestrate immune responses by enabling cell to cell communication and recruitment of immune cells to infection sites. Cytokines can be further subdivided into interleukins (IL), interferons (IFN), chemokines and tumor necrosis factors (TNF), which may promote either pro-inflammatory or anti-inflammatory responses. They have the capacity to stimulate and modulate the immune system and are therefore great indicators of normal immunological processes, pathological processes or responses to treatment.

Cytokines are key players in homeostasis and immune responses and thus hold great potential for becoming biomarkers of disease and response to treatment. Despite current limitations, numerous successful examples exist, both in human and veterinary medicine, of cytokine biomarkers that help diagnosis and monitoring of a wide range of diseases.

Changes in the levels of these biomarkers along with changes in lymphocyte subset activity can provide important prognostic value by reflecting underlying disease conditions. Clinical usefulness of these biomarkers depends upon: 1) their ability to account for a significant portion of the disease being evaluated; 2) the ability to be accurately, reproducibly, and reliably measured; and 3) the availability of the assay for widespread application. Since blood levels of immunological biomarkers differ widely between individuals based on their gender, age, and other factors, baseline concentrations of biomarkers should be established for healthy individuals.

Biological variation is often the most important source of variation over time for certain biomarkers and marked changes can occur during the neonatal, childhood, puberty, menopause, and aging process. In addition, certain biomarkers have biological rhythms that can vary diurnally, monthly, or seasonally. There are only a limited numbers of studies examined the biological variation of immunological biomarkers and lymphocyte phenotype.

2.2 Specific Cells of the Innate Immune System

Blood leukograms are much useful clinically since the white blood cell counts as well as morphology are fairly stable and consistent in healthy animals, which may be altered dramatically in various pathological conditions. Leukogram findings are scarcely pathognomonic for a particular disease condition, which can furnish the clinical information to reach a set of differential diagnoses, to evaluate the response to treatment, and to hint a prognosis.

2.2.1 Neutrophils

The major function of neutrophils is destruction of the bacteria, but they may also have deleterious effects against fungi, parasites, and viruses. Further, they are also involved in the augmentation of acute inflammatory responses and elimination of transformed or infected cells. Toxic neutrophils refer to the presence of azurophilic dark coarse granules found in the cytoplasm of neutrophils (Fig. 2.1), especially during inflammatory conditions of any cause and severe enough to increase the neutrophil production. Toxic changes in neutrophils are morphologic abnormalities acquired during Gram-negative sepsis and endotoxemia. Toxic granulation is attributed to acid mucopolysaccharide retention and increased permeability of primary granules to Romanowsky stains.

Fig. 2.1 Toxic granulation in neutrophil of human. Presence of large, more numerous purple or dark blue cytoplasmic granules (primary granules) in neutrophils (red arrow) and megakaryocytes (black arrow). 100×, oil

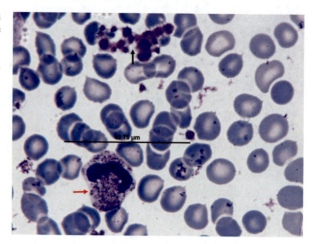

Neutrophilia (higher neutrophil count in the blood) can be most commonly associated with physiological response and corticosteroid-induced or in association with infection and/or inflammation. Physiological neutrophilia is most often observed in young animals due to the endogenous release of catecholamines as a result of fright, excitement, or arduous exercise (Stockham and Scott 2008). This change in leukogram will be transitory and usually diminishes within 10 to 20 minutes. The mechanism behind this phenomenon is presumed to be the rapid increase in blood flow through the pulmonary microvasculature due to epinephrine release, which further leads to the release of the marginal neutrophil pool into the general circulation. Corticosteroid-induced neutrophilia is associated with the endogenous release of glucocorticoids due to extreme stress or disease or due to administration of exogenous corticosteroids, and the underlying mechanism is the accelerated rate of release of neutrophils from the bone marrow. In case of infection or inflammation neutrophilic leukocytosis is observed and the counts usually range between 20,000 and 30,000 cells per microliter; rarely even a count more than 50,000 cells per microliter is observed in association with localized infections like abscesses (Fig. 2.2), pyometra, peritonitis, and pleuritis (Culp et al. 2009; Shah et al. 2017).

Neutropenia is commonly associated with decreased neutrophil production from the bone marrow, neutrophil sequestration in microvasculature, and massive consumption of neutrophils in the tissues exceeding their replacement rate from the bone marrow to the blood. Since the most abundant leukocyte in canine and feline blood is neutrophils, neutropenia generally led to leucopenia and the major clinical outcome of leucopenia is bacterial infections (Brown and Rogers 2001). Decreased neutrophil production from the bone marrow can be associated with hematopoietic stem cell death due to ionizing radiations (Clermont et al. 2012), drugs (Sontas et al. 2009), or pathogenic agents. Quickly progressing severe neutropenia is often associated with Gram-negative septicemic shock, which is due to the sequestration of neutrophils in microvasculature or shift of neutrophils from general circulation to marginal pool.

2.2 Specific Cells of the Innate Immune System

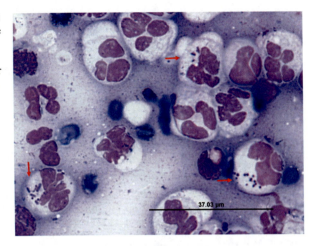

Fig. 2.2 Fine needle aspirate from abscess of dog. Presence of more number of activated neutrophils with phagocytosed bacteria in their cytoplasm (red arrow). 100×, oil

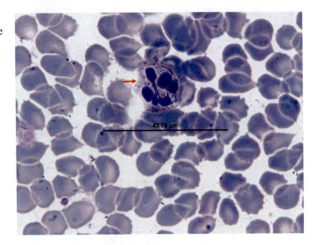

Fig. 2.3 Hypersegmented neutrophil of human. Presence of six or more nuclear lobes (red arrow), commonly seen during megaloblastic anemia. 100×, oil

Neutropenia due to massive consumption of neutrophils is usually observed in localized bacterial infections involving the uterus, integumentary system, gastrointestinal tract, or lungs. Hypersegmented neutrophil can be defined as the presence of six or more nuclear lobes, which are seen in combination with macrocytic or megaloblastic anemia caused by vitamin B12 or folic acid deficiency; but, may also be present in myelodysplastic syndromes and rarely in congenital conditions (Fig. 2.3).

2.2.2 Monocytes

Blood monocytes are the precursor pool to replace tissue macrophages (Fig. 2.4). The major functions of monocytes and macrophages are phagocytosis (Fig. 2.5) and destruction of certain bacteria (Fig. 2.6), protozoa, fungi, and viruses, removal of tissue debris by phagocytosis, destruction of transformed cells and virus-infected cells, tissue repair, and secretion of various bioactive molecules (Richards et al. 2013; Wynn and Vannella 2016).

Monocytosis (higher monocyte count in the blood) is often observed along with neutrophilia in many acute and chronic diseases of dogs and cats. Monocytosis as a primary leukogram abnormality is often observed in bacterial endocarditis (MacDonald et al. 2004). Exogenous and endogenous corticosteroids usually result in monocytosis and concurrent neutrophilia especially in dogs and cats (Kritsepi-

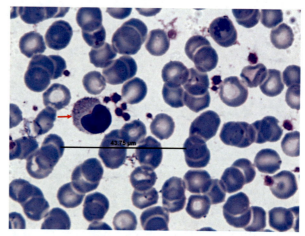

Fig. 2.4 Monocyte of dog in a blood smear. Largest mononuclear leukocyte has large eccentrically placed kidney bean-shaped nucleus with abundant cytoplasm (red arrow). 100×, oil

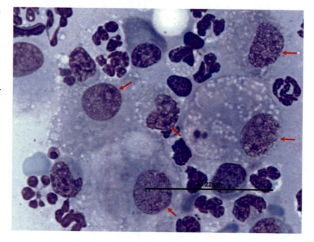

Fig. 2.5 Fine needle aspirate from a mass of dog. Presence of activated macrophages has large eccentrically placed nucleus with abundant vacuolated cytoplasm and phagocytosed material in their cytoplasm (red arrow) and neutrophils. 100×, oil

2.2 Specific Cells of the Innate Immune System

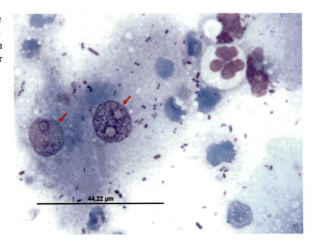

Fig. 2.6 Fine needle aspirate from a mass of dog. Presence of activated macrophages with phagocytosed bacteria in their cytoplasm (red arrow) and neutrophils. 100×, oil

Konstantinou and Oikonomidis 2016). Extreme monocytosis can be observed often in monocytic leukemias of dogs and cats (McManus 2005).

2.2.3 Lymphocytes

Lymphocytes are the most numerous blood leukocytes in bovine and the second most numerous in dogs (Fig. 2.7) and cats; they are the indispensable constituents of both humoral and cell-mediated immune systems. The number of blood lymphocytes in animals can be promptly varied in various pathological conditions, drug administration, and physiological states.

Pseudolymphocytosis or physiological lymphocytosis (higher lymphocyte count in the blood) in response to epinephrine release is common in young ones especially

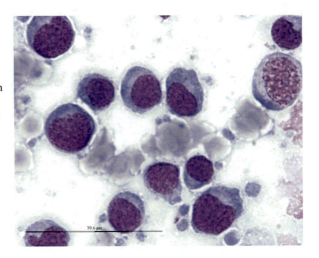

Fig. 2.7 Lymphocytes of dog in an aspirate from prescapular lymph node. Lymphocytes have a regular, spherical nucleus and high nuclear:cytoplasmic ratio with scanty, pale blue, agranular rim of cytoplasm. 100×, oil

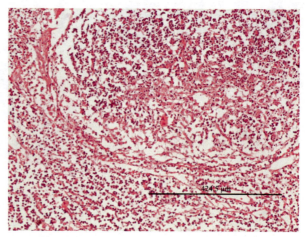

Fig. 2.8 Lymph node of dog infected with canine distemper virus (CDV). Lymph node showed marked lymphocytic depletion in cortex. H&E ×100

in cats, which is often transient in nature (Kritsepi-Konstantinou and Oikonomidis 2016). Chronic infectious diseases and inflammatory conditions are the major differentials enlisted in case of lymphocytosis in dogs and cats (Avery and Avery 2007; Kritsepi-Konstantinou and Oikonomidis 2016). Extreme lymphocytosis can be observed often in lymphocytic leukemias of dogs and cats (McManus 2005).

Corticosteroid-induced lymphopenia is often observed in extreme stress or after corticosteroid administration. Following corticosteroid therapy, lymphopenia appears within 4 to 6 h and lasts during the course of drug administration. Restoration of baseline lymphocyte counts takes place within 24 to 72 h of cessation of drug. Stress-related lymphopenia is also as a result of a release of endogenous corticosteroids (Bodnariu 2008). Viral infections like feline panleukopenia virus (FPV), canine parvovirus (CPV), and canine distemper virus (CDV) produce marked lymphopenia (Fig. 2.8) due to bone marrow suppression and atrophy of lymphoid tissue.

2.3 Receptors for Microbial Ligands

Immune cells and some parenchymal cells of the body expressing a group of receptor molecules targeting specific epitopes on various pathogenic organisms are called as pattern-recognition receptors (PRRs) and the corresponding target epitopes are termed as pathogen-associated molecular patterns (PAMPs) (Takeuchi and Akira 2010). These PRRs act as a first line of defense against invasion of pathogens and they may trigger both innate and adaptive immune responses.

2.3.1 Transmembrane PRRs

Transmembrane PRRs detect PAMPs present in the extracellular sites and phagosomes; they constitute mainly two families: Toll-like receptors (TLRs) and dectin-1. The ligands detected by TLRs are mainly bacterial cell wall constituents and viral nucleic acids and they can induce humoral (especially IgG2) and $CD8^+$ T-cell immune responses (Iwasaki and Medzhitov 2004; Pasare and Medzhitov 2005). The dectin-1 detects fungal cell wall constituents and β-glucans of fungal pathogens like *Candida albicans* and induce innate and adaptive immune responses (Brown and Gordon 2001; LeibundGut-Landmann et al. 2007).

2.3.2 Cytosolic PRRs

The TLRs play an important role in recognizing microbes and in triggering inflammation. These receptors are expressed in antigen-presenting cells (APCs) like macrophage and dendritic cells, mast cells, eosinophils, and the epithelium of the respiratory tract and intestines (Akira 2003). The TLRs do not seem to be capable of identifying intracellular cytosolic pathogens and derivatives, since they are expressed on either the cell surface or the luminal aspect of endo-lysosomal membranes. The TLR-independent pathogen recognition is carried out by an extensive array of cytosolic PRRs, which can be split into retinoid acid-inducible gene I (RIG-I)-like receptors (RLRs) and nucleotide-binding oligomerization domain (NOD)-like receptors (NLRs).

The RLRs are RNA virus-sensing TLRs localized inside the cytoplasm and it encompasses three members, RIG-I, melanoma differentiation-associated protein 5 (MDA5), and laboratory of genetics and physiology 2 (LGP2). The IFN-inducible RNA helicases are present in RIG-I and MDA5, which plays a critical role in prolonged induction of IFN cytokines against viral particles. The NLR family constituting NOD1 and NOD2 is recognizing bacterial invasion through detecting bacterial peptidoglycan components in the cytoplasm and inducing innate immune responses (Medzhitov 2009). There are 22 known NLRs in humans, and their critical involvement in host defense is shown by the relationship of mutations and single nucleotide polymorphisms (SNPs) in their genes with human diseases. The NLRs play a role in reproduction and embryonic development in addition to immunity (Tong et al. 2000; Murdoch et al. 2006; Fernandes et al. 2012).

2.4 Inflammatory Mediators

The term "inflammation" derives from the Latin word "inflammare," which means "to burn" (de oliveira). Inflammation is one of the most important mechanisms in animal cells defense against damage and microbial infections (Isailovic et al. 2015; Todd et al. 2015). Nevertheless, inflammation regularly progresses to acute or chronic. It is characterized by a series of well-organized, dynamic responses that include both cellular and vascular processes as well as distinct humoral discharges. Changes in the physical location of white blood cells (monocytes, lymphocytes, basophils, eosinophils, and neutrophils), plasma, and fluids at the inflamed site are involved in these processes (Huether and McCance 2015). Immune defense cells release a collection of secreted mediators (cytokines, interleukins, and chemokines) and other signaling molecules (e.g., histamine, prostaglandins, leukotrienes, oxygen- and nitrogen-derived free radicals, and serotonin) as part of a mechanism that can trigger inflammatory process (Anwikar and Bhitre 2010).

2.4.1 Cytokines

Cytokines are small secreted proteins released by the cells and have a specific effect on the interactions and communications between cells. Other names for cytokines are lymphokines (cytokines produced by lymphocytes), monokines (cytokines produced by monocytes), chemokines (cytokines with chemotactic activity), and interleukins (cytokines produced by the interleukins and cytokines made by one leukocyte and acting on other leukocytes). Cytokines can act on the cells that release them (autocrine action), on neighboring cells (paracrine action), and on the distant cells (paracrine or endocrine action) (Zhang and An 2007). They are made up of many cell populations, but the predominant producers are helper T cells (Th) and macrophages. Following an injury, macrophage cells gather around the injured site and secrete cytokines and specific growth factors required for regeneration (Watkins et al. 2003; Xie et al. 2006).

Due to the effect of cytokines in the context of an inflammatory disease, they can be divided into inflammatory and anti-inflammatory (Goldring and Goldring 2004). An inflammatory cytokine is a type of signaling molecule that can promote inflammation and is released by the immune cells and some other cell types. Pro-inflammatory cytokines are produced predominantly by activated macrophages and T-helper cells (Th) and are involved in the upregulation of inflammatory reactions (Zhang and An 2007). Inflammatory cytokines include interleukin-1 (IL-1), IL-12, IL-18, tumor necrosis factor-alpha (TNF-α), interferon-gamma (IFN-γ), and granulocyte-macrophage colony-stimulating factor (GM-CSF) (Cavaillon 2001).

On the other hand, anti-inflammatory cytokines are a group of immunoregulatory molecules that regulate the production of pro-inflammatory cytokines. Cytokines act in concert with specific cytokine inhibitors and soluble cytokine receptors to regulate the immune responses. Major anti-inflammatory cytokines include IL-1 receptor antagonist, IL-4, IL-6, IL-10, IL-11, and IL-13. Specific cytokine receptors for IL-1, TNF-α, and IL-18 also function as pro-inflammatory cytokine inhibitors (Opal and DePalo 2000).

2.4.2 Interleukins

Interleukins are a type of cytokines that was once considered to be produced only by leukocytes, but has now been discovered to be produced by a variety of different body cells. They are involved in immune cell activation and differentiation, as well as proliferation, maturation, migration, and adhesion (Table 2.1). They have anti-inflammatory and pro-inflammatory effects as well (Akdis et al. 2011). So far around 40 interleukins were identified and each has a unique function in their target cells.

2.4.3 Chemokines

Chemokines (also known as chemotactic cytokines) are a broad class of small secreted proteins that signal through G protein-coupled heptahelical chemokine

Table 2.1 List of known interleukins and their functions

Interleukin (cytokine)	Source	Target cell	Effect
IL-1	Macrophage, lymphocytes, endothelium, fibroblasts, astrocytes	T-cells, B-cells, macrophages, endothelium, tissue cells	Lymphocyte activation, leukocyte-endothelial adhesion, fever, regulates sleep
IL-2	T-cells	T-cells	T cell growth factor I
IL-3	T-cells	Bone marrow cells	Stimulates bone marrow growth
IL-4	T-cells	B- and T-cells	B-cell growth factor
IL-5	T-cells	B-cells	B-cell growth factor
IL-6	T- and B-cells, macrophages, fibroblasts	B-cells and hepatocytes	B-cell differentiation and synthesis of acute phase reactants
IL-7	Lymphocytes	B- and T-cells	Stimulates proliferation of immature cells
IL-8	T-cells, macrophages	Granulocytes, endothelium	Stimulates the activity of neutrophils, acts as chemotaxin, inhibitor of endothelial cell-leukocyte adhesion
IL-9	T-cells	T-cells	T-cell and mast cell growth enhancement
IL-10	T-cells	Macrophage	Suppresses the development of T-cell subpopulations (TH1) by inhibition of macrophage IL-12 production
IL-11	Bone marrow stromal cells	Hepatocyte	Induces synthesis of acute phase proteins
IL-12	Macrophage	T-cells	Enhances the B-cell expression of IFN-γ during T-cell activation; stimulates lymphocyte subpopulation (NK cells)

receptors on cell surfaces. They are well known for their capacity to induce cell migration, particularly leukocytes migration (Charo and Ransohoff 2006). Chemokines are divided into four distinct subfamilies: CXC, CC, CX3C, and C. All these proteins have biological effects via interacting with chemokine receptors, which are G protein-linked transmembrane receptors present on the surfaces of their target cells (Mélik-Parsadaniantz and Rostène 2008). Certain chemokines are expected to play a pro-inflammatory role, attracting cells to an infection site during an immune response, whereas others are thought to play a homeostatic role, regulating cell migration as part of normal tissue growth and maintenance. Nineteen types of chemokine receptor have so far been identified in mammals and they are found predominantly on the surface of leukocytes. Inflammatory chemokines include CCL2, CCL3, CCL5, CXCL1, CXCL2, and CXCL8. The chemokine CXCL-8 works as a chemoattractant for neutrophils (Graham and Locati 2013).

2.5 Anti-microbial Molecules

2.5.1 Complement

The complement system, also known as the complement cascade, is an innate immune system component that boosts (complements) antibodies and phagocytic cells to eliminate the pathogens and damaged cells from an organism, stimulate inflammation, and damage the pathogen's cell membrane (Janeway Jr et al. 2001). More than 30 soluble plasma and bodily fluid proteins, as well as a variety of cell receptors and regulatory proteins found in blood and tissues, are together referred to as "complement system." Complement activation acts as a "cascade" defense against bacteria, viruses, virus-infected cells, parasites, and tumor cells (Walport 2001). The complement system can be activated by the classical, alternative, or lectin pathways. At the point of C3 cleavage, all three pathways converge, resulting in the formation of the membrane attack complex C5b-9, which leads to cytolysis (Rus et al. 2005).

2.5.2 Lysozyme

Lysozyme (also known as muramidase or N-acetylmuramic acid hydrolase) is a cellular enzyme, which exerts antibacterial activity by hydrolyzing peptidoglycans found in Gram-positive bacterial cell wall (Ferraboschi et al. 2021). Lysozyme has been regarded as an endogenous antibiotic due to its ability to destroy the bacterial cell wall. Due to the ability to hydrolyze the 1,4-glycosidic bond present in the polysaccharide layer of bacterial cell walls, its antibacterial action is especially effective against Gram-positive bacteria. Action against Gram-negative bacteria is significantly reduced due to the existence of protective lipopolysaccharide layer on the outer membrane (Ferraboschi et al. 2021).

2.5.3 Anti-microbial Peptides

Antimicrobial peptides (AMPs) are essential components of the innate immune system in humans, animals, and plants, and they serve as the first-line of defense against foreign invaders (Kosciuczuk et al. 2012; Starr et al. 2018). In the 1980s, AMPs or host defense peptides were discovered and they displayed their broad-spectrum and potent antimicrobial efficacy against bacteria, fungi, and viruses (Zanetti 2004; Bahar and Ren 2013). The AMPs were identified in a variety of organisms (bacteria, fungi, mammals, and plants) and thousands of AMPs have been discovered so far (Jenssen et al. 2006; Kosciuczuk et al. 2012). Most of these AMPs are cationic and they serve key antimicrobial property. These positively charged AMPs interact with negatively charged cell membranes through electrostatic interactions and undergo membrane adsorption and conformational change in the microbes (Chen et al. 2007; Som et al. 2008).

2.5.4 Cathelicidins

Cathelicidins are small amphiphilic, cationic peptides consisting of 12–97 amino acids. They were first identified by Zanetti and collaborators in bovine neutrophils in the early 1990s (Zanetti 2004). Cathelicidins are antimicrobial peptides that include proteins like pig protegrins and cattle indolicidins, which have been used as templates for some of the most advanced antimicrobial peptide medicines (Tomasinsig and Zanetti 2005; Nijnik and Hancock 2009). Cathelicidin is primarily stored in the lysosomes of macrophages and polymorphonuclear leukocytes (PMNs) and it exerts antimicrobial activity through disintegration (damaging and puncturing) of cell membranes (Kosciuczuk et al. 2012). The LL-37 is the only peptide in the cathelicidin family found in the human body (Dürr et al. 2006).

2.5.5 Defensins

Defensins are a large class of peptides that are primarily found in neutrophils and epithelial cells (Xu and Lu 2020). The first mammalian defensin (also known as microbicidal cationic protein) was identified from rabbit lung macrophages in 1980 (Patterson-Delafield et al. 1980). Their broad antibacterial properties and complex immunomodulatory actions have been extensively studied, solidifying their significance in innate immunity as a key component of host defense against bacterial, viral, and fungal diseases, and also they possess anti-tumor activity (Xu and Lu 2020).

Defensins directly inactivate and inhibit the replication of a variety of viruses. They prevent host-virus interactions from numerous enveloped viruses and inhibit the fusion mechanism (Yasin et al. 2004; Hazrati et al. 2006; Wang et al. 2013). Defensins have a range of antimicrobial mechanisms that can kill bacteria or impede their development, including direct membrane disruption (Lehrer and Lu 2012) and inhibition of bacterial cell wall synthesis (de Leeuw et al. 2010; Munch and Sahl

2015). The β-defensins are expressed differently in normal tissues and malignancies. Defensins exhibit anti-tumor activity through upregulation of human β-defensin protein-1 (HBD1), which confers tumor cell apoptosis (Bullard et al. 2008; Han et al. 2014). In contrast, HBD3 is frequently overexpressed in various carcinomas (Shuyi et al. 2011; Xu et al. 2016), and its upregulation has been linked to human papillomavirus (HPV) co-infection-induced p53 degradation (DasGupta et al. 2016) and resistance of tumor cells to apoptosis (Mburu et al. 2011), and it promotes tumorigenesis.

2.5.6 Collectins

Collectins (collagen-containing C-type lectins) are soluble mammalian C-type lectins that serve diverse functions in the innate immune system and represent an important group of pattern-recognition molecules. They are known to use calcium-dependent carbohydrate recognition domains (CRDs) to mediate pathogen recognition.

Each collectin subunit is composed of a cysteine-rich domain, a collagen-like domain, and C-terminal globular C-type lectin domain, also called the CRDs (Uemura et al. 2006). Binding of collectins to microbes can accelerate microbial clearance through aggregation, complement activation, opsonization and activation of phagocytosis, and inhibition of microbial growth. Moreover, collectins can influence apoptotic cell clearance and modulate the adaptive immune responses, as well as modulate inflammatory and allergic reactions (van de Wetering et al. 2004). The following nine collectins have been identified to date: mannan-binding lectin (MBL), three bovine serum collectins, conglutinin, CL-43, CL-46, lung surfactant proteins SP-A and SP-D, and more recently discovered collectins including collectin kidney 1 (CL-K1, also called CL-11), collectin liver 1 (CL-L1, also called CL-10), and collectin placenta 1 (CL-P1 also called CL-12) (Murugaiah et al. 2020).

2.6 Conclusion

The biomarkers were defined as a molecule that can be consistently and objectively measured and evaluated qualitatively and/or quantitatively as an indicator of normal biological processes, pathologic processes, or pharmacologic responses to a therapeutic intervention. Biomarkers may consist of nucleic acids, proteins, metabolites etc. Biomarkers have been extensively used in the veterinary medicine to evaluate the health status, risk, diagnosis, prognosis, progression of disease, to predict and monitor response to therapy, and to measure the toxicity or failure of organs. Immune biomarkers may have an interaction with immune system and other systems of the body, hence, they play a significant role as an immune biomarker in disease progression and prognosis for many diseases. Blood, urine, or tissues can be measured as samples for biomarkers evaluation. Assessing the health and disease through the quantification of cytokines present in the plasma or serum is mainly useful due to the ease, safety, and feasibility of the method. Acute phase proteins (APPs) have been used as biomarkers of inflammation, infection, and trauma for decades in veterinary and human medicine. Autoantibody biomarkers are valuable tools for the diagnosis and management of autoimmune diseases in animals.

References

Akdis M, Burgler S, Crameri R, Eiwegger T, Fujita H, Gomez E, Klunker S, Meyer N, O'Mahony L, Palomares O, Rhyner C, Ouaked N, Quaked N, Schaffartzik A, Van De Veen W, Zeller S, Zimmermann M, Akdis CA (2011) Interleukins, from 1 to 37, and interferon-γ: receptors, functions, and roles in diseases. J Allergy Clin Immunol 127(3):701–21. e1–70

Akira S (2003) Mammalian toll-like receptor. Curr Opin Immunol 15:5–11

Anwikar S, Bhitre M (2010) Study of the synergistic anti-inflammatory activity of *Solanum xanthocarpum* Schrader and Wendl and *Cassia fistula* Linn. Int J Ayurveda Res 1(3):167

Avery AC, Avery PR (2007) Determining the significance of persistent lymphocytosis. Vet Clin N Am Small Anim Pract 37(2):267–282

Bahar AA, Ren D (2013) Antimicrobial peptides. Pharmaceuticals (Basel) 6:1543–1575

Bodnariu ALINA (2008) Indicators of stress and stress assessment in dogs. Lucr Stiint Med Vet 41: 20–26

Brown GD, Gordon S (2001) A new receptor for β-glucans. Nature 413(6851):36–37

Brown MR, Rogers KS (2001) Neutropenia in dogs and cats: a retrospective study of 261 cases. J Am Anim Hosp Assoc 37(2):131–139

Bullard RS, Gibson W, Bose SK, Belgrave JK, Eaddy AC, Wright CJ et al (2008) Functional analysis of the host defense peptide human beta defensin-1: new insight into its potential role in cancer. Mol Immunol 45:839–848

Cavaillon JM (2001) Pro- versus anti-inflammatory cytokines: myth or reality. Cellular and Molecular Biology 47(4):695–702

Charo IF, Ransohoff RM (2006) The many roles of chemokines and chemokine receptors in inflammation. N Engl J Med 354(6):610–621

Chen Y, Guarnieri MT, Vasil AI, Vasil ML, Mant CT, Hodges RS (2007) Role of peptide hydrophobicity in the mechanism of action of alpha-helical antimicrobial peptides. Antimicrob Agents Chemother 51:1398–1406

Clermont T, Leblanc AK, Adams WH, Leblanc CJ, Bartges JW (2012) Radiotherapy-induced myelosuppression in dogs: 103 cases (2002–2006). Vet Comp Oncol 10(1):24–32

Culp WT, Zeldis TE, Reese MS, Drobatz KJ (2009) Primary bacterial peritonitis in dogs and cats: 24 cases (1990–2006). J Am Vet Med Assoc 234(7):906–913

DasGupta T, Nweze EI, Yue H, Wang L, Jin J, Ghosh SK et al (2016) Human papillomavirus oncogenic E6 protein regulates human β-defensin 3 (hBD3) expression via the tumor suppressor protein p53. Oncotarget 7:27430–27444

de Leeuw E, Li C, Zeng P, Li C, Diepeveen-de Buin M, Lu WY et al (2010) Functional interaction of human neutrophil peptide-1 with the cell wall precursor lipid II. FEBS Lett 584:1543–1548

Dürr U, Sudheendra U, Ramamoorthy A (2006) LL-37, the only human member of the cathelicidin family of antimicrobial peptides. Biochim Biophys Acta Biomembr 1758(9):1408–1425

Fernandes R, Tsuda C, Perumalsamy AL, Naranian T, Chong J, Acton BM et al (2012) NLRP5 mediates mitochondrial function in mouse oocytes and embryos. Biol Reprod 86(138):131–110. https://doi.org/10.1095/biolreprod.111.093583

Ferraboschi P, Ciceri S, Grisenti P (2021) Applications of lysozyme, an innate immune defense factor, as an alternative antibiotic. Antibiotics 10(12):1534

Goldring SR, Goldring MB (2004) The role of cytokines in cartilage matrix degeneration in osteoarthritis. Clin Orthop Relat Res 427(Suppl):S27–S36

Graham GJ, Locati M (2013) Regulation of the immune and inflammatory responses by the 'atypical' chemokine receptor D6. J Pathol 229(2):168–175

Han Q, Wang R, Sun C, Jin X, Liu D, Zhao X et al (2014) Human beta-defensin-1 suppresses tumor migration and invasion and is an independent predictor for survival of oral squamous cell carcinoma patients. PLoS One 9:e91867. https://doi.org/10.1371/journal.pone.0091867

Hazrati E, Galen B, Lu W, Wang W, Ouyang Y, Keller MJ et al (2006) Human α- and β-defensins block multiple steps in herpes simplex virus infection. J Immunol 177:8658

Huether SE, McCance KL (2015) Understanding pathophysiology. Elsevier, Förlag

Isailovic N, Daigo K, Mantovani A, Selmi C (2015) Interleukin-17 and innate immunity in infections and chronic inflammation. J Autoimmun 60:1–11

Iwasaki A, Medzhitov R (2004) Toll-like receptor control of the adaptive immune responses. Nat Immunol 5(10):987–995

Janeway CA Jr, Travers P, Walport M et al (2001) The complement system and innate immunity. Immunobiology: the immune system in health and disease. Garland Science, New York. Retrieved 25 February 2013

Jenssen H, Hamill P, Hancock RE (2006) Peptide antimicrobial agents. Clin Microbiol Rev 19:491–511

Kosciuczuk EM, Lisowski P, Jarczak J, Strzalkowska N, Jozwik A, Horbanczuk J, Krzyżewski J, Zwierzchowski L, Bagnicka E (2012) Cathelicidins: family of antimicrobial peptides. A review. Mol Biol Rep 39(12):10957–10970

Kritsepi-Konstantinou M, Oikonomidis IL (2016) The interpretation of leukogram in dog and cat. Hellenic J Compan Anim Med 5(2):54–68

Lehrer RI, Lu W (2012) Alpha-Defensins in human innate immunity. Immunol Rev 245:84–112

LeibundGut-Landmann S, Grob O, Robinson MJ, Osorio F, Slack EC, Tsoni SV, Reis e Sousa C (2007) Syk-and CARD9-dependent coupling of innate immunity to the induction of T helper cells that produce interleukin 17. Nat Immunol 8(6):630–638

Linde A, Ross CR, Davis EG, Dib L, Blecha F, Melgarejo T (2008) Innate immunity and host defense peptides in veterinary medicine. J Vet Intern Med 22(2):247–265

Llibre A, Duffy D (2018) Immune response biomarkers in human and veterinary research. Comp Immunol Microbiol Infect Dis 59:57–62

MacDonald KA, Chomel BB, Kittleson MD, Kasten RW, Thomas WP, Pesavento P (2004) A prospective study of canine infective endocarditis in northern California (1999–2001): emergence of Bartonella as a prevalent etiologic agent. J Vet Intern Med 18(1):56–64

Mburu YK, Abe K, Ferris LK, Sarkar SN, Ferris RL (2011) Human β-defensin 3 promotes NF-κB-mediated CCR7 expression and anti-apoptotic signals in squamous cell carcinoma of the head and neck. Carcinogenesis 32:168–174

McManus PM (2005) Classification of myeloid neoplasms: a comparative review. Vet Clin Pathol 34(3):189–212

Medzhitov R (2009) Approaching the asymptote: 20 years later. Immunity 30:766–775. https://doi.org/10.1016/j.immuni.2009.06.004

Mélik-Parsadaniantz S, Rostène W (2008) Chemokines and neuromodulation. J Neuroimmunol 198(1–2):62–68

Munch D, Sahl HG (2015) Structural variations of the cell wall precursor lipid II in Gram-positive bacteria - impact on binding and efficacy of antimicrobial peptides. Biochim Biophys Acta 1848(11 Pt B):3062–3071

Murdoch S, Djuric U, Mazhar B, Seoud M, Khan R, Kuick R et al (2006) Mutations in NALP7 cause recurrent hydatidiform moles and reproductive wastage in humans. Nat Genet 38:300–302

Murugaiah V, Tsolaki AG, Kishore U (2020) Collectins: innate immune pattern recognition molecules. In: Lectin in host defense against microbial infections, pp 75–127

Nijnik A, Hancock REW (2009) The roles of cathelicidin LL-37 in immune defences and novel clinical applications. Curr Opin Hematol 16:41–47

Opal SM, DePalo VA (2000) Anti-inflammatory cytokines. Chest 117(4):1162–1172

Pasare C, Medzhitov R (2005) Toll-like receptors: linking innate and adaptive immunity. In: Mechanisms of lymphocyte activation and immune regulation X, pp 11–18

Patterson-Delafield J, Martinez RJ, Lehrer RI (1980) Microbicidal cationic proteins in rabbit alveolar macrophages: a potential host defense mechanism. Infect Immun 30:180–192

Richards DM, Hettinger J, Feuerer M (2013) Monocytes and macrophages in cancer: development and functions. Cancer Microenviron 6(2):179–191

Rus H, Cudrici C, Niculescu F (2005) The role of the complement system in innate immunity. Immunol Res 33(2):103–112

Shah SA, Sood NK, Wani BM, Rather MA, Beigh AB, Amin U (2017) Haemato-biochemical studies in canine pyometra. J Pharmacogn Phytochem 6(4):14–17

Shuyi Y, Feng W, Jing T, Hongzhang H, Haiyan W, Pingping M et al (2011) Human beta-defensin-3 (hBD-3) upregulated by LPS via epidermal growth factor receptor (EGFR) signaling pathways to enhance lymphatic invasion of oral squamous cell carcinoma. Oral Surg Oral Med Oral Pathol Oral Radiol Endodontol 112:616–625

Som A, Vemparala S, Ivanov I, Tew GN (2008) Synthetic mimics of antimicrobial peptides. Biopolymers 90:83–93

Sontas HB, Dokuzeylu B, Turna O, Ekici H (2009) Estrogen-induced myelotoxicity in dogs: a review. Can Vet J 50(10):1054

Starr CG, Maderdrut JL, He J, Coy DH, Wimley WC (2018) Pituitary adenylate cyclase-activating polypeptide is a potent broad-spectrum antimicrobial peptide: structure-activity relationships. Peptides 104:35–40

Stockham SL, Scott MA (2008) In: Stockham SL, Scott MA (eds) Leukocytes. In: fundamentals of veterinary clinical pathology, 2nd edn. Blackwell Publishing, Ames, pp 53–106

Takeuchi O, Akira S (2010) Pattern recognition receptors and inflammation. Cell 140(6):805–820

Todd I, Spickett G, Fairclough L (eds) (2015) Lecture notes: immunology. Wiley, New York

Tomasinsig L, Zanetti M (2005) The cathelicidins—structure, function and evolution. Curr Protein Pept Sci 6:23–34

Tong ZB, Gold L, Pfeifer KE, Dorward H, Lee E, Bondy CA et al (2000) Mater, a maternal effect gene required for early embryonic development in mice. Nat Genet 26:267–268

Uemura T, Sano H, Katoh T, Nishitani C, Mitsuzawa H, Shimizu T, Kuroki Y (2006) Surfactant protein a without the interruption of Gly-X-Y repeats loses a kink of oligomeric structure and exhibits impaired phospholipid liposome aggregation ability. Biochemistry 45(48):14543–14551

van de Wetering JK, van Golde LM, Batenburg JJ (2004) Collectins: players of the innate immune system. Eur J Biochem 271(7):1229–1249

Walport MJ (2001) Complement. First of two parts. N Engl J Med 344:1058–1066

Wang A, Chen F, Wang Y, Shen M, Xu Y, Hu J et al (2013) Enhancement of antiviral activity of human alpha-defensin 5 against herpes simplex virus 2 by arginine mutagenesis at adaptive evolution sites. J Virol 87:2835–2845

Watkins LR, Milligan ED, Maier SF (2003) Glial proinflammatory cytokines mediate exaggerated pain states: implications for clinical pain. Adv Exp Med Biol 521:1–21

Wynn TA, Vannella KM (2016) Macrophages in tissue repair, regeneration, and fibrosis. Immunity 44(3):450–462

Xie WR, Deng H, Li H et al (2006) Robust increase of cutaneous sensitivity, cytokine production and sympathetic sprouting in rats with localized inflammatory irritation of the spinal ganglia. Neuroscience 142:809–822

Xu D, Lu W (2020) Defensins: a double-edged sword in host immunity. Front Immunol 11:764

Xu D, Zhang B, Liao C, Zhang W, Wang W, Chang Y et al (2016) Human beta-defensin 3 contributes to the carcinogenesis of cervical cancer via activation of NF-κB signaling. Oncotarget 7:75902–75913

Yasin B, Wang W, Pang M, Cheshenko N, Hong T, Waring AJ et al (2004) Theta defensins protect cells from infection by herpes simplex virus by inhibiting viral adhesion and entry. J Virol 78: 5147–5156

Zanetti M (2004) Cathelicidins, multifunctional peptides of the innate immunity. J Leukoc Biol 75: 39–48

Zhang JM, An J (2007) Cytokines, inflammation, and pain. Int Anesthesiol Clin 45(2):27–37

Hypersensitivity

Key Points

1. As an immunological malfunction, hypersensitivity is characterized by excessive or inappropriate immune responses, which is frequently directed towards normal tissue antigens resulting in tissue damage.
2. There are four categories of hypersensitivity reactions: type I (immediate), type II (antibody-mediated), type III (immune complex-mediated), and type IV (cell-mediated or delayed-type).
3. The first three types I to III are immunoglobulin-dependent reactions involving a humoral B-lymphocyte-mediated response. Conversely, type IV is a T-cell-mediated hypersensitivity reaction.
4. Type I hypersensitivities are acute inflammatory reactions that are mediated by cytotropic IgE antibody bound to activated mast cells and basophils resulting in the release of biologically active substances.
5. Acute systemic anaphylaxis, drugs and vaccine allergies, milk allergy, food allergy, and allergies to parasitic antigens are examples of type I hypersensitivity.
6. Antibody-mediated destruction of cells is the basic mechanism involved in type II hypersensitivity reactions.
7. Incompatible blood transfusion and hemolytic diseases of newborn are examples of type II hypersensitivity.
8. Serum sickness, systemic lupus erythematosus (SLE), and Arthus reaction are examples of type III hypersensitivity.
9. Type IV hypersensitivity is mediated by sensitized T-cells and inflammatory reaction takes several hours (24 to 72 h) to develop.
10. Tuberculin reaction, Johnin reaction, and allergic contact dermatitis are examples of type IV hypersensitivity.

3.1 Hypersensitivity

It is known that the adaptive immune response is a significant constituent of host defense against infections and hence essential for maintaining normal health. The immune responses in the form of either cell mediated or humoral mediated, sometimes elicited by antigens not associated with infectious agents, are inappropriate and this may lead to causation of serious disease. The inappropriate immune response, rather than providing exemption or safety to the affected animal, can produce severe and occasionally fatal results. These are known as "hypersensitivity reactions" and the diseases caused are known as hypersensitivity diseases. Coombs and Gell in 1963 defined four types of hypersensitivity based on immunologic mechanisms involved. The first three types I to III are immunoglobulin-dependent reactions involving a humoral B-lymphocyte-mediated response. Conversely, type IV is a T-cell-mediated hypersensitivity reaction. Overreaction to antigen is also described as "allergy," the term originally coined by Von Pirquet early in the twentieth century. Allergy is defined as the altered reactivity of an animal following exposure to a foreign antigen and included both immunity and hypersensitivity. The term, however, is now restricted to refer only to the hypersensitivity, which may be associated with the development of the immune response to a foreign substance. The essential basis of these hypersensitivity reactions is briefly summarized here and then each will be described separately in greater detail (Table 3.1)

Allergic reactions occur when an already sensitized animal is re-exposed to the same allergen. These responses may range from a localized reaction to systemic anaphylaxis, which may even result into death. Allergic responses do not occur when naive animals are first exposed to an allergen; instead initial response takes time to produce specific antibody or T-cells that react with the allergen, and usually does not produce any symptoms. Any further re-exposure of such animal will produce symptoms. Immune responses to allergens (innocuous substances) are identical to the offending pathogen. In allergic reactions, foreign substances are non-harmful and thus the pathology induced is purely the result of immune response. Hypersensitivity reactions thus demonstrate that immune response itself can cause significant pathology, as it does in some responses to infection. The type of hypersensitivity reaction depends on the nature of antigen and its immune responses. The antibody-mediated hypersensitivity can be classified into three classes. Most common allergies occur due to the production of IgE and are kept in type I hypersensitivity. This is regarded as the classic hypersensitivity reaction, which occurs within seconds or minutes of the antigen contact. IgE antibody-bound mast cells or basophils are activated to release vasoactive amines, leukotrienes, and cytokines in the same fashion as mast cells respond to an infection.

Some hypersensitivity reactions are mediated by antibody isotypes other than IgE. When the allergen is cell found, the antibody activates complement and Fc-mediated effector reactions, and cells are attacked in the same way as bacteria. This type of reaction is classified as type II hypersensitivity. When the antigen is soluble, immune complexes formed at the sites of antigen deposition induce local

3.1 Hypersensitivity

Table 3.1 Features of different types of hypersensitivity reactions

	Type I	Type II		Type III	Type IV
Descriptive name	IgE-mediated hypersensitivity	Antibody-dependent cellular cytotoxicity (ADCC)		Immune complex-mediated hypersensitivity	Cell mediated (Delayed-type hypersensitivity)
Antibody/cell involved	IgE, Th2 cell	IgG antibody		IgG antibody	Th1 cells	CTL
Nature of antigen	Soluble antigen	Cell or matrix-associated antigen	Cell surface receptors	Soluble antigen	Soluble antigen	Cell-associated antigen
Initiation time	1–30 min	5–8 h	–	2–8 h	24–72 h	–
Effector mechanism	Activation of mast cells and basophils following antigen-induced cross-linking of IgE receptors	Antibody to cell surface antigen mediates cell destruction via complement or ADCC (FcR+ cells, phagocytes, NK cells)	Alteration in antibody signaling	Antigen-antibody complexes activate complement to release C_3a and C_5a resulting in local inflammatory response (FcR+ cells, complement)	Cytokines secreted by sensitized T-cells (T_{DTH}) activate macrophages that mediate damage (Macrophage activation)	T cytotoxic cell (Tc) mediate cell cytotoxicity
Clinical manifestation	Acute systemic anaphylaxis, milk allergy, food allergy, allergic rhinitis, asthma, etc.	Blood transfusion reaction, autoimmune hemolytic anemia, Hemolytic disease of newborn (HDNB) in foal	Grave's disease (agonist), myasthenia gravis (antagonist)	Arthus reaction, serum sickness, rheumatoid arthritis, glomerulonephritis, SLE	Tuberculin reaction, contact dermatitis, graft rejection	Contact dermatitis, graft rejection

inflammation and are classified under type III hypersensitivity reaction. While type I reaction occurs within minutes of allergen contact, type II and type III reactions are observed within a few hours of exposure.

In type IV reactions, the allergen may be a foreign protein or a chemical substance that reacts with self-proteins. Once the animal is sensitized to a modified protein, re-exposure with the same antigen leads to T-cell response that evolves over several days; hence, these reactions are also called delayed-type hypersensitivity. Such reactions occur in infections with intracellular bacteria and after contact with certain chemicals (contact hypersensitivity reaction).

Thus, it is evident from the foregoing that the class of antibody or T-cell produced in response to an allergen determines the type of a hypersensitivity reaction that will occur following its re-exposure.

3.2 Type I Hypersensitivity

Type I hypersensitivities are acute inflammatory reactions that occur as a result of the release of biologically active substances from activated mast cells and basophils. The reaction is mediated by cytotropic IgE antibody bound to these cells. Antigen that stimulates allergy is called the *allergen*. An allergen generates plasma cells and memory cells that secrete IgE. This class of antibody binds with high affinity to Fc receptors on the surface of mast cells and basophils. The IgE-bound mast cells and basophils are referred to as sensitized. Subsequent exposure to the same allergen cross-links the membrane-bound IgE on sensitized mast cells and basophils causing their degranulation. The allergic reactions occur immediately after the antigen contact, hence called as *immediate hypersensitivity* reactions. The reaction may be either systemic and severe (*anaphylaxis*) or localized to certain organs or tissues.

The IgE antibody, which mediates type I hypersensitivity, is synthesized predominantly in lymphoid tissues associated with skin and gastrointestinal and respiratory tracts. Most allergic IgE responses occur on mucosal surfaces in response to allergens that enter the body either by inhalation or ingestion. These allergens include proteins from parasite helminths, insects, foreign serum, vaccine, plant pollens, drugs, food, mold spores, etc. The production of IgE against parasitic antigens suggests that IgE evolved specifically to produce resistance against parasites. The self-cure phenomenon is the best example of the beneficial effects of type I hypersensitivity. A normal individual produces only small amount of IgE. But some individual who produces high level of IgE is said to be *atopic*. The condition is called *atopy*.

3.2.1 Components of Type I Hypersensitivity

3.2.1.1 Mast Cells and Basophils

Mast cells are large, stellate, or round cells with a diameter of 15–20 μm. They are widely distributed in connective tissue closely associated with blood vessels and lymphatics. It possesses a bean or oval-shaped nucleus and contains numerous granules with eccentric distribution. The liver in dogs and mesentery in chickens have large numbers of mast cells. The blood basophils, though present in extremely small numbers (0.5–2%), play a very important function in the body. It is round in shape with a diameter of 10–15 μm and has a multilobed nucleus and relatively evenly distributed less numerous granules. Some of the morphological characteristics such as number, size, and stainability of granules vary among domestic species. It is believed that basophils are derived from promyelocytes in the bone marrow. Morphologically, it resembles with mast cells and share similar functions. Granules of mast cells and basophils stain metachromatically at low pH with certain dyes such as alcian blue, toluidine blue, etc.

Significant variation has been noted in the mast cell population at different sites with regard to the types and amount of allergic mediators they contain and their sensitivities to activating stimuli and cytokines. Precursors of mast cells are formed in the bone marrow and are carried to virtually all vascularized peripheral tissues, where they differentiate into mature cells. Two types of mast cells have been identified in rodents and humans; one type is found in the connective tissues and the other is associated with mucosal surfaces. Connective tissue mast cells contain many uniform granules and are rich in histamine and heparin. On the contrary, mucosa-associated mast cells have few variable-sized granules that contain chondroitin sulfate, not heparin. They contain little histamine and produce different prostaglandins and leukotrienes as well as platelet-activating factor (PAF). Mucosal mast cells can proliferate in response to IL-3 and IL-4, which are secreted from T-cells. They are also activated in response to parasitic helminth antigens.

Mast cells and basophils possess a variety of biologically active preformed mediators and are capable of synthesizing several other pharmacologically active substances upon immunologic and non-immunologic stimulations. These mediators are released in a sequential fashion and are important mediators of allergic and other inflammatory reactions. Both the cells have receptors for IgE, IgG, β-adrenergic catecholamines, prostaglandins, and histamine. In comparison to IgE, IgG binding is less effective in inducing degranulation. Cell surface receptor density for IgE is more on the basophil (15,000–600,000 receptors/cell) than on the mast cells (3000–600,000). Comparative features of mast cells and basophils are summarized in Table 3.2.

3.2.1.2 Immunoglobulin E (IgE)

C.R. Reicherts' findings for the first time suggested that some constituent of serum was responsible for hypersensitivity in dog. Systemic anaphylaxis could be produced in an unsensitized dog by injecting serum from a sensitized dog. Similar component in the human serum was demonstrated and was later identified as IgE antibody. It is found in the serum in very small quantity (9 to 700 μg/ml in dog), which made its physiochemical characterization difficult. The discovery of an IgE myeloma in 1967 led to a comprehensive chemical analysis of IgE. It is a heat-labile immunoglobulin and composed of two heavy and two light chains with a molecular weight of 190,000. The increase in the molecular weight is due to an additional

Table 3.2 Comparison of mast cells and basophils

Criterion	Mast cells	Basophils
Anatomic distribution	Connective tissues especially near the blood and lymph vessels, mucosal surfaces; occasionally in bone marrow	Blood and bone marrow; infiltrate in tissues during hypersensitivity and other inflammatory reactions
Size (diameter)	Mucosal mast cell—9–10 µm Connective tissue mast cell—19–20 µm	12–15 µm
Origin	Not precisely known; undifferentiated mesenchymal connective tissue cell; bone marrow is suggested	Bone marrow
Morphology	Large round to oval or stellate cell; round- or bean-shaped nucleus; cytoplasm packed with darkly stained granules	Small round cell with bi- or trilobed nucleus; large loosely packed intense reddish violet granules
Scanning electron microscopy	Long and prominent microvilli with the presence of villous processes	Villi short and some smooth folds; uropod seen in mobile cell
Biochemical composition	Relatively high	Relatively low
	More species variation	Variable amounts
Histamine	Present	Absent
Heparin	Present	Absent
Acid phosphatases	Fast	Slow
Acid hydrolases	Large quantity	Small quantity
Degranulation process		
Arachidonic acid metabolites		
Life span	Several weeks to months	In blood: 6 h; in tissues: few days
Major cytokines produced in type I hypersensitivity reactions	IL-3, IL-4, IL-5, IL-6, IL-13, IL-16, IL-22, IL-25, GM-CSF, and TNF-α	IL-4 and IL-6

conformation of Fc portion of the molecule. It enables IgE to bind to glycoprotein receptors on the surface of mast cells and basophils. The half-life of IgE in the serum is only 2–3 days, but when bound to mast cells, it is stable for a few weeks. The serum IgE level is found to be related with the parasite burden of the animal. Though affinity of IgG_1 to mast cell is extremely low, it has been found to mediate atopic dermatitis in dogs.

IgE Binding Fc Receptors

The reaginic activity of IgE is dependent upon its ability to bind to receptors specific for the Fc portion of heavy chain. Two types of receptors have been identified: a high-affinity (FcεRI) and a low-affinity (FcεRII, CD23) receptor. They are expressed by different types of cells, including mast cells, basophils, and

3.2 Type I Hypersensitivity

eosinophils. The affinity of FcεRI for IgE is 1000 times more than FcεRII, which enables it to bind IgE almost irreversibly despite the very low concentration of IgE in serum.

The FcεRI receptor consists of four polypeptide chains; an α and a β-chain and two γ-chains linked with disulfide bond. The extracytoplasmic portion of the α-chain binds with CH_3 domain of IgE molecule via its two immunoglobulin-like molecules. The β-chain acts as a linker between α-chain and γ-homodimer. The two γ-chains extend deeper into the cytoplasm and contain immunoreceptor tyrosine activation motif (ITAM), which interacts with protein tyrosine kinase (PTK). PTK is responsible for tyrosine phosphorylation and this initiates the process of mast cell degranulation.

FcεRII (CD23) is another receptor with lower affinity for IgE in comparison to FcεRI and does belong to the immunoglobulin superfamily. The FcεRII receptor plays a variety of functions in regulating the intensity of IgE response. It is found on NK cells, eosinophils, platelets, macrophages, and dendritic cells and on nearly one third of the population of B-cells.

Molecular Mechanism of IgE-Mediated Degranulation

The mechanism leading to degranulation remains the same for both the mast cells and the basophils. The first step is the binding of allergens to the IgE and cross-linking the receptor-bound IgE on the surface of basophils and mast cells. The binding of IgE alone on the mast cells does not trigger the degranulation process. Thus, monovalent allergens cannot initiate the process. Experimental studies have shown that cross-linkage of two or more FcεRI receptors is necessary for degranulation to occur, which can be achieved by bindings with allergens or other cross-linking methods (anti-IgE antibody, anti-receptor antibody, and anti-idiotype antibody). It has also been seen that the ratio of IgE to allergen should be 2:1 or more to induce degranulation (Fig. 3.1).

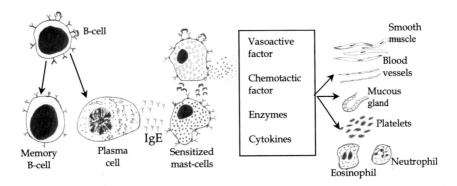

Fig. 3.1 The mechanism of type I hypersensitivity reaction. Following allergen contact, specific IgE molecules secreted from B-cell-derived plasma cells bind to mast cells or basophils and cause their sensitization. Re-exposure with the same allergen leads to cross-linking of the bound IgE, resulting in degranulation of mast cells and basophils

Intracellular Events

Intracellular events consist of several sequential steps involving receptor cross-linkage, activation of protein tyrosine kinase, methylation of membrane phospholipids, influx of Ca^{++}, change in the cAMP levels, and the fusion of granules with plasma membrane (Fig. 3.2).

Cross-linkage of IgE by allergen results into aggregation of FcεRI receptors and activation of PTKs associated with cytoplasmic domains of β- and γ-chains. PTKs subsequently phosphorylate phospholipase C, which converts phosphatidylinositol-4,5 biphosphate into diacylglycerol (DAG) and inositol triphosphate. These in turn increase intracellular calcium level and activate protein kinases (PKC). Activated PKC phosphorylate myosin light chain necessary for microtubular assembly and fusion of granules with the plasma membrane and releasing their content into extracellular fluid. Simultaneously, FcεRI cross-linkage also activates phospholipases, which acts on the membrane phospholipids to produce arachidonic acid. Two classes of potent mediators are produced from arachidonic acid: the prostaglandins and the leukotrienes. Finally, protein kinases promote translation and expression of genes encoding several cytokines such as IL-4, IL-5, IL-6, and tumor necrosis factor alpha (TNF-α). Degranulation of mast cells and basophils occurs within seconds of binding of allergen to IgE on the cell surface. Degranulated

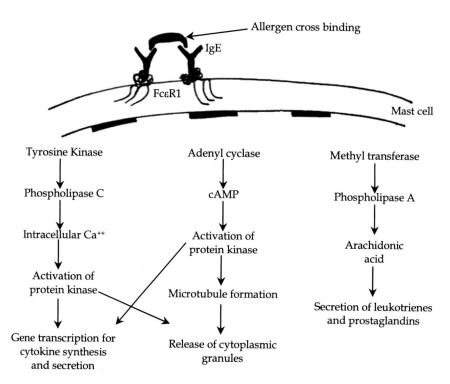

Fig. 3.2 Diagrammatic presentation of signal transduction pathways in mast cell degranulation

mast cells do not die, but their identification becomes difficult due to the changed morphology.

3.2.2 Mediators of Type I Hypersensitivity Reaction

Following cross bridging of FcεRI receptors by allergen on the surface of mast cells, several pharmacologically active agents are released in the extracellular fluid. The clinical manifestation of type I hypersensitivity in fact results from biological effects of these agents, which can be classified into primary and secondary mediators. The primary mediators are those which are produced before degranulation and stored in the granules. These include histamine, serotonin, proteases, chemotactic factors for eosinophil and neutrophil, and heparin (Table 3.3). The secondary mediators are synthesized following activation of mast cells and include platelet-activating factors (PAF), leukotrienes, prostaglandins, bradykinins, and various cytokines. The difference in the clinical manifestation of the type of reaction among different species of animals may partly reflect variation in the primary and secondary mediator secretions.

3.2.2.1 Primary Mediators

Histamine and serotonin are the most important vasoactive amines, which are formed in high concentration in granules of mast cells. Its biological effects are observed within minutes of mast cell activation. Histamine exerts its effects by binding with H1 receptors present on different tissues. It includes contraction of smooth muscle in bronchi, gastrointestinal tract, uterus, and bladder and increased permeability of vessels. Histamine stimulates mucus secretion by goblet cells,

Table 3.3 Major mediators of type I hypersensitivity

Mediators	Major action
A. Preformed	
Histamine	Enhanced vascular permeability, smooth muscle contraction, itching, increased glandular (exocrine) secretion
Serotonin	Smooth muscle contraction, vasospasm
ECF—A	Eosinophil chemotaxis
PAF	Platelet aggregation factor
NCF—A	Neutrophil chemotaxis
B. De novo synthesis	
Prostaglandins	Very complex; influence vascular and smooth muscle tone, aggregation, and immune reactivity
Leukotrienes B	Neutrophil and eosinophil chemotaxis
Leukotrienes C, D	Smooth muscle contraction, vascular permeability
Bradykinin	Smooth muscle contraction, vascular permeability
Serotonin	Smooth muscle contraction, vasospasm
Cytokines, IL-1, TNF-α	Systemic anaphylaxis, increased expression of cell adhesion molecules on venular endothelium

lacrimation, and salivation. Tryptophan-derived serotonin (5-hydroxytryptamine) is released from mast cells of rodents and the large ruminants. Its main function is vasoconstriction that results in the rise of the blood pressure. In cattle, however, serotonin is a vasodilator. It has only minor effects on vascular permeability except in rats and mice. Other mediators, which are rapidly released from mast cells, include eosinophilic chemotactic factor (ECF) and neutrophilic chemotactic factor (NCF). Infiltration of eosinophils is often related with type I reaction. In addition to these, more than 50% of the protein content of granules are made up of neutral proteases such as trypsin and chymotrypsin. The complement components C_3 and C_5 are cleaved by these proteases to generate anaphylatoxin (C_3a and C_5a). Mast cell granules also contain kallikreins, which act on kininogen to produce kinins.

3.2.2.2 Secondary Mediators

These include lipid mediators and cytokines. Lipid mediators prostaglandins and leukotrienes are produced as a result of enzymatic cascade. Activated phospholipases act on the membrane phospholipids to produce arachidonic acid. The latter leads to the production of prostaglandins, prostacyclins, and thromboxanes via cyclooxygenase pathway. Prostaglandins cause intense bronchospasm and increased mucus secretion. Leukotrienes are potent vasoactive and spasmogenic agents. They increase vascular permeability and cause bronchial smooth muscle contraction several thousand times more than histamine. Leukotrienes (B4, C4, and D4) were earlier collectively called as slow-releasing substances of anaphylaxis (SRS-A). In addition, leukotriene B4 is highly chemotactic for neutrophils, eosinophils, and monocytes.

Cytokines

Mast cells and basophils secrete cytokines, which further complicate the inflammatory process. Some of these cytokines are involved in the clinical manifestation of type I hypersensitivity reaction. IL-4, IL-5, IL-6, IL-13, and TNF-α change the local microenvironment leading to the recruitment of several inflammatory cells such as neutrophils and basophils.

3.2.3 Clinical Manifestations

The consequences of type I reaction in an animal depend on several factors including genetic constitution of the animal, nature and amount of allergen, tissue distribution of mast cells and its content in the target organs, and most importantly the route of administration of the allergen. The clinical manifestation may range from serious life-threatening condition such as acute systemic anaphylaxis to localized allergic reaction of limited consequence.

3.2.3.1 Acute Systemic Anaphylaxis

Systemic anaphylaxis occurs within minutes of type I reaction and usually fatal if not attended. This type of reaction was observed for the first time in 1839 in dogs

3.2 Type I Hypersensitivity

Table 3.4 Comparative features of anaphylaxis in animals and humans

Species	Shock organs	Predominant clinical signs	Pathological findings	Major mediators
Avian	Respiratory tract	Dyspnea, convulsions	Lung edema	Serotonin, Leukotrienes
Canine	Hepatic veins	Dyspnea, diarrhea, vomiting, collapse	Hepatic engorgement visceral hemorrhage	Histamine, Leukotrienes
Feline	Respiratory tract intestinal tract	Dyspnea, cough, vomiting, diarrhea, pruritus	Edematous lung Edematous intestine	Histamine, Leukotrienes
Swine	Respiratory tract intestinal tract	Cyanosis Pruritus	Systemic hypotension	Histamine
Equine	Respiratory tract intestinal tract	Cough, dyspnea, diarrhea	Lung emphysema Intestinal hemorrhage	Histamine Serotonin Kinins
Bovine	Respiratory tract	Dyspnea, cough collapse	Lung edema, emphysema, hemorrhage	Serotonin Kinins Leukotrienes
Ovine	Respiratory tract	Dyspnea, cough	Lung edema, emphysema	Histamine, Serotonin, Leukotrienes, Kinins
Human	Respiratory tract	Dyspnea, urticaria	Laryngeal and lung edema, emphysema	Histamine, Leukotrienes

following repeated injections of egg albumin. The importance of the findings was, however, realized only in 1902, when two French physicians were attempting to develop antitoxin to protect swimmers from painful stings of jelly fish and sea anemone. They found that after primary immunization of dog with sublethal dose of extract of sea anemone, the second injection after several weeks caused rapid development of symptoms like vomiting, bloody diarrhea, asphyxia, unconsciousness, and death. They named this phenomenon anaphylaxis (from Greek, *ana*—against; *phylaxis*—protection) in context with their findings as they were looking for a prophylactic but in return got anaphylactic. Clinical and pathologic features of acute anaphylaxis differ among domestic species and humans and are summarized in Table 3.4.

Cattle

Major mediators of anaphylaxis in cattle are serotonin, kinins, and the leukotrienes. Histamine is of little significance. The main shock organ is the lungs, which show hypertension due to constriction of pulmonary veins resulting in dyspnea and pulmonary edema. Hypersecretion of mucus further aggravates the respiratory difficulty. Affected animals show urination, defecation, and bloating, which result from smooth muscle contraction of urinary bladder and intestines. Dopamine enhances histamine and leukotriene secretion from bovine lungs in acute anaphylaxis. The α- and β-adrenoceptors on mast cells of cattle behave differently in comparison to other species. Drugs that stimulate β-receptor potentiate histamine release from leucocytes, whereas drugs that stimulate α-receptor inhibit histamine release. The mechanism of these peculiar effects is not yet clear.

Sheep
Acute anaphylaxis in sheep presents almost similar symptoms as seen in cattle. Pulmonary signs predominate as a result of the constriction of bronchi and blood vessels. Smooth musculature of intestines and urinary bladder are also affected with expected results. Histamine is the major mediator besides serotonin, leukotrienes, and kinins.

Horse
In equines, lungs and intestines are the main organs to be affected in systemic anaphylaxis. Clinical signs consisting of cough and dyspnea leading to apnea are the consequences of histamine- and serotonin-mediated bronchial and bronchiolar constriction. On postmortem examination, pulmonary emphysema and peribronchiolar edema are consistently seen. The animal may also show diarrhea and hemorrhagic enterocolitis.

Pig
In pigs also, the major shock organ is the lungs and the principal features of acute anaphylaxis include systemic and pulmonary hypertension, which are mostly histamine mediated. The animal dies due to respiratory distress. Intestines are infrequently involved.

Dogs and Cats
Acute anaphylaxis in dogs, particularly in respect to shock organs, differs from those of domestic species. Hepatic vein in liver is the major site of action for mediators such as histamine, prostaglandins, and leukotrienes. Clinical symptoms in anaphylactic dog include initial excitement, followed by vomiting, defecation, and urination. With the progress of reaction, the dog shows muscular weakness, depressed respiration, and convulsions and becomes comatose and dies within 45–60 min. Postmortem examination reveals severe engorgement of liver and intestines holding more than 60% of the total blood volume. These occur as a result of hepatic vein occlusion due to smooth muscle contraction and swelling of hepatic cells. In cats, the major shock organ is the lungs and mediators of anaphylaxis are histamine and the leukotrienes. The animal shows scratching of face and head, dyspnea, salivation, vomiting, incoordination, and collapse. Pulmonary emphysema, hemorrhage and edema, bronchial constriction, and edema of glottis are the significant lesions observed at necropsy.

3.2.3.2 Localized Specific Allergic Conditions

Localized allergic reactions are more commonly seen than the acute anaphylaxis. Organs affected reflect the route of entry of the allergen. For example, hay fever results from fluid exudation from nasal mucosa as inhaled antigen acts on the upper respiratory tract, trachea, and bronchi. Asthma in humans occurs due to tracheobronchial constriction in response to inhaled antigen. Similarly, allergic conjunctivitis, urticaria, diarrhea, and hemorrhagic enteritis may occur as a result of antigen contact to respective organs. The following are some of the specific localized allergic conditions in animals.

Milk Allergy

Certain breed of high-yielding cows such as Jersey mounts immune response to its own α-casein of milk, which is synthesized in the udder. This protein does not get access to blood circulation if the cow is milked regularly that avoids increased intramammary pressure. Delay in milking causes undue increase in the intramammary pressure, which allows seepage of milk protein in circulation and production of cytotropic IgE antibody. Subsequent release of α-casein protein results in type I reaction, which may vary from mild discomfort with urticarial skin lesions to acute systemic anaphylaxis and death. Regular milking prevents the occurrence of such condition in high-yielding cows.

Food Allergy

Food allergy in dogs and cats is a common condition and causes allergic dermatitis and gastrointestinal disorders. Protein-rich foods such as milk and milk products, wheat meal, fish, chicken, beef and egg may cause allergy. About 15% of dogs suffering from food allergy show gastrointestinal involvement. The clinical signs include vomiting, cramps, and loose fetid stool, and in the severe cases hemorrhagic diarrhea may be seen soon after intake of the food. Skin lesions in food allergy have been found in about 50% of the affected dogs. Eyes, ears, feet, axillae, and perianal areas are usually involved and show reactions consisting of erythematous papules. The lesions are highly pruritic because of histamine and are frequently complicated with self-inflicted injuries and secondary bacterial or fungal infections. In chronic cases, skin is further thickened, hyperpigmented, and secondarily infected. In pigs, fish meal and alfalfa and in horses, wild oats, white clover, and alfalfa have been incriminated as potential food allergens. Treatment of food allergies includes correct identification of food responsible for allergy and replacing it with hypoallergenic diets. Dietary elimination of the food components one by one is the best means of diagnosis. Intradermal skin testing is not very much useful in detecting allergy to food components or ingredients.

Respiratory Allergy

Inhalant allergy is most commonly manifested as atopic dermatitis in dogs and cats. The major inhalant allergens identified are mold, weed, and pollen grains especially those which are very small, light, and produced in large quantities. Erythema and edema of the face, axilla, and foot are observed in uncomplicated cases. However, any part of body can be affected. Secondary complication leads to crusting, scaling, hyperpigmentation, and pyogenic infection of the skin. Some dogs may also suffer with otitis externa and conjunctivitis. Allergic rhinitis and conjunctivitis induced by pollens are less frequently observed in inhalant allergy. It is characterized by excessive lacrimation and watery nasal discharge.

Cattle
Allergic rhinitis occurs in cattle as a result of inhalation of antigen from a number of plants and fungi. Clinically, the affected animal shows excessive lacrimation, mucoid nasal discharge, and intense pruritus at the nasal region. In chronic cases, nodular growth is formed in the nasal mucosa, which consists of large numbers of mast cells, eosinophils, and plasma cells.

Equines
Chronic obstructive pulmonary disease (COPD) in horses is analogous to asthma in humans. It is thought to be a broncho-pulmonary mold allergy with the involvement of type I hypersensitivity in its pathogenesis. As seen in allergic asthma in humans, the major component of late-phase reaction is the leukotrienes causing sustained smooth muscle contraction. The ineffectiveness of anti-histamines in the treatment of this disease suggests the role for the late-phase reactivity. COPD-affected horses exhibit positive skin reaction to extract from several actinomycetes and fungi including *Micropolyspora faeni*, *Aspergillus* spp., and *Cladosporium* spp. But horses without COPD also show positive skin reaction. Also, there has been no correlation between circulating mast cell mediators and severity of COPD. This indicates that precise etiopathogenesis of the condition is unclear.

3.2.3.3 Allergies to Parasitic Antigens in Animals
IgE-mediated reaction to parasitic antigens plays a significant role in resistance to helminth infection. The helminth's infection stimulates IgE production, which is responsible for allergy and even anaphylactic reaction. The beneficial role of type I hypersensitivity was first observed in the form of self-cure phenomenon in helminth infection. A variety of parasitic infections have been identified to cause type I reaction in animals. Animals infected with cestodes sometimes show symptoms of respiratory distress and urticaria. In dogs, rupture of hydatid cysts during surgical manipulation or due to other reasons may cause anaphylaxis. Transfusion of blood from dog infected with heartworm (*Dirofilaria immitis*) to already sensitized dog may result in anaphylaxis.

Antigens from certain arthropod parasite have been shown to cause allergies in humans and animals. Acute anaphylaxis in sensitized humans due to insect stings is commonly observed. Cattle infected with *Hypoderma bovis* (warble fly) may exhibit anaphylaxis as a result of rupture of pupal stage during its physical removal from the back of the animal. The release of pupal coelomic fluid in the sensitized animal may cause acute reaction and occasionally death of the animal.

Biting of cattle and horses by certain insects such as midges (*Culicoides* spp.) and black flies (*Simulium* spp.) causes allergic dermatitis popularly known as Gulf coast itch, Queensland itch, or sweet itch. Saliva-associated antigens of these parasites cause the formation of urticaria that is intensely pruritic.

Mites can also stimulate IgE production and hence lesions produced by them show features of type I hypersensitivity. Mange in dogs and cats caused by *Sarcoptes scabiei* and *Otodectes cyanotis*, respectively, is an example. Dermal lesions consist of infiltration with mast cells, lymphocytes, and plasma cells. The affected animals show an immediate wheal and flare response following intradermal injection of mite antigens. Type III reaction-mediated immune complex formation may also be associated with the lesion development.

Other helminth parasites such as *Ascaris suum* in pigs and *Fasciola hepatica* in calves have been shown to induce type I hypersensitivity reaction. Apart from a damaging role, IgE antibodies play a significant protective role in several parasitic infections.

3.2.3.4 Drugs and Vaccine Allergies

Some drugs and vaccines elicit IgE response and cause discomfort to humans and animals mediated by type I hypersensitivity reaction. Among drugs, penicillin allergy is the most notable one. The animal may be exposed to penicillin either through therapeutic dosage or ingestion of contaminated milk. The penicillin molecule is degraded into several compounds including penicilloyl. This binds to protein in the body and mounts IgE response. Re-exposure of such sensitized animal may lead to acute anaphylaxis or milder form of allergy. Antibodies and hormones may also cause allergies in domestic animals. The induction of IgE response leading to severe allergies has been reported in cattle with the use of killed FMD vaccines, rabies vaccine, and contagious bovine pleuropneumonia vaccine.

3.2.4 Detection of Type I Hypersensitivity

The most simple method to assess and identify type I reaction is the intradermal skin testing. Small amount of potential or suspected allergen is applied at specific skin site by intradermal injection or superficial scratching. If the animal is hypersensitive to the allergen, local mast cells will degranulate and the release of histamine and other mediators will produce edema (wheal) and erythema (flare) within minutes. This acute inflammatory reaction reaches its maximum intensity in 30 minutes and then disappears within the next few hours. The advantage of skin testing is that it is inexpensive and simple to perform and allows screening of several allergens.

Passive cutaneous anaphylaxis (PCA) test is another in vivo method that is used to detect IgE antibody in the serum of hypersensitive animals. In this test, several dilutions of serum from affected animals are injected into the skin of normal animal and the allergen is inoculated intravenously after 24–48 h. In positive reaction, acute inflammatory response develops at the injection sites. Sometimes, skin reactions are too mild to detect clearly. In such cases, Evans blue dye is injected intravenously into the test animal, which binds to albumin. Due to the increased permeability at the site, dye-labeled albumin comes out in the tissue fluid and produces a striking blue patch. The size of the patch is proportional to the intensity of the inflammatory reaction.

In vitro method of assessing type I hypersensitivity involves determination of total serum IgE antibody by radio-immunosorbent test (RIST). The assay is highly sensitive and can detect nanogram level of total IgE. A similar test, called radio-allergosorbent test (RAST), allows detection of serum IgE specific to a given allergen. In this technique, allergens bound to beads are allowed to react with the test serum. The concentration of specific IgE bound to solid-phase allergen is then measured by adding ^{125}I-labeled anti-IgE and counting the bound radioactivity. Enzyme-linked immunosorbent assay (ELISA) has also been used to measure specific IgE antibody in atopic dogs. However, total serum IgE level does not always correlate well with clinical severity. For example, a heavily parasitized dog may reveal elevated level of IgE antibody. Therefore, assessment of allergen-specific IgE is more advantageous.

3.3 Type II Hypersensitivity

Antibody binding to cell surface antigens causes destruction of cells through a mechanism called the type II hypersensitivity. This type of reaction is best exemplified by incompatible blood transfusion, where antibodies present in the recipient serum destroy donor red blood cells. Certain glycolipids are an integral part of erythrocyte plasma membrane and act as antigen. They are water soluble. Physiological functions of most of these antigens are not known, except for the ABO system of humans, which act as glucose transporter proteins. These antigens found on the surface of erythrocytes are known as blood group antigens. Erythrocytes of humans and animals are provided with different blood group antigens. They vary among different species with regard to their structure, antigenicity, and complexity. Some blood group antigens such as "B" system in cattle and "A" antigen in cat are more important from the clinical point of view and are widely distributed in the population.

Blood group antigen may be simple (J antigen in cattle) or may be complex (B antigen of cattle). These antigens are not unique to erythrocytes. They have also been identified in several secretions, saliva, and body fluids and are passively absorbed onto the erythrocytes.

Natural antibodies (isoantibodies) to red blood cells are formed in humans and animals without any previous exposure to foreign blood group antigens via blood transfusion or other means. Isoantibody is usually of IgM type. Experimental evidence suggests that many of the blood group antigenic epitopes are shared by bacterial and plant cells. Hence, exposure to these antigens occurs during neonatal period that leads to antibody formation. Isoantibody formation is commonly seen in human ABO blood group system.

3.3.1 Mechanism of Type II Hypersensitivity

Antibody-mediated destruction of cells is the basic mechanism involved in type II hypersensitivity reactions. Examples include incompatible blood transfusion, hemolytic diseases of the newborn, and cellular dysfunction. Antibody can mediate destruction of cells in three ways. First, combination of antibody with the cell surface antigen activates full complement system generating membrane attack complex and formation of pores in the foreign cells. Second, antibody can mediate killing of cells by antibody-dependent cellular cytotoxicity (ADCC) mechanism. A number of cells including NK cells, macrophages, monocytes, neutrophils, and basophils express receptors for Fc region of antibody on their surfaces. These effector cells bind to the target cells through Fc receptor and initiate lysis of antibody-coated target cells. Cytotoxicity mechanism of these cells includes the release of lytic components, tumor necrosis factor, perforin, etc. Third, antibody bound to the foreign red cell antigen acts as opsonin enabling phagocytic cells with Fc or C_3b receptor to bind and phagocytose the antibody-coated cells (Fig. 3.3).

In incompatible blood transfusion, rapid destruction of large number of erythrocytes results from type II reaction. In severe reaction, there is massive hemolysis and complement activation. This results into the release of a large amount of hemoglobin in the blood and urine. Lysed red blood cells also activate blood-clotting system, which leads to disseminated intravascular coagulation (DIC). Activated complements cause the formation of anaphylatoxin and release of vasoactive agents due to mast cell degranulation. These substances provoke vicious cycle, where animals show circulatory hypotension, bradycardia, and apnea. The affected animals exhibit sweating, salivation, lacrimation, diarrhea, and vomiting. Blood transfusion should be immediately stopped and diuretic therapy may be resorted to maintain urine flow and to prevent hemoglobin-induced tubular necrosis.

3.3.1.1 Blood Groups and Hemolytic Disease

Dog
Eleven independent blood group systems—A, B, C, D, F, J, K, L, M, and N—have been identified in dogs. Most of these antigens are inherited as simple Mendelian dominant traits. Blood typing in dogs is carried out by agglutination, hemolysis, and Coombs or antiglobulin tests. Before transfusion, blood typing is generally required in dogs, because many dogs contain natural antibody. Out of 11 blood group systems, "A" system is highly immunogenic and is of clinical significance. About two third of dogs have "A" blood group system. Only a minority of dogs shows the presence of natural antibodies to "A" antigen in A-negative dogs. Spontaneous hemolytic disease in newborn pups has been rarely reported.

Cattle
In cattle, blood group system is very complex, and so far, 11 blood groups—A, B, C, F, J, L, M, R, S, Z, and T—have been identified. Of these, B and J groups are most important. The B blood group in cattle was first described in 1950 and has been

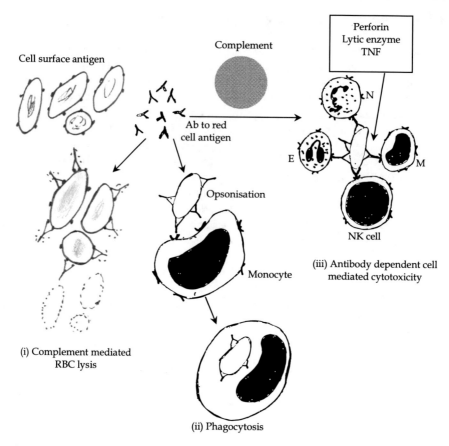

Fig. 3.3 Three mechanisms of cell destruction in type II hypersensitivity including complement-mediated lysis, opsonization-phagocytosis, and antibody-dependent cellular cytotoxicity (ADCC)

extensively studied since then. At least 600 alleles have been identified in this group. The polymorphic character of its alleles has been widely used by breed registries for parentage confirmation and for maintaining identification of animals. These antigens are inherited in combinations, known as phenogroup.

In C blood group, there are 10 antigens, which in combination form 90 phenogroups. The J antigen is actually a soluble lipid that is adsorbed onto the surface of erythrocytes. It may be found in high concentration or in extremely low concentration. The J-negative cattle possess anti-J antibodies and its concentration varies with seasonal variation. Transfusion of blood from J-positive cattle to J negative cattle may cause transfusion reaction. However, transfusion reaction in bovine is of minor consequence.

Hemolytic disease of newborn in calf is rarely encountered, but may occur as a result of vaccination of cattle against anaplasmosis or babesiosis. Both the vaccines contain blood components, as these are prepared from the blood of cattle infected with *Anaplasma* or *Babesia*. While vaccine confers immunity in recipient animals against these protozoal diseases, it produces antibodies against blood group antigens present in the vaccine. This is of little consequence to animal itself; however, it often produces severe disease in suckling calves. Such vaccinated cow when mated with bull carrying the same blood antigen eventually transfers isoantibodies against red cell antigen to the newborn calf via colostrum causing hemolytic disease. A and F systems have been frequently implicated in HDNB in calves.

The severity of HDNB in calves depends on the amount of colostrum ingested. Calves are usually born healthy but soon show symptoms of respiratory difficulty and hemoglobinuria as a result of erythrolysis. In acute cases, death may occur after 24 h. In less severe cases, the calf develops anemia and jaundice and may succumb during the first week of life. Postmortem changes consist of splenomegaly, pulmonary edema, and dark kidneys. The affected calves show antibodies on their red cells in antiglobulin test. Death is due to massive erythrolysis and eventual disseminated intravascular coagulation (DIC).

Horse

In horses, seven internationally accepted blood group systems—A, C, D, K, P, Q, and U—have been identified so far, in addition to few others without official recognition (Table 3.5). As with other species, simple blood transfusion is of little significance in equines. Hemolytic disease of newborn, however, is relatively common as compared with other species. In the mule foal, the condition has been reported more frequently (10%) than in the horse foal (up to 2%).

Information on blood groups in equines is helpful in predicting whether hemolysis will occur in the foal. Foals born out of mare sensitized by incompatible blood transfusion may suffer from hemolytic disease. But most commonly, the syndrome is initiated when fetal red blood cells expressed antigens derived from stallion, whose blood group differs from the mare. The pregnant mare devoid of these antigens produces isoantibodies against them. The mechanism, how fetal erythrocyte antigen reaches to the mare, is not precisely known, but it is assumed that fetal erythrocytes gain access to the maternal circulation as a result of transplacental hemorrhage.

Table 3.5 Blood groups in domestic animals

Species	Number	Blood group systems	Detection method(s)
Horse	7	A/EAA, C, D, K, P, Q, U	Agglutination, hemolysis
Dog	11	A, B, C, D, F, J, K, L, M, N, Tr (DEA 1.1, 1.2, 3, 4, 5, 6, 7^a, 8)	Agglutination, hemolysis, antiglobulin
Cattle	11	A/EAA, B, C, F, J^a, L, M, R^a, S, Z, T	Hemolysis
Sheep	7	A/EAA, B, C, D, M, R^a, X	Agglutination (D only), hemolysis
Pig	16	A/EAA^a, B, C, D, E, F, G, H, I, J, K, L, M, N, O, P	Agglutination, hemolysis, antiglobulin
Cat	1	AB	Agglutination, hemolysis
Goat	6	A, B, C, R, E, F	Hemolysis

^{a}Soluble blood group substances

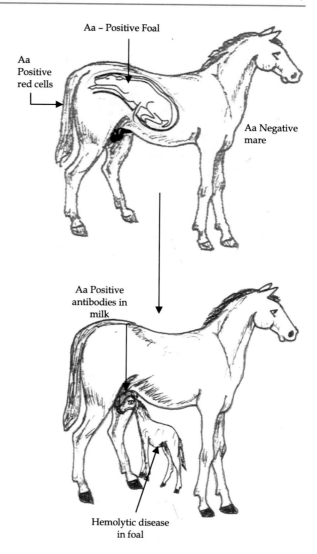

Fig. 3.4 Diagram showing type II hypersensitivity (hemolytic disease in foal)

During the last trimester of pregnancy and during parturition, the possibility of leakage of erythrocytes is enormous. The first pregnancy is usually without any adverse effect in foals. However, repeated pregnancies from the same or other stallion with like blood group will cause further sensitization of dam and predisposes the newborn foal to isoerythrolysis. Antibodies produced by the sensitized mare do not cross placenta to reach the foal. Foal receives them through the colostrum. Antibodies are absorbed by gastrointestinal mucosa and reach in the blood circulation. A type II hypersensitivity reaction ensues with resultant erythrolysis. Hence, foal is born healthy and becomes sick only after ingestion of colostrum (Fig. 3.4).

Clinical signs depend on the amount of antibodies absorbed by the foal and usually appear after 6–48 h. It includes anemia, depression, weakness, and slow and shallow respiration. Foals surviving beyond 48 h show icterus of the mucous membrane and sclera. Hemoglobinuria, if present, is considered pathognomonic. Postmortem examination of the affected foals reveals anemia and icterus. The spleen and liver are enlarged.

Characteristic clinical signs can readily diagnose HDNB in foals. Laboratory confirmation is done by agglutination test using foal's or stallion's erythrocytes and mare's serum or colostrum. Hemolysis test is carried out by addition of fresh normal rabbit serum as a source of complement. Erythrocytes from the affected foal spontaneously agglutinated in vitro are Coombs positive. As the disease is common in horses, mares with history of neonatal erythrolysis should be tested to adopt preventive measures. Pregnant mare serum is tested for antibodies by indirect antiglobulin test. A rising antibody titer indicates in utero sensitization. Newborn foal born from such mare should not be allowed to suckle colostrum and given frozen isoantibody-free colostrum.

Sheep and Goat

The blood group systems of sheep resemble to those of cattle. Seven blood groups—A, B, C, D, M, R, and X—are recognized. Blood group B of sheep is also complex and is reported to have more than 50 different alleles. Ovine R system is analogous to bovine J system.

In goats, six genetic systems of erythrocyte antigen have been identified. These are A, B, C, R, E, and F. Like sheep, B system is complex and contains at least 21 different alleles. The E system has only two alleles, but has four phenotypes due to codominance. Hemolytic disease of newborn has been rarely reported in sheep and goats. Hemolysis test is used for identification of erythrocyte antigens.

Pig

Fifteen blood group systems, A to O, have been identified in pigs. Of these, A blood group is the most important. Two blood group systems A and O require a gene S (secretor) for their expression. When the secretor gene is in homozygous recessive state, A and O antigens are not produced. These antigens are found in the serum and passively adsorbed onto the erythrocytes after birth. A-negative pig harboring anti-A antibody may show transfusion reaction after getting blood from A-positive pig.

Hemolytic disease of newborn piglets is an iatrogenic disease, which occurs as a result of vaccination of pigs with crystal violet-inactivated hog cholera vaccine. Since this old-fashioned vaccine is prepared from the pooled blood of viremic pigs (infected with hog cholera), it contains erythrocyte antigens. Sensitization with the vaccine also leads to isoantibody production, which in turn causes hemolytic disease in the progeny. The affected piglets show progressive weakness and icteric mucous membrane. Surviving piglets may show jaundice and hemoglobinuria. Along with the hemolytic anemia, antibodies against platelets cause thrombocytopenia.

Cat

AB is the only major blood group system identified in cats. The population of cat, thus, has three blood antigens: A, B, and AB. A blood group is dominant and distributed in 75–95% of the cat population. B group is prevalent in 5–25% of cats and AB in less than 1% of cats. This distribution, however, differs in different geographical region and purebred cat breeds. Severe transfusion reactions have been reported especially in B cats, because majority of B cats possess anti-A of IgM class. Even very small amount of blood transfusion from A cat to B cat causes fatal shock. The affected cat shows hypotension, apnea, and atrioventricular block within few minutes of transfusion.

Hemolytic disease of kitten has been reported rarely in Persian or Himalayan breeds. Kittens born from B-positive queen mated with A-positive sire suffer from hemolytic disease. Affected kittens are anemic as a result of intravascular hemolysis. Hemoglobinuria may be noticed after several hours. Icteric mucous membrane and splenomegaly are observed at postmortem. The queen serum contains antibodies to kitten's or sire's erythrocytes. The blood typing in cats is carried out by agglutination and hemolysis tests.

3.3.1.2 Hemolytic Disease of the Newborn in Humans

In humans, HDNB occurs as a result of crossing of the maternal IgG antibodies to fetal erythrocyte antigen to the fetus via placenta, causing erythrocyte destruction. Severe hemolytic disease, also called as erythroblastosis fetalis, is caused by Rhesus incompatibility. It develops in Rh^- mother carrying Rh^+ fetus. During pregnancy fetal erythrocytes are separated from the maternal circulation by a layer called trophoblast. At the time of delivery, however, fetal red cells gain access to the maternal circulation due to placental separation from the uterine wall. Rh^+ fetal erythrocytes stimulate Rh^+-specific B-cells, which transform into plasma cells and memory cells. Plasma cells secrete IgM antibodies, which kill fetal cells, but memory cells remain. Subsequent pregnancy with Rh^+ fetus results in the activation of memory cells and formation of anti-Rh-IgG antibodies, which cross the placenta and damage the fetal erythrocytes. Mild to severe anemia develops, which if overlooked may become fatal. The breakdown product of hemoglobin, the bilirubin, which is lipid soluble, may accumulate in the brain and cause damage there. Hemolytic disease of newborn can be prevented by the administration of antibodies to Rh antigens within 24–48 h of delivery.

3.3.1.3 Blood Transfusion Reactions

Blood transfusion reactions have been reported in the dogs, cats, horses, cows, pigs, and goats. As naturally occurring isoantibodies to most of the erythrocyte antigens are absent in animals, first transfusion does not cause any discomfort or clinical reaction. Hence, crossmatching or blood typing before first transfusion is not required. However, if the donor erythrocyte antigen is not identical to that of the recipient, it does stimulate antibody formation. The second blood transfusion from the same animal or other animal with identical antigens would induce type II reaction mediated by circulating isoantibodies, which are usually of IgG type. There is rapid agglutination of erythrocytes and intra- and extravascular erythrocyte destruction.

The severity of transfusion reaction depends on the immunogenicity of the blood group antigens involved. The animal may suffer generalized anaphylactic shock, hemoglobinemia, and disseminated intravascular coagulation. Incompatible blood transfusions involving minor antigens have a longer course (4–14 days) and cause progressive anemia and icterus. Direct antiglobulin test can be used for the diagnosis. Crossmatching using the donor's red blood cells and the recipient's serum will result in positive slide agglutination test.

There are some practical tips to avoid the occurrence of acute blood transfusion reaction. For example, transfusion of A-positive red cells in dogs, cats, and horses, T-positive red cells in cattle, and R-positive red cells in sheep should be avoided. These blood group antigens provoke strong isoimmune response in animals, thus causing severe reaction following subsequent exposure. Weak blood group antigens such as B, D, and E in dogs elicit formation of low titer isoantibodies and thus are of little clinical significance. However, such sensitized animal may give positive antiglobulin test.

Blood Groups and Transfusion Reaction in Human

Four blood group phenotypes A, B, AB, and O are found in humans (Table 3.6), besides others such as Rh, Kidd, Kell, and Duffy. Incompatible blood transfusions, such as infusion of type A blood into a type B recipient, result in type II hypersensitivity reaction. Anti-A antibody present in the recipient blood recognizes A antigen on transfused erythrocytes as foreign and initiates complement-mediated erythrolysis. The clinical manifestation may have immediate or delayed onset. ABO incompatibilities are most commonly associated with immediate reaction in which complement-mediated lysis is triggered by IgM antibodies. Hemoglobinemia and hemoglobinuria appear within 1–2 h of transfusion. Patients show respiratory distress, disorientation, and cardiovascular collapse that may be fatal.

Delayed transfusion reactions occur as a result of blood group antigen incompatibilities other than ABO incompatibilities. The patients receiving repeated transfusion of ABO-compatible blood produce antibodies against other antigens such as Rh, Kida, Kell, and Duffy. The antibody is of IgG type, which is less efficient than IgM in activating complement-mediated lysis. Hence, many of donor red cells are destroyed extracellularly by agglutination, opsonization, and subsequent phagocytosis by macrophages. The reaction develops within 2 to 6 days of transfusion, reflecting the secondary nature of the response. Symptoms are fever, low hemoglobin content, anemia, and mild jaundice. There may not be hemoglobinuria as most of erythrocytes are killed at extracellular sites.

Table 3.6 ABO blood group systems in humans

Genotypes	Phenotypes	Antigens on erythrocytes	Serum antibodies (isoantibodies)
AA or AO	A	A	Anti-B
BB or BO	B	B	Anti-A
AB	AB	A and B	None
OO	O	None	Anti-A and anti-B

3.3.2 Type II Hypersensitivity to Drugs

Certain drugs are capable of inducing type II reaction and cause hemolytic anemia. There are three mechanisms by which drugs destroy erythrocytes. First, drugs such as penicillin, phenacetin, quinine, etc. are passively adsorbed onto the surface of erythrocytes and render them immunologically foreign. In horses, penicillin-induced hemolytic anemia has been reported. Antibodies to penicillin or penicillin-coated red cells can be demonstrated in the affected animals. A few drugs such as sulfonamides and phenylbutazone can cause agranulocytosis. Similarly, drug-induced thrombocytopenia is also reported. Second, drugs and antibody bind together and activate complement, which in turn cause hemolysis of the nearby cells. Thus, erythrocytes are killed as innocent bystanders. Third, the mechanism involves drug-induced modification of the cell membrane, allowing antibodies to be absorbed on the red cells for subsequent opsonization by phagocytes.

3.3.3 Type II Hypersensitivity in Infectious Diseases

During infection, bacterial lipopolysaccharides, viruses of equine infectious anemia and Aleutian disease, anaplasma, trypanosomes, and *Babesia* may alter erythrocytes, making them immunologically foreign. Such erythrocytes are then eliminated by antibody- and complement-mediated lysis or phagocytosis by mononuclear cells.

3.4 Type III Hypersensitivity

Immune complex diseases occur in animals and humans due to antigen-antibody complex-induced pathological alterations including inflammation (Table 3.7). Immune complexes are formed normally and are removed by phagocytic cells from the system. But occasionally, the formation of antigen and antibody complexes is enhanced, which may get deposited in tissues and leads to type III hypersensitivity diseases. Broadly, the diseases of immune complex origin can be classified into three groups:

1. In persistent infection, the low-grade persistent infection (antigen) is present in the body and combines with antibodies produced against them, leading to immune complex formation and damage in tissue wherever it gets deposited, e.g., viral hepatitis.
2. Certain autoimmune diseases also lead to immune complex-mediated inflammations. However, it requires a continuous production of autoantibodies against self-antigens. The immune complexes, thus formed, are deposited in various tissues leading to pathological implications. e.g., systemic lupus erythematosus (SLE).
3. The formation of immune complexes in tissues due to repeated exposure of antigen and formation of antibodies. The antibodies produced are of IgG class,

3.4 Type III Hypersensitivity

Table 3.7 Infectious diseases causing type III hypersensitivity reactions in animals

Organism or disease	Major type III hypersensitivity lesion
Cattle	
Bovine virus diarrhea	Glomerulonephritis
Staphylococcus aureus	Dermatitis
Mycobacterium johnei	Enteritis
Pig	
Erysipelothrix rhusiopathiae	Arthritis
Hog cholera	Glomerulonephritis
African swine fever	Glomerulonephritis
Horse	
Streptococcus equi	Purpura
Equine viral arteritis	Arteritis
Equine infectious anemia	Anemia and glomerulonephritis
Dog	
Borrelia burgdorferi	Glomerulonephritis
Ehrlichiosis	Glomerulonephritis
Canine adenovirus-1	Uveitis and glomerulonephritis
Canine adenovirus-2	Glomerulonephritis
Visceral leishmaniasis	Glomerulonephritis
Dirofilaria immitis	Glomerulonephritis
Cat	
Feline leukemia	Glomerulonephritis
Feline infectious peritonitis	Peritonitis and glomerulonephritis
Other animals	
Aleutian disease	Glomerulonephritis, anemia, and arteritis

e.g., farmer's lung. Due to inhalation of molds/fungal spores, local immune complexes are formed in lung alveoli leading to alveolitis/pneumonia.

Immune complexes are formed at two places:

1. In blood circulation/stream; they circulate to lodge in vascular channel such as capillaries, renal glomerulus, choroid plexus, and/or synovial membrane.
2. In tissues, which remain localized to the site of immune complex formation.

The size and characteristics of the antibody are more important than the nature of antigen. Small-sized immune complexes remain in the circulation and are not trapped in blood vessels/capillaries, while large-sized immune complexes are insoluble and are quickly removed by phagocytic cells. However, the medium-sized immune complexes remain in the circulation for a longer period; they can fix the complement and are trapped in small capillaries and renal glomeruli leading to inflammatory process.

Immune complex may induce a variety of inflammatory lesions. The binding of antibody to antigen also interacts with the complement system leading to the generation of C3a and C5a which are having anaphylatoxin and chemotactic properties and cause the release of vasoactive amines from mast cells and basophils. These chemical mediators of inflammation act on the blood vessels and cause an increase in vascular permeability and attract phagocytic cells. Immune complex also interacts with Fc receptors of platelets leading to their aggregation and microthrombus formation, which further facilitate an increase in vascular permeability through the action of vasoactive amines. The phagocytic cells present at the site of immune complex deposition may attempt to phagocytose the complexes and are unable to do so because of their trapping in tissues. Thus, these phagocytic cells release lysosomal enzymes at the site of immune complex deposition leading to further tissue damage (Fig. 3.5).

The class of immunoglobulin can influence the deposition of immune complexes. In experiments with systemic lupus erythematosus (SLE) models in mice, it has been observed that IgM and IgG_{2a} participate in the immune complex formation. However, once complexes are deposited in the tissues, complement makes them soluble again. The solubilization appears to occur by the insertion of complement C3b and C3d fragments into the complex. The complexes are continually being deposited in normal individuals and are removed by solubilization process. But in cases of hypocomplementemic, the solubilization process is either absent or decreased, leading to prolonged deposition of immune complex. The solubilization defects have been observed in sera from patients with systemic immune complex diseases.

The experimental models of all the three classical types of immune complex are as follows.

3.4.1 Serum Sickness

In serum sickness, circulating immune complexes deposit in tissues and initiate inflammatory process leading to glomerulonephritis and arthritis. It has been observed as a complication of serum therapy. For example, in diphtheria, anti-diphtheria horse serum is given in humans, which is recognized as foreign protein and the body initiates an immune response against horse serum. Thus, the immune complexes are formed leading to serum sickness. The serum sickness can also be produced in rabbits by administering intravenous injection of a foreign soluble protein such as bovine serum albumin (BSA). After 1 week, antibodies are formed, which enter the circulation and bind with antigen to make immune complexes. These immune complexes are removed by mononuclear phagocyte system slowly and persist in the circulation. The formation of immune complexes leads to the fall in total complement level in blood. The clinical signs of serum sickness can be observed as the antigen-antibody and C_3 deposits on glomerular basement membrane and in small vessels. As the complexes are removed from there either by phagocytes or solubilization by complement, animals recover, and the disease may take a chronic course by continued daily administration of antigen.

3.4 Type III Hypersensitivity

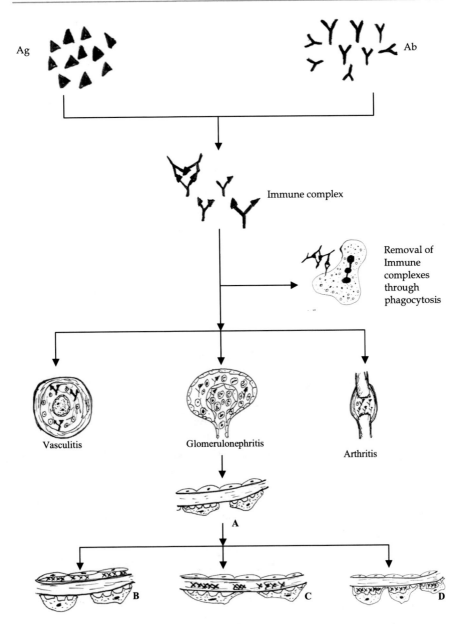

Fig. 3.5 Diagram showing type III hypersensitivity reaction. (**a**) Normal architecture of glomeruli. (**b**) Type I. C. Type II. D. Type III membranoproliferative glomerulonephritis (MPGN)

3.4.2 Autoimmune Complex Disease

In SLE, a range of autoantibodies can be detected such as anti-RBC, anti-nuclear, anti-DNA, etc. The deposition of immune complexes is observed in glomeruli and choroid plexus.

3.4.3 Arthus Reaction

Arthus reaction takes place at a local site in and around the wall of small blood vessels and can be demonstrated in the skin. It can be observed in animals by administration of repeated injection of antigen until an appreciable amount of precipitating IgG antibody appears. Then on subcutaneous or intradermal injection of antigen it gives inflammatory reaction within 4–10 h of administration. There is marked edema and hemorrhage at the site of injection, which disappears after 48 h. Antigen/antibody/complement can be demonstrated around the wall of small blood vessel in the lesion, which is also infiltrated by neutrophils followed by mononuclear cells. There is intravascular clumping of platelets leading to occlusion of blood vessel and necrosis.

3.4.4 Diseases Associated with Immune Complexes

3.4.4.1 Glomerulonephritis

Immune complex-mediated glomerulonephritis was considered as a rare disease entity till the 1970s, but now with the advancement of immunopathology, it accounts for substantial morbidity and mortality not only in animals but also in humans. In immune complex-mediated glomerulonephritis, the antigen-antibody complexes are deposited in glomerulus leading to alteration in structure and function.

It has been reported in middle-aged dogs specially associated with chronic skin disease, neoplasia, and hyperadrenocorticism. In animals, the immune complex-mediated glomerulonephritis has been found to occur in various other disease conditions listed below (Table 3.8).

Table 3.8 Diseases causing immune complex-mediated glomerulonephritis

Animal	Diseases associated with immune complex-mediated glomerulonephritis
Bovine	Bovine viral diarrhea
Ovine	Campylobacteriosis
Porcine	Swine fever
Equine	Equine infectious anemia and strangles
Canine	Brucellosis, lymphosarcoma, mastocytoma, adenovirus infection, pyometra, systemic lupus erythematosus

3.4.5 Pathogenesis

Immune complexes are formed through either endogenous or exogenous antigenic determinants in host tissue. The antigen implanted in host tissue is recognized by the circulating antibodies, which binds with antigen, and the process is known as in situ immune complex formation. This type of immune complex-mediated glomerulonephritis has been observed in most cases of humans and animals (Fig. 3.6).

In another type, the immune complexes are formed in circulation and they get deposited in the wall of medium- or small-sized blood vessels such as glomerular capillaries. Such complexes require a high level of antigen as seen in certain persistent viral infections.

Immune complexes are deposited within glomerulus in either of the four anatomical locations (Fig. 3.5).

1. Sub-epithelial—beneath the visceral epithelial cells
2. Sub-endothelial—beneath the endothelial cells
3. Intramembranous—in lamina densa of the basement membrane
4. Mesangial cells—outside the glomerular basement membrane in mesangial cells

3.4.5.1 Sub-epithelial

The immune complexes are deposited in sub-epithelial region when they are composed of cationic charged antigen or complexes of low avidity. The immune complexes having high cationic charge may cross glomerular basement membranes and bind with the anionic charged epithelial cell cytoplasm. In immune complexes with low avidity, antibody dissociates at the inner part of the glomerular basement membrane. The antigen then may diffuse across the membrane and is trapped on epithelial cell cytoplasm and subsequently rebind to its antibody. Thus, sub-epithelial immune complexes may result from either in situ or formation of circulating antigen-antibody complexes.

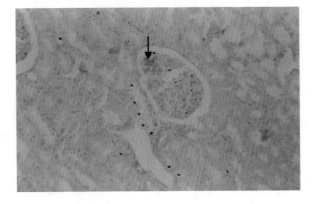

Fig. 3.6 Photomicrograph showing immune complexes in glomerulus through immunoperoxidase technique

3.4.5.2 Sub-endothelial

Those immune complexes are deposited in sub-endothelial area, which are having neutral or anionic charged antigen and thus cannot penetrate the barrier of the glomerular basement membrane. Antibodies having high avidity may also tend to localize in sub-endothelial area. The immune complexes localized in sub-endothelial area have been found to be associated with more intense inflammation.

3.4.5.3 Intramembranous

This is a very rare pathological condition. In intramembranous deposition of immune complexes, there is an autoimmune humoral response against glomerular basement membrane in which indigenous structural glomerular antigen acts as autoantigen.

3.4.5.4 Mesangium

The mesangium is composed of specialized cells and extracellular matrix and is constantly perfused by macromolecules such as infectious agents or immune complexes. Immune complexes accumulate in matrix after ultrafiltration and subsequently localize in mesangial cells through endocytosis. It results in the proliferation of mesangial cells and production of excess mesangial matrix.

3.4.6 Clinical Findings

Immune complex-mediated glomerulonephritis has been well studied in canines. Initially, there are no clinical symptoms even after the disease started with glomerular injury but it is not sufficient to produce increased capillary permeability. However, one can detect the high protein level in the urine of patients as about 200 mg of protein may pass through urine per day. This leads to hypoproteinemia, edema, ascites, and hypercholesterolemia. The low level of albumin in blood circulation may also result into hypovolemia. There are elevated levels of serum cholesterol and triglycerides leading to hyperlipidemia.

In advanced cases, blood urea nitrogen level increases, resulting in azotemia and uremia characterized by anorexia, vomiting, diarrhea, melena, polydipsia, polyuria, dehydration, anemia, convulsions, and weakness. These signs occur with a functional loss of about 75% nephrons. Reduced glomerular blood flow and filtration rate may lead to hypoxia, cell necrosis, interstitial inflammation, and fibrosis. Renal osteodystrophy can also be observed in patients with immune complex-mediated nephritis because of increased renal retention of phosphorus and ineffective renal conversion of the active form of vitamin D, which leads to hypocalcemia, increased production of parathormone, and eventually decalcification of bone.

3.4.7 Lesions

On necropsy, pale and firm kidneys are seen with little fibrosis along the capsule, which is difficult to remove from kidney parenchyma. There is loss of a clear line of demarcation between the cortex and medulla. There is a high level of protein in urine present in the urinary bladder. Microscopically, four basic types of changes can be observed in kidneys:

1. Proliferation of mesangial cells
2. Thickening of basement membrane
3. Infiltration of leucocytes in injured glomeruli
4. Hyalinization and sclerosis

Based on the lesions described above, the glomerulonephritis of immune complex origin is divided into four categories.

3.4.7.1 Proliferative Glomerulonephritis

This form of immune complex-mediated glomerulonephritis is characterized by an increase in the number of cells within the glomerulus such as epithelial cells, endothelial cells, and mesangial cells, of which mesangial cell proliferation is the most markedly seen. It is also known as mesangio-proliferative in medical sciences. In this type of glomerulonephritis, adhesions between Bowman's capsule and glomerular tufts are seen as subacute or chronic lesion in horses and ruminants. Immunofluorescence or immunoperoxidase staining techniques revealed the presence of immune complexes with IgG or IgM in capillary walls and in mesangium.

3.4.7.2 Membranous Glomerulonephritis

Membranous glomerulonephritis is characterized by the marked thickening of glomerular basement membrane. Immunofluorescence or immunoperoxidase staining of kidney sections may reveal the presence of uniformly coarse granular deposits of host immunoglobulin (IgG) or complement (C_3) within the wall of glomerular capillaries. Chronic membranous glomerulonephritis is commonly seen in cats and dogs.

3.4.7.3 Membranoproliferative Glomerulonephritis

This is a composite form of proliferative and membranous glomerulonephritis, in which both types of lesions are recorded. In this form, glomerular tufts and capillary wall become thickened along with increased infiltration of leucocytes. Irregular granular accumulations of immune complexes can be demonstrated in the wall of glomerular capillaries and within the expanded mesangial matrix. The type of glomerulonephritis is most commonly seen in dogs.

3.4.7.4 Mesangiosclerotic Glomerulonephritis

It can be observed due to prolonged glomerular injury, which occurs after either of the three types described above. In this form, glomerular tufts are extensively hyalinized, which becomes avascular and adhere to Bowman's capsule. There is complete destruction of glomerular cytoarchitecture and immune complexes can be seen in capillary walls and within the mesangium.

Besides, the pathological lesions are intraglomerular space; there are significant tubulointerstitial lesions on chronic glomerulonephritis; the type and extent of lesion depends on the quality and quantity of immune complexes and their site of deposition. However, there are some lesions overlapping to each other, needing confirmation through immunofluorescence test (IFT) or immunoperoxidase staining.

3.4.7.5 Rheumatoid Arthritis

Rheumatoid arthritis is a bilateral erosive polyarthritis caused by deposition of immune complexes within the synovial tissue. This type of arthritis occurs in humans and dogs. Rheumatoid arthritis is an intra-articular deposition of immune complexes due to the production of autoantibodies against self-immunoglobulins (antigen). Thus, the altered immunoglobulins of host act as antigen and the antibody to these immunoglobulins is known as rheumatoid factor (RF), which is an autoantibody.

The autoantibody (RF) binds with the Fc portion of host immunoglobulins (Ag) and thus the formed complexes are deposited in synovium leading to complement activation chemotaxis of inflammatory cells and proliferation of synovial cells. There is configurational change in the Fc portion of host IgG after its binding to an unknown antigen. These changes in immunoglobulin render it foreign to the host and initiate the production of autoantibodies. It may also happen through a breach of self-tolerance owing to abnormalities of immunoregulation. In some cases of men with rheumatoid arthritis, decreased mitogenic responsiveness of lymphocytes leads to anergy. Once there is defect in host immunoglobulin and immunoregulation is established, the plasma cells/activated B-cells within the synovium and regional lymph nodes produce a large amount of autoantibodies (RF). These autoantibodies form immune complexes with host immunoglobulins and deposit in synovium leading to inflammation and pannus formation.

The inflammation in synovial membrane occurs due to fixation of complement with immune complex and the release of C3a and C5a. The pannus is the intra-articular formation of granulation tissue, which arises from inflamed synovium and extends across the articular cartilage. The inflammatory cells including proliferating synoviocytes, fibrin, and lectin are the main components of the pannus.

Clinically, the rheumatoid arthritis is characterized by bilaterally symmetric progressive polyarthritis most commonly affecting the carpal-metacarpal and tarsal-metatarsal joints. The other joints, which are involved in rheumatoid arthritis, include interphalangeal, stifle, elbow, and intervertebral joints. The patients suffer from joint pain, stiff gait, and periarticular swelling along with fever, depression, and anorexia. On clinical examination, such joints are found to be swollen and painful.

Diagnosis can be made by demonstration of rheumatoid factor in the serum of the patients. Immune complex-mediated polyarthritis commonly occurs in humans, dogs, and cats, and other animals; it has not been documented so far.

For treatment of immune complex-mediated disorders in humans and animals immunosuppressive and anti-inflammatory drugs are given. Treatment with corticosteroids has been found to have a recovery of about 90% in arthritis patients.

However, it may have its other side effects also which should be looked into before the start of the treatment.

3.5 Type IV Hypersensitivity

We have learned that antibody mediates the first three types of hypersensitivity reactions (type I, II, and III), which occur within few minutes to few hours of re-exposure to allergens. Another type of hypersensitivity also occurs, which is known as type IV hypersensitivity and is mediated by sensitized T-cells. When some antigens are injected into the skin of sensitized animal, acute inflammatory reaction takes several hours to develop and becomes clinically obvious between 24 and 72 h. Hence, this type of hypersensitivity reaction is also called as delayed-type hypersensitivity (DTH). It results from interaction between the allergen, macrophages, and the T-cells. The reaction is characterized by a red indurated painful swelling in which macrophage is the principal component. Historically, Robert Koch first observed the phenomenon about a century ago. He found that individual infected with *Mycobacterium tuberculosis* showed local inflammatory reaction when injected intradermally with mycobacterial culture filtrate. The reaction was named as tuberculin reaction, which has now been considered as the most classical example of DTH. Subsequently, it was found that a variety of bacterial and other agents could cause this phenomenon. As the term suggests, type IV hypersensitivity is detrimental and at times causes extensive tissue damage, but in many instances especially against intracellular pathogens and contact antigens, it plays an important protective role.

3.5.1 The Tuberculin Reaction

Tuberculin in the antigenic extract is derived from *M. bovis*, *M. tuberculosis*, and *M. avium*. In the past, several types of tuberculin were prepared as a reagent for the diagnosis of tuberculosis in animals. But currently, a purified protein derivative (PPD) of tuberculin is the most commonly used. Normal healthy animal, when injected with tuberculin, does not show any reaction. On the other hand, when tuberculin is injected into an animal already infected with tuberculous bacilli or sensitized with mycobacterial antigens, an acute indurated swelling develops at the site of injection after 24 h. The swelling reaches maximum size within 48–72 h. The skin reaction may persist for several weeks before it disappears. If the animal is highly sensitized, a severe reaction consisting of tissue destruction and necrosis occurs in the dermis. Histologically, the reaction is characterized by engorgement of blood vessels, edema, and heavy infiltration with lymphocytes and macrophages. The presence of neutrophil in significant numbers may be seen in the early stages.

3.5.1.1 Mechanism of DTH Reaction

It is evident from the classical tuberculin reaction that for DTH reaction to occur, as for other hypersensitivity reactions, in the first step the animal has to be sensitized. Following re-exposure with the same antigen clinically obvious skin reaction occurs only after 24 h, which indicates effector function of the sensitized T-cells. Thus, the mechanism of DTH reaction can be explained in two phases; the first phase is the sensitization and the second phase is the effector phase.

In the **sensitization phase**, the offending antigen causes activation of Th cells in 1–2 weeks. The antigen is processed by the antigen-presenting cells (APC) such as Langerhans cells and macrophages and is presented to T-helper cell subpopulations in association with MHC class II molecules. The antigen-presenting cells are thought to pick up the antigen from the site of infection or injection and bring them to the regional lymph nodes, where T-cells are activated and clonally expanded. Usually, $CD4^+$ T-cells are activated and participate in the DTH reaction. These cells are specifically called as T_{DTH} cell. In some cases, cytotoxic T-cells are also activated. Activated T-cells may be present at the site of infection or circulate in the blood.

The **effector phase** is induced by subsequent exposure with the similar antigen. Following intradermal injection, a part of the antigen is taken by the dendritic cells, which migrate to the draining lymph node to activate sensitized T_{DTH} cells. Antigens are also locally absorbed and come in contact with circulating T_{DTH} cells, which in turn adhere to the endothelial cells and migrate to the antigen deposition site. Locally, antigens also attract neutrophils and monocytes (Fig. 3.7).

Macrophage functions as the principal effector cells in DTH reaction. The cytokines secreted by the activated T_{DTH} cells cause increased expression of adhesion and MHC class II molecules. This results in the migration of blood monocytes in the surrounding tissues. They are differentiated into activated macrophages equipped with enhanced capability of phagocytosis and destruction of the microorganisms. These activated macrophages also express increased levels of MHC class II and cell adhesion molecules, so as to function more effectively as antigen-processing cells. It has been observed in cattle by 24 h; the injection site is mainly infiltrated with $\gamma\delta+$ and WC+ T-cells along with few neutrophils. The reaction is apparently visible by 24 h, and its intensity may reach peak level within 48 h. Vasoactive substances are released by T-cells and also from basophils and mast cells, which are attracted to the site in response to cytokines. More and more T-cells are attracted to the site in response to T-cell-derived molecules (autocrine function). Only about 5% of the infiltrated T-cells are antigen-specific T_{DTH} cells and the rest are non-specific to the inducing antigen. At the peak of response, phenotypically, lymphocytes are TCR $\alpha/\beta+$, CD4+, and CD8+ T-cells. Proteases and reactive oxygen metabolites released from the activated macrophages cause tissue destruction. The area is swollen and indurated due to massive infiltration of macrophages and lymphocytes, fibrin deposition, and inflammatory edema. The injected antigens are eventually ingested and destroyed and the swelling gradually disappears in several weeks (Fig. 3.7).

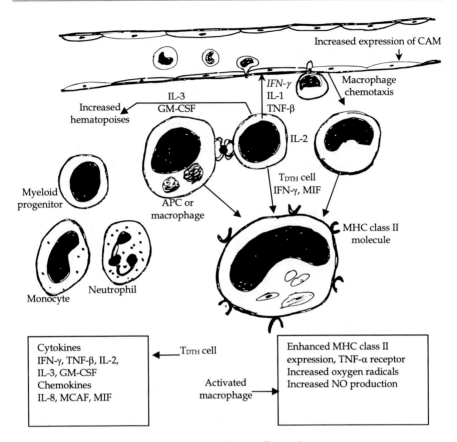

Fig. 3.7 The mechanism of type IV hypersensitivity (effector phase)

3.5.1.2 Mediators of DTH Response

A variety of cytokines and chemokines secreted by activated lymphocytes and macrophages mediate DTH response. The pattern of cytokines secreted suggests that T_{DTH} cells are derived from T-helper cell population. Interferon-gamma (IFN-γ) is the most important of all and activates macrophages and promotes increased expression of MHC class II molecules on them. IFN-γ and tumor necrosis factor-beta (TNF-β) along with TNF-α and IL-1 act on the endothelium of the neighboring blood vessels and facilitate extravasation of monocytes and other non-specific inflammatory cells. The process involves increased expression of the adhesion molecules on the endothelium and increased vascular permeability. Neutrophils appear early in the reaction and are maximum by 6 h, after which the number declines. Monocytes start appearing at about 12 h post-injection and attain peak number between 24 and 48 h. Monocytes are attracted to the area of reaction by monocyte chemotactic and activating factor (MCAF) and IFN-γ. T_{DTH} cells also secrete another chemokine, the macrophage migration inhibition factor (MIF) that prevents macrophages to migrate from the reaction site. These macrophages are further activated by T_{DTH}-derived IFN-γ and TNF-β, which in turn activate more T-cells. Thus, these self-perpetuating cycles occur during type IV hypersensitivity. This response may turn out to be beneficial and protective, destroying foreign antigen or microorganisms, or becomes detrimental, causing extensive tissue damage.

3.5.1.3 Protective and Pathological Role of DTH Responses

Humoral immune response is of little significance in offering protection to intracellular bacteria, because of the inability of antibodies to reach the bacteria. Type IV hypersensitivity plays an important role in host defense against such bacteria. Lytic enzymes and oxygen metabolites of activated macrophages that infiltrate at the site of reaction kill cells harboring intracellular bacteria. Immunity to mycobacterial infection is a DTH response in which activated macrophages wall off the organisms to form a granuloma. If the DTH response is appropriate, organisms are killed and infection eliminated. The protective role of DTH in mycobacterial diseases such as tuberculosis, Johne's disease or paratuberculosis, and leprosy is well known. Strong DTH response is elicited in animals with early lesions in tuberculosis and paratuberculosis. Similarly, persons with tuberculoid leprosy with less number of bacilli show strong DTH response and those with lepromatous leprosy show poor response.

The significance of hypersensitivity in the pathogenesis of tuberculosis was first demonstrated by Koch, which was later named as Koch's phenomenon. Generalized tuberculosis develops if a normal guinea pig is injected subcutaneously with tubercle bacilli. At the site of inoculation, hard nodule formed, which breaks down to form an ulcar. Guinea pig dies within 2 to 3 months. If, however, a tuberculous guinea pig is injected similarly, an acute response consisting of exudation and necrosis develops at the inoculation site. The necrotic tissue soon sloughs and heals within a short period. There is no generalization of infection and bacteria are killed rapidly. This is due to DTH response operating in the sensitized guinea pig.

Beneficial and harmful effects of hypersensitivity depend on the circumstances. Hypersensitivity to a small number of bacilli results in tubercle formation that enhances the killing of organisms by the activated macrophages. This helps in the prevention of re-infection and also dissemination of infection. Hypersensitive responses to a large number of bacilli result into extensive necrosis and tissue damage. Liquefaction caused by lytic enzymes of macrophages is considered most harmful in the pathogenesis of tuberculosis. Mycobacteria resist intracellular destruction by the macrophages until T-cells activate them. Bacteria being rich in poorly metabolizable wax are not easily removed and hence are present for a prolonged time, causing more and more accumulation of macrophages. The macrophages in this location change into epithelial-like cells known as epithelioid cells. An aggregation of epithelioid cells surrounded by lymphocytes is referred to as granuloma. Several of the macrophages are fused to form giant cells (Langhans type), a characteristic feature of tuberculosis lesion (Fig. 3.8). Foreign body-type giant cells can also be formed. If the reaction is sustained, granuloma may be

3.5 Type IV Hypersensitivity

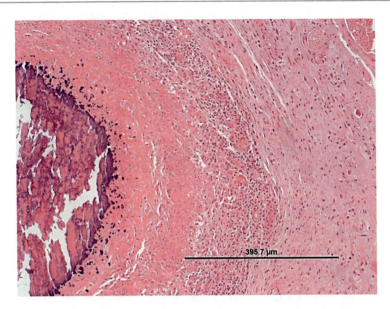

Fig. 3.8 Bovine tuberculosis (*Mycobacterium bovis*): tuberculin reaction (type IV hypersensitivity)—central area of caseous necrosis with calcification (blue color), surrounded by epithelioid cells, Langhans giant cells, lymphocytes, and plasma cells with a fibrous capsule. H&E ×100

surrounded by a thin rim of connective tissues under the influence of platelet-derived growth factor (PDGF) and transforming growth factor-beta (TGF-β) secreted from activated macrophages. This type of granuloma is also called as hypersensitivity granuloma.

3.5.2 Johnin Reaction

Animals (cattle, sheep, and goat) infected with *M. paratuberculosis* show DTH response following intradermal injection of Johnin PPD. The maximum reaction reaches after 48 h of inoculation. Intravenous Johnin test is sometimes used for the diagnosis of Johne's disease. A rise in temperature of 1 °C or neutrophilia recorded after 6 h of inoculation is suggestive of positive reaction.

3.5.3 Other Intracellular Pathogens Showing DTH

Besides mycobacterial infections, positive DTH response may be observed in several infectious diseases caused by intracellular pathogens. Microbial extract is prepared from these pathogens for intradermal skin testing. Brucellin prepared from *Brucella abortus* is sometimes used for the diagnosis of brucellosis with some limitation. Culture filtrate of *Pseudomonas mallei*, known as mallein, is used for skin testing in horses suspected to be suffering from glanders. A number of modifications of mallein test have evolved, but the most commonly used method is the intradermopalpebral test. In this test, mallein is injected into the skin of the lower eyelid. Positive reaction appearing after 24 h is characterized by edematous swelling of the eyelids, lacrimation, and ophthalmia. Certain fungal diseases such as histoplasmosis and coccidioidomycosis can be diagnosed by skin testing using histoplasmin and coccidioidin, respectively. Toxinoplasmin is used for the diagnosis of toxoplasmosis. Most of these tests are considered non-specific, and because of being an in vivo method, they also induce antibody production, which hinders serological monitoring.

3.5.4 Allergic Contact Dermatitis

Several chemicals and other substances have been found to cause allergic dermatitis, which are mediated by type IV hypersensitivity. These include formaldehyde, trinitrophenol, dinitrochlorobenzene, picric acid, aniline dyes, nickel, turpentine, various cosmetics and hair dye, poison oak, poison ivy, etc. Most of these substances are small molecules that can complex with the skin protein when applied on the skin. These complexes are internalized by Langerhans cells (antigen-presenting cells) processed and along with MHC class II molecules are presented to T-cells. Subsequent exposure with the same chemical causes infiltration of a large number of mononuclear cells in the dermis within 24 h. Intra-epithelial vesicles are produced as a result of killing of Langerhans cell containing the chemical-protein complex by the activated T-cells. The skin lesion is highly pruritic and hence known as allergic contact dermatitis. Pathologists working with formaldehyde develop allergic contact dermatitis. In dogs, allergic contact dermatitis of ear may occur following neomycin treatment of otitis externa and ventral abdomen, scrotum, etc. following contact with carpet dye. The clinical findings in contact dermatitis include the appearance of mild erythema (red patches) to severe erythematous vesicle formation, which are intensely pruritic. Self-inflicted injuries may lead to excoriation and ulceration. Secondary infections with staphylococci often lead to pyoderma. Chronic exposure to these allergens causes hyperkeratosis, acanthosis, and dermal fibrosis of the skin. A large number of mononuclear cell infiltration and vesiculation of the epidermal layer characterize the microscopical lesions. Closed or open patch test employing suspected allergen is carried out for the identification of the offending chemical allergens.

3.5.5 Detection of Type IV Hypersensitivity

Techniques used for the measurement of cell-mediated immunity are also applied to detect type IV hypersensitivity. The in vivo methods are intradermal skin test and dinitrochlorobenzene (DNCB) test. The classical examples of intradermal skin test are tuberculin and Johnin tests. Cell-mediated immunity can also be roughly measured by applying sensitizing chemical such as DNCB.

In vitro methods are used to measure either proliferation of T-cells in response to antigen or their ability to produce cytokines. Lymphocyte proliferation assay is carried out by incubating purified peripheral blood mononuclear cells (PBMCs) with the antigen followed by measuring the uptake of incorporated tritiated thymidine by dividing lymphocytes. The assay can also be performed using 3-(4,5-dimethylthiazol-2-yl)-2,5-diphenyltetrazolium bromide (MTT) dye. IFN-γ release assay (IGRA) is another in vitro method to measure cell-mediated immunity. In this test, PBMCs or whole blood is incubated with the antigen, and after 72 to 96 h, supernatant is collected for estimation of IFN-γ. Estimation of IFN-γ is carried out either by bioassay or preferably by sandwich ELISA using mAb. The advantage of this test is that it does not interfere with the immune status of the animal. Thus, animals can be tested any number of times. IFN-γ-based sandwich ELISAs are being used currently for the diagnosis of tuberculosis and paratuberculosis in cattle.

Further Reading

Askenase PW, Van Loveren M (1983) Delayed type hypersensitivity: activation of mast cells by antigen specific T-cell factors initiates the cascade of cellular interactions. Immunol Today 4: 259–264

Auer L, Bell K, Gates S (1962) Blood transfusion reactions in the cat. Am J Veter Med Assoc 180: 729–730

Bailey E (1982) Prevalence of anti-red blood cells antibodies to neonatal isoerythrolysis. Am J Vet Res 43:1917–1921

Befus AD, Bienenstock J, Denburg JA (1985) Mast cell differentiation and heterogenicity. Immunol Today 6:281–284

Borish L, Mascali JJ, Rosenwasser J (1991) IgE-dependent cytokine production by human peripheral blood mononuclear phagocytes. J Immunol 146:63–67

Chauhan RS (1998) An introduction to immunopathology. G.B. Pant University, Pantnagar

Chauhan RS (1998) Immune complex mediated pathological lesions in man and animals. In: Chauhan RS (ed) An introduction to immunopathology. G.B. Pant University, Pantnagar, pp 114–121

Coe Clough NE, Roth JA (1995) Methods for assessing cell-mediated immunity in infectious disease resistance and in the development of vaccines. J Am Veter Med Assoc 206:1208–1216

Conrad DH (1990) FceRII/CD23, the low affinity receptor for IgE. Annu Rev. Immunol 8:623–645

Dannenberg AM (1991) Delayed-type hypersensitivity and cell-mediated immunity in the pathogenesis of tuberculosis. Immunol Today 12:228–233

Dimmock CK, Webster WR, Shiels IA, Edwards CL (1982) Isoimmune thrombocytopenic purpura in piglets. Aust Vet J 59:157–159

Doherty ML, Bassett HF, Quinn PJ et al (1996) A sequential study of the bovine tuberculin reaction. Immunology 87:9–14

Gershwin LJ, Krakowka S, Olsen RG (1995) Immunology and immunopathology of domestic animals, 2nd edn. Mosby, St. Louis

Grant DI, Thoday KL (1980) Canine allergic contact dermatitis: a clinical review. J Small Anim Pract 21:17–27

Halliwell REW, Longino DJ (1985) IgE and IgG antibodies to flea antigen in differing dog population. Vet Immunol Immunopathol 8:215–224

Henderson WR, Chi EY, Klebanoff SJ (1980) Eosinophil peroxidase- induced mast cell secretion. J Exp Med 152:265–279

Jackson HA, Miller HRP, Halliwell REW (1996) Canine leucocyte histamine release: response to antigen and to anti IgE. Vet Immunol Immunopathol 53(3–4):195–206

Janeway CA, Travers PC (1994) Immunology: the immune system in health and diseases, 2nd edn. Churchill Livingstone

Jarrett EE, Haig DM (1984) Mucosal mast cells *in vivo* and *in vitro*. Immunol Today 5:115–118

Jonson NN, Pullen C, Watson ADJ (1990) Neonatal isoerythrolysis in Himalayan kittens. Aust Vet J 67:416–417

Khurana, R., Mahipal, S.K. and Chauhan, R.S. (1995). Pesticide induced glomerulonephritis in sheep. In: Second annual conference of IAAVR and national symposium on "modern trends in animal health and production research and its impact on rural development, Jan 24–25, 1995, Hisar, India

Khurana R, Mahipal SK, Chauhan RS (1999) Effects of pesticides on delayed type hypersensitivity reaction in sheep. Indian J Anim Sci 69:880–881

Khurana SK, Chauhan RS, Mahipal SK (1999) Immunotoxic effect of cypermethrin on delayed type hypersensitivity (DTH) reaction in chickens. Indian Veter J 76:1055–1057

Killingsworth CR (1984) Use of blood and blood components for feline and canine patients. Journal of American Veterinary Medical Association 185:1452–1454

Kuby J (1997) Hypersensitivity reactions. In: Immunology. W.H. Freeman and Company, New York, pp 413–439

Linklater K (1977) Post-transfusion purpura in a pig. Res Vet Sci 22:257–258

McClure JJ, Kohh C, Traub-Dargarz JL (1994) Characterization of a red cell antigen in donkeys and mules associated with neonatal isoerythrolysis. Anim Genet 25:119–120

McConnico RS, Roberts MC, Tompkins M (1992) Penicillin induced immune-mediated hemolytic anemia in a horse. J Am Veter Med Assoc 201:1402–1403

McEwen BJ (1992) Eosinophils: a review. Vet Res Commun 16:11–44

Norsworthy GD (1992) Clinical aspects of feline blood transfusions. Compar Contin Educ Pract Veterin 14:469–475

Olivry T (2001) The ACVD task force on canine atopic dermatitis. (XVII): histopathology of skin lesions. Veterin Immunol Immunopathol 81:305–309

Olivry T (2001) The American College of Veterinary Dermatology (ACDV) task force on atopic dermatitis. Special Issue, Veter Immunol Immunopathol 81:143–388

Symons M, Bell K (1992) Canine blood groups: description of 20 specificities. Anim Genet 23: 509–515

Tizard I (1998) Red cell antigen and type II hypersensitivity. In: Veterinary immunology-an introduction. Harcourt Brace and Company, Asia Pvt. Ltd, pp 359–367

Weller PF (1991) The Immunobiology of eosinophils. N Engl J Med 324:1110–1118

Whyte A, Haskard DO, Binns RM (1994) Infiltrating T-cells and selection endothelial ligands in the cutaneous phytohemagglutinin-induced inflammatory reaction. Vet Immunol Immunopathol 41:31–40

Wood PR, Corner LA, Plackett P (1990) Development of simple, rapid *in vitro* cellular assay for bovine tuberculosis based on the production of γ-interferon. Res Vet Sci 49:46–49

Autoimmunity

Key Points

1. Autoimmunity defines a state in which loss of natural immunologic tolerance or unresponsiveness to self-antigens happens. As a result, immune responses against self-antigens induce pathology, known as autoimmune diseases.
2. Failure to maintain tolerance to self-antigens is the primary cause of the majority of autoimmune disorders.
3. Autoimmunity is not always pathological.
4. Antigens that emerge as a result of the creation of novel molecular configurations, antigens that are hidden inside cells, and antigens that evolve late in life can all be the targets of autoimmune reactions.
5. Some microorganisms and parasites have antigenic epitopes, which are similar to tissue components of the host and antibodies or T-cell responses against these organisms may react with the host tissue components and cause autoimmune disease, known as a molecular mimicry.
6. Rheumatoid factors are autoantibodies, directed against the Fc portion of the immunoglobulin (IgG).
7. Systemic lupus erythematosus (SLE) results from the production of autoantibodies against a variety of antigens present in the host such as red blood cells, platelets, leukocytes, and nuclear antigens.
8. Sjogren's syndrome is the simultaneous occurrence of keratoconjunctivitis sicca (KCS), xerostomia, and rheumatoid factors in dogs.
9. Addition's disease (autoimmune adrenalitis) is an adrenal insufficiency (hypoadrenocorticism) due to autoimmune destruction of the adrenal cortex.
10. Pemphigus vulgaris causes acantholytic epidermal lesions which result from the production of autoantibodies against a protein called desmoglein-3, which is an intercellular cement substance responsible for squamous cell adhesion.
11. Pemphigus foliaceus is a milder but more common disease than pemphigus vulgaris which results from the production of autoantibodies against desmoglein-1.

12. Bullous pemphigoid is a self-limited blistering disease characterized by the formation of autoantibodies against desmoplakins.
13. Myasthenia gravis is an autoimmune disease of neuromuscular junction that results from the production of autoantibodies against acetylcholine receptor, characterized by skeletal muscle fatigue and weakness.
14. Immune stimulants such as viral infections, vaccinations, and some medications can cause several autoimmune diseases.

4.1 General Concept

Since the beginning of the twentieth century, it has been believed that the immune system does not normally react to self. This phenomenon is now described as immunologic tolerance to the self-components and obviously an important necessity for maintaining the normal health. **Autoimmunity** defines a state in which the natural immunologic tolerance or unresponsiveness to self-antigen terminates. As a result, immune responses against the self- antigens induce pathology, known as **autoimmune diseases**. These are now considered a major medical problem of today's industrialized societies. With major advances in veterinary immunology, autoimmune disorders are being identified in animals and birds too.

The term autoimmunity was first introduced by Paul Ehrlich to convey immunity against self. In spite of a few preliminary evidences, the concept of autoimmunity was rejected for more than 50 years. The development of acute disseminated encephalitis in monkeys following immunization with foreign nervous tissue was a significant discovery in 1933. This finding was also not widely accepted because there was no correlation between brain-specific autoantibodies and the occurrence of encephalomyelitis. However, the work of Ernest Witebsky and Noel Rose in 1956 gave a new turn to the concept of autoimmunity. They found that rabbits immunized with rabbit thyroglobulin not only had thyroid lesions identical to those seen in human thyroiditis but also produced antithyroglobulin antibodies. Further, demonstration of antiglobulin antibodies in human cases of thyroiditis amplified the impact of result in rabbit. Studies on autoimmune hemolytic anemia and thrombocytopenia contributed significantly to the field of autoimmunity. Antiglobulin test developed by Coombs in 1945 provided a tool for detection of antierythrocyte autoantibodies. The most notable experiment, which unequivocally proved the ill effects of autoimmunity, was the daring experiment of the hematologist William Harrington on himself. He volunteered to receive plasma infusion from a patient with thrombocytopenia. His platelet count dropped to a dangerous level and he collapsed with seizure and developed purpura. Harrington's bone marrow showed no signs of damage to megakaryocytes and his platelet counts became normal within a week. This was the first experiment, which established that autoantibody can cause human illness.

In spite of all these observations, doubts and reservations on autoimmunity persisted until the discovery of New Zealand Black (NZB) mouse that develops spontaneous autoimmune hemolytic anemia. While on one hand this finding legitimizes the research on autoimmunity, it also provided the genetic basis of autoimmunity. It must be borne in mind that autoimmunization is not similar to an immune response to a foreign antigen. Autoimmunization needs all the components and mechanism of the immune system, but to cause self-destruction in the host, it requires to overcome all those mechanisms that prevent the harmful effects of the autoimmunity. In autoimmunity, the problem does not lie in autoantibodies or T-cells that cause the lesions in the disease but lie in the complex network of components that stimulate the event. The complexity of the problem was further compounded by the fact that autoimmunity is an inherent property of the normal immune system. Therefore, despite the major development in the field of immunology, a unifying concept to explain the origin and pathogenesis of various autoimmune disorders is yet to be established. Experimental evidences are, however, accumulating in favor of the opinion that autoimmune disease may result from a wide variety of genetic, environmental, and immunological factors.

4.2 Mechanism of Induction

4.2.1 Physiological Autoimmunity

Autoimmune responses are not always harmful. Controlled immune responses to self-antigen have certain physiological functions. Control of antibody production and removal of aged cells involve autoimmune process.

Immunoglobulin molecules have antigen-binding sites, which act as epitopes (idiotype) and generate autoantibodies (anti-idiotype). The anti-idiotype antibody also contains epitopes that can generate an anti-idiotype antibody. Each anti-idiotype has its negative action on the preceding response and then the ultimate result of this network is to regulate and terminate antibody production. Regulation of T-cell response also involves similar mechanism.

Removal of old erythrocytes from the vascular system is necessary and is accomplished by the autoimmune process. Band-3 protein is a constituent of normal plasma membrane of erythrocytes and other cells such as platelets, lymphocytes, neutrophils, hepatocytes, and kidney cells. When erythrocyte approaches its life span, band-3 protein is cleaved into new epitopes that provoke IgG autoantibody formation. The autoantibody binds to the aged cell and triggers its phagocytosis by macrophages in the spleen. Similar mechanism may be involved in the removal of other types of cells bearing band-3 protein.

4.2.2 Pathological Autoimmunity

A number of autoimmune diseases have been described in man and animals. However, the precise mechanism involved in the breakdown of the self-tolerance is hardly known for any of them. It is suggested that many different environmental, genetic, and immunological factors may contribute to the failure of development of tolerant T-cells to self-antigen. A variety of mechanisms has been proposed to account for T-cell-mediated generation of autoimmune diseases. Experimental evidences exist for some of them. It is likely that autoimmune diseases may result from interaction of a number of factors rather than only one factor.

4.2.2.1 Release of Sequestered or Hidden Antigens

Induction of self-tolerance in self-reactive T-cells is thought to be due to exposure of immature lymphocytes to the self-antigens and their subsequent clonal deletion during the embryonic development. Certain tissue antigens are placed in such a way that they are sequestered from the circulation and therefore are not encountered by the developing T-cells in the thymus. Such hidden antigens normally do not induce self-tolerance. However, when these antigens are revealed and exposed to mature T-cells, autoimmune response develops and cause tissue injuries. There are several examples of induction of autoimmune response against hidden antigens.

In the brain, myelin basic protein (MBP) is sequestered from the immune system by blood-brain barrier. Following accidental damage or damage caused by bacterial infection, MBP is released in the circulation. Autoimmune encephalitis develops after stimulation of non-tolerant T-cells. The disease can be produced experimentally by injection of MBP directly into the animal. Trauma to tissues may also expose certain antigens to the circulating T-lymphocytes. Most notable among these is the autoantibody production against sperm antigens. Spermatogenesis in the testes occurs long after the development of T-cells. Thus, self-tolerance does not develop against sperm antigen. During vasectomy some sperm antigens are released into the circulation, which provoke autoantibody production in some men. Similarly, the release of cardiac muscle protein from the heart during myocardial infarction and lens protein after eye damage has been shown to induce autoantibody formation. Hidden antigens are also found inside the cells. For example, chronic hepatitis in dogs causes the release of liver membrane protein against which autoantibody is formed. Diseases, such as tuberculosis and trypanosomiasis cause widespread tissue damage, and autoantibodies to various tissue antigens may be detected in the serum.

Recent experimental studies suggest that injection of normally hidden antigens in the thymus prevents the occurrence of tissue-specific autoimmune disease. For example, injection of MBP directly in the thymus prevents the development of autoimmune encephalitis in susceptible rats.

4.2.2.2 Antigens Generated by Molecular Changes

It has been observed that the appearance of new epitopes on the normal protein may cause autoantibody formation. There are two well-known autoimmune diseases where autoantibodies are generated in this way. These include production of rheumatoid factors (RFs) and immunoconglutinins (IK).

Rheumatoid factors are the autoantibodies, directed against the Fc portion of the immunoglobulin (IgG). In fact, following the binding of antibody to antigens, the complex is stabilized in such a way that new epitopes are exposed in the Fc portion. In the immune complex-mediated disease, such as rheumatoid arthritis and systemic lupus erythematosus (SLE), RFs are produced.

4.2 Mechanism of Induction

Autoantibodies directed against the complement component are called as immunoconglutinins. During activation of complement components such as C2 and C4 and particularly C5, new epitopes are formed on them, which stimulate IK production. Increased level of IK may be found in animals suffering from infectious diseases.

4.2.2.3 Molecular Mimicry

A variety of microorganisms and parasites have been shown to possess antigenic epitopes, which are similar to tissue components of the host. In such situation antibody or T-cell response mounted against the organism also reacts with the host tissue components and causes autoimmune disease. This phenomenon is known as a molecular mimicry and is fairly common. One of the best examples of this type of autoimmunity is the development of post-rabies vaccine encephalitis that occurs in some individuals after inoculation of rabies vaccine prepared from rabbit brain cell culture. Antibodies and activated T-cells to rabbit brain antigens cross-react with the recipient brain cells leading to encephalitis. In children, suffering from rheumatic arthritis, antibodies to cell wall M protein of *Streptococcus* spp. cross-react with cardiac myosin, producing heart disease.

Encephalitogenic MBP has been shown to be molecularly mimicked by proteins of several other organisms. The MBP peptides are highly homologous to P3 protein of measles virus. Homology of MBP peptides has also been reported with many of the animal viruses including adenovirus, influenza, polyoma, Rous sarcoma, poliomyelitis, Epstein-Barr, and hepatitis B viruses. Antibodies to certain antigens of *Trypanosoma cruzi* cross-react with nervous and cardiac tissues leading to nervous disorders and heart diseases. In mycoplasmal pneumonia in pigs, caused by *Mycoplasma hyopneumoniae*, and in cattle by *M. mycoides*, antibodies produced against these organisms react with lung tissue antigens. However, their role in the pathogenesis of the disease is not well known.

4.2.2.4 Inappropriate Expression of MHC Class II Molecules

The MHC class II molecules are generally expressed on antigen-presenting cells such as macrophages, which help in the presentation of processed antigen to T-cells. These molecules are normally not present on other cells. However, it has been observed that pancreatic beta cells of individual with insulin-dependent diabetes mellitus (IDDM) express a high level of MHC class I and II molecules. Similarly in autoimmune thyroiditis or Grave's disease (in human), thyroid acinar cells express MHC class II molecules on their surfaces. This inappropriate expression of class II MHC molecules may serve to sensitize T-helper cell to protein molecules derived from beta cells or thyroid cells.

It has also been shown that certain agents such as phytohemagglutinin (PHA) induce MHC class II expression in cells that normally do not express. IFN-γ also induces class II molecules on non-antigen-presenting cells. In such situation inappropriate T-helper cell activation may follow with autoimmune consequences. It is worth to mention that a high level of IFN-γ occurs in the serum of patients with SLE.

4.2.2.5 Virus-Induced Autoimmunity

The occurrences of virus infections in autoimmune diseases suggests that virus may induce autoimmunity. Reovirus infection of mice leads to the development of autoimmune diabetes mellitus. The infected mice reveal autoantibody against tissues such as pituitary, pancreas, gastric mucosa, glucagon, growth hormones, etc. Similarly, chronic infection of NZB mice with type C RNA virus stimulates the production of autoantibodies against nucleic acid and erythrocytes. Conclusive evidence, however, is not forthcoming regarding the association of the virus in spontaneously occurring autoimmune diseases in animals.

Type C retrovirus and *Paramyxovirus* have been isolated from dogs with SLE. In Sjogren's syndrome in humans, Epstein-Barr virus (EBV) gene has been demonstrated in the salivary gland. The onset of IDDM in children appears to be initiated by Coxsackie virus infection.

4.2.2.6 Genetic Factor

It has been generally accepted that genetic factor plays an important role in autoimmune diseases. Occurrence of some autoimmune diseases in humans and animals shows familial pattern, suggesting the involvement of genetic factor. No single gene has been identified as autoimmune gene. But genes determining the susceptibility to autoimmunity are generally located within MHC genes and the immunoglobulin genes that code for the major region of immunoglobulin molecules. Both these genes have a profound effect on the immunoresponsive capability of the host. In humans, it has been shown that almost all autoimmune diseases are associated with possession of certain MHC class II genes. Certain diseases such as diabetes mellitus, myasthenia gravis, and SLE may be linked with a combination of MHC genes (HLA-A1, B8, and DR3). In dogs, diabetes mellitus is associated with DLA-3, A7, A10, and DLA-B4; antinuclear antibodies with DLA-12; and SLE with DLA-A7, and autoimmune polyarthritis is associated with class III genes of C4.

4.2.2.7 Polyclonal B-Cell Activation

A mechanism by which autoantibody is produced by autoantigen-specific B-cells without the help from T-cell is known as polyclonal B-cell activation. A variety of viruses, bacteria, and substances such as lipopolysaccharides, proteolytic enzymes, and certain cytokines can induce widespread non-specific polyclonal B-cell activation. Gram-negative bacteria, cytomegalovirus, and Epstein-Barr virus are all known polyclonal activators that induce proliferation of numerous clones of B-cells expressing IgM without the help of T-cells. If autoantigen specific B-cells are activated by chance in this mechanism, autoantibodies will appear. In EBV-induced infectious mononucleosis, a variety of autoantibodies are produced against T- and B-cells and rheumatoid factor. Polyclonally activated lymphocytes from SLE patients produce a large quantity of IgM in culture.

4.2.2.8 Failure of Regulatory Control

The immune system functions in a controlled manner in the healthy animals. Autoimmune response occurs as a result of the failure of the normal control mechanism. Only triggering of autoimmune response is not necessary but it should sustain for occurrence of clinically obvious autoimmune disease.

If a mouse is inoculated with rat red blood cells, it produces antibody not only against rat cells but also against its own blood cells. This autoimmune response is however controlled by the mouse. If similar experiment is done in NZB mouse, where regulatory mechanism is impaired, autoantibody production is sustained, which causes significant red blood cell destruction resulting in severe anemia.

Certain autoimmune diseases have been found to be associated with lymphoid tumors. Myasthenia gravis, an autoimmune disease affecting the motor end plate of striated muscle, is commonly associated with thymoma. The incidence of rheumatoid arthritis increases four-fold in human patients with malignant lymphoid tumors.

Many of the lymphoid tumors result from the failure in immunological control mechanisms and it is possible that similar failure may occur in self-tolerance.

During developmental process, self-reactive lymphocytes are destroyed in the thymus by apoptosis initiated by the cell surface receptor CD95. It has been seen that defects in CD95 protein cause autoimmunity by preventing negative selection and permitting these cells to survive and cause disease.

4.2.3 Mechanisms of Tissue Injury

Tissue injuries in autoimmune diseases, irrespective of whether they are organ specific or generalized, are brought about by any or a combination of the three basic pathways. These include complement-mediated cell lysis (type II hypersensitivity), immune complex-mediated (type III hypersensitivity), and effector cell-mediated lysis (type IV hypersensitivity). Type I hypersensitivity plays a role only in the milk allergy.

4.2.3.1 Complement-Mediated Lysis (Type II Hypersensitivity)
Autoantibodies directed against normal or slightly altered cell surface antigens may cause target cell lysis either with the help of complement or cytotoxic cells. The binding of autoantibodies with the antigens on the cell surface results in the activation of the complement (C5–C9), which causes lysis of the cells. Autoantibodies directed against erythrocytes cause autoimmune hemolytic anemia and, against platelets, cause thrombocytopenia. Myasthenia gravis occurs as a result of complement-mediated lysis of acetylcholine receptors (Ach-R) following their binding with anti-Ach-R autoantibodies. Autoantibodies produced against thyroid-stimulating hormone (TSH) receptors stimulate thyroid response (hyperthyroidism) rather than mediate thyroid destruction. Complement fixation and activation also cause tissue injury and inflammation by recruiting inflammatory cells. Glomerular basement membrane disease (Goodpasture's syndrome) and bullous pemphigoid are examples of complement-mediated autoimmune reactions.

4.2.3.2 Immune Complex-Mediated Injuries (Type III Hypersensitivity)

Autoantibody and autoantigen bind together to generate immune complex which under appropriate condition may subsequently be deposited in the blood vessels usually at filtration sites. Glomerulus, synovium, and choroid plexus are prone to immune complex deposition, which causes complement activation, local inflammation, and tissue injuries. This is the principal mechanism involved in several autoimmune diseases such as glomerulonephritis, systemic lupus erythematosus, polyarthritis, vasculitis, etc.

4.2.3.3 Effector Cell-Mediated Lysis (Type IV Hypersensitivity)

The histological lesions in several autoimmune diseases show heavy infiltration with mononuclear cells and lymphocytes, suggesting their role in producing pathology. Specifically sensitized cytotoxic T-cells and their secretary products may cause the death of individual cells. Cytotoxic T-cells cause demyelination in experimental allergic encephalitis and multiple sclerosis. In insulin-dependent diabetes mellitus, destruction of beta cells of Langerhans is mediated by cell-mediated autoimmune response.

Cytokines also cause tissue damage in autoimmune diseases. Cytokines produced by Th cells such as IL-2 and IFN-γ will tend to promote cytotoxic effects and activated macrophages. IL-1 and TNF-alpha secreted by macrophages further add in the tissue damage by upregulating adhesion molecules to facilitate neutrophil emigration. If Th2 response is triggered, it will promote antibody production.

4.3 Autoimmune Diseases

4.3.1 Systemic Autoimmune Diseases

In the previous chapter, we have seen that a number of diseases occur due to autoimmune response directed to target antigen that is unique to a single organ or tissue and manifestations are largely confined to that organ. However, in systemic autoimmune diseases, the response is directed against a broad range of antigens found in the different organ systems. One of the most classical examples is the systemic lupus erythematosus (SLE), a devastating autoimmune disease of man and animal. Other examples of systemic autoimmune diseases are rheumatoid arthritis, canine dermatomyositis, Sjogren's syndrome, and vasculitides. The diseases reflect a generalized failure in immune regulation that results in the generation of autoreactive T-cells and B-cells. Tissue injury occurs in several organs as a result from cell-mediated immune response and from direct cellular damage caused by autoantibodies or accumulation of immune complexes.

4.3.1.1 Systemic Lupus Erythematosus (SLE)

The term lupus was originally used to describe horrible facial rash that affects patients. Systemic lupus erythematosus in man and animal results from the production of autoantibodies against a variety of antigens present in the host. Two types of autoantibodies are produced. The cell- or tissue-specific autoantibodies include those directed to red blood cells, platelets, and leukocytes. The cell- or tissue-non-specific autoantibodies are directed to nuclear antigens and hence caused widespread tissue damage. Canine SLE affects adult dogs without any gender bias. However, in few reports female dogs were found to be more susceptible to the disease.

Pathogenesis
The immunologic mechanism responsible for autoantibody production is poorly understood. However, three hypotheses can be considered to explain the induction of autoimmune response. Structural alteration in the self-antigen at molecular level, exposure of the sequestered antigen to host immune response, and more likely a fundamental defect in normal immunoregulation mechanism could be possible reasons for the initiation of the disease in genetically predisposed animal. Defects in immunoregulation mechanism may cause a decrease in the population of T suppressor (Ts) cells, which ultimately disturb the normal balance between Ts and Th cells. Certain B-cells may escape the immunoregulation step and cause uncontrolled production of autoantibody.

Autoantibodies thus produced cause tissue damage in the host through mechanism of type I, type II, and type III hypersensitivities.

Type I reactions are triggered by the binding of IgE autoantibody to the surface of mast cells and basophils. Cross-linking of IgE antibody by the autoantigen results in the release of vasoactive amines, which increase vascular permeability. This facilitates the deposition of antigen-antibody complex in the wall of blood vessels of glomerulus causing glomerulonephritis.

Autoantibodies produced against the cell surface antigens of erythrocytes and platelets mediate destruction of these cells by type II hypersensitivity reaction. The clinical consequences of these two types of antibodies are hemolytic anemia and thrombocytopenia.

A major part of the tissue damage caused by parenchymatous organs in SLE is type III hypersensitivity mediated. Antigen and antibody complexes are formed and deposited in the walls of blood vessels and basement membrane, which activate complement C3, and the release of soluble mediators leads to local inflammatory response and tissue injury. In SLE, autoantigens are nucleic acids and other nucleoproteins against which autoantibodies are directed. Thus, antinuclear antibodies (ANAs) are responsible for causing glomerulonephritis and generalized vasculitis. Though type IV hypersensitivity reaction does not appear to have any precise role, it may involve in the synergistic mechanism in the pathogenesis of SLE.

Autoantigens in SLE
Two types of autoantigens are found in animals with SLE (Table 4.1). Some cell- or tissue-specific antigens are found on the surface of certain cells such as erythrocytes, platelets, and leukocytes. Other antigens may be present in the secretory products of cell such as thyroglobulin.

Cell- or tissue-non-specific antigens are ubiquitous native molecules, which include nucleic acid, nucleoproteins, cytoplasmic organelles, and phospholipids.

Table 4.1 List of antigens against which autoantibodies are produced in SLE in dogs

A. Cell- or tissue-specific antigens
1. Erythrocytes (autoimmune hemolytic anemia)
2. Platelets (immune-mediated thrombocytopenia)
3. Granulocytes (neutropenia)
4. Lymphocytes (lymphopenia)
5. Thyroglobulin (thyroiditis)
6. Clotting factors (bleeding diathesis)
B. Cell- or tissue-non-specific antigens
1. Nuclear antigens including DNA and histones
2. Cytoplasmic antigens
3. Mitochondrial antigens
4. Microsomal antigen
5. Lysosomal antigen

These molecules can trigger autoantibody formation in SLE-affected animals. Out of these, antinuclear antibodies are the most important and considered as the hallmark of SLE, because when present in high titer, they are unique to this disease. About 16 different nuclear antigens have been described in humans. However, in dogs, autoantibodies develop against a restricted group of nuclear antigens that include mostly histones especially H1, H2A, H3, and H4. The presence of anti-DNA antibody in canine lupus is not yet settled. These ANAs can combine with free antigen to form immune complexes, which if deposited in glomeruli cause glomerulonephritis and if deposed in blood vessel wall cause vasculitis or in synovia to provoke arthritis. Autoantibodies are also produced against certain cytoplasmic antigens associated with mitochondria, microsomes, and lysosomes more commonly in human than in canine SLE.

Clinical Signs

Canine SLE patients may manifest clinical signs referable to single organ or cell type or multiple organ system. The disease tends to be progressive. The dog may become normal for a short period but usually followed by exacerbation of similar or additional clinical signs of illness.

In canine SLE, the most characteristic clinical sign is symmetrical non-erosive polyarthritis, characterized by shifting leg lameness and swollen painful joints. About 75% of dogs with SLE develop arthritis at some stage during the course of the disease. Other clinical signs observed in 20% to 50% of SLE-affected dogs are due to glomerulonephritis, peripheral lymphadenopathy, dermatologic disease, hemolytic anemia, thrombocytopenia purpura, and central nervous system disease. Other less commonly visible clinical features include polymyositis, pericarditis, thyroiditis, and leukopenia evidence by recurrent infections.

In equine SLE, generalized skin disease is spectacular, which may be accompanied by hemolytic anemia, glomerulonephritis, synovitis, and lymphadenopathy.

The SLE in cat has been rarely reported. It usually occurs as hemolytic anemia. Other clinical manifestations are fever, skin disease, thrombocytopenia, polyarthritis, and renal failure.

Diagnosis

Antinuclear Antibody (ANA) Tests
Demonstration of ANAs in the serum of patients is confirmative. Immunohistochemistry, latex agglutination, gel diffusion, ELISA, or radioimmunoassay may be used depending on the facility available in the laboratory. The most common test, however, is an indirect immunofluorescence assay, in which the serum of the animal is incubated with frozen section of rat liver, followed by the addition of anti-dog immunoglobulins conjugated with FITC. Different nuclear staining patterns have been described for humans. In animals, however, staining patterns have been less thoroughly investigated and their significance is yet to be assessed. The pattern may be diffuse homogenous, indicating autoantibodies to DNA histones. The rim pattern staining represents autoantibody to native dsDNA. The speckled staining pattern indicates autoantibody against extractable nuclear antigens. Nucleolar fluorescence may also be obtained that indicates autoantibody specificity to ribonucleoprotein.

LE Cell Test
Lupus erythematosus (LE) cell formation is an important event in SLE of humans and dogs, and its demonstration is considered diagnostic. Antinuclear antibody binds to the degenerated nuclei (opsonization), which stimulate its phagocytosis. Such phagocytic cells, containing opsonized nuclei, are called as LE cells and are usually found in the bone marrow and less commonly in the blood. The LE cell phenomenon can be demonstrated in vitro, which sometimes becomes necessary for diagnostic purposes. This can be carried out by allowing the blood from the affected animals to clot and then incubating it at 37 °C for 1–2 h. During this period polymorphonuclear cells will phagocytose the dying nuclei bound with ANAs. The clot is broken into a fine mesh and centrifuged and buffy coat smear is prepared, stained, and examined. The finding of several LE cells constitutes a positive test result.

Direct Immunofluorescence Test of Skin (Lupus Band Test)
In SLE, antibodies are also produced against skin components, which cause dermatitis. The lesions are characterized by the thickness of epidermis, focal mononuclear cell infiltration, collagen degeneration, and deposition of immunoglobulin along the basement membrane zone at the dermo-epidermal junction in the skin. This deposition is known as lupus band. Skin lesions occur frequently in human and canine SLE; hence, the demonstration of lupus band (deposition of immunoglobulin) by direct immunofluorescence test could be a valuable diagnostic test. However, this test is not specific for SLE, because similar fluorescence can be seen in other autoimmune skin disease such as bullous complex.

Due to a diversity of clinical manifestation, diagnosis of SLE is not easy. For the sake of proper and standard diagnosis, certain criteria have been fixed for humans

Table 4.2 Diagnostic criteria for canine SLE

Major clinical findings	Minor clinical findings	Serology
Polyarthritis (symmetric, non-erosive)	Fever of unknown origin	ANA demonstration
Polymyositis	Pleuritis	LE test
Glomerulonephritis (proteinuria)	Oral ulcers	
Bullous dermatitis	Depression/seizure	
Coombs positive hemolytic anemia	Myocarditis/pericarditis	
Immune-mediated thrombocytopenia	Peripheral lymphadenopathy	
Leucopenia		

and dogs. Gorman and Werner (1986) reported a scheme for the diagnosis of SLE in dogs, which is outlined in Table 4.2. Positive diagnosis should always include one major finding and positive serologic evidence. The presence of two major findings in the absence of demonstrable ANAs and LE cells also warrants SLE diagnosis.

Classic SLE
1. Two major findings and positive serology
2. One major and two minor findings and positive serology

Probably SLE
1. One major finding and positive serology
2. Two minor findings and positive serology

Discoid lupus erythematosus is a disease of dogs, cats, horses, and humans and considered a variant of SLE. Lesions are usually restricted to facial skin without the involvement of other organ systems. ANAs and LE cells are not detected. There is deposition of immunoglobulins (IgG, IgM, or IgA) and C3 component of the complement in the skin basement membrane. A typical lupus band is formed, which can be detected by direct immunofluorescence test. In dogs, nasal dermatitis is most common, which is morphologically characterized by depigmentation, erythema, erosion, ulceration, scaling, and crust formation. The lesions are exacerbated by sunlight. Hence, animals should be kept away from intense sunlight.

4.3.1.2 Sjogren's Syndrome
Sjogren's syndrome is the simultaneous occurrence of keratoconjunctivitis sicca (KCS), xerostomia, and rheumatoid factors in dogs. The disease is frequently reported in English bulldogs and West highland white terriers, which suggests a genetic predisposition for the disease. In this syndrome, keratoconjunctivitis and xerostomia occur as a result of autoimmune attack on the lacrimal gland and salivary gland, respectively. Clinically, there is dryness of conjunctiva and mouth. The syndrome is usually associated with SLE, rheumatoid arthritis, polymyositis, and autoimmune thyroiditis. Majority of dogs are hypergammaglobulinemic and 40–50% of them also show ANAs and RFs.

The KCS may occur alone in dogs and is regarded as the most common ophthalmic condition where lacrimal secretion is substantially reduced. The affected dog shows corneal dryness that results in abrasion and inflammation. Ocular discharge is mucoid or mucopurulent. The dog shows blepharitis and conjunctivitis, which may be secondarily infected with bacteria. This may lead to corneal ulceration and occasionally perforation in the absence of appropriate treatment. A case of KCS has been reported in horse with bilateral ulcerative keratoconjunctivitis.

4.3.1.3 Arthritides

Arthritis is the inflammation of joints and constitutes an important group of diseases of man and animals. Two major types of diseases have been identified; first, those associated with inflammatory lesions and the second associated with non-inflammatory lesions (degenerative, traumatic, and neoplastic). Inflammatory arthritides may be infectious or may be immunologically mediated. Most of the immunologically mediated arthritis occurs as a result of deposition of immunoglobulin or immune complex within joint tissues. Immunologically mediated arthritis may be further categorized into two: based on the inflammatory process leading to erosion and loss of articular cartilage. Rheumatoid arthritis is the best example of erosive arthritis. Non-erosive arthritis includes polyarthritis, plasmacytic-lymphocytic synovitis, arthritis associated with polyarteritis nodosa, etc.

4.3.1.4 Rheumatoid Arthritis

Rheumatoid arthritis is a bilaterally symmetric erosive polyarthritis and is most common of all immune-mediated arthritis. It is characterized by deposition of immune complexes within synovial tissue. It is a common crippling disease of humans and has also been reported in domestic animals particularly dogs. Although all breeds of dogs may be affected, small and toy breeds are frequently affected. Familial occurrence suggests genetic basis of the disease.

Pathogenesis

The pathogenesis of arthritis is very clear, but the mechanism of induction of immunologic defects still remains obscure. In this disease, autoantibody is produced against altered immunoglobulin. The autoantibody is called as rheumatoid factor, which is directed against Ch2 domain of antigen-bound IgG. Thus, rheumatoid factor is the pathogenic autoantibody that mediates the disease. Certain hypotheses that show normal IgG molecules become immunologically foreign have been considered.

These include steric configurational change in the IgG molecule after its binding to antigen and altered immunoregulation or both. Once the autoimmune process takes off, plasma cells and B-cells within the synovium and regional lymph nodes produce large quantities of RF, which may also appear in the circulation. Bacterial, mycoplasmal, and viral infections for possible initiation of configurational change in the IgG could not be convincingly demonstrated. The RF produced both locally and systemically is crucial to the development of disease and it initiates the process of disease by forming complex with the autologous IgG. The IgG in rheumatoid arthritis patients is less glycosylated than the normal IgG, which may possibly be responsible for autoantigenicity of the abnormal IgG. Rheumatoid factor, either IgG or IgM type, has a significant effect on the pathogenesis of the disease. RF complexed with IgG is smaller in size and escapes degradation by phagocytes. They are deposited in the synovium and activate complement. On the contrary, immune complexes of RF with IgM subclass being larger in size are vulnerable to phagocytosis and do not deposit in the synovium easily. Thus, immune complexes consisting of RF-IgM are less pathogenic.

Immune complex formation followed by complement fixation and activation results in two important events, i.e., inflammation and pannus formation. Inflammatory process begins as a result of the release of macrophage cytokines and a series of chemotactic, enzymatic, and vasoactive substances. The presence of C5a, leukotrienes B4, and platelet-activating factor (PAF) causes infiltration of large numbers of neutrophils within the synovial fluid. Proteases and free radicals are released from macrophages after phagocytosis of immune complexes. This, together with activated kinins and plasmin, leads to intense inflammation. The proteases released from neutrophils cause degradation of articular cartilage.

Other even more important event is the pannus formation in RA. It is characterized by intra-articular formation of granulation tissue, which emanates from inflamed synovium and invades articular cartilage. Hence, the pannus consists of inflammatory cells, synoviocytes, and fibronectin. Ingestion of RF-IgG immune complex by type A synoviocytes causes their activation and proliferation. Enzymes and mediators released from these synoviocytes and other cells such as lymphocytes, monocytes, and neutrophils cause the destruction of bones and cartilage. The IL-1-activated collagenases and peptidases released by synoviocytes cause resorption of endochondral bone and erosion of articular cartilage (erosive arthritis). Type A synoviocytes have all the characteristics of macrophages including Fc receptors and MHC class II molecules. Another important component of the pannus formation is the fibronectin, which stimulates fibroblast proliferation during the healing process of the rheumatoid lesions.

In RA patients, autoantibody to collagen is also detected. Studies have shown that type II collagen molecules are found hidden in the articular cartilage. They are exposed to circulating T-cells after removal of proteoglycans during the inflammatory process. Thus, autoantibody formed against collagen also participates in cartilage damage. Cell-mediated immunity also contributes in the pathogenesis of RA as agammaglobulinemic patient, devoid of RF, develops seronegative RA.

Clinical Signs

The affected dogs suffer from chronic, bilaterally symmetric, progressive erosive polyarthritis. Carpal-metacarpal and tarsal-metatarsal joints are most commonly affected. In addition, interphalangeal, stifle, elbow, and intervertebral junctions are also affected. The joints are swollen and painful with stiff gait. Dogs with RA develop depression, anorexia, and pyrexia, besides lameness, which tends to be severe after a long rest especially in the morning. RA is a progressive disease, which eventually leads to joint erosion and deformities. In advanced cases, bony ankylosis causes fusion of joints. Radiological examination, though variable, reveals swelling of soft tissues, subchondral rarefaction, cartilage erosion, and narrowing of the joint space.

Clinical Pathology
Hematological and serum biochemical analyses reveal only leukocytosis and polyclonal hyperglobulinemia. Increased protein content and neutrophil count and decreased C3 complement are observed on examination of synovial fluid, which is less viscous than normal.

Pathology
Apart from gross swelling and deformities seen clinically, on opening, joint capsule and periarticular tissue are thickened and fibrotic. Exuberant synovium protrudes in the joint space. The erosive lesions are most prominent towards the periphery of the joints and are associated with villous proliferation of the neighboring synovium. The articular cartilage shows red brown erosion and the pannus may be found adhered with it. Histological lesions in soft tissue include villous hypertrophy and hyperplasia of synovium, pannus formation, and periarticular fibrosis. Pannus consists of proliferating synoviocytes infiltrated with lymphocytes, plasma cells, and neutrophils. Pannus infiltrates from the surface of the articular cartilage and from beneath the subchondral bone. This infiltration produces a pincher effect in which microcavitation occurs as a result of fusion of erosive surface cartilage and lysed subchondral bone. In rheumatoid arthritis, early lesions are edema, congestion, and hemorrhage and deposition of fibrin are variably present. In advanced cases, lesions are usually fibrotic. Thus, most characteristic histological lesions in RA are the proliferative synovitis and pannus formation.

Diagnosis
The diagnosis of RA is usually carried out by characteristic clinical signs, radiological examination, and demonstration of RF in the serum of the affected animal. Mucin clot test, examination of the synovial biopsy, and histological section may also be used depending on the availability of the material. The demonstration of RF is performed by the agglutination test. The test uses particulate carrier on which isologous IgG is chemically adsorbed. In this test, isologous IgG is chemically bound to a particulate carrier, which may be latex beads or sheep red blood cells. This process exposes the Fc portion of IgG. If RF (anti-IgG) is present in the serum, it will agglutinate the particle, indicating a positive reaction. In the Rose-Waaler test, in place of latex beads sheep erythrocytes coated with canine anti-sheep red blood cell IgG are used as a source of antigen. This is the most sensitive and reliable method for detection of RF in canines.

Mucin clot test is an indirect test, which can be used as an aid in the diagnosis of RA. Normal synovial fluid contains mucin, which on addition of diluted glacial acetic acid causes the formation of firm rope like non-friable clot. The synovial fluid of RA patient lacks mucin, and hence on addition of glacial acetic acid, it does not form non-friable clot. Diagnosis of RA in canines sometimes presents a confusing

Table 4.3 Criteria for the diagnosis of canine rheumatoid arthritis[a]

1. Morning stiffness
2. Pain on motion
3. Soft tissue swelling
4. Swelling of at least one joint in a 3-month period
5. Symmetrical swelling with bilateral involvement of the same joint
6. Nodules in subcutaneous tissue
7. Characteristic radiographic findings
8. Positive rheumatoid test result
9. Characteristic synovial histology
10. Poor mucin precipitate from synovial fluid
11. Characteristic histologic findings of subcutaneous nodule

[a] Five of the 11 along with negative ANA and LE cell test results constitute a definitive diagnosis of rheumatoid arthritis in dogs

Table 4.4 Classification of immune-mediated hemolytic anemias

Class	Predominant antibody	Activity	Optimal temperature (° C)	Site of red cell removal	Clinical effect
I	IgG >> IgM	Agglutinin	37	Spleen	Intravascular agglutination
II	IgM	Hemolysin	37	Liver	Intravascular hemolysin
III	IgG	Incomplete	37	Spleen	Anemia
IV	IgM	Agglutinin	4	Liver	Cyanosis and infarction of extremities
V	IgM	Incomplete	4	Liver	Anemia

picture; hence, a list of criteria made for human patients is also used for the canine patients (Table 4.3). At least five of the major criteria should be present in the dog and at least one of the five should persist in the dog for 6 weeks. RA should be differentiated from other immune-mediated arthritis and infectious arthritis.

4.3.1.5 Organ-Specific Autoimmune Diseases

In this type of diseases, immune reaction is directed to antigens that are specific to a single organ or tissue. Hence, clinical manifestations are confined to that particular organ, which result from cellular damage by humoral or cell-mediated mechanism.

4.3.1.6 Autoimmune Hemolytic Anemia

Autoimmune hemolytic anemia (AIHA) is a serious hematologic disorder, characterized by the production of autoantibodies to erythrocyte antigens, which cause intravascular or extravascular destruction of erythrocytes (Table 4.4). The disease is well recognized in humans and dogs and has also been reported in cats, horses, cattle, mice, rabbits, and raccoons (Fig. 4.1).

4.3 Autoimmune Diseases

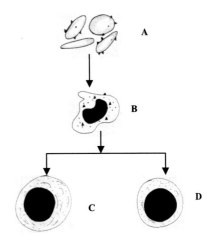

Fig. 4.1 Diagram showing autoimmunity. (**a**) RBC showing the presence of autoantigens. (**b**) Recognition of autoantigen by APC and their processing. (**c**) B-cells for antibody production. (**d**) T-cells for cytotoxicity

The occurrence of the disease more frequently in certain breeds of dog such as German shepherd, Irish setter, English sheepdog, and American cocker spaniel suggests a genetic predisposition. Middle-aged dogs (4–5 years) usually manifest the disease. Female dogs are affected 3–4 times more frequently than the males. AIHA is a distinct entity; hence, it may occur independently. But, it has been observed that about one third of the AIHA-affected dogs shows multiple immunologic disorders such as autoimmune thrombocytopenia, SLE, and lymphoid tumors. The disease is well characterized in dogs and has been classified in five classes (class I to class V) depending on the type of autoantibody produced, the thermal range for the optimal activity of the antibody, and the mechanism of hemolysis (Table 4.5). The characteristics of each type of anemia are necessary for proper diagnosis, prognosis, and treatment.

Pathogenesis

The underlying factors responsible for causation of AIHA are not well understood; however, it may involve two processes. Firstly, there may be alteration in the biochemical characteristics of the plasma membrane of erythrocyte, which is brought about by drugs, chemicals, viruses, and bacteria. These may alter the antigenicity of red cells evoking the production of antierythrocyte antibodies, which ultimately cause elimination of erythrocytes. Secondly, there may be defect in the normal immunoregulatory mechanism leading to loss of self-tolerance or to hyperactivity of the latent clones of B-cells. The antibody thus produced may cause destruction of erythrocytes in three ways including intravascular agglutination, intravascular hemolysis, and extravascular hemolysis.

In class I and IV AIHA, erythrocytes are agglutinated by autoantibodies, followed by their removal from the circulation by phagocytosis in the spleen and liver. High titer of IgG and/or low titer of IgM autoantibodies is required to initiate the process. Intravascular hemolysis does not occur because IgG is not a good activator of the complement. In class I AIHA, when a drop of the blood is placed on the slide at 37 °

Table 4.5 Comparative features of various classes of autoimmune hemolytic anemia

Class	Antibody type	Activity	Optimal temp. for activity (°C)	Site of erythrocyte destruction	Mechanism of erythrocyte destruction	Pathology
I	IgG (high titer)	Agglutinin	37	Extravascular (spleen)	Intravascular agglutination followed by phagocytosis	Hepatosplenomegaly, lymphadenopathy, hyperplastic bone marrow
II	IgM	Hemolysin (in vivo)	37	Intravascular	Intravascular hemolysis, i.e., complement mediated	Dark red urine, hemoglobinuric nephrosis
III	IgG	Incomplete agglutination	37	Extravascular	Phagocytosis	Splenomegaly
IV	IgM	Cold hemagglutinin	4	Extravascular	Intravascular agglutination followed by phagocytosis	Necrosis of extremities
V	IgM	Cold autoimmune incomplete or non-agglutinating	4	Intravascular	Intravascular hemolysis, i.e., complement mediated	Dark red urine, icterus

4.3 Autoimmune Diseases

C, it agglutinates. Intravascular agglutination in class IV AIHA differs from class I AIHA in that the IgM antibody mediates agglutination at 4–10 °C. Hence, it is also called as cold hemagglutinin disease. Thus, agglutination occurs in vivo in distal extremities after exposure to cold. Direct agglutination test is carried out at 4–10 °C at which clumping of erythrocytes occurs. Increasing the temperature can reverse this clumping. Anemia, acrocyanosis, and peripheral thrombosis are characteristic features of class IV AIHA.

The second major mechanism causing autoimmune destruction of erythrocytes is the intravascular hemolysis, which is complement mediated. This mechanism operates in AIHA classes II and V. Erythrolysis occurs as a result of binding of complement fixing antierythrocyte autoantibody to the circulating red cells. In this reaction, IgM predominates, because it is more efficient in complement fixing than IgG antibody. Activation of complements (C5 to C9) generates membrane attack complex leading to osmotic lysis. Massive intravascular hemolysis resulting in hemoglobinemia, hemoglobinuria, and icterus is a typical feature of class II AIHA. Positive direct antiglobulin test (DAT) at 37 °C along with prominent spherocytosis and reticulocytosis characterizes class II AIHA.

In class V AIHA, intravascular hemolysis is mediated by cold reactive agglutinating IgM autoantibody; hence, it does not occur at normal body temperature. Patients subjected to cold environment develop this type of anemia. Positive DAT occurs at 4 °C. In class III AIHA, erythrocytes are killed by another mechanism, i.e., extravascular hemolysis, which is accomplished by non-agglutinating and incomplete complement fixing IgG autoantibody. This is the most common type of anemia seen in dogs and cats. In this type of anemia, IgG autoantibodies are neither capable of completely agglutinating red blood cells nor fixing complement for erythrocyte destruction in the circulation. These opsonize erythrocytes for their phagocytosis at extravascular sites, i.e., spleen and liver. The complement is activated to only C3b level, which also opsonizes the red blood cells. Extravascular elimination of such opsonized red cells is accomplished by macrophages bearing Fc and C3b receptors in the spleen. Thus, splenomegaly is a significant finding in class III AIHA. Spherocytosis and reticulocytosis may occur depending on the severity of the anemia.

Clinical Signs
Clinical signs are consistent with anemia and vary from animal to animal. It includes weakness, pallor of mucous membrane, lethargy, and exercise intolerance. Fever, icterus, and peripheral lymphadenopathy may be additionally seen in some animals. Approximately one third of AIHA cases in dogs and cats are associated with other immunological disorders such as SLE, autoimmune thrombocytopenia (AITP), and lymphoid tumor. In such complicated cases, clinical signs referable to these ailments are also seen in the animals.

Clinical Pathology
Hematological changes include reduced packed cell volume, hemoglobin content, and total erythrocyte counts. Peripheral blood smear examination reveals

macrocytosis, reticulocytosis, and the presence of nucleated red blood cells, which are indicative of bone marrow regenerative response. Spherocytosis and anisocytosis are morphological abnormalities and are considered the hallmark of immune-mediated anemias. Their percentage counts are useful in making prognosis of the disease. A high percentage of spherocyte with low count of reticulocyte suggests a grave diagnosis. On the contrary, low spherocytes and high reticulocyte counts indicate a favorable prognosis.

Pathology
Pathological lesions depend on the type of hemolysis that has occurred. In intravascular hemolysis, pallor, icterus, and dark red kidneys are observed grossly. In extravascular hemolysis, gross lesions consist of hepatosplenomegaly, peripheral lymphadenopathy, and hyperplastic bone marrow. In anemia mediated by cold hemagglutinin, thrombosis and necrosis of extremities may be seen. Histological findings in intravascular hemolytic anemia are hemoglobinuric nephrosis, centrilobular fatty infiltration, and extramedullary hematopoiesis. Lesions in AIHA due to extravascular hemolysis are mainly confined to reticuloendothelial system. It consists of hyperplasia, hemosiderosis, and erythrophagocytosis. Organ-wise lesions are reticuloendothelial cell hyperplasia in the red pulp of the spleen, Kupffer cell hyperplasia in the liver, and histiocytosis in lymph nodes. Hemosiderosis is prominently seen in the liver, spleen, bone marrow, lymph nodes, and alveolar macrophages. In addition, myeloid and erythroid hyperplasia are also observed in the bone marrow.

Diagnosis
Characteristic clinico-pathological changes referable to anemia are observed. Blood smear examination shows spherocytes. Direct antiglobulin test (DAT) is done to confirm the diagnosis of class II, III, and V AIHA, where non-agglutinating or incomplete agglutination causing autoantibodies are present on the patient's erythrocytes. Erythrocytes are collected from the animal, washed, and incubated with Coombs reagent. The Coombs reagent is anti-canine IgG, IgM, and complement prepared in heterologous host. DAT is conducted at 4 °C and 37 °C to discriminate between different causes of anemia and to confirm the diagnosis.

Indirect antiglobulin test (IAT) allows detection of free circulating antierythrocyte antibodies in the blood of affected animals. Samples are collected and incubated with a panel of canine erythrocytes followed by addition of the Coombs reagent. This test is not considered reliable because of incomplete knowledge on the blood groups and the presence of isoantibodies in the serum of dogs. DAT positivity is also observed in hemolytic anemia caused by non-infections and infectious agents. This secondary immune-mediated hemolytic anemia should be differentiated from AIHA by acid elution test.

4.3.1.7 Autoimmune Thrombocytopenia
Autoimmune thrombocytopenia (AITP) occurs as a result of destruction of platelets and its precursor, the megakaryocytes by antiplatelet autoantibody. The disease has

been reported in cats, dogs, and horses. The first documented proof of AITP was given by Harrington et al. (1951) in which thrombocytopenic factor was found in the serum of human with clinical purpura. This factor agglutinated normal human platelets in vitro. AITP has been found commonly associated with AIHA, SLE, and rheumatoid arthritis. Other immune-mediated thrombocytopenia called the secondary immunopathic purpura is not caused by antiplatelet antibody.

Pathogenesis
Factors provoking antiplatelet autoantibody production are not precisely known. As for other autoimmune diseases, modification in the cell membrane antigens or loss of immunoregulation could be the possible factors. Irrespective of the initiating factors, the affected animal produces antiplatelet antibodies, which are mostly non-complement fixing IgG. It opsonizes platelets in the circulation and megakaryocytes in the bone marrow, which are rapidly eliminated by phagocytosis in the spleen. IgM or IgA antibodies are rarely involved in the process. Destruction of megakaryocytes results in reduced thrombopoiesis. A regenerative bone marrow response leads to a compensatory increase in thromboplastin level, which stimulates megakaryocytosis. Thus, mature and immature megakaryocytes may be seen in the affected animals.

Clinical Signs
The clinical signs in AITP are due to the inability of the animal to repair minor damage caused by capillaries during the course of normal hemostasis. Hence, the patient with AITP shows widespread petechiae on the mucous membrane and skin. Massive hemorrhage is not the feature of the disease but may occur. Epistaxis, hematuria, and hyphema are occasionally observed in the affected dogs. Though purpura of the external body surfaces is common, internal bleeding may occur. In dogs, gastrointestinal hemorrhage may be the cause of death.

Hematological examination reveals a precipitous drop in the platelet numbers ($<20,000/\mu l$) that induced purpura. In stained blood smear, platelets are very few and many of them are fragmented and immature. Aspirates from bone marrow show both mature and immature megakaryocytes without any significant reduction in their counts.

Pathology
The macroscopic lesions are characterized by the presence of petechiae and ecchymoses of the skin, mucosal surfaces, and internal organs. A severe trauma during the course of the disease causes extensive hemorrhages, which may be fatal. The spleen may be slightly enlarged. The bone marrow is apparently normal but shows characteristic changes on histology. The degree of hyperplasia of megakaryocytes depends on the length of illness. Immature megakaryocytes with bizarre hyperchromatic nuclei are frequently seen in the bone marrow. Vacuolated cytoplasm, karyolysis, and decreased cytoplasmic granularity are other morphological changes seen in the megakaryocytes.

Diagnosis

Tests commonly employed for the diagnosis of AITP in dogs and other animals are platelet factor-3 test (PF-3 test) and direct fluorescent antibody test. The PF test is performed by incubating animal's serum with normal isologous platelet-rich plasma. Antiplatelet antibody present in the serum will cause damage to the normal platelet resulting in the release of a phospholipid (PF-3, thromboplastin) in the test medium. The procoagulant property of the released PF-3 is assessed. PF-3 test can also be applied to secondary drug-induced ITP. In this case, positive test should come only after addition of the suspected drug.

Direct immuoflourescent antibody test is carried out on the bone marrow aspirate from the AITP-affected animal. Megakaryocytes coated with antiplatelet autoantibodies react positively when incubated with FITC-conjugated anti-species (anti-canine if the patient is a dog) immunoglobulin. The test is very specific, but not popular because of the invasive nature of the procedure.

4.3.1.8 Autoimmune Endocrine Diseases

Autoimmune diseases in animals usually involve single organ or tissue in comparison to humans where multiple endocrine glands are involved. Occasionally more than one endocrine gland may be involved in dogs.

Autoimmune Thyroiditis

Naturally occurring autoimmune thyroiditis has been reported in humans, dogs, and chickens. Antibodies to thyroglobulin antigens of the thyroid gland were demonstrated long back in the 1950s. It has now been established that there are several types of antigens found in the thyroid gland, against which antibodies are produced. These are thyroglobulin, microsomal antigen, colloidal antigen, a cell surface antigen, thyrotropin receptor, thyroxine, and triiodothyronine. Autoantibodies are formed against these antigens, which subsequently interfere with the synthesis of thyroid hormone.

The disease in dogs may occur either in asymptomatic form or in clinical form. The latter appears only when more than 75% of the thyroid gland is destroyed. The disease is more common in certain breeds of dog such as Great Dane, Doberman, golden retriever, cocker spaniel, etc. A strong genetic component appears to be involved in certain strain of beagle dogs and rats, and obese strain (OS) of chicken has a strong tendency to develop thyroiditis spontaneously.

The clinical signs in autoimmune thyroiditis in dogs are referable to hypothyroidism. The animal may be dull, depressed, fat, and inactive. Skin changes are conspicuous and are characterized by dry, dull, and coarse coat, hypotrichosis, hyperpigmentation, myxedema, and pyoderma. In addition, animals may be lethargic and may suffer from hyperlipidemia, hypothermia, and anestrous.

Histologically, thyroid glands are infiltrated with lymphocytes, plasma cells, and macrophages. These findings are more suggestive of cell-mediated than of antibody-mediated immunological reactions. The affected dogs exhibit delayed hypersensitivity to intradermally injected thyroid extract. It has also been proven experimentally that thyroid cells are killed by antibody-dependent cell-mediated cytotoxicity, which is responsible for the induction of pathologic changes in the thyroid. Immune complexes have also been found in the thyroid basement membrane in a few patients with thyroiditis.

Diagnosis of autoimmune thyroiditis includes the presence of characteristic lymphocytic infiltration in the thyroid biopsy and antithyroid autoantibody in the serum of the affected animals. An ELISA can also be used for the detection of autoantibodies to thyroid microsomal and colloid antigens.

Autoimmune Thyroiditis in Chickens
Autoimmune thyroiditis occurs naturally in the OS (obese strain) of white leghorn chickens. Among OS chickens, defects in three different types of genes seem to predispose the bird to the development of thyroiditis. One gene is linked to the MHC and is probably similar to the Ir genes of mouse. A second gene controls the maturation of the thymus, particularly the emigration of helper and suppressor T-cells. Finally, the third gene regulates thyroid function. Autoantibodies are directed against thyroglobulin and the affected birds show sign of hypothyroidism. Histologically, the thyroid tissue is heavily infiltrated with lymphocytes and plasma cells, which may organize to form follicles with germinal center. Birds affected with thyroiditis have been shown to produce antibodies against the adrenal gland, exocrine pancreas, and proventricular cells.

Insulin-Dependent Diabetes Mellitus
The human equivalent of insulin-dependent diabetes mellitus (IDDM) also occurs in dogs and rarely in other animals. The disease is associated with atrophy of the pancreatic islets and a complete loss of beta cells. In both humans and dogs, diabetes mellitus has a familial pattern of inheritance. In humans, a relationship between human leukocytic antigens (HLAs) and IDDM has been recognized. IDDM in humans is an autoimmune disease where autoantibodies are produced against an islet cell enzyme called glutamic acid decarboxylase. It is presumed that similar mechanism exists in IDDM of dogs also. The autoimmune attack causes destruction of beta cells, resulting in the decreased production of insulin and consequently increased blood glucose levels. There is insulitis in which a large number of T_{DTH} cells infiltrate the islet of Langerhans. A cell-mediated DTH develops as a result of the infiltration and activation of numerous macrophages. It is thought that beta cells are subsequently destroyed by cytokine released during the DTH response. The lytic enzymes of activated macrophages also add in the destruction of beta cells. IFN-γ, TNF-α, and IL-1 have been implicated in the destruction process. Autoantibody to beta cells can also mediate cell killing by complement-induced lysis or by antibody-dependent cell cytotoxicity (ADCC) mechanisms.

Addition's Disease (Autoimmune Adrenalitis)
Hypoadrenocorticism (adrenal insufficiency) or Addition's disease due to autoimmune destruction of the adrenal cortex has been reported in humans and dogs. Clinically affected animals show depression, weak pulse, abdominal pain, bradycardia, vomiting, diarrhea, and hypothermia. The animal may develop hypovolemia and

acidosis, which results in circulating shock and hyperkalemia. There is strong evidence of involvement of autoimmune process in the pathogenesis of the disease. Adrenal glands of affected man and dogs have shown infiltration with lymphocytes and plasma cells. In human patients, autoantibodies to cell surface and cytoplasmic antigens of adrenal cells have been demonstrated frequently. Cell-mediated immune response to adrenal antigen in human patients with Addition's disease suggests its role in the gland destruction. In the affected dogs circulating antibodies reactive with the cells of the adrenal cortex can be demonstrated by immunofluorescence test.

4.3.1.9 Autoimmune Dermatologic Diseases

Immune-mediated bullous disorders of skin are collectively called as the pemphigus or pemphigoid. This is basically a vesicle or blister formation in the skin.

The Pemphigus Complex

This includes four rare skin diseases that have been described in humans, dogs, horses, and cats. The most severe of these and first reported in a domestic species is pemphigus vulgaris. Other three forms, namely, pemphigus foliaceus, pemphigus vegetans, and pemphigus erythematosus, are variants and generally of less severe nature. All these variants can be differentiated by their histological appearance with regard to the site of vesicle formation.

In pemphigus vulgaris, bullae develop around mucocutaneous junctions such as nose, lips, eyes, prepuce, and anus. They also develop on the tongue and inner surface of the ear. The vesicles are fragile and rupture easily leaving weeping denuded areas that may be secondarily infected. Microscopical examination of an intact bulla reveals separation of the skin epithelial cells (acantholysis) in the lower epidermis. The acantholytic epidermal lesions result from autoantibody formation against a protein called desmoglein-3, which is an intercellular cement substance responsible for squamous cell adhesion. Though both pemphigus antibody (IgG) and complement have been demonstrated in the skin lesion by direct immunofluorescence method, experimental evidence exists that acantholytic dermal lesion can be produced without complement. The binding of antibody to desmoglein-3 provokes keratinocytes to secrete certain proteases such as plasminogen activator. This leads to the digestion of adhesion protein and separation of keratinocytes from each other. The epidermal detachment eventually leads to bullae formation, the location of which depends on the dissolution of specific adhesion protein involved.

Pemphigus foliaceus is a milder but more common disease than pemphigus vulgaris and has been reported in humans, cats, dogs, goats, and horses. In dogs, it occurs as scaling eruptive dermatitis. Autoantibody is formed against desmoglein-1, a protein found in the squamous cell desmosomes. On histological examination, vesicle formation occurs superficially in the subcorneal region.

Pemphigus erythematosus is a milder variant of bullous diseases and may be an early stage of pemphigus foliaceus. The lesions tend to be confined to the face and ear and appear similar to those of SLE. Other very rare and mild variant of pemphigus vulgaris is pemphigus vegetans. In this form, vesicles or pustules are formed and papillomatous proliferation of the base occurs on healing. The confirmatory diagnosis of pemphigus is achieved by examination of histological sections. Skin biopsy stained with fluorescein-conjugated anti-IgG or anti-C_3 reveals the deposition of immunoglobulin and complement in an intercellular pattern (chicken wire pattern) in the epidermis. It is important to differentiate between pemphigus vulgaris and pemphigus foliaceus from the prognosis point of view. Pemphigus vulgaris has grave prognosis.

Bullous Pemphigoid
It is a rare bullous skin disorder that resembles pemphigus vulgaris. It has been reported in humans, dogs, cats, and horses. Bullous pemphigoid is a self-limited blistering disease characterized by the formation of tense bullae under the subepidermal region. Bullae are filled with fibrin and leukocytes and develop mostly at mucocutaneous junctions and in the groin or axillae. In this disease, autoantibodies are directed against desmoplakin, a protein found in hemidesmosomes. The latter attach cells to the basement membrane of the skin. Direct immunofluorescence staining shows deposition of IgG at the dermal epidermal junctions (linear fluorescence) rather than an intercellular epidermal fluorescence seen in pemphigus vulgaris.

4.3.1.10 Autoimmune Neuromuscular Disorders
Immune-mediated muscle diseases are myasthenia gravis, polymyositis, and masticatory myopathy. While myasthenia gravis is a proven autoimmune disease, etiopathogenesis of others is yet to be established and needs more investigations.

Myasthenia Gravis
Myasthenia gravis (MG), an autoimmune disease of neuromuscular function, has been reported in humans, dogs, and cats. The disease is clinically characterized by skeletal muscle fatigue and weakness. Two types of disease have been recognized in dogs. The congenital form of the disease occurs in Jack Russell terrier, Springer spaniels, and fox terrier due to deficiency of autosomal recessive genes for acetylcholine receptor at the molar end plate. It is primarily a disease of young dogs. The acquired MG occurs in adult dogs in which autoantibodies are produced against cell surface receptors of acetylcholine present on the cytoplasmic membrane of the molar end plate. These autoantibodies prevent the neuromuscular transmission at the synaptic junction (Fig. 4.2).

Pathogenesis
Autoantibody to acetylcholine receptor (Ach-R) is the principal factor that mediates loss of motor function in MG. Several mechanisms have been proposed in the immunopathogenesis of this disease. The autoantibody cross binds the Ach-R, which prevents the activation of adenylate cyclase and normal muscle contraction. Cross-linkage of receptors by autoantibodies may also cause aggregation, internalization, and accelerated degradation of receptors, the rate of which is three times more than that normally seen. The physical binding of autoantibodies to Ach-R also blocks the access of acetylcholine to its receptor and thus inhibiting the physiologic

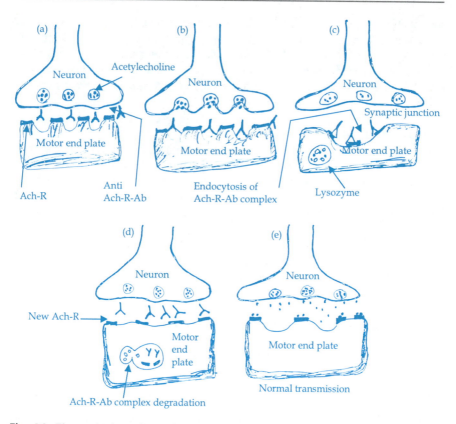

Fig. 4.2 The mechanism of myasthenia gravis: (**a**) anti-Ach-R autoantibody present in the myoneural junction, (**b**) anti-receptor antibody that blocks the Ach-R and prevents transmission, (**c**) endocytosis of Ach-R antibody complex, (**d**) internalization and degradation of the complex and appearance of new Ach-R, and (**e**) normal neuromuscular transmission

effect of the neurotransmitter at the motor end plate. This mechanism, however, is reported to have only a minor role in the decreased motor function. It has also been suggested that the affected muscle fibers may reveal decreased synthesis of new receptors, which may be seen in chronically sick dogs. The binding of autoantibody may also trigger complement-mediated destruction of Ach-R.

Occurrence of thymic diseases such as thymitis, thymic follicular hyperplasia, thymoma, etc., in more than 75% of human patients with MG, suggests the critical role of thymus in the causation of the disease. In normal neuromuscular transmission, Ach binding to its receptors results in the generation of localized end plate potential, which if sufficient will generate an action potential that causes muscle contraction. In MG, the release of Ach is normal but an insufficient generation of action potential at the end plate fails to cause a contraction of muscle fibers, resulting into muscle weakness. Repeated stimulus causes a progressive increase in the muscle weakness. After some time, the reduced release of Ach coupled with reduced availability of receptors causes the progressive loss of the muscle function.

Clinical Signs
The affected animals show progressive weakness and fatigue of skeletal muscles that increase in severity with exercise. The muscle strength is regained after rest. Initial clinical signs develop insidiously or suddenly and generally involved muscles, which are in continuous use such as muscle of eyelids, tongue, pharynx, etc. Consequently, animals show drooping of eyelids, sluggish movement of tongue (dysphagia), difficulty in swallowing, and choking. As the disease advances, other muscles are affected leading to generalized muscular weakness. There is no change in the hemoglobin and serum biochemicals. Even enzymes specific to muscle are normal throughout the course of the disease.

Pathology
No gross lesion is found as MG is considered more a functional than structural disorder. However, some lesions may be present that result from complication of MG. Thus, dogs may show aspirated bronchopneumonia and ingesta-filled esophagus (megaesophagus) at necropsy. Thymoma may be present. Histological examination of the affected muscle shows minimum non-inflammatory lesions, which consist of focally infiltrated lymphocytes, myofiber atrophy, and scattered necrotic foci in the skeletal muscle. However, these lesions are not consistent. Ultrastructural changes are specific and consistent with the pathogenesis of the disease. Degeneration and formation of secondary cleft and significant reduction in the number of Ach-R on the cytoplasmic membrane are observed. The remaining Ach-Rs of myocytes are complexed with immunoglobulins.

Diagnosis
The principle of diagnosis is based on the demonstration of progressive decline in the action potential of the skeletal muscle after exercise. This can be achieved by electromyographic analysis and pharmacologic test (Tensilon test) involving the administration of anticholinesterase drugs. Tensilon test is the most important test for diagnosing muscle diseases. In this test, following administration of anticholinesterase agent such as edrophonium chloride (Tensilon), patient regained the muscle strength quickly. The improved tone of the muscle does not last long and that depends on whether the agent is short or long acting. Electromyography in response to repetitive nerve stimulation shows progressive decline in the muscle action potential. The result of the Tensilon test and electromyography confirms the diagnosis of MG. Serological test includes the demonstration of anti-Ach-R antibody by radioimmunoassay. Autoantibody to Ach-R can also be detected by indirect immunofluorescence test where the serum of myasthenic dog reacts with the frozen section of normal canine skeletal muscle. Fluorescence of cross-striated bands indicates a positive test result.

Polymyositis

It is a generalized inflammatory myositis of large breeds of dogs of both sexes. The etiopathogenesis of the condition is poorly understood. The disease has been commonly reported in German shepherds. Clinical signs appear acutely or develop progressively. Dogs exhibit progressive weakness of muscles of the head, trunk, and limbs, which is not associated with the exercise. Laryngeal muscle weakness may cause change in the voice of the dog. Other clinical signs include dysphagia, weakness of facial muscles, pain on palpation, shifting-leg lameness, and megaesophagus. Examination of blood reveals leukocytosis and eosinophilia. Serum biochemical analysis shows elevated levels of alanine aminotransferase (ALT), aspartate aminotransferase (AST), lactate dehydrogenase, and aldolase due to muscle damage. These findings differentiate polymyositis from myasthenia gravis. Histological findings on collected multiple biopsies of muscles consist of vacuolation, degeneration, and focal to diffuse necrosis. The affected muscle shows infiltration with lymphocytes and plasma cells.

Presently, specific immunological test is not available for diagnosis. The disease is confirmed by muscle biopsy examination. Electromyography of the affected muscle may be used to analyze the extent of muscle damage. Antinuclear antibody (ANA) and/or antisarcolemmal antibody has been demonstrated by immunofluorescence test in about 50% of the affected dogs. The significance of ANA and at times occurrence of polymyositis as one of the components of SLE are not precisely understood. The treatment of canine polymyositis is currently achieved by administration of corticosteroids.

Autoimmune Masticatory Myopathy

Masticatory myopathy refers to the disease involving muscles associated with mastication and is the most common type of myositis reported in dogs. The muscles include masseter, temporalis, and pterygoid. On the basis of clinico-pathological findings, two forms of the disease have been identified: an acute eosinophilic type and a chronic atrophic type. Though these forms appear to be distinct, most consider them to be the two stages of the same disease. Some evidence suggests that the disease is immunologically mediated.

Eosinophilic myositis is a serious clinical disorder primarily affecting young adult German shepherd and Doberman pinscher. Occasionally, it also occurs in other breeds. The affected dogs exhibit firm, swollen, and painful masseter, temporalis, and pterygoid muscles, which are manifested by difficulty in opening and closing of jaw. During acute pain, dog may show jaw partially open or signs of lockjaw (trismus).

Examination of peripheral blood reveals moderate leukocytosis and significant eosinophilia that may reach up to 70% of the circulating leukocytes.

The etiopathogenesis of disease is yet to be elucidated. Lesions confining only to masticatory muscles suggest that these muscles may be different from other skeletal muscle. They are derived from cranial mesoderm rather than myotomes and contain unique myofibrillar proteins. Recently, autoantibodies have been demonstrated against four myofibrillar proteins. However, this finding is not sufficient for accepting autoimmune basis of the disease.

Grossly, the acutely inflamed muscles are firm and red and show streaks of hemorrhage. Histopathological examination of the affected muscle shows degeneration, necrosis, and infiltration with eosinophils, lymphocyte, and plasma cells.

In atrophic myositis, masticatory muscles exhibit fibrous atrophy. The condition has been reported in all ages of dogs. The affected dog does not evince pain and exhibits sunken eyes and trismus. Several investigators believe that it is the chronic form of eosinophilic myositis. Histopathological examination of biopsy material reveals increased perimysial connective tissue, focal myodegeneration, and lymphocytic infiltration. The disease can be diagnosed by clinical signs emanating from the involvement of masticatory muscles and histological examination of affected muscles.

4.3.2 Autoimmune Ocular Disease

4.3.2.1 Periodic Ophthalmia

Equine periodic ophthalmia or recurrent uveitis is a common disease in horses and occurs as a result of recurrent autoimmune attacks of ocular tissues.

It has been shown that some of the corneal antigens are molecularly mimicked by antigenic epitopes of *Leptospira interrogans*. Therefore, horses in *Leptospira* infection or immunization by killed *L. interrogans* produce antibody, which cross-reacts with the corneal antigens. Antigen-antibody complex activates complement and leads to the development of corneal opacity. The affected animals show high titer of antibody to *L. interrogans*. Acutely affected horses show blepharospasm, lacrimation, and photophobia. The severity of the disease increases with each attack and involves the iris and other tissues in the eyes. Recurrent attacks may cause some horses to become blind. The iris and ciliary body are infiltrated with lymphocytes and neutrophils with extensive fibrin and C_3 deposition. Horses infected with other related bacteria, i.e., *Borrelia burgdorferi*, or with nematode *Onchocerca cervicalis* have also been shown to suffer from periodic ophthalmia, suggesting antigenic relatedness of these organisms with the cornea.

References

Coombs RRA, Mourant AE, Race RR (1945) A new test for the detection of weak and incomplete Rh agglutinin. Br J Exp Pathol 26:255

Gorman NT, Werner LL (1986) Immune-mediated diseases of the dog and cat. I. Basic concept on the systemic immune-mediated diseases. Br Vet J 142:395

Harrington WJ, Minnich V, Hollingsworth JW, Moore CV (1951) Demonstration of a thrombocytopenic factor in the blood of patients with thrombocytopenia purpura. J Lab Clin Med 38:1–10

Further Reading

Bennett D (1987) Immune based non-erosive inflammatory joint disease in the dog. 3. Canine idiopathic polyarthritis. J Small Anim Pract 28:909–928

Charron D (1990) Molecular basis of human leukocyte antigen class II disease associations. Adv Immunol 48:107–159

Drachman DB (1994) Myasthenia gravis. N Engl J Med 330:1797–1809

Fauci AS (1980) Immunoregulation in autoimmunity. J Allergy Clin Immunol 66:5–17

Geor RJ, Clark EG, Haines DM, Napier PG (1990) Systemic Iupus erythematous in a filly. J Am Veter Med Assoc 197:1492–1498

Gilmour MA, Morgan RV, Moore FM (1992) Masticatory myopathy in the dog: a retrospective study of 18 cases. J Am Anim Hospit Assoc 28:300–306

Gosselin SJ, Capen CC, Martin SL, Krakowka S (1982) Autoimmune lymphocytic thyroiditis in dogs. Vet Immunol Immunopathol 3:185–201

Grindem CB, Johnson KH (1983) Systemic lupus erythematosus: literature review and report of 42 new canine cases. J Am Anim Hosp Assoc 19:489–503

Harris ED (1990) Rheumatoid arthritis: pathophysiology and implications for therapy. N Engl J Med 322:1277–1289

Hoenig M, Dawe DL (1992) A qualitative assay for beta cell antibodies. Preliminary results in dogs with diabetes mellitus. Vet Immunol Immunopathol 32:195–203

Ibrke PJ, Stannard AA, Ardans AA, Griffin CE (1985) Pemphigus foliaceus in dogs: a review of 37 cases. J Am Veter Med Assoc 186:59–66

Indrieri RJ, Creighton SR, Lambert EH, Lennon VA (1983) Myasthenia gravis in two cats. J Am Veter Med Asso. 182:57–60

Janeway C (1982) Beneficial autoimmunity. Nature 299:396–397

Kaswan RL, Salisbury MA (1988) Canine keratoconjunctivitis sicca: etiology, clinical signs, diagnosis and treatment. Part II. Diagnosis and treatment with cyclosporine. J Veter Aller Clin Immunol 2:8–12

Kennedy RL, Thoday KL (1988) Autoantibodies in feline hyperthyroidism. Res Vet Sci 45:300–306

Kuby J (1997) Autoimmunity. In: Immunology. W.H. Freeman and Company, New York, pp 485–505

Levis RM (1972) Animal model of human disease: systemic lupus erythematosus. Am J Pathol 69:537

Levis RM, Picut CA (1989) Veterinary clinical immunology, from classroom to clinics. Lea and Febiger

Madison JB, Scarratt WK (1988) Immune-mediated polysynovitis in four foals. J Am Veter Med Assoc 192:1581–1584

May C, Hughes DE, Carter SD, Bennett D (1992) Lymphocyte populations in the synovial membranes in dogs with rheumatoid arthritis. Vet Immunol Immunopathol 31:289–300

McVey DS, Shuman WS (1989) Detection of antiplatelet immunoglobulin in thrombocytopenic dogs. Vet Immunol Immunopathol 22:101–112

Monestier M, Novick KE, Karam ET et al (1995) Autoantibodies to histone, DNA and nucleosome antigens in canine systemic lupus erythematous. Clin Exp Immunol 99:37–41

Parma AE, Santisteban CG, Villalba JS, Bowden RA (1985) Experimental demonstration of an antigenic relationship between Leptospira and equine cornea. Vet Immunol Immunopathol 10:215–224

Schwartz RS (1993) Autoimmunity and autoimmune diseases. In: Paul WE (ed) Fundamental Immunology. Raven Press, New York, pp 1033–1150

Schwartz RS (1982) Viruses and systemic lupus erythematosus. N Engl J Med. 307:1499–1507

Scott DW, Walton DK, Manning TO, Smith CA, Lewis RM (1983) Canine lupus erythematosus. I. Systemic lupus erythematous. J Am Anim Hosp Assoc 19:461–479

Shoenfeld Y, Schwartz RS (1984) Immunologic and genetic factors in autoimmune diseases. N Engl J Med 311:1015–1029

Sinha AA, Lopez MT, McDevitt HO (1990) Autoimmune disease: the failure of self-tolerance. Science 248:1380–1386

Stanley JR (1995) Autoantibodies against adhesion molecules and structures in blistering skin disease. J Experim Med 181:1–4

Taniyama H, Shirakawa T, Furuoka H (1993) Spontaneous diabetes mellitus in young cattle. Histologic, immunohistochemical and electron microscopic studies of the islets of langerhans. Vet Pathol 30:46–54

Trogdon-Hines M (1984) Immunologically mediated ocular disease in the horse. Veter Clin North Am Large Anim Pract 6-3:501–512

Immunodeficiency 5

Key Points

1. Immunodeficiency in animals can be broadly classified into congenital (primary) and acquired (secondary) immunodeficiencies.
2. Congenital or primary immunodeficiency is the defect in immunity, which is genetically determined and present in animals, since their birth.
3. Severe combined immunodeficiency syndrome occurs in animals due to inherited gene defect. The syndrome is characterized by recurrent infection since birth, agammaglobulinemia, and absence of T- and B-lymphocytes.
4. In Chediak-Higashi syndrome, phagocytic cells contain large granules and chemotaxis, and phagocytosis and killing of bacteria are abnormal due to defective assembly of cytoplasmic microtubules responsible for degranulation and release of lysosomal enzymes.
5. Pelger-Huet anomaly is characterized by failure of neutrophilic nuclei to segment into lobes, and the nucleus remains rounded just like immature cells.
6. Acquired or secondary immunodeficiency may occur as a result of the suppression of the immune system due to drugs, diseases, deficiency of nutrition, neoplasm, or environmental pollution, which is clinically manifested by increased susceptibility to infectious diseases.
7. Acquired immunodeficiency is more common than congenital immunodeficiency.
8. Many infectious agents are known to cause immunosuppression in animals and poultry like bovine immunodeficiency virus, bovine viral diarrhea virus, feline leukemia virus, infectious bursal disease virus, feline immunodeficiency virus, feline leukemia virus, feline panleukopenia virus, simian immunodeficiency virus, bovine herpesvirus-1, canine distemper virus, and bluetongue virus.
9. Diagnosis of immunodeficiency diseases can be made by detection of immune responses against any kind of antigen or non-specifically by measuring gamma globulins and antibody levels in the serum.

5.1 Immunodeficiency

The struggle for existence is the law of nature, and acquisition of the efficient weaponry paves the way for the survival of the fittest. The immune system is one of the most complex, ubiquitous, sensitive, and specific arsenal acquired by living creatures to sustain the onslaughts of the physical, chemical, biological, and environmental adversities. The alterations which decrease the effectiveness or destroy the capabilities of the system to respond to various antigens, are collectively designated as immunodeficiency disorders. The prevalence of the immunodeficiencies varies extensively according to the type of disease, and some of such diseases are rare in occurrence. During the last few years, it has been observed that in spite of good management practices, various infectious diseases raise their ugly heads even after the implementation of proper vaccination schedule. This precarious situation may be attributed to poorly developed immunocompetence or depressed immune system as a result of environmental factors, genetic defects, drugs, infections, environmental pollution, etc. The immunodeficiencies in animals can be broadly classified into congenital (primary) and acquired (secondary) immunodeficiencies.

5.1.1 Congenital Immunodeficiency

In this type of immunodeficiency, the defect in immunity is genetically determined and is present in animals since their birth. It is also known as primary immunodeficiency. The congenital immunodeficiency is very rare in animals and has been reported due to defect in basic cellular components at the time of development. Although the exact cause of such defects is not fully understood, such alterations are expected due to defective genes. These defects may occur during differentiation and maturation of bone marrow elements derived from stem cells and are clinically characterized by the symptoms related to the affected cell line and the stage of differentiation at the time of expression of cellular defects. The congenital immunodeficiency diseases are recognized early in life by the appearance of recurrent infections, increased susceptibility to even mild pathogens, poor response to treatment, and occurrence of systemic diseases after vaccination with live attenuated vaccines. Most of the immunodeficiency problems are species or breed specific, and it is very difficult to treat them at later stages. Since these problems are not curable, an early diagnosis helps in segregation and elimination of the animal from the herd. The various types of congenital immunodeficiencies are described as follows:

5.1.1.1 Severe Combined Immunodeficiency Syndrome

The combined immunodeficiency syndrome occurs in animals due to inherited gene defect. In this syndrome, the stem cells are absent or unable to differentiate into T- and B-lymphocytes. The syndrome is characterized by recurrent infection since birth, agammaglobulinemia, and absence of T- and B-lymphocytes and has been reported in Arabian foals.

The combined immunodeficiency syndrome occurs due to an autosomal recessive gene causing abnormal purine metabolism, and about 3 percent of all Arabian foals die due to this syndrome before attaining the age of 5–6 months. The absence of adenosine deaminase and purine nucleoside phosphorylase leads to accumulation of adenosine nucleotides, which are toxic to lymphocytes. The defective development of T- and B-lymphocytes leads to lymphoid hypoplasia in the thymus, spleen, and lymph nodes causing agammaglobulinemia and lymphopenia. The other cells in the blood, e.g., erythrocytes, neutrophils, and monocytes, are normal. Death occurs due to recurrent infection, such as *Pneumocystis carinii* and adenovirus infection, within 4–6 months.

In dogs, a similar syndrome characterized by hypoplasia of the thymus, lymph nodes, and spleen occurs due to combined immunodeficiency. The occurrence of listeriosis in an Arabian foal has also been reported due to combined immunodeficiency. Affected foals do not have functional T- or B-lymphocytes and have very low circulating lymphocyte count. The maternal antibodies are catabolized within 2–4 months, and then foals begin to fall sick in the absence of antibodies. Severe bronchopneumonia with adenovirus and *Rhodococcus equi* infection is the predominant finding on postmortem examination. The spleen of such foals is hypoplastic and lacks in germinal centers and periarteriolar lymphoid cells. The lymph nodes also show lack of lymphoid follicles and germinal centers with the depletion of lymphoid cells in the paracortex region. There is hypoplasia of the thymus.

5.1.1.2 Defects in T-Lymphocytes

In animals, three types of syndromes occur due to T-cell defects, which are associated with production or maturation of the cells.

1. Thymic hypoplasia occurs in pups and leads to defective T-cell function with normal B-cells and adequate levels of immunoglobulins in the serum. The pups have increased susceptibility to various infections, and death occurs within a few weeks of life. A similar syndrome, "DiGeorge" syndrome, occurs in man due to failure of development of the third and fourth pharyngeal pouches leading to aplasia of the thymus.
2. In black pied Danish cattle, exanthema, alopecia, crusting, and parakeratosis occur due to T-cell defects as a result of lethal trait A-46. The affected calves are susceptible to various viral, bacterial, and fungal infections. Death occurs within 4 months of age. A similar syndrome has also been reported in Holstein calves. The clinical features are lymphopenia, deficiency of zinc, and normal level of immunoglobulins in the serum. On necropsy, the hypoplasia of the thymus and T-dependent regions of the lymph nodes, spleen, and gut-associated lymphoid tissue (GALT) have been observed. These animals are deficient in T-cells and have depressed cell-mediated immunity with normal antibody titers.

3. A third syndrome due to T-cell defect occurs in dogs as a result of lethal trait A-46. This is also known as "lethal acrodermatitis" and is characterized by hypoplasia of T-dependent lymphoid tissue and normal level of immunoglobulins in the serum. The affected animal does not show any deficiency of zinc and die within a few months.

5.1.1.3 Defects in B-Lymphocytes

The primary immunodeficiency due to B-cell defect occurs in equines and is known as "equine agammaglobulinemia." This is characterized by normal count of T-cells, absence of B-cells, and absence of all classes and subclasses of immunoglobulins. This defect is thought to be due to "X" linked, as it mostly occurs in males. The pathological investigations revealed the absence of primary lymphoid follicles and germinal centers in the spleen and lymph nodes. The main defect is considered to be the maturation arrest in B-precursor cells. The absence of plasma cells in the lymph nodes and spleen can be demonstrated. However, such animals possess circulating lymphocytes in the blood, which show reaction to phytohemagglutinin and produce migration inhibitory factor. Type IV hypersensitivity reaction is unaffected in animals, indicating intact cell-mediated immunity. Such foals can survive up to 1.5 years and show high rate of recurrent bacterial infections and absence of B-lymphocytes.

Selective IgA deficiency has been recorded in dogs, which is characterized by recurrent dermatitis and respiratory disease. The IgA deficiency predisposes the mucosa of respiratory and gastrointestinal tract for bacterial and viral infections. It is mainly due to maturation arrest from B-cells to IgA-secreting plasma cells. The serum level of IgA is absent, while that of IgM and IgG is normal. The deficiency of IgA is associated with the presence of rheumatoid factor in the serum of dogs. Such dogs are unusually susceptible to chronic small intestinal disorders caused by *Microsporum canis*.

Selective IgM deficiency is characterized by very low levels of serum IgM and presence of recurrent respiratory and joint infections in Arabian horses. The clinical manifestations appear at about 1–2 months of age, and both sexes of foals do suffer from IgM deficiency. The foals suffer from septicemia caused by *Klebsiella pneumoniae* or *Rhodococcus equi*. Except the low IgM levels, all other immune responses are normal.

IgG deficiency has been reported in the Danish red cattle, and clinically, it is characterized by increased susceptibility to pyogenic infections, gangrenous mastitis, bronchopneumonia, and peritonitis. A case with extremely low IgG level was also reported in the foal which had normal IgA and IgM levels but absence of germinal centers, lymphoid follicles, and periarteriolar lymphoid sheath. The diagnosis can be made by quantitative radial immunodiffusion test to demonstrate the missing isotype of antibody.

Transient hypogammaglobulinemia in newborns occurs at 4–6 months of age. The maternal immunoglobulins are catabolized slowly, and the levels of these antibodies fall down drastically. The production of immunoglobulins from neonatal lymphoid tissue is delayed, resulting into low levels of immunoglobulins in the blood of patients. Normally, the production of immunoglobulins starts at 4–6 months of age. This condition has been reported in lambs, foals, and dogs. During the period of transient hypogammaglobulinemia, the neonate is susceptible to various opportunistic bacterial and viral infections. As the normal production of immunoglobulins resumes, this condition disappears.

5.1.1.4 Partial Defects in T- and B-Lymphocytes

Partial maturational defects in T- and B-lymphocytes are characterized by the presence of recurrent infections, eczema, and purpura. This condition is considered to be "X" chromosome linked. The eczematous condition occurs due to increased level of IgE in the blood with low IgG level. The purpura is often associated with poor platelet aggregation and thrombocytopenia. It can be cured through bone marrow transplantation from a suitable donor.

5.1.1.5 Deficiency of Complement

The congenital deficiency of complement is very rare in animals. However, the deficient complement components are associated with abnormal regulation of immunological responses leading to autoimmunity. The complement components C1, C2, and C4 are deficient and are usually associated with systemic lupus erythematosus, polyarteritis nodosa, glomerulonephritis, and rheumatoid arthritis. The deficiency of complement components C5, C6, C7, and C8 may lead to the occurrence of recurrent infections. The absence of deficiency of C3 component is usually found to be associated with increased susceptibility to bacterial infections. It has been reported in spaniel dogs and is transmitted as an autosomal recessive gene. The level of C3 becomes as low as 10% of the normal value and is usually associated with bacterial infections due to lack of complement-mediated opsonization, chemotaxis, and phagocytosis.

5.1.1.6 Defects in Phagocytosis

It includes defects in neutrophils, monocytes, platelets, melanocytes, and eosinophils. The defective phagocytic disorders are usually characterized by neutropenia or defective neutrophil function with regard to chemotaxis, phagocytosis, and bactericidal activity leading to persistent pyogenic bacterial infections. The cyclic leukopenia is the most sensitive indicator of maturational arrest of granulopoiesis and is of diagnostic significance. Such neutrophils also exhibit ineffective bactericidal activity. The other defects in neutrophils, platelets, melanocytes, and renal tubular epithelium are associated with autosomal recessive defect and are designated as "Chediak-Higashi syndrome." In this syndrome, the phagocytic cells contain large granules stainable by peroxidase. Chemotaxis, phagocytosis, and killing of bacteria are abnormal and associated with defective assembly of cytoplasmic microtubules responsible for degranulation and release of lysosomal enzymes. The depression of superoxide anions, an indication of defective respiratory burst, has been detected through nitroblue tetrazolium (NBT) reduction test in dogs with persistent bacterial infections. Transient neutropenia may be observed in neonates of animals characterized by reduced chemotaxis and impaired phagocytosis by neutrophils. This is of shorter duration and has little clinical significance.

Chediak-Higashi syndrome is an inherited disease of cattle and is associated with dilution of hair pigmentation, ocular abnormalities, and increased susceptibility. This may be diagnosed either by examination of blood smear for the presence of large granules within phagocytic cells or by examining hair shafts for enlarged melanin granules. The enlarged neutrophil granules result from fusion of primary and secondary granules, while in monocytes and eosinophils, these are formed due to the presence of large abnormal lysosomes. The large granules of these phagocytic cells are more fragile and liable to cause tissue damage. Such phagocytic cells have defective chemotaxis, motility, and intracellular killing. In animals with Chediak-Higashi syndrome, there is defective development of natural killer cells leading to increased occurrence of cancers.

Pelger-Huet anomaly is characterized by failure of neutrophilic nuclei to segment into lobes, and the nucleus remains rounded just like that in the immature cells present in shift to left. Though it does not affect the health status of animals, the blood picture shows persistent shift to left. Such cells are docile and show poor and slow migration. B-lymphocytes are also found defective, and this combination of neutrophilic and lymphocytic defect causes sufficient suppression of body defenses and reduced survival of such animals.

An autosomal recessive gene has been found responsible for integrin deficiency in Holstein calves. The disease is characterized by recurrent bacterial infections, delayed wound healing, peripheral lymphadenopathy, and persistent neutrophilia and death within 2–7 months. Such animals show the presence of large number of neutrophils in the vascular system, but these cells are scarce in the interstitium or extravascular locations even in the presence of bacteria. This defect occurs in neutrophils as a result of defective genes of CD18 molecule due to point mutation. As a result of absence or defective integrins, the neutrophils are not able to firmly adhere with the endothelium of blood vessel wall and migrate into extravascular spaces. Such calves also show defective T-cell responses in DTH reaction because CD18 molecule is also responsible for the migration of T-cells to the sites of antigen. The defective neutrophils are shown to have reduced responsiveness to any chemotactic stimuli and decreased superoxide production. However, such cells have increased receptors for Fc portion of IgG but with poor binding leading to reduced endocytosis and killing of bacteria.

5.1.2 Acquired Immunodeficiency

The animal may acquire the suppression of the immune system due to drugs, diseases, deficiency of nutrition, neoplasm, or environmental pollution, which is clinically manifested by increased susceptibility to infectious diseases. Acquired immunodeficiency, also known as secondary immunodeficiency, is more common than congenital immunodeficiencies. The animals may come in contact with several xenobiotics present in the environment that may be toxic to the immune system

5.1.2.1 Drugs

Several drugs are known to cause immunosuppression in man and animals; these include corticosteroids, azathioprines, alkylating agents, cyclophosphamide, cyclosporine A, and many antibiotics having intracellular actions and are listed in Table 5.1.

The *corticosteroids* bind with the receptors present on the surface of lymphocytes, and thus, the T-helper cell function is reduced (Table 5.2).

Table 5.1 Drugs causing immunodeficiency

Corticosteroids-dexamethasone
Cyclophosphamide
Azathioprine
Methotrexate
Chlorambucil
Busulfan
Melphalan
Cyclosporine
Tacrolimus (rapamycin)
Gentamicin
Aspirin
Analgesic and anti-inflammatory drugs

Table 5.2 Effects of corticosteroids on the immune system

Immune component	Mechanism of action
Neutrophils	• Neutrophilia • Reduced chemotaxis • Reduced margination • Reduced phagocytosis • Reduced antibody-dependent cellular cytotoxicity (ADCC) • Reduced bactericidal activity • Stabilization of membranes • Inhibition of phospholipase A2
Macrophages	• Reduced chemotaxis • Reduced phagocytosis • Reduced bactericidal activity • Reduced IL-1 and IL-6 production • Reduced antigen processing
Lymphocytes	• Reduced proliferation • Reduced T-cell responses • Impaired T-cell-mediated cytotoxicity • Reduced IL-2 production • Reduced lymphokine production
Immunoglobulins	• Decreased production
Complement	• No effect

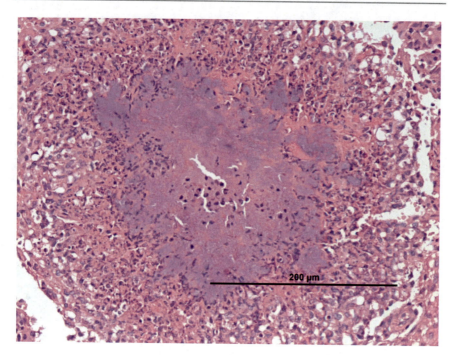

Fig. 5.1 Dexamethasone-induced toxicity in the spleen of rats: the spleen showed severe necrosis of lymphocytes in white pulp area with basophilic bacterial colonies, karyolysis, and karyorrhexis. H&E ×200

Long-term therapy with steroids leads to decreased antibody level in the serum. Exogenous administration of corticosteroids is toxic to immature T-cells, including thymocytes and lymphoblasts. Further, corticosteroids have been shown to suppress IL-2-mediated T-cell proliferation and cytokine production. Dexamethasone-mediated T-cell suppression diminishes naïve T-cell proliferation and differentiation by attenuating the CD28 co-stimulatory pathway (Figs. 5.1 and 5.2). Azathioprine is mostly used to reduce the graft rejection in the case of transplantation of tissues or organs. This drug acts as purine analogue and inhibits synthesis of DNA, RNA, and protein in lymphoid cells leading to suppression of antibody synthesis particularly IgG in animals. *Cyclophosphamides* and *chlorambucil* are used to treat malignancy, which affect the DNA reduplication in T- and B-lymphocytes leading to alteration of surface markers and defective functional activity. However, the macrophage functions are not altered.

Cyclosporine A is a fungal metabolite, which has antibacterial activity. It is used to depress the cell-mediated immune response in order to accept the bone marrow or renal transplant. It affects the T-lymphocytes leading to maturation arrest and altered response of T-cells to growth factors and interleukins. Several anti-inflammatory agents are used in animals in order to reduce swelling and to check the allergic reactions. These drugs inhibit lysosomal enzyme activity and decrease phagocytosis

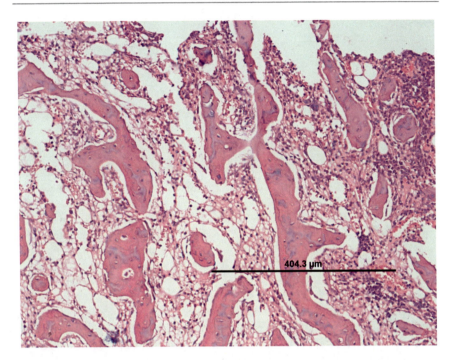

Fig. 5.2 Dexamethasone-induced toxicity in the bone marrow of rats: the femur showed hypocellular bone marrow cavity with significantly decreased varying populations of hematopoietic cells with prominent reticular stroma and adipocytes. H&E ×100

and local inflammatory reaction. These drugs also inhibit the growth of lymphocytes and cause immunosuppression.

Aspirin is used to treat the rheumatoid arthritis in dogs. It has some adverse effects like reduced platelet aggregation, decreased phagocytic activity of neutrophils, and suppression of lymphocyte functions. Phenylbutazone also acts like aspirin and causes immunosuppression.

5.1.2.2 Infections

Many infectious agents are known to cause immunosuppression in animals and poultry either by directly acting on immunocytes or through action on cytokines and activation of suppressor T-cells (Table 5.3 and 5.4). *Bovine herpesvirus-1* (BHV-1) infection is known to cause abortion in cattle, balanoposthitis in bulls, and pneumonia and meningoencephalitis in calves. This virus also causes decrease in peripheral blood CD4+ and CD8+ T-lymphocytes. The reduction in cytotoxic T-lymphocytes has been reported in calves infected with BHV-1. Likewise, *equine herpesvirus-1* (EHV-1) is also found to be associated with suppression of non-specific T-cell functions in horses. This is clinically characterized by leukopenia, neutropenia, and/or lymphopenia. *Marek's disease virus* suppresses the mitogen-induced lymphocyte proliferation. It acts as a lymphocytolytic agent in

Table 5.3 Viral infections causing immunodeficiency in animals

Bovine immunodeficiency virus
Human immunodeficiency virus
Measles virus
Bovine viral diarrhea virus
Infectious bursal disease virus
Feline immunodeficiency virus
Feline leukemia virus
Feline panleukopenia virus
Simian immunodeficiency virus
Equine herpesvirus-1 (EHV-1)
Bovine herpesvirus-1 (BHV-1)
Canine distemper virus
African swine fever virus
Mouse thymus herpesvirus
Ranikhet disease virus
Bluetongue virus
Infectious laryngotracheitis virus

lymphoid follicles of the bursa, spleen, and thymus in poultry. The virus affects both T- and B-lymphocytes. The immunosuppressive activity is mediated by glycoproteins present on the virion envelope.

Bovine viral diarrhea virus causes reduction of CD4+ and CD8+ T-lymphocytes, B-lymphocytes, and neutrophils in cattle. In vitro studies indicated that the virus inhibited production of interleukin-2 by lymphocytes. Respiratory syncytial virus infection in lambs makes them more susceptible to secondary bacterial infection by *Pasteurella multocida*. This virus is known to inhibit live antigen-specific lymphoproliferative responses in sheep and cattle. It also reduces production of CD4+ (T-helper cells) in the peripheral blood of sheep.

Bluetongue virus infects the CD4+ and CD8+ T-lymphocytes and causes their destruction. The border disease virus is known to depress the T-helper and cytotoxic T-lymphocyte responses in lambs. *Canine parvovirus* also infects immunocytes and causes their destruction, which leads to the depletion of lymphoid tissue in the body. *Canine distemper virus* activates the suppressor T-cells, which are responsible for immunosuppression.

Infectious bursal disease virus selectively infects pre-B-lymphocytes in the bursa of Fabricius (Figs. 5.3 and 5.4). The immunosuppressive effect is associated with IgM-bearing cells in the spleen and blood (Figs. 5.5 and 5.6). It depresses MHC class II molecule Ia expressing cells in the bursa and spleen with no alteration in the bone marrow lymphocytes (Figs. 5.7 and 5.8). Infectious laryngotracheitis virus infects macrophages and replicates in them leading to their destruction.

Feline leukemia virus infection is associated with lymphoid depletion, glomerulonephritis, defective macrophages, and deficient complement. The viral DNA present in the bone marrow, lymphoid tissues, and intestines has been considered to be the cause of virus-mediated cytotoxicity of lymphocytes. It also suppresses

5.1 Immunodeficiency

Table 5.4 Infectious and non-infectious causes of immunosuppression in poultry

Causal agent	Genus and family	Host	Disease	Target immune cells	Atrophy of lymphoid organs
Infectious bursal disease virus	*Avibirnavirus* and *Birnaviridae*	Chicken	Infectious bursal disease	T-cells and B-cells	Bursa of Fabricius, thymus, GALT
Gallid alphaherpesvirus 2	*Mardivirus* and *Herpesviridae*	Chicken	Marek's disease	B-cells and CD4+ T-cells	Bursa of Fabricius, thymus, GALT
Avian orthoreovirus	*Orthoreovirus* and *Reoviridae*	Chicken, turkeys	Infectious tenosynovitis	B-cells	Bursa of Fabricius, thymus, GALT
Avian leukosis virus	*Alpharetrovirus* and *Retroviridae*	Chicken, turkeys	Avian lymphoid leukosis	T-cells and B-cells	Bursa of Fabricius, thymus, GALT
Reticuloendotheliosis virus	*Gammaretrovirus* and *Retroviridae*	Chicken, quail, geese, duck, turkey	Runting disease syndrome, chronic neoplasia of lymphoid tissues, and acute reticulum cell neoplasia	T-cells and B-cells	Bursa of Fabricius, thymus, GALT
Chicken anemia virus	*Gyrovirus* and *Anelloviridae*	Chicken	Chicken infectious anemia	All cell lines	Bursa of Fabricius, thymus, GALT, bone marrow
Avian orthoavulavirus 1	*Orthoavulavirus* and *Paramyxoviridae*	Chicken	Newcastle disease	Macrophages	Bursa of Fabricius, GALT
Avian influenza virus	*Influenzavirus A* and *Orthomyxoviridae*	Chicken, turkeys	Avian influenza	Macrophages	Bursa of Fabricius, GALT
Mycoplasma gallisepticum	*Mycoplasma* and *Mycoplasmataceae*	Chicken, turkeys	Chronic respiratory disease (CRD) in chickens and infectious sinusitis in turkeys	T-cells and B-cells	Bursa of Fabricius, thymus, GALT
Ammonia	–	Chicken, quail, geese, duck, turkey	–	T-cells and B-cells	Bursa of Fabricius, GALT
Mycotoxin	–		Mycotoxicosis		

(continued)

Table 5.4 (continued)

Causal agent	Genus and family	Host	Disease	Target immune cells	Atrophy of lymphoid organs
		Chicken, quail, duck, turkey		T-cells and B-cells	Bursa of Fabricius, thymus, GALT, spleen
Heat stress	–	Chicken, quail, duck, turkey	–	T-cells and B-cells	Thymus, GALT, spleen

5.1 Immunodeficiency

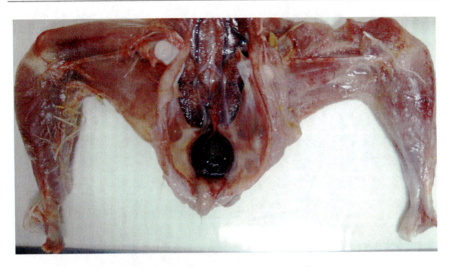

Fig. 5.3 Photograph showing hemorrhage in the bursa of Fabricius in Gumboro disease

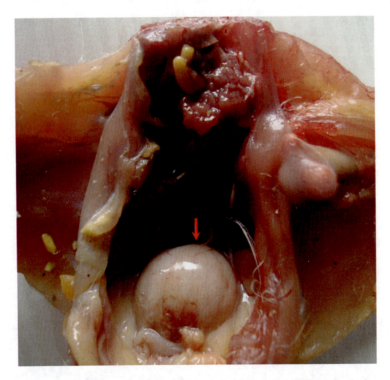

Fig. 5.4 Photograph showing edema and enlargement of the bursa of Fabricius (red arrow) in Gumboro disease

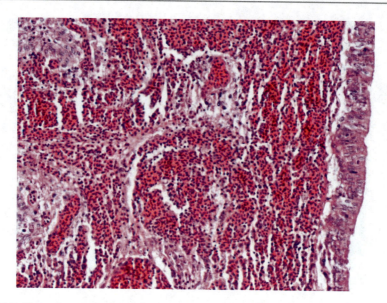

Fig. 5.5 Photomicrograph of the bursa of Fabricius showing hemorrhage in Gumboro disease

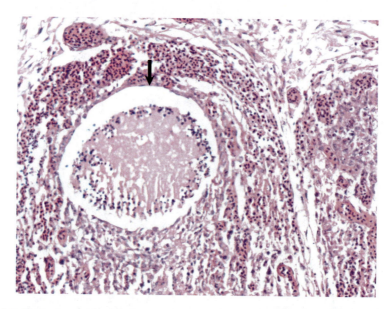

Fig. 5.6 Photomicrograph of the bursa of Fabricius showing depletion of lymphoid tissue (black arrow) in Gumboro disease

production of IL-2 because the viral protein binds with CD4+ lymphocytes. *Feline immunodeficiency virus*, a lentivirus, is known to cause neutropenia and lymphopenia. The immunosuppression caused by this virus is due to inhibition of

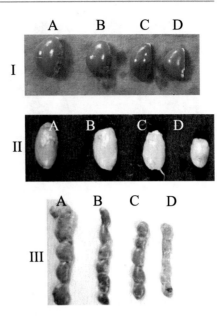

Fig. 5.7 Photograph of the (I) Spleen, (II) Bursa of Fabricius and (III) Thymus showing atrophy and fibrosis (A. Normal, B–D. progressive atrophic changes) due to environmental pollution

T- and B-cell cooperation. The virus selectively infects CD4+ cells and kills them by poorly understood mechanism.

Bovine immunodeficiency virus (BIV) is also a *lentivirus* of *Retroviridae* family. The virus is exogenous and non-oncogenic and causes persistent infection in cattles. The virus replicates in macrophages and CD4+ lymphocytes and causes their destruction and immunosuppression. The virus can be transmitted horizontally by intravenous inoculation in calves. On the entry of the virus into these cells, it may remain latent even up to its whole life without causing any clinical illness. However, sometimes, it causes lymphadenopathy, lymphocytolysis, progressive weakness, and emaciation. The immune response to the virus starts initially at about 3 weeks after infection; antibodies can be easily detected by Western blot technique. NK cells and antibody-dependent cell-mediated cytotoxicity mechanisms also operate simultaneously, but none of these mechanisms succeeds in controlling the BIV infection. The immune response declines shortly after the onset of clinical disease due to necrosis of antigen-presenting cells (macrophages and dendritic cells), reduction in B-lymphocytes, reduction in lymphokine production, supervisor factors, and genetic variation affecting critical viral epitopes.

5.1.2.3 Trauma or Surgery

The physical trauma or surgical operation may also lead to reduction in specific immune response and the functional capacity of phagocytic cells particularly macrophages. Such defects are transient and may become normal after healing of trauma or surgery. The depression of macrophage function is due to reduction of lymphokines, monokines, and other chemotactic factors. It also increases the number of suppressor T-cells and depresses the T-cell function. Corticosteroids,

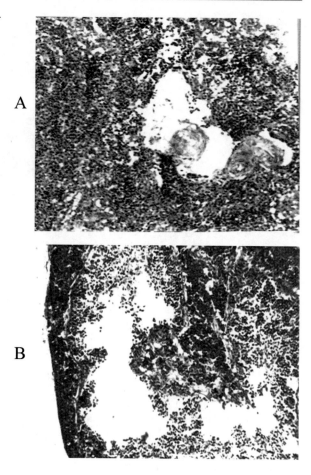

Fig. 5.8 Photomicrograph of the (**a**) thymus and (**b**) spleen showing depletion of lymphoid tissue due to environmental pollution

prostaglandins, suppressive peptides, etc. released during trauma or surgery cause immunosuppression affecting mainly T-cells and macrophages. B-cell functions are usually normal. It leads to impairment of type IV hypersensitivity reaction, allograft rejection, and T-dependent antibody responses. There is reduction of IL-1 and IL-2 production.

5.1.2.4 Environmental Pollution

Rapid advancement in the human civilization has introduced in our environment a large number of synthetic chemicals such as pesticides, heavy metals, etc. Pesticides are widely distributed and used in agriculture, animal husbandry, and public health operations throughout the world. Majority of these compounds are beneficial when used judiciously. However, many of them become contaminants due to their persistence in the ecosystem, i.e., in soil, water, plant, and animal tissues. The residues have been found in human and animal food and dairy products of animal origin. On

5.1 Immunodeficiency

eating such food, the residual compounds reach the tissues of man and animals and produce deleterious effects.

Tens of thousands of new chemicals are being synthesized each year and disseminated to various degrees into the population. The immune mechanism is highly susceptible to these chemicals present in the environment leading to immunosuppression. Pesticides are classified as insecticides, weedicides, herbicides, rodenticides, and fungicides. Of these, insecticides assume greater significance because of having much higher share (77%) in the total pesticide application in agriculture. Insecticides are further grouped as organochlorines, organophosphates, carbamates, and synthetic pyrethroids and have been shown to exert deleterious effects on macrophage functions, DTH reactions, and serum biochemical attributes. Similarly, endosulfan and cypermethrin were also found to severely alter macrophage functions.

The immune system is considered to be a more sensitive indicator of toxicity assays especially for environmental pollutants, which may have residual effects in the ecosystem. The organochlorine and organophosphate groups of pesticides are more immunotoxic than carbamates and synthetic pyrethroids. Many of *organochlorine compounds* (DDT, mirex, endosulfan, lindane, aldrin, and dieldrin) are known to cause reduction in the humoral as well as cell-mediated immune response in animals and poultry. These pesticides appear to be more potent, but many have residual effects in the ecosystem and comparatively more harmful to non-target animals. Endosulfan may cause immunosuppression and reduction in macrophage functions in poultry. Lindane, a gamma isomer of BHC, has been found to cause reduction in NBT-positive cells in lambs. Organochlorine pesticides are also known to cause immune complex-mediated glomerulonephritis in lambs and poultry.

The *organophosphate* group of pesticides are increasingly used due to occurrence of resistance to organochlorines in insects and pests. The immunosuppressive effect of low level of parathion, malathion, sumithion, and monocrotophos has been reported in animals and poultry. The suppression of cell-mediated immune response has been observed due to low doses of malathion in poultry. Monocrotophos is found to have depressive effect on bactericidal activity of macrophages in lambs. *Carbamate* group of pesticides are being used in various agricultural and animal husbandry practices due to their high efficiency and greater safety. However, even in "no observable effect levels" (NOEL), these pesticides cause immunosuppression in animals and poultry. Carbaryl was found to affect cell-mediated immune response in chickens when given at NOEL doses for 2 months. Carbofuran affects both humoral and cell-mediated immune responses in lambs. It is also found to have adverse effect on macrophage functions in lambs after oral feeding for a period of 6 months.

The *synthetic pyrethroid* pesticides are considered to be stable and highly toxic to insects and relatively less toxic to animals and do not accumulate in the environment. However, immunosuppression in goats has been recorded when fed with low doses of cypermethrin. It exerts immunosuppressive effect on both the wings of the immune system. A synthetic pyrethroid d-trans allethrin, a common pesticide used as mosquito repellent in most of the commercial mats, was also found to have immunotoxic effect on humoral and cell-mediated immune responses in mice.

Cypermethrin was found to suppress the humoral immune response and DTH reaction in chickens at very low doses.

Besides, there are many *heavy metals* like lead, mercury, copper, cadmium, etc. found in the environment as pollutants, which also produce immunotoxic effects on non-targeted animal species and man. Lead, when given to chickens at "NOEL" dose for 8 weeks in water, exerted depressive effect on humoral as well as cell-mediated immune responses. Also, it was found to decrease the macrophage functions. Likewise, mercury is also known to cause immunosuppressive effects on both the wings, i.e., humoral and CMI in poultry. The study on immunopathological effects of cadmium in bovine calves includes its immunosuppressive effect on humoral and cell-mediated immunity. It reduces the number of CD4+ and CD8+ cells in bovine calves.

The immunosuppressive effect of environmental pollutants on animals and man is not yet fully investigated. Many pollutants do affect the immune system slowly, and after a longer period or even after many generations, the resistance of the body gets lowered and the individual becomes more susceptible to various infectious diseases. In spite of vaccination and good management conditions, disease outbreaks do occur in population exposed to environmental pollutants.

Mycotoxins present in the food may produce their toxic effects on lymphoid organs leading to immunosuppression and occurrence of disease outbreaks in animals and man. Aflatoxin, the main culprit in this series, is mostly present in poultry feed causing hepatotoxicity and immunosuppression in birds.

5.2 Diagnosis of Immunodeficiency

The diagnosis of immunodeficiency diseases can be made by detection of immune responses against any kind of antigen or non-specifically by measuring gamma globulins and antibody levels in the serum. For the detection of humoral immune response, serum globulins and gamma globulins can be measured by electrophoretic and spectrophotometric methods. However, more precise and accurate results can be obtained by ELISA using the sera of patients. Isotype-specific conjugates are available commercially, which can be used in indirect ELISA to measure the titers of IgA, IgG, IgM, and IgE. If the facility of ELISA reader is not available, dot-immunobinding assay using dipsticks can be used. This assay is comparatively less expensive and quick, and results can be read by naked eyes. The dipsticks can be stored for a longer period without any deterioration. The B-lymphocyte response can be observed by culturing lymphocytes from the peripheral blood, spleen, lymph nodes, or bursa of Fabricius. Using the mitogen LPS, the lymphocyte transformation or blastogenesis can be observed, which will be helpful for the detection of B-cell activity.

The cell-mediated immunity (CMI), as evidenced by T-cell functions, can be measured by culturing the lymphocytes from the peripheral blood or spleen in the presence of mitogens (Con-A, PHA), and their transformation is detected by thymidine or MTT dye method. The transformation of lymphocytes in the presence of

PHA or Con-A is directly correlated with the cytotoxic action of T-lymphocytes. However, if monoclonal antibodies (mAbs) for CD4 or CD8 molecules are available, one can measure the helper or cytotoxic T-cell-mediated immune responses specifically using peripheral blood or tissue sections of lymphoid organs by immunoperoxidase method. Another method of assessing cell-mediated immune response is the delayed-type hypersensitivity (DTH) reaction in which specific or non-specific antigen is applied on the skin and there is hot, painful, and indurated swelling after 48–72 h. If the CMI response is present, the increase in thickness can be measured by vernier caliper.

In order to assess the macrophage functions, macrophages can be collected from the peritoneal fluid after injecting some irritant. Monocytes can be directly collected from the peripheral blood. The functional activity of these cells is assessed by NBT reduction test or by their bactericidal activities.

The C3 component of complement can be easily quantitated by radial immunodiffusion test. The complete measurement of the complement is determined by the total hemolytic activity in which fresh serum from the patient is incubated with antibody-coated sheep red blood cells (SRBC). The lysis of SRBC due to the presence of complement in the serum is measured colorimetrically. However, to be more specific, the components of complement are measured using anti-species complement conjugates by ELISA and the titers correlated with quantitation of complement.

Abnormalities in lymphoid organs are determined grossly on necropsy examination. It is also helpful in determining the size, shape, and weight of lymphoid organs. The tissue reaction is assessed histopathologically. Tissue pieces from lymphoid organs like the spleen, bursa, thymus, lymph nodes, and mucosa-associated lymphoid tissue are processed and examined as per routine histopathological procedures of hematoxylin and eosin staining. The examination of tissue sections of the lymphoid organs for depletion, necrosis, congestion, hemorrhages, and fibrosis or any other significant alteration gives an idea of the damage and the structural and functional status of the organ. The interpretation of histopathological examination is quantitatively analyzed in relation to modifying factors such as age, sex, strain of animals, housing conditions, and nutritional status. A three-tier approach has been adopted for the assessment of immunodeficiency by the National Institute of Public Health and Environment Protection (NIPHEP), the Netherlands, and the US National Toxicology Program, which include hematological parameters such as total leukocyte count (TLC), differential leukocyte count (DLC), absolute lymphocyte count (ALC), absolute neutrophil count (ANC), body weight, thymus weight, and spleen, bursa, lymph nodes, and functional tests for CMI and humoral immune responses and NK cell activity.

Further Reading

Bartram PA, Smith BP, Holmberg C, Mandell CP (1989) Combined immunodeficiency in a calf. J Am Vet Med Assoc 195:347–350

Chauhan RS (1998a) Alphamethrin induced immunosuppression in calves and its modulation using herbal immunomodulator. Immunol Supp 1:496

Chauhan RS (1998b) An introduction to immunopathology. G.B. Pant University, Pantnagar, p 339

Chauhan RS (2001) Immunopathological effects of environmental pollutants in animals. Pantnagar News 4:3–4

Chauhan RS, Agarwal DK (1999a) Immunopathology of alphamethrin in bovine calves. Indian J Anim Sci 69:556–559

Chauhan RS, Agarwal DK (1999b) Immunopathology of cadmium in calves. J Immunol Immunopathol 1:31–34

Chauhan RS, Chandra R (1997) Environmental pollution and immunodeficiency in animals. Livestock International 1:6–11

Chauhan RS, Singh GK (2000) Congenital and acquired immunodeficiency disorders of man and animals. J Immunol Immunopathol 2:1–14

Chauhan RS, Mahipal SK, Kumar S, Jindal N (1997) Aflatoxicosis in animals and man. Galgotia Publishers, Delhi, p 86

Dowling PM (1995) Immunosuppressive drug therapy. Can Vet J 36:281–283

Gonda MA (1992) Bovine immunodeficiency virus. AIDS 6:759–776

Guilford WG (1988) Primary immunodeficiency diseases in dogs and cats. Friskies Res Digest 24:1–13

Gupta S (1990) New concepts in immunodeficiency diseases. Immunol Today 11:344–346

Hoffman Goetz L, Pederson BK (1994) Exercise and the immune system: a model of stress response? Immunol Today 15:382–387

Kakkar BB, Mahipal SK, Chauhan RS (1996) Effect of carbaryl and malathion on cell mediated immune response in chickens. Int J Anim Sci 11:231–233

Khurana SK, Mahipal SK, Chauhan RS, Rishi N (1996) Effect of cypermethrin on serum biochemical attributes in chickens. Int J Anim Sci 11:235–257

Khurana R, Chauhan RS, Mahipal SK (1997a) Effect of insecticides on peritoneal macrophages in sheep. Indian J Vet Res 6(32):36

Khurana R, Mahipal SK, Chauhan RS (1997b) Insecticides induced biochemical alternations in sheep. Indian J Vet Res 8(31):38

Khurana R, Mahipal SK, Chauhan RS (1998a) Effect of carbofuran on cell mediated immunity in sheep. Indian J Toxicol 5:1–6

Khurana SK, Chauhan RS, Mahipal SK (1998b) Immunotoxic effect of cypermethrin and endosulfan on macrophage functions of broiler chicks. Indian J Anim Sci 68:105–106

Khurana SK, Mahipal SK, Chauhan RS (1998c) Immunotoxic effect of cypermethrin on humoral immune response in chickens. Indian J Toxicol 5:137–140

Khurana R, Mahipal SK, Chauhan RS (1999a) Effects of pesticides on delayed type hypersensitivity reaction in sheep. Indian J Anim Sci 69:880–881

Khurana SK, Mahipal SK, Chauhan RS (1999b) Immunotoxic effect of cypermethrin on delayed type hypersensitivity reaction in chickens. Indian Vet J 76:1055–1057

Kumar A, Chauhan RS, Singh NP (1998) Immunopathological effect of lead on cell mediated immunity in chickens. Indian J Vet Pathol 22:22–25

Kumar A, Chauhan RS, Singh NP (1999a) Immunosuppressive effect of lead on humoral immune response in chickens. Indian J Toxicol 6:27–31

Kumar A, Chauhan RS, Singh NP (1999b) Effect of subchronic lead intoxication on IBD vaccine induced humoral immune response in poultry. J Immunol Immunopathol 1:60–62

Kumar A, Chauhan RS, Singh NP (1999c) Immunopathological effect of mercury on humoral immune response in chickens. Indian J Anim Sci 69:550–552

Kumar A, Chauhan RS, Singh NP (1999d) Immunopathological effects of mercury on cell mediated immune response in poultry. Indian Vet J 76:779–783

Roseh FS, Cooper MD, Wedgewood RJP (1995) The primary immunodeficiencies. N Engl J Med 333:431–439

Saminathan M, Singh KP, Maity M, Vineetha S, Manjunathareddy GB, Dhama K, Malik YS, Ramakrishnan MA, Misri J, Gupta VK (2021) Pathological and immunological characterization of bluetongue virus serotype 1 infection in type I interferons blocked immunocompetent adult mice. J Adv Res 31:137

Thompson AW (1983) Immunobiology of cyclosporin a: a review. Aust J Exp Biol Med Sci 61: 147–172

Immunomodulation

Key Points

1. Immunomodulation is the manipulation of the immune system by augmenting or decreasing the immune responses.
2. Augmentation of immune response is known as immunostimulation or immunopotentiation.
3. Suppression of immune responses is termed as immunosuppression.
4. Neuroendocrine system controls the immune mechanisms through neuropeptides and hormones.
5. Neuropeptides or neurotransmitters are secreted by nerve cells, which maintain the communication between the nerve cells.
6. Cytokines are hormonelike small, low-molecular-weight polypeptides, which maintain constant communication among cells to coordinate the immune responses.
7. Cytokines may act synergistically or antagonistically by enhancing or suppressing their own production.
8. Cytokines are produced by lymphocytes, monocytes, fibroblasts, mast cells, eosinophils, vascular endothelial cells, etc.
9. Cytokines include interleukins, interferons, cytotoxins, chemokines, growth factors, etc.
10. Chemical immunomodulators are levamisole, thiabendazole, imuthiol, avridine, isoprinosine, glucan, indomethacin, ascorbic acid derivatives, biostim, dihydroheptaprenol, etc.
11. Probiotics are live microorganisms, which when supplemented in adequate amounts enhance the growth of other organisms and provide a health benefit to the host.
12. Probiotics exert immunostimulatory action in a strain-specific manner by stimulating the cell-mediated immunity, increasing the immunoglobulin and interferon production, and activating macrophages, lymphocytes, and NK cells.

13. Adjuvant is a term derived from the Latin word *adjuvare*, meaning to help or to aid.
14. Adjuvants are defined as any substances which act as a hapten or antigen and enhance the immune responses.
15. Cow therapy consists of five materials (panchgavya) received from Indian Zebu cow including milk, curd, ghee, urine, and dung extract, which enhances the resistance of body and makes body refractory to infections.

6.1 Immunomodulation

Immunomodulation is the manipulation of the immune system; it may augment or decrease the magnitude of immune responsiveness. The augmentation of immune response is known as *immunostimulation or immunopotentiation*, while suppression of immune responsiveness is termed as *immunosuppression*. The necessity of suppression of the function of the immune system is well recognized in the areas of transplantation and immunopathological disorder like autoimmunity. Conversely, augmentation of immune response has been a matter of considerable interest among the scientists of veterinary as well as medical sciences in order to increase the host's resistance to diseases. Specific immunomodulation is limited to a single antigen such as vaccine, i.e., immunopotentiation used, for development of resistance in body against a particular disease. Non-specific immunomodulation implies for a more generalized change in the immune responsiveness leading to altered host reactivity to many different antigens (Mulcatiy and Quinn 1986; Quinn 1990).

6.2 Need of Immunomodulation

Prevention and treatment of diseases in animals and man are of primary concern of veterinarians and medicos. A wide range of antibacterial, antiparasitic, and antifungal agents and vaccines have been developed during the last few decades for the control of diseases in animals and man. The impact of chemotherapy and vaccination on many complex diseases has reached a plateau, and if further progress is to be made, different strategies have to be developed. Immunomodulation is one of the most important alternatives in order to control diseases with additional advantages of amplifying specific responses to vaccines. The immunomodulatory compounds also offer prospects of reversing immunosuppression caused by stress, viruses, or environmental pollution (Mulcatiy and Quinn 1986; Quinn 1990). A brief history of immunomodulators is summarized in Table 6.1.

It has been well said, "Prevention is better than cure." Therefore, efforts are being made to reduce the incidence of diseases in animals and man, and one of the important means of decreasing the impact of diseases is to accelerate the host's immune functions towards a specific antigen, e.g., vaccination. However, emphasis is being given on the development of products, which can heighten the immunological capabilities of hosts, when they are exposed to pathogens. The non-specific

6.2 Need of Immunomodulation

Table 6.1 History of immunomodulators

Year	Scientists	Contribution
1865	T. Bilroth	Endotoxin (LPS)
1894	W. Coley	Erysipelas toxin
1936	J. Freund	Mycobacterium adjuvant (BCG)
1941	L. Pillemer and E.E. Ecker	Zymosan
1942	J. Freund and D. McDermott	Freund's complete adjuvant (FCA)
1957	A. Isaacs and J. Lindenmann	Interferon
1961	Alec Douglas Bangham and R.W. Horne	Liposomes
1963	A.R. Prevot, B.N. Halpern, and G. Biozzi	*Corynebacterium parvum*
1964	J. Maisin	Thymic hormones
1967	J. Vilcek	Double stranded polynucleotides
1968	N.R. DiLuzio and S.J. Riggi	Yeast glucan
1969	G. Chihara	Lentinan
1971	G. Renoux	Levamisole
1975	E. Lederer	Muramyl dipeptide
1980	Kendall A. Smith	IL-1 and IL-2
1989	E.J. Leonard, T. Yoshimura, and M. Baggiolini	Discovery of first chemokines (IL-8 or NAP 1)
1995	S. Sakaguchi	CD25 as a marker of natural Treg cells
2002	R.S. McHugh and coworkers	Glucocorticoid-induced TNF receptor (GITR)
2008	E. Ortiz-Sánchez	Antibody-cytokine fusion protein
2012	M. H. Yazdi	Biogenic selenium nanoparticles

immunomodulation is also required during the neonatal period (immune system is not fully developed) and during periods of stress, infection, and environmental pollution-induced immunotoxicity leading to immunosuppression (Chauhan 1998a; Quinn 1990).

The main objectives of the immunostimulation are as follows:

1. To induce effective and sustained immune response against infections including both humoral and cell-mediated immunity.
2. To speed up the maturation of non-specific and specific immunity during neonatal period.
3. To enhance local immunity.
4. To overcome the immunosuppressive effects of stress and environmental pollution.
5. To maintain immune surveillance in order to remove neoplasia.

Most of the immunomodulators were discovered fortuitously that limit their prophylactic or therapeutic application. So far, no such single immunomodulator has been shown to have absolute selectivity at all levels of the immune response. An ideal immunomodulator is yet to be discovered, developed, and validated. There is an obvious need for immunomodulator that can safely and selectively enhance the specific class or subclass of immunocyte in animals and man. Such compounds will have to conform to defined criteria to ensure the safety of the consumer, compatibility, and minimal deleterious effects in host (Chauhan 1998b). An ideal immunomodulator should meet the following criteria:

1. It should be non-toxic for animals and man even at high doses.
2. It should not have teratogenic, carcinogenic, or any other side effects.
3. It should have a short withdrawal period with low tissue residues. It should not be secreted in milk or come in eggs.
4. It should stimulate both specific and paraspecific immune responses in the body.
5. It should act as adjuvant when given with vaccines.
6. The immunomodulator or its breakdown products should be either inactive or readily biodegradable in the environment.
7. It should be active through oral route and should be stable in its natural state even after incorporation into food and water.
8. It should be compatible with other drugs.
9. It should not be antigenic.
10. It should be of defined chemical composition or biological activity.

The compounds fulfilling the above criteria have yet to be discovered and synthesized. A complete understanding of the activation and suppression of the immune response may pave the way towards the development of certain compounds with known and predictable activity for either augmenting the humoral or cell-mediated immune response or lowering the undesirable and deleterious immune reactions in particular organ or tissue (Quinn 1990).

The immunomodulatory property of physiological products with their mechanism of action is described here (Mulcatiy and Quinn 1986).

6.3 Physiological Products

6.3.1 Neuroendocrine Hormones

The neuroendocrine system controls immune mechanisms through neuropeptides and hormones. Neuropeptides, secreted by nerve cells, maintain communication between nerve cells. They are also known as neurotransmitters. Neuropeptides are thought to exert control over differentiation of lymphocytes and macrophages from their progenitors. The arrangement of genes during the course of antibody synthesis is mediated by neuropeptides. These peptides are also responsible for the expression of T-cell receptors in the thymus. Similarly, the cytokines secreted by leukocytes affect the neuroendocrine system and change the animal behavior. Lymphocytes and macrophages have a wide variety of receptors on their surfaces for a number of hormones and neuropeptides; stimulation of these receptors may alter the functional status of these cells. It has been observed that during the development of brain lesions, the immune system does not work properly. Besides, the spleen, thymus, bone marrow, lymph nodes, bursa, etc. are innervated with autonomic noradrenergic sympathetic neurons, which exert their effect on the immune mechanisms through neurotransmitters and hormones (Kelley 1988; Kelley and Dantzer 1990). In this chapter, the emphasis has been given on the effect of neuroendocrine system on immune mechanisms and its manipulation through medication or by other means for positive modulation of immunity to control diseases (Table 6.2).

6.4 Neuropeptides

Many noradrenergic neurons are in close contact with lymphocytes and reticular cells in the spleen. The release of norepinephrine by the nerve terminals acts at postsynaptic receptor on lymphocytes and macrophages. Noradrenergic innervations in the parenchyma of the spleen parallel the migration of lymphocytes into the periarteriolar lymphatic sheath and the density of these neurons declines with aging. The autonomic nor-adrenergic innervations in spleen have a great role in the development of T-lymphocytes in young animals and decline in T-dependent immune functions in old age. The mucosal mast cells present in the lamina propria are in close contact with peripheral nerves, which may be activated during psychological problems to cause intestinal disorders.

There are receptors for interleukin-1 in many locations of the brain. Leukocytes possess a wide variety of receptors for neuroendocrine peptides such as proopiomelanocortin (POMC) and adrenocorticotropic hormone (ACTH), β-endorphin, substance-P, somatostatin, vasoactive intestinal peptide, and nerve growth factor (Kelley 1988; Kelley and Dantzer 1990). The epithelial cells of the thymus have receptors for acetylcholine. Insulin-specific receptors can be detected on activated lymphocytes. Leukocytes are also provided with receptors for growth hormone and prolactin. Porcine spleen cells possess receptor for β-adrenergic hormone and α-1 and α-2 adrenoceptors are found on bovine macrophages.

The presence of specific receptors on leukocytes for a wide variety of neuropeptides clearly establishes a biochemical means for transducing the binding of a ligand into some type of second signal that can deliver a message to the nucleus of the cell. Adrenocorticotropic hormone (ACTH) inhibits antibody synthesis but stimulates proliferation of B-lymphocytes. It also suppresses the synthesis of gamma interferon by T-cells and also inhibits the activity of gamma interferon to generate tumoricidal macrophages. ACTH may exert its effect directly on lymphocytes and through its action on the adrenal cortex and production of glucocorticoids, which further suppresses the cell-mediated immunity. Glucocorticoids inhibit synthesis of IL-1, IL-2, and TNF-α and expression of class II genes of major histocompatibility complex. Glucocorticoids suppress proliferation of Con A-stimulated lymphocytes in vitro in pigs, poultry, and cattle. The phagocytic activity of neutrophil is also inhibited by glucocorticoids. During stress, the secretion of glucocorticoid suppresses activities of T-lymphocytes and phagocytic cells, which can be corrected through immunomodulatory therapy using cytokines (Cupps and Fanci 1982).

Table 6.2 Neuroendocrine hormones having immunomodulatory properties

Products	Sub-products	Action on the immune system
Autonomic nervous system (ANS)	Sympathetic	• Decrease macrophage activity • Increase B- and T-cell activity
	Parasympathetic	• Increase B- and T-cell function
Hypothalamic-pituitary (H-P) hormones	Oxytocin and vasopressin	• Increase T-lymphocyte growth
	Growth hormone (GH) and prolactin	• Increase T-lymphocyte growth • Augment antibody synthesis, activity of cytotoxic T- lymphocytes, and NK cells • Maintains the size of the thymus and induces the production of super oxide anion
	Thyrotropin-releasing hormone (TRH) and thyroid-stimulating hormone (TSH)	• Increase B- and T-lymphocyte function
	Sex hormones	• Generally inhibitory to leukocyte action
H-P-adrenal	Adrenocorticotropic hormone (ACTH)	• Decrease macrophage activity • Increase B- and T-cell function • Immunosuppression, decreases blastogenic responses of lymphocytes, and inhibits antibody synthesis
	Glucocorticoids (dexamethasone)	• Inhibitory action on leukocytes • Inhibits IL-2 production
Neuropeptides	Substance-P	• Stimulatory action on leukocytes
	Somatostatin	• Inhibitory action on leukocytes
	Endogenous opioid peptides	• Mainly stimulatory on leukocytes • Immunosuppression and atrophy of the spleen
	Vasoactive intestinal peptide (VIP)	• Potent endogenous anti-inflammatory agent
	Nerve growth factor (NGF)	• Increase T-lymphocyte function
Pineal gland	Melatonin	• Increases antibody production and the number of cells in the spleen • Inhibit the synthesis of prostaglandins, thromboxanes, and leukotrienes • Decrease the circulating lymphocytes and eosinophils • Decreased chemotaxis • Depletion of monocytes and decreased NK cell activity
Endogenous ligand	Enkephalins	• Proliferation of lymphocytes

6.5 Growth Hormone and Prolactin

Experimental studies in rats indicate that growth hormone and prolactin augment antibody synthesis. It has been observed that low level of plasma prolactin is responsible for decreased activity of tumoricidal macrophages. The inability of T-lymphocytes in prolactin-deficient mice to synthesize and secrete IFN-γ leads to the inhibition of activated macrophages. Growth hormone is also responsible for the growth of the thymus, production of thymulin, increase in the synthesis of antibodies, and generation of cytotoxic T-cells. It also enhances granulopoiesis synergistically with colony-stimulating factors. Therapy with growth hormone and prolactin can restore the size of the thymus, its structure, and cytokine production (Narnaware et al. 1998). Growth hormone is a potent primer of macrophages as assessed by the production of superoxide anions to cause respiratory burst for destruction of opsonized targets. It has been observed that recombinant bovine growth hormone augments the number of circulating neutrophils, increases the production of reactive oxygen intermediates, and reduces the clinical symptoms of acute mastitis induced experimentally with *E. coli* (Narnaware et al. 1998).

Thyroid-stimulating hormone (TSH) is known to augment antibody synthesis. The TSH is synthesized by T-lymphocytes and is controlled by adenohypophysis and acts as a cytokine at antibody producing sites to control antibody production.

Supplementary dietary triiodothyronine (T-3) also increases the number of splenic IgG plaque-forming cells and induces the proliferation of thymic epithelial cells. Triiodothyronine and thyroxine augment the plasma level of a thymic hormone known as thymulin. The excess of T4 suppresses the activity of NK cells.

6.6 Opioid Peptides

Opioid peptides are the endogenous analogues of opiates, which are elevated during acute stress and cause immunosuppression during stress (Dantzer and Kelley 1989). It is also responsible for the inhibition of NK cells. Alpha-endorphin suppresses the primary antibody synthesis by lymphocytes by inhibiting the production of an antigen-specific T-cell helper factor. β-Endorphin also indirectly inhibits the production of toxic oxygen intermediates in mononuclear phagocytic cells. Leukocytes possess all four types of opioid receptors like mu, delta, kappa, and epsilon.

Other neuropeptides including substance-P, somatostatin, and vasoactive intestinal peptide cause immunomodulatory action in the body. Substance-P is released from afferent sensory nerve endings which causes the release of IL-1, IL-6, and TNF-α by monocytes, proliferation of fibroblasts, infiltration of granulocytes, and degranulation of mast cells and increases the respiratory burst in neutrophils.

6.7 Thymic Products

The thymus gland has a central role in the development and maintenance of the immune system. Involution of the thymus is associated with aging and a corresponding decline in the immune reactivity, particularly of T-cells. More than 20 thymic products have been identified, of which thymosin fraction 5, thymosin α-1, thymosin β-4, thymulin, thymopoietin, and thymic humoral factor are important as they play an active role in the immunity (Table 6.3). Thymosin fraction 5 is made up of 30 polypeptides, which induces T-cell markers on bone marrow cells, enhances migration inhibitory factor, and increases antibody production and interferon production following virus infection. It also induces T-suppressor cells. Thymosin α-1 increases mitogenic responses of lymphocytes and interferon production. Thymopoietin is responsible for T-cell differentiation. Thymulin enhances the generation of effector cytotoxic T-cells in vivo as well as in vitro. Thymic humoral factor increases the cytotoxic reactivity of lymphoid cells against syngeneic tumors. It has been observed that both thymopoietin and thymosin fraction 5 increase cGMP, which is consistent with their immunostimulatory activity especially in T-cell-deficient animals. The thymic products act on developing cells like thymocytes and prothymocyte rather than on mature cells. These hormones are particularly responsible for the maintenance of an active population of circulating precursor of lymphocytes, which have blastogenic properties throughout their life. Some of these thymic products are chemically synthesized and used as immunomodulatory products. They enhance primary and secondary antibody response and have depressing effects on different types of hypersensitivity reactions. Low doses of synthetic thymulin increase NK cell activity and polymorphonuclear leukocytes, while its high doses increase the suppressor T-cells (Quinn 1990).

Table 6.3 Thymic products having immunomodulatory properties

Thymic products	Action on the immune system
Thymosin α-1	Increases mitogenic responsiveness of lymphocytes and interferon production
Thymopoietin	T-cell differentiation
Thymulin	Key player during interaction of immune system to neuroendocrine system; generates effector cytotoxic T-lymphocytes; increases NK cell activity
Thymosin fraction 5	Increases cGMP; induces T-cell markers on bone marrow; enhances migration inhibitory factor; increases antibody production and interferons
Thymic humoral factor	Increases cytotoxic reactivity of lymphoid cells against synergic tumors
Splenopentin (SP-5, Arg-Lys-Glu-Val-Tyr) and thymopentin (TP-5, Arg-Lys-Asp-Val-Tyr)	Affects the neuromuscular transmission and subsequently affects T-cell differentiation and function

6.8 Cytokines

Cytokines are hormonelike small, low-molecular-weight polypeptides, which maintain constant communication among cells to coordinate the immune response. Cytokines may act synergistically or antagonistically, thereby enhancing or suppressing their own production. Cytokines are produced by lymphocytes, monocytes, fibroblasts, mast cells, eosinophils, vascular endothelial cells, etc. They include interleukins, interferons, cytotoxins, chemokines, and growth factors (Table 6.4). They differ from hormones, which are specifically produced by endocrine glands to maintain homeostasis through endocrine action, while cytokines are produced by many different cell types and act on different cells of the body with very high functional activity. They have autocrine, paracrine, or endocrine in action and cause tissue repair and provide resistance to infection (Mulcatiy and Quinn 1986; Kelley 1988).

Prophylactic and therapeutic uses of cytokines are limited because of difficulties with their production and purification. However, recombinant cytokines are now being used in several ailments. Polyinosinic:polycytidylic acid [poly I:C or poly(I:C)] is used as interferon inducers in mice. It restores NK cell activity in immunocompromised animals. Gamma interferon produced by recombinant technique in mice induces high levels of NK cell activity against the target cells. Synthetic IFN-γ is also a potent activator of peritoneal macrophages. It protects mice challenged with virus infections. Recombinant IL-2 increases production of neutralizing antibody in calves against BHV-1 virus infection and induces LAK cells. Recombinant IFN-γ protected calves against challenge with vaccine virus and also protected bovine cells in vitro. Treatment with interferon reduced temperature responses, clinical signs of disease, and mortality in calves infected with BHV-1 virus.

6.9 Microbial Products

The products of *Mycobacterium phlei* are used as adjuvants to enhance immune responses non-specifically. The microbial products are known for their non-specific activation of macrophages and stimulation of NK cell activity. Well-established microbial products having immunomodulatory properties are *Propionibacterium acnes* and lentinan.

6.9.1 *P. acnes* (Corynebacterium Parvum)

Heat-killed or formaldehyde-treated suspension of *P. acnes* is used for immunotherapy. It activates macrophages and clears particulate material from circulation. Products of *P. acnes* enhance the humoral and cell-mediated immune response and alter the liver enzyme levels. The ability of *P. acnes* to introduce tumor regression has been known for many years. It increases resistance to bacterial, viral, and protozoal infections. It enhances chemotaxis to phagocytic cells. It increases

Table 6.4 Cytokines having immunomodulatory properties

Name of cytokine	Source	Action on the immune system	Therapeutic application
Interleukin-1 (IL-1)	Monocyte, lymphocyte, and endothelium	Hematopoiesis, T- and B-cell activation, fibroblast proliferation, and acute phase response	Blockage of IL-1 activity
Interleukin-2 (IL-2)	Activated T-cells	Proliferation and differentiation of T-cells, cytotoxic T-cells, B-cells; Ig secretion and cytolytic activity	Treatment of cancer, infectious diseases, and bone marrow transplantation
Interleukin-3 (IL-3)	Activated T-cells, mast cells, and NK cells	Proliferation and differentiation of myeloid progenitor stem cells, increased macrophages, leukocyte count and spleen weight, and prevention of apoptosis induction in macrophages	Bone marrow transplantation
Interleukin-4 (IL-4)	T-cells, mast cells, eosinophils, and basophils	Proliferation and differentiation of B-cells and Ig switching	Anti-tumor agent and immune stimulator
Interleukin-5 (IL-5)	Activated CD4+ T-cells of Th2 subset, mast cells, and eosinophils	Stimulates growth and differentiation of eosinophil precursor cells	Suppress the eosinophil inflammation
Interleukin-6 (IL-6)	T-cells, monocyte, endothelial cells, and mast cells	Stimulate B-cells for antibody (IgM and IgA) production, T-cell growth, and CTL differentiation	Anti-tumor activity
Interleukin-7 (IL-7)	Stromal cells in bone marrow and thymus and dendritic cells	Formation of lymphokine-activated killer (LAK) cells and cytotoxic T-cells	Anti-tumor activity
Interleukin-8 (IL-8)	Monocyte, lymphocyte, and endothelial cells	Chemotactic for neutrophils, basophils, and T-lymphocytes and chemokine function	None
Interleukin-9 (IL-9)	Mast cells, NKT cells, Th2, Th17, Treg, ILC2, and Th9 cells	Growth of T-helper cells	Allergic and autoimmune diseases
Interleukin-10 (IL-10)	Monocyte, lymphocyte, and endothelial cells	Inhibition of pro-inflammatory cytokines by monocyte and granulocytes, inhibition of IL-2 production by antigen-specific T-cells, stimulation of B-cells and thymocytes	Anti-inflammatory and immunosuppressive, used in autoimmune disease

(continued)

6.9 Microbial Products

Table 6.4 (continued)

Name of cytokine	Source	Action on the immune system	Therapeutic application
Interleukin-11 (IL-11)	Bone cells, fibroblasts, epithelial cells, and endothelial cells	Stimulates B-cell growth	Idiopathic pulmonary fibrosis
Interleukin-12 (IL-12)	Monocyte and B-cells	Proliferation of T- and NK cells, CTL response to tumor cells, increased IFN-γ production by T- and NK cells, inhibit IgE production	Anti-metastatic, anti-tumor, vaccine adjuvant
Interleukin-13 (IL-13)	Activated T- and B-cells	B-cell growth and differentiation factor and stimulates B-cells for IgG$_4$ production	Anti-tumor and anti-inflammatory agent
Interleukin-14 (IL-14)	T-cells and some B-cell tumors	B-cell proliferation	Mediator of renal transplantation
Interleukin-15 (IL-15)	Mononuclear cells	Stimulation and proliferation of activated B-, T-, LAK, and NK cells, chemoattractant	Anti-tumor and rheumatoid arthritis
Interleukin-16 (IL-16)	Cytotoxic T-cells and eosinophils	Chemotaxis for CD4 T-lymphocytes	Anti-HIV
Interleukin-17 (IL-17)	Activated CD4 T-cells	Promotes IL-6 and IL-8 production	Psoriasis, psoriatic arthritis, and ankylosing spondylitis
Interleukin-18 (IL-18)	Macrophages	Anti-tumor and anti-microbial activity	Immunotherapy for cancer
Interferon-alpha (IFN-α)	Leukocyte	Anti-proliferative action, immunoregulatory action, enhances NK cells, macrophages, and T-cell activities	Cancer, hepatitis B and C, AIDS, Kaposi sarcoma, multiple sclerosis
Interferon-beta (IFN-β)	Fibroblast, epithelial cells, and endothelial cells	Anti-viral, MHC antigen upregulation, NK-cell-enhanced cytotoxicity, antimicrobial	Cancer and multiple sclerosis
Interferon-gamma (IFN-γ)	Monocyte, macrophages, dendritic cells, T-cells, and B-cells	MHC class II expression, macrophage and NK cell activation, Ig isotype selection	Used as adjuvant
G-CSF	Stromal cells and endothelial cells	Proliferation and differentiation of immunocytes, macrophages, and progenitor cells	After bone marrow transplantation

(continued)

Table 6.4 (continued)

Name of cytokine	Source	Action on the immune system	Therapeutic application
M-CSF	Fibroblast, endothelial cells, T-cells, monocyte, and neutrophil	Monocyte proliferation, differentiation, and activation, development of bone marrow precursor cells	Anti-tumor, anti-infection, myelosuppression
GM-CSF	T-cells, macrophages, endothelial cells, and B-cells	Inhibit apoptosis of target; proliferation, differentiation, and activation of granulocyte and macrophage lineage	Recruitment of peripheral blood stem cells, stimulation of APC for immunotherapy
Chemokines	Monocyte, neutrophil, endothelial cells, epithelial cells, and fibroblast	Neutrophil, eosinophils and T-cell chemotaxis and adherence, IL-6 secretion, monocyte and basophil activation, NK cell cytolysis	None yet
RANTES	T-cells, monocyte, NK cells, fibroblast, epithelial cells, and endothelial cells	T-cells, monocyte, and NK cell chemotaxis and proliferation; modulation of macrophages, eosinophils, and T-cells	Suppression of HIV replication
TNF-α	Macrophages and T-cells	Cytotoxic for tumor cells, anti-viral, anti-bacterial, and anti-parasitic activity, apoptosis of tumor cells	Cancer and autoimmune disease
TNF-β	Mast cells, platelet, and fibroblast	Wound repair, cell growth regulation, tissue remodeling, immunosuppression	Inhibition of inflammatory cells and treatment of breast cancer

macrophage number in the spleen, lungs, liver, and lymph nodes with lymphoid hyperplasia in the thymus, lymph nodes, and mucosa-associated lymphoid tissue. An increase in the bacterial clearance has been observed after *P. acnes* therapy. Oral administration of P-40, a fraction of *P. acnes*, protected mice from viral infection. Stimulation of cytotoxic T-cells is also observed in tumor-bearing mice. The generalized stimulation of T- and B-lymphocytes, NK cells, and macrophages appears to be the method whereby *P. acnes* produces its immunomodulatory effect. It has a very limited role in antibody production. However, anti-tumor activity of *P. acnes* and its products appear to be due to its paraspecific activation of NK cells, macrophages, and T-lymphocytes (Collins and Scott 1974).

6.10 Lentinan

Lentinan is a neutral polysaccharide isolated from mycelia of *Lentinus edodes*, an edible mushroom. It is β-1,3-glucan with high molecular weight and a triple helix structure. This is water-soluble, heat and acid stable, but liable to alkalies. It has antitumor activity. It stimulates pinocytosis in macrophages. Lentinan also stimulates cytokine production including IL-1. It augments antigen-specific cellular immune responses as well as non-specific immune responses against neoplastic cells. It enhances the activity of giant cells and activates complement through classical and alternate pathways. Immunomodulatory properties of lentinan are thought to be due to its activity on precursor effector cells, cytotoxic T-lymphocytes, NK cells, and macrophages and increased antibody production.

6.11 Probiotics

Antibiotics and immunosuppressive therapy can alter the normal microflora of the gastrointestinal tract. The introduction of beneficial microflora into the system will help to prevent the establishment of disease. The word "probiotic" was first introduced by Lilly and Stillwell in 1965. Probiotics are live microorganisms, which when supplemented in adequate amounts enhance the growth of other organisms and provide a health benefit to the host. The word "probiotics" was obtained from the Greek word meaning "for life."

Probiotics or direct fed microbials (DFM) are often accomplished by their ability to alter the intestinal microbial balance in a beneficial manner, which in turn improves the health of animals, birds, or human beings (Dhama et al. 2015). Probiotics include bacteria, fungi, and yeast. Commonly, apathogenic live bacterial strains consisting of the genera *Enterococcus*, *Streptococcus*, and *Lactobacillus* are mainly utilized in poultry and livestock. As growth promoters, probiotics increase the feed conversion efficiency, growth performance, and immune responses in poultry and livestock (Dhama et al. 2015). Probiotics stimulate the immune system of human, animals, and birds to fight against infectious agents, tumors, and other stress factors (Dhama et al. 2015).

Probiotics exert immunostimulatory action by stimulating the cell-mediated immunity, increasing the immunoglobulin and interferon production, and activating macrophages, lymphocytes, and natural killer (NK) cells (Dhama et al. 2015). Probiotics stimulate the immune responses in a strain-specific manner. Thus, a combination of strains should be used to get the beneficial effect of probiotics (Dhama et al. 2015). *Lactobacillus* spp. increase the intra-epithelial lymphocytes of intestinal lymphoid tissue, which responds to microbes by secreting IgA and thereby providing local immunity (Dhama et al. 2015).

Various strains of probiotic bacteria such as *Lactobacillus casei*, *L. delbrueckii* subsp. *bulgaricus*, *L. acidophilus*, *L. plantarum*, *L. paracasei*, *L. fermentum*, *L. rhamnosus*, *L. brevis*, *L. helveticus*, *L. reuteri*, and *Bifidobacterium animalis* are used for immunomodulation (Dhama et al. 2015). The mechanisms of action of

Table 6.5 Probiotics having immunomodulatory properties

Probiotic bacteria	Species	Assessment	Effect
Lactobacillus casei	Rodent	Infection and antibody production in malnourished animals	Increased serum IgA and reduced enteric infections caused by Salmonella
L. acidophilus and Peptostreptococcus	Rodent	Translocation of Escherichia coli and serum total anti-E. coli IgG, IgE, and IgM	Decreased translocation and increased anti-E. coli IgM and IgE
Bifidobacterium bifidus	Human	Total IgA and response to polio virus	Increased serum IgA
Bacillus subtilis natto	Calf	Stimulation of humoral immunity	Increased production of IgG, IgM, and IgA
Lactobacillus plantarum DK119	Rodent	Stimulation of host innate immunity	Increase in dendritic cells, macrophages, and cytokine production
Lactococcus lactis BFE920	Olive flounder (fish)	Stimulation of host innate immunity	Increased lysosomal activities and production of IL-12 and IFN-γ

immunomodulation for these probiotics are increased secretion of immunoglobulins (IgG, IgM, and IgA), induction of cell-mediated immunity, absorption of antigens released from dead microbes, increased phagocytic activity of granulocytes and macrophages, and increased expression of activation marker (CD25) on T-cells and NK cells, cytokine production, etc. (Dhama et al. 2015). Strains of *Leuconostoc* and *Streptococcus* are potent enhancers of Th1 cytokines. *Propionibacterium* and *Bifidobacterium* genera are potent anti-inflammatory probiotics that induce IL-10 secretion. Lactocepin produced by *Lactobacillus casei* and *Lactobacillus paracasei* selectively degrade pro-inflammatory chemokines and thus may be useful for the control and treatment of inflammatory diseases like IBD, allergic skin inflammation, and psoriasis (Dhama et al. 2015).

Interaction of prebiotics like *Agave fructans* (*Agave salmiana*) with probiotics *Lactobacillus casei* and *Bifidobacterium lactis* is helpful in the activation and selective differentiation of immune cells. *Saccharomyces boulardii* has stimulatory effect on secretory IgA and other secretory components of immunoglobulins in small intestine against diarrhea (Dhama et al. 2015). Encapsulated *Bifidobacterium bifidum* enhances intestinal IgA secretion. Modulation of humoral and cell-mediated immunity by probiotics and its effects on cytokine production are depicted in Table 6.5.

6.12 Chemical Compounds

Various chemical compounds have been reported in the literatures that possess immunomodulatory properties. Chemicals having immunomodulatory properties should also be seen from the viewpoint of their residues in animal products such

Table 6.6 Synthetic chemical compounds with immunomodulatory properties

Synthetic compound	Immunomodulatory action
Levamisole	Increases T-cell and macrophage activity
Thiabendazole	Enhances lymphocyte blastogenic responsiveness to mitogens
Imuthiol	Increases lymphocyte blastogenesis and IL-2 production
Avridine	Increases bactericidal activity of neutrophils
Isoprinosine	Increases T-helper cells and increases NK cell cytotoxicity
Glucan	Enhances chemotaxis for neutrophils
Indomethacin	Increases blastogenic responses to T-cells
Ascorbic acid	T-lymphocyte proliferation, lymphokine production, and increased antibody production
Biostim	Improves DTH reaction
Thalidomide	Decrease cytokine production (TNF-α, IL-6, and IL-8) during tumor
Glatiramer acetate	Alters Th1 response to Th2 response during multiple sclerosis
Ciclosporin	Inhibition of calcineurin
Dapsone	Inhibition of folic acid

as milk, meat, eggs, etc. Chemicals with any carcinogenic or teratogenic effects on long-term use or with residual effect should be avoided. Chemical immunomodulators have an advantage of oral administration for large population (Kehrli Jr and Roth 1990; Quinn 1990). Chemical immunomodulators are levamisole, thiabendazole, imuthiol, avridine, isoprinosine, glucan, indomethacin, ascorbic acid derivatives, biostim, and dihydroheptaprenol, etc. (Table 6.6).

6.12.1 Levamisole

Levamisole is a phenylimidathiazole antihelminthic drug and also has immunomodulatory effects on T-lymphocyte and macrophages. The effectiveness of this antihelminthic preparation is variable depending upon dose, timing of administration in relation to disease or stress, and host immunocompetence. It increases the immune activity of cells whose functions are impaired. Levamisole does not affect primary immune response to vaccination or prevent infections by boostering innate immune mechanisms. At high doses, levamisole causes immunosuppression in animals. It enhances phytohemagglutinin (PHA)-stimulated peripheral blood lymphocytes in poultry. Levamisole could not be able to reverse the immunosuppression caused by Marek's disease. It stimulates development of memory T-lymphocytes in pigs. Mammary gland-derived macrophages are also known to be activated by levamisole as determined by increased Fc receptor activity. It increases the blastogenic capacity of bovine lymphocytes in vitro induced by PHA and increases interferon production by mononuclear cells. It has no effect on bovine leukemia virus (BLV) replication or BLV antibody titers in persistently infected sheep or cattle. Weekly administration of levamisole for 6 weeks caused reduction in the incidence of mastitis, fetal death, and endometritis in cattle. Levamisole reduces the incidence of mastitis in dairy cows and this effect is due to the increased level of potentially opsonic antibody in the normal milk, which activates normal paraspecific defense mechanisms. It does not alter the acute and severe inflammatory responses to the presence of pathogens in lacteal secretions (Kehrli Jr and Roth 1990; Mulcatiy and Quinn 1986).

6.12.2 Thiabendazole

Thiabendazole is also an anthelmintic chemical compound, which has been exploited for its immunomodulatory properties. It was found to reverse the dexamethasone-induced and stress-induced immunosuppressions in animals. However, it failed to prevent or overcome dexamethasone-induced suppression of neutrophil functions or antibody production. It enhances blastogenic capacity of lymphocytes in response to mitogens. Stress caused by weaning, vaccination, or castration could not be reversed by thiabendazole (Kehrli Jr and Roth 1990; Lovet and Lundy 1977).

6.12.3 Imuthiol

Imuthiol (sodium diethyldithiocarbamate) restores T-lymphocyte proliferation, IL-2 production, and NK cell activity. However, at higher doses imuthiol significantly reduces lymphocyte blastogenesis and IL-2 production. One of the major disadvantages of low and high doses of imuthiol is the reduction of growth of animals (Kehrli Jr and Roth 1990).

6.12.4 Isoprinosine

Isoprinosine, N,N-dimethylamino-2-propanol, P-acetamidobenzene, and inosine enhance the PHA-induced blastogenic responses of the peripheral blood lymphocytes. It does not restore immune responsiveness of mononuclear cells suppressed by cyclosporine A. This drug was tested for its antiviral effects. It modulates T-helper cells and antigen-presenting macrophages leading to humoral and cell-mediated immune responses. Isoprinosine decreases T-suppressor cells (Kehrli Jr and Roth 1990).

6.12.5 Indomethacin

Indomethacin is an irreversible inhibitor of the cyclooxygenase pathway, which converts arachidonic acid to various other products such as prostacyclin, thromboxane, and other prostaglandin metabolites. It enhances blastogenic responses of peripheral blood lymphocytes by 30% (Kehrli Jr and Roth 1990; Kingston et al. 1984).

6.12.6 Ascorbic Acid Derivatives

Ascorbic acid is known to cause immunopotentiation in animals and man. High dose of ascorbic acid is able to reverse the immunosuppression caused by dexamethasone. It increases the phagocytic activity of neutrophils. One of the derivatives of ascorbic acid and methylfurylbutyrolactones (MFBL) makes T-lymphocytes sensitive to respond to antigenic or polyclonal stimulation to produce more lymphokines such as interleukins and interferons. It also increases antibody production. The derivatives also possess properties related to enhanced neutrophil adherence, chemotaxis, phagocytosis, and intracellular microbial killing (Kehrli Jr and Roth 1990).

6.12.7 Dihydroheptaprenol

Dihydroheptaprenol, a synthetic polyprenol derivative, is known to increase the number of peripheral blood polymorphonuclear leukocytes with increased phagocytic and intracellular killing activities in calves. It also enhances resistance of body against *E. coli* infection in claves.

The imidazole structure is present in several synthetic chemicals that have been reported to regulate the immune mechanisms. Imidazole elevates GMP levels in lymphocytes in vitro and enhances their proliferative response to mitogens or foreign cells. The imidazole ring seems to be one of the active moieties of levamisole responsible for the functional increase of peripheral T-cells and macrophages. Levamisole or its products appear to have thymomimetic properties and one of its metabolites dl-2-oxo-3 [2-mercaptoethyl]-5-phenyl imidazolidine (OMPI) is believed to have a direct effect on the immune system through its oxygen radical scavenging properties. Levamisole and OMPI restore cell functions by inhibition of peroxide formation and accordingly it is proposed that either levamisole or OMPI produces an antioxidant effect by preventing accumulation of peroxides and free radicals that limit metabolism of immunocytes (Kehrli Jr and Roth 1990).

6.13 Adjuvants

Adjuvant is a term derived from the Latin word *adjuvare*, meaning to help or to aid. The term was coined by Ramon in 1920. Adjuvants, defined as any substances, act as a hapten or antigen and enhance the immune responses. Vaccine adjuvants are a group of structurally heterogeneous compounds that may stimulate or modulate the immune system, thereby enhancing the specific immune responses of co-administered antigens without having any specific antigenic effect itself. There are a wide array of adjuvants that are being developed and used, from a variety of sources (Table 6.7). Only aluminum salts have gained wide acceptance in human and veterinary vaccine adjuvants (Dhama et al. 2015). Adjuvants increased the humoral and cell-mediated immune responses by enhancing the antigen presentation, activating dendritic cells, increasing the inflammatory cytokine production, etc (Mulcatiy and Quinn 1986; Quinn 1990).

Immunostimulatory property of aluminum salts is dendritic cell-dependent. Crystals of monosodium urate and aluminum-containing adjuvants activate the differentiation and recruitment of inflammatory monocytes and antibody secretion. Saponin-based adjuvants are obtained from the bark of the quillaja tree and possess immunomodulatory properties and activation of a balanced TH1/TH2 response with cytotoxic CD8+ lymphocyte production. Cationic liposome formulations (CAF) having positive surface charge with lipid bilayer vesicles cannot be adequately immunostimulatory and thus can be administered along with immunostimulators, viz., α, α-trehalose 6, 6′-dibehenate (TDB). TDB (adjuvant CAF01) is a synthetic mycobacterial cord factor analogue and acts as a stabilizing agent on liposomes. Muramyl dipeptide (MDP; synthetic adjuvant) showed pyrogenic and somnogenic activities (Quinn 1990).

A widely used vector is adenovirus serotype (Ad) 5 as an adjuvant. In some instances, vector immunity can lead to a decrease in vaccine efficacy. To avoid pre-existing immunity due to Ad5 vaccination, diverse vaccination strategies are used such as prime-boost approaches and increased vaccine doses. F3 is a high-molecular-weight polysaccharide extract of *Ganoderma lucidum* and has been comprehensively analyzed for adjuvant and immunomodulatory activities both in vitro and in vivo. TLR agonists are commonly used as immunostimulatory agents, for example, imiquimod, an agonist of TLR7, is approved for use against human papillomavirus topically. The most common adjuvants, which are used for veterinary vaccine production, are depicted in Table 6.7.

Adjuvants can be used to enhance the host immune responses against vaccine antigens in many different mechanisms that include:

- Enhance the immunogenicity of weak antigens.
- Increase the duration and speed of the immune responses.
- Modulate avidity as well as specificity, and isotype or subclass distribution of antibodies.
- Enhance strong cell-mediated immunity.
- Stimulate the mucosal immunity.
- Increase the immune responses in immunologically immature (newborn) or senescent and compromised individuals.
- Reduce the dose of antigen or number of immunizations needed for protective immunity to reduce the vaccine costs.
- Help to avoid antigen competition in combination vaccines.
- Increase the total antibody titer or functional titers.
- Induce broader immune response (cross-protection).

Table 6.7 Commonly used adjuvants in veterinary vaccines with immunomodulatory properties

Type		Adjuvant	Mode of action
Depot adjuvants	Aluminum salts	Aluminum phosphate	Slow-release antigen depot
		Aluminum hydroxide	Slow-release antigen depot
		Alum	Activate DAMPs
	Water-in-oil emulsion	Freund's incomplete adjuvant	Slow antigen release depot
Microbial adjuvants		Anaerobic corynebacteria	Macrophage stimulator
		BCG	Macrophage stimulator
		Muramyl dipeptide	Macrophage stimulator
		Bordetella pertussis	Lymphocyte stimulator
		Lipopolysaccharide	Macrophage stimulator
Immune stimulators	Surface active agents	Saponin	Stimulates antigen processing
		Lysolecithin	Stimulates antigen processing
		Pluronic detergents	Stimulates antigen processing
	Complex carbohydrates	Acemannan	Macrophage stimulator
		Glucans	Macrophage stimulator
		Dextran sulfate	Macrophage stimulator
Delivery systems		Liposomes	Stimulates antigen processing
		ISCOMS	Stimulates antigen processing
		Microparticles	Stimulates antigen processing
Mixed adjuvants		Freund's complete adjuvant	Depot plus immune stimulant

6.14 Herbal Products

In Indian ancient literature many herbs are described for strengthening of body and to keep away diseases. "Nakul samhita," the first treatise on the treatment of animals with herbs written about 5000 years B.C., has described many herbs with immunomodulatory properties (Table 6.8). Since time immemorial, reaching back to the distant past of human history, natural ingredients, chiefly herbs, were used extensively for treating various ailments (Singh et al. 2001). In our country, the ancient medicinal system of Ayurveda is a vast repository of knowledge in herbals as well as minerals with medicinal properties. In Ayurveda, the life describes four types of therapeutic approaches, namely, Prakriti Sthapanam (maintenance of health),

Table 6.8 Plants having immunomodulatory properties

Plant	Immunomodulatory action	Clinical application
Acorus calamus (bach)	• Inhibits the proliferation of phytohemagglutinin • Stimulate the human peripheral blood mononuclear cells (PBMCs) • Inhibition of production of nitric oxide (NO), IL-2, and tumor necrosis factor-α (TNF-α) • Downregulation of CD25 expression	Immunosuppressant
Azadirachta indica (Neem)	• Stimulate the phagocytic and antigen-presenting ability of macrophages	Allergic disorders, psoriasis, and anti-leprotic action
Allium sativum	• Augment NK cells • Stimulates T-cells and IL-2 boosts IL-4 and IL-10 production	Inhibit tumor development and treat psoriasis
Aloe vera	• Carboxypeptidase and salicylate showed anti-inflammatory effect	Improves wound healing
	• Acemannan enhances the production of IL-1 and TNF-α from macrophages	Antiretroviral therapy
Ocimum sanctum (tulsi/queen of plants/mother medicine of nature)	• Tulsi leaves are regarded as an "adaptogen" or anti-stress agent • It inhibits tumor development in mice • Aqueous extract of *O. sanctum* showed immunotherapeutic potential	Bovine sub-clinical mastitis and viral encephalitis
Emblica officinalis (amla/aonla)	• Adaptogenic • Improve both cell-mediated and humoral response and help to reduce inflammation and edema	Potent immune suppressant in arthritis
Evolvulus alsinoides	• Causes mild synovial hyperplasia • Decrease in nitric oxide synthase activity of mononuclear phagocytes • Causes immunosuppression	Anti-inflammatory and immunosuppressant like corticosteroids
Panax ginseng	• Saponins and glycosides—causes macrophage migration and antibody plaque-forming cells • Stimulate lymphocytes and cytokines	Immunomodulatory action
Tinospora cordifolia (giloy)	• Increases the number of macrophages and its phagocytic activity • Inhibits myelosuppression induced by cyclophosphamide	Hepatoprotectant, anti-neoplastic, and anti-tuberculosis activities
Withania somnifera (ashwagandha)	• Anti-carcinogenic effects in animal and cell cultures by decreasing the expression of nuclear factor-kappa B and suppressing intercellular tumor necrosis factor • Potentiating apoptotic signaling in cancerous cell lines • Adaptogen or vitalizer	Anti-carcinogenic action

(continued)

6.14 Herbal Products

Table 6.8 (continued)

Plant	Immunomodulatory action	Clinical application
Piper longum (pippali), *Asparagus adscendens* (safed musli), *Terminalia arjuna* (arjun), *Solanum nigrum* (makoy), *Agaricus* sp. (mushroom), *Xanthium strumarium* (chhota gokhru), *Syzygium aromaticum* (clove), *Populus alba* (safeda), *Phyllanthus niruri* (jar-amla), *Andrographis paniculata* (kirayat), *Curcuma longa* (turmeric), *Foeniculum vulgare* (Saunf), *Cichorium intybus* (kasni), and *Curcuma zedoaria* (kali haldi)		Immunomodulatory action

roganastiani chikitsa (cure of disease), naishtiki chikitsa (spiritual therapy), and rasayana chikitsa (herbal product therapy). The rasayana therapy is useful for preventing diseases. The rasayana drugs are endowed with multiple properties like delaying aging, improving mental functions, and preventing diseases (Chauhan 1998c; Chauhan 1998d; Mulcatiy and Quinn 1986).

There are many herbs known to have immunomodulatory properties. Of these, some of them are studied scientifically but most are yet to be scientifically validated. *Tinospora cordifolia, Withania somnifera, Allium sativum, Asparagus racemosus, Emblica officinalis, Piper longum, Terminalia chebula, Boerhavia diffusa, Acorus calamus, Ocimum sanctum, Azadirachta indica, Terminalia arjuna*, etc. are found to be immunostimulant in different models of immunosuppression or infection (Godhwani et al. 1988; Karande et al. 1991; Kuttan 1996; Tiwari et al. 2014; Verma et al. 2020). *Tinospora cordifolia* prevented cyclophosphamide-induced immunosuppression as well as immune response in suppressed mice. These herbs exhibit an array of diverse biological activities such as antistress, adaptogenic, antiaging, and immunomodulation (Karande et al. 1991; Singh et al. 2001).

The extract of *Azadirachta indica* (neem) stimulates phagocytic activity and antigen-presenting ability of macrophages and enhances the mitogenic response of splenocytes to Con-A. Besides, it is also effective against allergic disorders and desensitizes the host to specific allergens limiting the danger of anaphylactic reactions. *Piper longum* (pippali) is found to be effective in the prevention and control of giardiasis in man. *Withania somnifera* is known to positively modulate the immune system of man and animals (Tiwari et al. 2014). *Tinospora cordifolia, Ocimum sanctum, Allium sativum*, and *Emblica officinalis* along with *Withania somnifera* have immunomodulatory properties (Godhwani et al. 1988; Karande et al. 1991; Kuttan 1996; Tiwari et al. 2014; Verma et al. 2020). The herbal preparation (Immuplus containing these four herbs) was found to stimulate the blastogenesis in B- and T-lymphocytes and increases the antibody titers in dogs, poultry, and mice (Chauhan 1999; Chauhan 2001b). Another preparation Immu-21 has been found to increase the phagocytic activity of peritoneal macrophages and microbicidal activity of neutrophils (Table 6.9). *Curcuma longa* is commonly known as turmeric (haldi) and is used in Indian spices. It is considered to have anti-inflammatory properties along with bactericidal effects. *Annona squamosa* (sitaphal)

Table 6.9 Commercial herbal preparation having immunomodulatory activities

Name of preparation	Composition of plants	Clinical application
Immuplus	*Tinospora cordifolia*, *Ocimum sanctum*, *Emblica officinalis*, and *Withania somnifera*	• It stimulates the blastogenic capacity of B- and T-lymphocytes • Increases the antibody titers in dog, poultry, and mice • Widely used for immunomodulatory activities in treating diseases of domestic animals and poultry
Immu-21	*Ocimum sanctum, Emblica officinalis,* and *Withania somnifera*	• Increase the phagocytic activity of peritoneal macrophages
Immusarc	*Withania somnifera* and *Emblica officinalis*	• Helps to achieve optimum immune effectiveness
Septilin	*Balsamodendron mukul, Tinospora cordifolia, Rubia cordifolia, Glycyrrhiza glabra,* and *Emblica officinalis*	• Stimulates phagocytosis by macrophages and polymorphonuclear cells • Stimulates humoral immunity and antibody production

have a high content of tannin in leaves and possess anti-inflammatory properties and contain high levels of vitamin, which helps in healing and enhances immunity. *Terminalia arjuna* is a commonly available plant in Uttarakhand state, which contains arjunic acid, arjunantin, β-stilbesterol, and tannins, and is used for wound and fracture healing with immunopotentiation (Chauhan 1998c; Singh et al. 2001).

The effects of herbs have been seen mainly with their crude preparations: either the aqueous or alcoholic extracts or powders without identification of their active principles. It creates a problem in the quality control of such preparations. However, if the active principle is separated out and used as immunomodulatory preparation, it may not have its natural effect, while in natural preparation, crude extracts of herbs both types of compounds, i.e., for potentiating and inhibiting the immune mechanisms, are present. It is thus important to use only complete plant products as such to maintain homeostasis. It is imminent to decide certain parameters for the quality control in the preparation of these drugs, which can be enforced to meet the standards. The herbal preparations are said to be completely safe as their action on body consists of natural way. However, there are some reports on the presence of pesticide or heavy metal residues in these preparations, which needs further investigation. Scientific validation of herbs or their preparations requires sufficient data to prove their effectiveness and to make them popular in veterinary and medical sciences.

6.15 Vitamins

Vitamins are vital amines and play an important role in the regulation of the host immune defenses (Table 6.10). Vitamin A plays an important role in maintaining the integrity of mucosal surfaces in the respiratory and gastrointestinal tracts and in the regulation of innate and adaptive immune responses (Dhama et al. 2015). Vitamin A and its metabolites like trans retinoic acid and retinol play essential roles in both cell-mediated and humoral immunity. They enhance the phagocytic activity and regulate immune homeostasis via the peripheral induction of regulatory T-cells. Vitamin A deficiency results in decreased phagocytic activity and diminished oxidative burst activity of activated macrophages and NK cells (Dhama et al. 2015). Vitamin A deficiency strongly impairs the humoral immunity and provokes an inflammatory state in the body due to enhanced secretion of TNF-α and IL-12 (Mulcatiy and Quinn 1986; Quinn 1990).

Vitamin D (1,25-dihydroxycholecalciferol) is biologically active and is considered to be an important immunoregulator besides its role in calcium metabolism. Most cells of the immune system (except B-cells) express vitamin D receptors in significant concentrations (Dhama et al. 2015). Vitamin D performs immunomodulatory action by inhibiting the production of inflammatory cytokines and enhancing the oxidative burst activity of macrophages. It also induces the secretion of potent antimicrobial peptides. Deficiency of vitamin D leads to increased autoimmune and inflammatory diseases like multiple sclerosis and chronic rhinitis due to increased production of inflammatory substances. Vitamin D plays an important anti-neoplastic role and is used for anti-cancer immunotherapy. Vitamin D binding protein (DBP) is an essential precursor for macrophage activation and crucial for providing innate defense against cancer.

Vitamin E has a strong lipid-soluble antioxidant activity that scavenges free radicals and can enhance cytokine secretion from naive T-cells. Vitamin E can

Table 6.10 Vitamins and trace minerals having immunomodulatory properties

Vitamins and minerals	Animal	Immunomodulatory action
Vitamin E and selenium	Chicken	Act as immunomodulator in aflatoxicosis
Vitamin D3	Turkey	Act as immunomodulator during stress
Vitamin C	Pigs	Act as growth enhancer in newborn pigs and immunomodulator after weaning
Vitamin C	Cattle	Increased neutrophil oxidative metabolism and antibody-dependent cellular cytotoxicity
Vitamin A	Chicken	Increased innate immunity to enteric parasites
Vitamin E	Chicken	Modulates mucosal immunity
Folic acid	Poultry	Increased biochemical constituents, enhanced generation of total IgG, and exhibition of pleiotropic effects in inflammatory responses
Selenium	Pigs	Increased humoral immune responses

also suppress a variety of inflammatory processes by blocking the activity of transcription factor NF-kB, which is essential for the transcription of pro-inflammatory cytokines. Vitamin E favors the immune response, which is biased towards Th1 immunity.

Vitamin C is a major water-soluble vitamin and performs antioxidant activity by scavenging reactive oxygen species (ROS) generated during the process of phagocytosis by activated immune cells. Supplementation of vitamin C results in enhancement of immune responses. Vitamin C is essential to safeguard the host cells from free radicals produced during the respiratory burst from phagocyte cells. Administration of ascorbic acid enhanced the sensitivity of B-cells to the mitogen and DTH and prevention of T-cell apoptosis. Vitamin C acts as immunomodulator during *Pasteurella monodon* infection (Dhama et al. 2015).

Vitamin B complex deficiency in pregnant animals results in the defective formation of lymphoid organs, especially the thymus and spleen in their progeny. Further, vitamin B complex deficiency leads to reduced number of plasma cells and suppression of lymphocyte proliferation resulting in lowered DTH response. Vitamin B6 is essentially required as a cofactor in the biosynthesis of nucleic acid and proteins; hence, its role in immune function can be appreciated. The deficiency of vitamin B6 favors the Th2-mediated immunity and thus affects the cell-mediated immunity. Folate plays a significant role in protein and nucleic acid synthesis and folate deficiency significantly impairs the immune responses. Folate deficiency alters immune competence and protection against microbes and impairs cell-mediated immunity by decreasing the circulating T-lymphocytes. In *Helicobacter*-associated gastric cancer in mice, folic acid supplementation can be chemopreventive. Vitamin B12 may have an immunomodulatory influence on cell-mediated immunity. Vitamin B12 deficiency may influence the purine and thymidine synthesis and ultimately RNA and DNA synthesis that may lead to alterations in immune responses (Dhama et al. 2015).

6.16 Cow Therapy

Cow therapy consists of five materials (panchgavya) received from Indian Zebu cow including milk, curd, ghee, urine, and dung extract. Panchgavya plays an important role in Ayurveda system of medicine and it has been mentioned in ancient Indian literature that the panchgavya enhances the resistance of body and makes body refractory to infections. A preparation "Kamdhenu Ark" prepared by Govigyan Anusandhan Kendra, Nagpur, from the urine of Indian cows was tested for its immunomodulatory properties in mice (Chauhan et al. 2001). It has been observed that there was an increase in T- and B-lymphocyte blastogenesis and IgG, IgM, and IgA antibody titers in mice (Chauhan 2001a).

Immunomodulation is a very important area of Veterinary and Medical Science, which needs extensive research and development of compounds that can enhance the immunity in fast-changing environmental scenario. It needs utmost care while testing the immunomodulatory properties of herbs or the materials from cow for their stability, effectiveness, duration, effect of temperature, and/or moisture and the pesticide and heavy metal residues present in them (Chauhan 1998e). Besides, one should be cautious about the fungal toxins arising out of poor storage conditions.

References

Chauhan RS (1998a) Alphamethrin induced immunosuppression in calves and its modulation using herbal immunomodulator. Immunol Suppl 1:496

Chauhan RS (1998b) An introduction to immunopathology. G.B. Pant University of Agriculture and Technology, Pantnagar

Chauhan RS (1998c) Herbal immunomodulation: an approach towards eradication of infections. Eijkman Centennial on infections. The Hague, pp 42

Chauhan RS (1998d) Immunomodulators of herbal origin under Indian system of medicine: rationale of their use. In: Chauhan RS (ed) An introduction to immunopathology, pp 279–284

Chauhan RS (1998e) Laboratory manual of immunopathology. G.B. Pant University of Agriculture and Technology, Pantnagar

Chauhan RS (1999) Effect of immuplus on humoral and cell mediated immunity in dogs. J Immunol Immunopathol 1:54–57

Chauhan RS (2001a) Cow therapy: current status and future directions. In: Reforms in concept of rural development in Uttaranchal, Pantnagar. pp 21

Chauhan RS (2001b) Efficacy of herbal immuplus in enhancing humoral and cell mediated immunity. Livestock Int 5:12–18

Chauhan RS, Singh BP, Singhal LK (2001) Immunomodulation with Kamdhenu Ark in mice. J Immunol Immunopathol 3:74–77

Collins FM, Scott MT (1974) Effect of Corynebacterium parvum treatment on the growth of Salmonella enteritis in mice. Infect Immun 9:863–869

Cupps TR, Fanci AS (1982) Corticosteroid-mediated immunoregulation in man. Immunol Rev 65: 133–150

Dantzer R, Kelley KW (1989) Stress and immunity: an integrated view of relationship between the brain and immune system. Life Sci 44:1995–2008

Dhama K, Saminathan M, Jacob SS, Singh M, Karthik K, Amarpal, Tiwari R, Sunkara LT, Malik YS, Singh RK (2015) Effect of immunomodulation and immunomodulatory agents on health with some bioactive principles, modes of action and potent biomedical applications. Int J Pharmacol 11:253–290

Godhwani S, Godwani JL, Vyas DS (1988) Ocimum sanctum- a preliminary study evaluating its immunoregulatory profile in albino rats. J Ethnopharmacol 24:193–198

Karande SA, Thattes UM, Dhanukar SA (1991) Protective effect of Tinospora cordifolia against neutropenia induced by cytotoxic drugs. Indian J Pharmacol 23:34–35

Kehrli ME Jr, Roth JA (1990) Chemical induced immunomodulation in domestic food animals. Adv Vet Sci Comp Med 35:103–119

Kelley KW (1988) Cross talk between the immune and endocrine systems. J Anim Sci 66:2095–2108

Kelley KW, Dantzer R (1990) Neuroendocrine Immune interactions. Adv Vet Sci Comp Med 35: 283–305

Kingston AE, Ivanyl J, Kay JE (1984) The effect of indomethacin on T-lymphocyte stimulation. Immunolog Lett 8:310–305

Kuttan G (1996) Use of Withania somnifera dunal as an adjuvant during radiation therapy. Indian J Exp Biol 34:854–856

Lovet EJ, Lundy J (1977) The effect of thiabendazole in mixed leukocyte culture. Transplantation 24:93–47

Mulcatiy G, Quinn PJ (1986) A review of immunomodulators and their application in veterinary medicine. J Vet Pharmacol Ther 9:119–139

Narnaware YK, Kelly SP, Woo NYS (1998) Stimulation of macrophage phagocytosis and lymphocyte count by exogenous prolactin administration in silver sea bream (Sparus sarba) adapted to hyper- hypo-osmotic salinities. Vet Immunol Immunopathol 61:387–391

Quinn PJ (1990) Mechanism of action of some immunomodulators used in Veterinary Medicine. Adv Vet Sci Comp Med 35:43–99

Singh H, Sharma VK, Chauhan RS (2001) Herbal preparations and biostimulators in tissue repair. Research Bulletin. G.B. Pant University, Pantnagar, p 48

Tiwari R, Chakraborty S, Saminathan M, Dhama K, Singh SV (2014) Ashwagandha (*Withania somnifera*): role in safeguarding health, immunomodulatory effects, combating infections and therapeutic applications: a review. J Biol Sci 14:77–94

Verma M, Saminathan M, Sarah R, Rastogi SK (2020) Immunomodulatory effects of *Allium sativum* (garlic) in poultry: an overview. J Immunol Immunopathol 22:19–24

Immunopathology of Pneumonia in Animals

7

Key Points

1. Phagocytes (neutrophils and macrophages), dendritic cells, T-cells, natural killer T-cells, and epithelial cells lining the alveolar surface and conducting airways are the main components of innate immunity against respiratory infections.
2. Lysozyme, lactoferrin, IgA, IgG, defensins, and antimicrobial peptides are important innate immune molecules against respiratory infections.
3. IgG is the most prevalent immunoglobulin in alveolar fluid and serves as microbial opsonins, complement protein and surfactant-associated protein.
4. Surfactant protein A (SP-A) and SP-D are collectin family members that encourage alveolar macrophages to phagocytose particles.
5. Viruses cause alteration of alveolar macrophage function, suppression of lymphocyte proliferation, induced apoptosis, and modified cytokine and other inflammatory mediator releases result in altered innate and adaptive immune responses.
6. Parainfluenza virus-3, bovine herpesvirus-1 (causes infectious bovine rhinotracheitis), bovine respiratory syncytial virus, and bovine viral diarrhea virus are considered to be the main respiratory viral pathogens of bovine respiratory disease complex.
7. Virulence factors of *M. haemolytica* are capsular polysaccharide, iron-binding proteins, protein adhesins, lipopolysaccharide (LPS), secreted enzymes, ruminant-specific RTX toxin, and leukotoxin (LKT).
8. Majority of *M. haemolytica* infection-related destructive lesions are caused by LPS and LKT. The LPS exhibits a typical endotoxic and pro-inflammatory characteristics.
9. Peste des petits ruminants (PPRV) infection in goats causes classical inflammatory responses characterized by marked increase in the expression of cytokines such as interferon-beta, interferon-gamma, IL-1, IL-4, IL-6, IL-8, IL-10, and IL-12.

10. Histopathologically, porcine reproductive and respiratory syndrome virus causes interstitial pneumonia with thickening of alveolar walls by macrophages and lymphocytes.
11. Recurrent respiratory infections in Arabian horses have been recorded due to selective IgM deficiency.
12. Ataxia-telangiectasia is a disorder associated with IgG deficiency.

7.1 Introduction

Being the largest surface of the body, the alveolar membrane is in constant contact with the outside environment. A diverse array of microorganisms, inorganic and organic particulate materials, are continuously exposed to the lungs. This exposure to pathogens leads to lower respiratory tract infections. Pulmonary immunity determines the outcome of these infections (Table 7.1). To protect against a great diversity of possibly disease-causing pathogens, the host immune system has evolved with a series of diverse mechanisms. Failure of these defenses may lead to development of pneumonia (Table 7.2). Pneumonia is an inflammation of the lungs that can cause mild to severe illness in animals of all ages. It stands among one of the leading causes of mortality due to infection in animals of younger ages worldwide. Those at high risk for pneumonia include the very young, older animals, and animals with underlying health problems or immunosuppression. Predisposing factors weaken the lung defenses and lead to infection with any pathogen including viruses, bacteria, and fungi. Microbes can interfere with different defenses of the respiratory

Table 7.1 Main defense mechanisms of the respiratory system in domestic animals

Regions of the respiratory system	Defense mechanisms
Transitional epithelium of bronchioles	Club cells, antioxidants, lysozyme, and antibodies
Conducting system (nostrils, trachea, and bronchi)	Mucus production, mucociliary clearance, antibodies, and lysozyme
Exchange system (alveoli)	Alveolar and intravascular macrophages, opsonizing antibodies, surfactant, and antioxidants
Cells or secretory products	
Alveolar and intravascular macrophages	Phagocytosis
Ciliated epithelial cells	Expel inhaled microbial pathogens along with mucus
Club (Clara) cells	Production of surfactant and detoxification of xenobiotics
Mucus	Physical barrier and traps microbial pathogens
Surfactant	Increases phagocytosis and safeguards alveolar walls
Lysozyme	Antimicrobial enzyme
Alpha1 (α1)-antitrypsin	Shields against the damaging effects of the proteolytic enzymes generated by phagocytic cells and inhibits Inflammation

7.1 Introduction

Table 7.2 Mechanisms by which viruses and bacteria impair the defense mechanisms of the respiratory tract

- Decreased mucociliary clearance extends bacteria's duration in residence, which is favorable to colonization
- Damaged epithelium hinders the physical removal of germs and mucociliary clearance
- Breakdown of antimicrobial barrier in mucus
- Some pathogenic organisms like *Mycoplasma* spp. cause ciliostasis
- Lung alveolar macrophages and lymphocyte dysfunction
- Hypoxia brought on by lung consolidation reduces phagocytosis
- Infected macrophages fail to release chemotactic factors for other cells
- Lysosomes fail to fuse with phagosome-containing bacteria
- Altered cytokines and secretory products impair phagocytosis of bacteria
- Virus-induced apoptosis of alveolar macrophages
- Altered CD4 and CD8 lymphocytes
- TLRs boost pro-inflammatory responses in virus-infected macrophages

system, allowing two or more microbes to colonize the lungs together when either of the pathogen alone would be unable to survive on their own. The host defense mechanism can be deviated from microbes towards the pathological inflammation due to the involvement of various internal and external factors such as the alteration of the host defense signals. Pathogen-associated molecular patterns (PAMPs) are exogenous signals from microbial invaders which are unique molecules. On the other hand, damage-associated molecular patterns (DAMPs) are endogenous signals consist of molecules released from dead or damaged cells. Pattern-recognition receptors (PRRs) are present on sentinel cells located throughout the body, which recognize the DAMPs and PAMPs (Table 7.3). After recognition, they activate the innate immune responses. The effectiveness and management of this tiered response can be changed by environmental factors, obesity, and aging, which increases pathology and mortality. The inhalants like microbes and environmental particles need to be eliminated quickly by the immune system, as failure to do so can lead to inflammatory responses that result in the swelling that closes the airways or infection results in increased incidence and severity of pneumonia in diverse populations of immunocompromised hosts (Sanders and Crystal 1997).

Before reaching the lungs, most of the viruses that cause bacterial pneumonia replicate in the nasal cavity (Viuff et al. 2002). When calves are experimentally subjected to *Mannheimia haemolytica* and then challenged with either bovine herpesvirus type 1 (BHV-1) or bovine parainfluenza virus type 3 (BPIV-3), more bacteria are found in nasal swabs, quiescent infections are reactivated, and the clinical signs of the infection are more severe (Frank et al. 1989). The viscosity of mucus increases as a result of dehydration. The viscosity of mucus prevents clearance, causing airway blockage, bacterial colonization, and reduced neutrophil migration and bactericidal activity (Matsui et al. 2005). Ciliary dysfunction is a consequence of viral infections in cattle (Yates 1982). Chronic structural changes in the airways such as chronic bronchitis and bronchiectasis can debilitate the

Table 7.3 Recognition of pathogen-associated molecular patterns (PAMPs) by pattern-recognition receptors (PRRs) on sentinel cells located in the body

Receptor	Location	Ligand
Toll-like receptor (TLR)		
TLR1	Cell surface	Triacylated lipoprotein of bacteria
TLR2	Cell surface	Lipoproteins of bacteria, viruses, and parasites
TLR3	Intracellular	dsRNA of viruses
TLR4	Cell surface	Lipopolysaccharide (LPS) of bacteria and viruses
TLR5	Cell surface	Flagellin of bacteria
TLR6	Cell surface	Diacylated lipoprotein of bacteria and viruses
TLR7	Intracellular	ssRNA of viruses and bacteria
TLR8	Intracellular	ssRNA of viruses and bacteria
TLR9	Intracellular	Cytosine-guanosine (CpG) DNA and dsDNA of viruses, bacteria, and protozoa
TLR10	Intracellular	Unknown
TLR 11	Cell surface	Toxoplasma profilin-like molecule
TLR12 and TLR13	Found in mice, not humans	Unknown
Retinoic acid-inducible gene I (RIG-I)-like receptors (RLRs)		
RIG-1	Intracellular	Short dsRNA of RNA viruses
Nucleotide-binding oligomerization domain (NOD)-like receptors (NLRs)		
NOD1	Cytoplasm	Peptidoglycans of bacteria
NOD2	Cytoplasm	Muramyl dipeptide of bacteria
C-type lectin receptors (CLRs)		
Dectins	Cell surface	Glucans of fungi
Others		
Mannose-fucose receptor	Cell surface	Glycoproteins of bacteria
CD14	Cell surface	LPS of bacteria
Peptidoglycan recognition proteins	Cell surface	Peptidoglycans of bacteria
CD1	Cell surface	Glycolipids of bacteria
CD36	Cell surface	Lipoproteins of bacteria
CD48	Cell surface	Fimbria of bacteria

functions of the mucociliary escalator and predispose to pneumonia. Dogs with bronchiectasis frequently develop secondary bacterial infections (Johnson et al. 2016). Secondary pneumonia is associated to congenital abnormalities such as broncho-esophageal defects and fistulas that enable fluid and food to reach the lungs (Kaminen et al. 2014). Foreign bodies in the airways may also cause secondary pneumonia (Cerquetella et al. 2013).

In dogs with a congenital or acquired immunological deficiency, bacterial pneumonia is frequent (Breitschwerdt et al. 1987; Trowald-Wigh et al. 2000). Dogs with immune system problems may exhibit atypical infections with minimal pathogenicity, such as *Pneumocystis carinii* (Kanemoto et al. 2015). Mucociliary clearance is impacted by particles. Particles inhaled by calves and pigs kept in close quarters are probably a factor in the poor air quality they experience. Increased ammonia levels are linked to crowded conditions and poor ventilation, which increases the risk of pneumonia. In mice, prolonged exposure to ammonia results in ciliary dysfunction, nasal epithelial deterioration, and rhinitis (Vogelweid et al. 2011). It also exacerbates the lesions of *Mycoplasma* infection in rats (Broderson et al. 1976). Numerous microorganisms have been shown to obstruct ciliary activity by attaching to cilia and secreting toxins. The pathogenesis of both *Mycoplasma hyopneumoniae* in swine and *Mycoplasma pneumoniae* in mouse models depends on ciliostatic actions. Viruses alter the mucosal surfaces which lead to enhanced adhesion of bacteria to these surfaces. They may lead to erosion of mucosa and colonization of bacteria occurs readily in such areas (Czuprynski 2009). Further, viruses lead to alteration of alveolar macrophage function, suppression of lymphocyte proliferation, induced apoptosis, and modified cytokine, and other inflammatory mediator releases resulted in the modification of innate and adaptive immune responses (Srikumaran et al. 2007). Inflammatory and immunosuppressive reactions to viruses may also increase the expression of molecules that bacteria may utilize as receptors (Peltola and McCullers 2004).

7.2 Ruminants

In terms of morbidity and mortality in dairy calves, bacterial pneumonia is second only to diarrheal illnesses. Parainfluenza virus-3 (PI-3), bovine herpesvirus-1 [BHV-1 causing infectious bovine rhinotracheitis (IBR)], and bovine respiratory syncytial virus (BRSV) are considered to be the main respiratory pathogens (Lopez 2007). Bovine coronavirus (BCV) is a newly recognized agent to cause pneumonia in young calves (Caswell et al. 2012). These viruses help to create an environment in the respiratory system that is conducive to the colonization and reproduction of a variety of pathogenic bacteria that cause pneumonia (Dabo et al. 2007; Rice et al. 2007; Confer 2009). The bacterial pathogens *Mycoplasma capricolum* subspecies *capripneumoniae* (formerly *Mycoplasma* strain F38) are the direct causes of respiratory disease in cattle, sheep, and goat (Figs. 7.1 and 7.2), *Mycobacterium bovis* (Figs. 7.3 and 7.4), *Mannheimia haemolytica* (Figs. 7.5 and 7.6), *Bibersteinia trehalosi*, *Histophilus somni*, *Pasteurella multocida*, *Mycoplasma bovis*, and *Trueperella* (formerly *Arcanobacterium*) *pyogenes* (Tables 7.4 and 7.5). Other infectious agents—including *Dictyocaulus viviparus*—cause pneumonia in cattle. BRSV infection can also be directly associated with fatal pneumonic lesions in adult cattle (Ames 1993). One of the pathogens causing the bovine respiratory disease (BRD) complex, also known as shipping fever, is the BHV-1. The respiratory form of IBR is associated with affection of upper respiratory tract; mainly, high death rate might sometimes rise as a result of a subsequent bacterial or viral infections. Animals may display symptoms of pneumonitis and bronchitis (Nandi et al. 2009). The widespread prevalence of IBR (BHV-1) in India and the association of the disease with respiratory and genital tract infections were studied (Kollannur et al. 2014). The

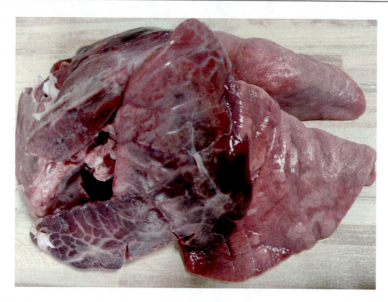

Fig. 7.1 Contagious caprine pleuropneumonia (CCPP): bilateral fibrinous pleuropneumonia, consolidation, and marbling of lungs due to marked thickening of interlobular septa with fibrin deposition

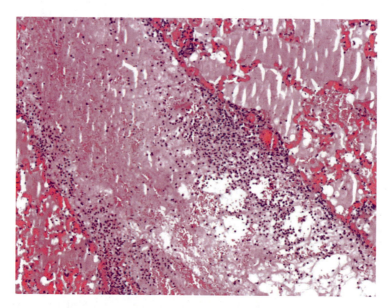

Fig. 7.2 Contagious caprine pleuropneumonia (CCPP): lungs showed marked thickening of interlobular septa due to hemorrhages, edematous serous fluid, fibrin deposition, and cellular infiltration. Alveoli are filled with protein-rich eosinophilic edematous fluid. H&E ×100

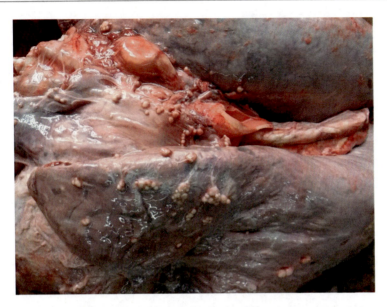

Fig. 7.3 Tuberculous bronchopneumonia in a buffalo: numerous variable-sized pearly tubercle nodules on dorsal surfaces of diaphragmatic lobes of lungs and enlarged mediastinal lymph nodes

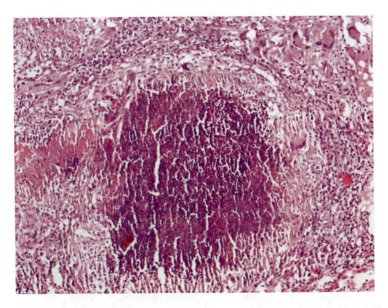

Fig. 7.4 Tuberculous bronchopneumonia: central area of caseous necrosis with calcification, surrounded by epithelioid cells, Langhans-type multinucleated giant cells, lymphocytes, and plasma cells with a fibrous capsule. H&E ×100

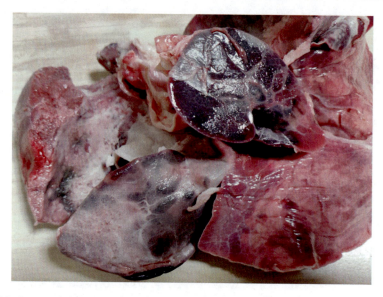

Fig. 7.5 Pneumonia in goat caused by *Mannheimia haemolytica*: congestion, marked hepatization, consolidation, and pneumonia of lungs with fibrin deposition and edema

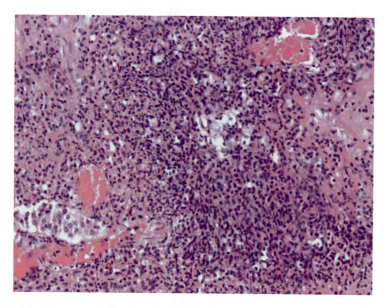

Fig. 7.6 Bronchopneumonia in goat caused by *Mannheimia haemolytica*: necrosis and infiltration of typical elongated and basophilic degenerated neutrophils known as oat cells with fibrin deposition and congestion of inter-alveolar blood vessels. H&E ×200

Table 7.4 Etiology of pneumonia in domestic animals

Disease	Etiologic agent
Cattle	
Pneumonic pasteurellosis (shipping fever pneumonia)	• *Mannheimia haemolytica* serotype A1 and A6 • *Pasteurella multocida* serotype A3
Contagious bovine pleuropneumonia (CBPP)/lung sickness	• *Mycoplasma mycoides* subsp. *mycoides* (small colony)
Mycoplasma bovis pneumonia associated with polyarthritis and mastitis	• *Mycoplasma bovis*
Enzootic pneumonia of calves	• *Major pathogen:* – Bovine respiratory syncytial virus (BRSV) – Bovine coronavirus (BoCV) – Parainfluenza-3 (PI-3) virus • *Less frequently:* – Bovine herpesvirus-1 (BHV-1) – *Mycoplasma bovis* • *Secondary opportunistic bacterial pathogens:* – *Pasteurella multocida* – *Mannheimia haemolytica*
Infectious bovine rhinotracheitis (red nose)	Bovine herpesvirus-1 subtypes: • BHV-1.1—Respiratory form • BHV-1.2a and 1.2b—Genital form • BHV-1.3 (renamed BHV-5)—Encephalitic form
Bovine virus diarrhea	• Bovine virus diarrhea virus (BVDV); Genus—*Pestivirus*; Family—*Flaviviridae*
Lungworm infestation	• Nematode *Dictyocaulus viviparous*.
Atypical interstitial pneumonia/acute bovine respiratory distress syndrome/acute pulmonary emphysema and edema	• D,L-tryptophan in forage • Inhalation of toxic gases and fumes • Hypersensitivity to molds • Mycotoxicosis • Plant poisonings or feed supplemented with melengestrol acetate
Pneumonia	• Bovine adenovirus (BAV) • *Histophilus somni* (formerly *Haemophilus somnus*) • *Mycoplasma bovirhinis* • *Mycoplasma dispar* • *Ureaplasma diversum*
Sheep and goat	
Contagious caprine pleuropneumonia (CCPP)	• *Mycoplasma capricolum* subsp. *capripneumoniae*
Chronic enzootic pneumonia of sheep/chronic non-progressive atypical pneumonia/summer pneumonia/proliferative exudative pneumonia	Multifactorial: • *Mycoplasma ovipneumoniae* • Viruses • Secondary bacterial infections
Ovine progressive pneumonia/maedi/maedi-visna	• Ovine retroviruses; Genus—*Lentivirus*; Family—*Retroviridae*
Ovine pulmonary adenocarcinoma/Jaagsiekte/ovine pulmonary adenomatosis	• • Jaagsiekte sheep retrovirus; Genus—*Betaretrovirus*; Family—*Retroviridae*

(continued)

Table 7.4 (continued)

Disease	Etiologic agent
Bluetongue	• Bluetongue virus; Genus—*Orbivirus*; Family—*Reoviridae*.
Peste des petits ruminants (PPR)	• Peste des petits ruminants virus (PPRV); Genus—*Morbillivirus*; Family—*Paramyxoviridae*
Nasal bots infestation of sheep and goats	• *Oestrus ovis*
Lungworm infestation in sheep and goats	• *Dictyocaulus filaria* • *Muellerius capillaris* • *Protostrongylus rufescens*
Equine	
Equine pleuropneumonia/equine pleuritis/equine pleurisy	Polymicrobial combination: • *Streptococcus equi* var. *Zooepidemicus* • *Actinobacillus* sp. • *Pasteurella* sp. • Enterobacteriaceae • Anaerobic bacteria—*Bacillus fragilis* • *Mycoplasma felis*
Acute broncho-interstitial pneumonia in foals	• Equine influenza virus • *Rhodococcus equi* • Equine herpesvirus-2 • Equine arteritis virus • *Pneumocystis carinii*
Interstitial pneumonia in adult horses	• Hendra virus • Equine influenza virus • Equine infectious anemia • *Rhodococcus equi* • *Aspergillus* sp., *Cryptococcus* sp., *Histoplasma* sp., *Pneumocystis carinii* • *Parascaris equorum* • *Dictyocaulus arnfieldi* • Intoxication with perilla ketone derived from *Perilla frutescens*—Acute restrictive lung disease of horses • Ingestion of *Eupatorium* sp.—Interstitial pneumonia in horses • Ingestion of *Crotalaria* spp.—Interstitial pneumonia in donkeys • Silicosis—Interstitial pneumonia in horses.
Rhodococcus equi pneumonia of foals	• Virulent strains of *Rhodococcus equi* (*Rhodococcus hoagie/Prescottella equi*)
Strangles	• *Streptococcus equi* subsp. *equi*
Glanders	• *Burkholderia mallei*
Equine influenza	• Influenza virus H3N8
Equine viral rhinopneumonitis	• Equid alphaherpesvirus 1 (formerly equine herpesvirus-1 (EHV-1)] • Equine herpesvirus-4 (EHV-4)
Pulmonary and systemic aspergillosis	• *Aspergillus* spp.
Rhinosporidiosis	• *Rhinosporidium seeberi*

(continued)

Table 7.4 (continued)

Disease	Etiologic agent
Lungworm in horses	• *Dictyocaulus arnfieldi*
Equine pneumonia	• Equine hendra virus infection
Swine	
Pleuropneumonia of pigs/fibrohemorrhagic and necrotizing pleuropneumonia	• *Actinobacillus pleuropneumoniae* (formerly known as *Haemophilus pleuropneumoniae*) • *Actinobacillus suis* • *A. porcitonsillarum*—completely non-pathogenic species
Porcine respiratory disease complex (PRDC) and mycoplasmal pneumonia of pigs	• *Mycoplasma hyopneumoniae* • Porcine reproductive and respiratory syndrome (PRRS) virus • Porcine circovirus type 2 (PCV2) • Swine influenza virus (SIV) • Secondary bacterial agents: • *Pasteurella multocida* • *Actinobacillus pleuropneumoniae* (APP) • *Haemophilus parasuis* (HPS) • *E. coli, Klebsiella, Trueperella pyogenes, Bordetella bronchiseptica, Streptococci* (alpha-hemolytic), and *Staphylococci* • *Actinomyces hyovaginalis*
Inclusion-body rhinitis/generalized cytomegalic inclusion-body disease of swine	• Porcine cytomegalic virus; Genus: *Cytomegalovirus*; Family: *Herpesviridae*; Subfamily: *Betaherpesvirinae*
Swine influenza	• Influenza A virus subtypes H1N1, H1N2, and H3N2; Family: *Orthomyxoviridae*
Lungworm in pigs	• *Metastrongylus apri (M. elongatus)* • *Metastrongylus salmi* • *Metastrongylus pudendotectus*
Pneumonia in pigs	• Porcine respiratory coronavirus
Dogs and cats	
Bacterial bronchopneumonia	• *Bordetella bronchiseptica* • *Streptococcus* spp. • *Pasteurella* spp. • *Staphylococcus* spp. • *Escherichia coli*

relative pathogenicity and lesions that are characteristic of a particular bacterial infection are caused by distinct virulence factors that are present in various bacterial species. Capsular polysaccharide, iron-binding proteins, protein adhesins, lipopolysaccharide (LPS), secreted enzymes, ruminant-specific RTX toxin, and leukotoxin (LKT) are the virulence factors of *M. haemolytica* (Rice et al. 2007). The majority of *M. haemolytica* infection-related destructive lesions are caused by LPS and LKT. The LPS of *M. haemolytica* exhibits a typical endotoxic and pro-inflammatory characteristics and interacts with LKT to increase the development of LKT receptors. Bovine leukocytes undergo a variety of alterations as a

Table 7.5 Different types of pneumonia and their etiological agents in domestic animals

Type of pneumonia	Etiological agents
Bronchopneumonia	• *Streptococcus pneumonia* • *Streptococcus suis* • *Mannheimia haemolytica* • *Pasteurella multocida* • *Bordetella bronchiseptica* • *Histophilus somni* • *Haemophilus parasuis* • *Rhodococcus equi* • *Staphylococcus* spp. • *Escherichia coli* • *Actinobacillus pleuropneumoniae* • *Actinobacillus suis* • *Klebsiella* spp.
Suppurative bronchopneumonia	• *Bordetella bronchiseptica* • *Pasteurella multocida* • *Trueperella (Arcanobacterium) pyogenes* • *Escherichia coli* • *Streptococcus* spp. • *Mycoplasma* spp.
Chronic suppurative bronchopneumonia	• *Trueperella pyogenes* in cattle
Fibrinous bronchopneumonia	• *Mannheimia (Pasteurella) haemolytica* • *Histophilus somni* • *Actinobacillus pleuropneumoniae* • *Mycoplasma bovis* • *Mycoplasma mycoides* ssp. *mycoides small colony type*
Fulminating hemorrhagic bronchopneumonia	• *Bacillus anthracis*
Interstitial pneumonia	• *Ascaris suum* • Endotheliotropic viruses—Canine adenovirus and classical swine fever • PRRS virus • Influenza virus
Acute interstitial pneumonia	• Equine and porcine influenza virus
Chronic interstitial pneumonia	• Ovine retroviruses • Pneumoconioses (silicosis and asbestosis) • Paraquat toxicity • Extrinsic allergic alveolitis (farmer's lung)
Bronchointerstitial pneumonia	• Bovine respiratory syncytial virus • Canine distemper virus • Influenza A virus in pigs and horses
Embolic pneumonia	• *Trueperella pyogenes* in cattle • *Fusobacterium necrophorum* in cattle and pigs • *Erysipelothrix rhusiopathiae* in pigs, cattle, and dogs • *Streptococcus suis* in pigs • *Staphylococcus aureus* in dogs • *Streptococcus equi* in horses
Granulomatous pneumonia	• Coccidioidomycosis—*Coccidioides immitis* • Cryptococcosis—*Cryptococcus neoformans* and

(continued)

Table 7.5 (continued)

Type of pneumonia	Etiological agents
	Cryptococcus gattii • Blastomycosis—*Blastomyces dermatitidis* • Histoplasmosis—*Histoplasma capsulatum* • Filamentous fungi—*Aspergillus* spp. or *Mucor* spp. • *Mycobacterium bovis* • *Rhodococcus equi* in horses • Aberrant parasites—*Fasciola hepatica* in cattle • Feline infectious peritonitis (FIP)
Lobar pneumonia	• *M. haemolytica* in cattle • *Actinobacillus pleuropneumoniae* in swine

result of LKT, including apoptosis, necrosis, membrane pore development, and the production of pro-inflammatory cytokines, free radicals, and cellular proteases (Confer et al. 1995). *N*-acetyl-D-glucosamine, a specific glycoprotein adhesin, aids in tracheal epithelial cell adhesion and activates the oxidative burst of bovine neutrophils. Fibrinogen-binding proteins have been identified (McNeil et al. 2002).

7.3 Mycoplasmal Diseases

Contagious bovine pleuropneumonia (CBPP) is an acute lobar pneumonia, which develops after localization of organisms in lungs from septicemia caused by *Mycoplasma mycoides* subsp. *mycoides* (Vegad and Katiyar 2015). *Mycoplasma bovis* primarily causes chronic pneumonic lesions and a significant etiologic factor in bovine respiratory infection. *Mycoplasma bovis* associated granulomatous pneumonia was observed in an adult cow characterized by caseous necrosis, fibrosis, and leucocytic infiltrations containing epithelioid cells, lymphocytes, plasma cells, macrophages, and Langhans-type giant cells (Lather et al. 2017). Lower respiratory tract infections are most common infectious diseases of sheep and goats and continue to be the leading cause of death. Gram-negative organisms such as *E. coli* and *Klebsiella* have been associated with purulent pneumonia. These organisms were found associated with interstitial pneumonia (Galav et al. 2017). Contagious caprine pleuropneumonia (CCPP) is a respiratory disease of goats similar to CBPP of cattle (Figs. 7.1 and 7.2). The etiological agent for this disease is *Mycoplasma mycoides* subsp. *capri*. *Mycoplasma ovipneumoniae*, which is a pathogen of sheep and goats associated with respiratory disease. *M. ovipneumoniae* has been reported in wildlife such as moose, mule deer, and caribou and its emergence has been observed in deer (Highland et al. 2018).

7.4 Peste des Petits Ruminants (PPR)

In India, PPR was first diagnosed in goats of Tamil Nadu (Shaila et al. 1989, 1996). Histopathology of lungs revealed pneumonic changes with infiltration of mononuclear cells in interstitial tissues. Infected animals usually develop acute pulmonary congestion and edema and die within a week. On the other hand, certain animals may experience a long-lasting, chronic illness that is characterized by giant cell pneumonia and may even be accompanied by bronchopneumonia. Pneumonia in goats caused by PPRV is characterized by multinucleated giant cells in alveoli with infiltration of mononuclear cells especially lymphocytes. Alveolar lumen contained infiltration of mononuclear cells especially alveolar macrophages with transformation of type-I pneumocytes into type-II penumocytes (Figs. 7.7a, b). A classical inflammatory response brought on by PPRV infection in goats is marked by increased expression of cytokines such as interferon-beta (IFN-beta), interferon-gamma (IFN-gamma), interleukin-1 (IL-1), IL-4, IL-6, IL-8, IL-10, and IL-12 (Baron et al. 2014; Wani et al. 2018). Immunosuppression is brought on by the severe harm that the *Morbillivirus* infection causes to the lymphoid organs. Immunosuppression and infection levels in lymphoid tissues and peripheral blood are directly related. Inhibition of IFN production, altered cytokine responses, suppression of the inflammatory responses, direct infection and subsequent leucopenia, inhibition of immunoglobulin synthesis (due to loss of B-cells), and cell cycle arrest following direct contact with viral glycoproteins can result in immunosuppression (Schneider-Schaulies et al. 2001; Wani et al. 2018).

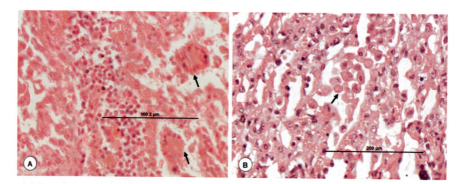

Fig. 7.7 Pneumonia in goat caused by peste des petits ruminants virus (PPRV): (**a**) Alveoli contained multinucleated giant cells (arrow) with infiltration of mononuclear cells especially lymphocytes. H&E ×400. (**b**) Alveolar lumen contained infiltration of mononuclear cells especially alveolar macrophages (arrow) with transformation of type-I pneumocytes into type-II pneumocytes. H&E ×200

7.5 Chlamydiosis

Chlamydiosis was probably first reported in India in sheep and goats by Jain et al. (1975). Asrani et al. (1996) conducted a comparative pathological study of chlamydial pneumonia among domestic animals in Himachal Pradesh. Occurrence of chlamydial pneumonia among sheep has been reported by several workers in India (Kharole 1973; Purohit and Paul Gupta 1980).

7.6 Parainfluenza-3

Parainfluenza-3 infects cattle, sheep, pigs and cats, and causes interstitial pneumonia. There is formation of multinucleated cells with both intranuclear and cytoplasmic inclusions. The bovine and ovine parainfluenza-3 predisposes to other respiratory pathogens such as *Pasteurella haemolytica*.

7.7 Equines

Equine influenza is an infectious respiratory disease caused by type A influenza virus. Death has been reported in young foals from a viral pneumonitis or from secondary pneumonia manifested as bronchopneumonia. Horses with pleuropneumonia often develop mixed anaerobic-aerobic infections and polymicrobial diseases. *Streptococcus equi* subsp. *zooepidemicus*, *Escherichia coli*, *Actinobacillus* spp., *Klebsiella* spp., *Enterobacter* spp., *Staphylococcus aureus*, and *Pasteurella* spp. are the most prevalent aerobic microorganisms (Tables 7.4 and 7.5). About 40–70% of horses with pleuropneumonia have anaerobic bacteria. The most prevalent bacteria are *Bacteroides* spp., *Clostridium* spp., *Peptostreptococcus* spp., and *Fusobacterium* spp.; however, *Mycoplasma felis* and Nocardial agents have been isolated from pleural effusions. Bacterial infections are typically the cause of pleural infections in horses.

7.8 Swine

One of the most prevalent respiratory conditions affecting pigs worldwide is swine enzootic pneumonia (SEP), which is caused by *Mycoplasma hyopneumoniae*. A common illness syndrome that is mainly caused by *Mycoplasma hyopneumoniae* is commonly referred to as "viral pneumonia" and "enzootic pneumonia". About 30–80% of the slaughtered pigs in most of pig farms showed pneumonic lesions linked with mycoplasmal infection of lungs. If pathogens such as influenza virus, porcine reproductive and respiratory syndrome (PRRS) virus, *Mycoplasma hyopneumoniae*, or virulent strain of *Actinobacillus pleuropneumoniae* enter a susceptible herd for the first time, severe outbreaks may occur in sows (Tables 7.4 and 7.5). Pleuropneumonia is a serious respiratory illness that usually affects young pigs under 6 months old. *Actinobacillus pleuropneumoniae* pathogen causes characteristic lesions like severe fibrinonecrotic and hemorrhagic pneumonia with associated fibrinous pleuritis.

7.9 Porcine Reproductive and Respiratory Syndrome (PRRS)

It is an important viral disease of pigs confronting the pig industry worldwide. Severe fever, high morbidity, and mortality are the main features of highly pathogenic PRRS, which first appeared in China in 2006. It is characterized by respiratory illness and reproductive failure in pigs (Rossow 1998). The consistent microscopic feature is interstitial pneumonia. This virus is a unique PRRSV strain that has a discontinuous deletion in non-structural protein (Nsp2) that spans 30 amino acids (Li et al. 2007; Tong et al. 2007). In India, first outbreak was reported in 2013 in pigs in Mizoram and following subsequent highly pathogenic PRRS outbreaks in 2015 and 2016 (Rajkhowa et al. 2016; Gogoi et al. 2017). In India, during an outbreak of PRRS, histopathologically, interstitial pneumonia was the most characteristic lesion observed in lungs besides thickening of alveolar walls by macrophages and lymphocytes infiltration (Shivashankar et al. 2017). In a study conducted on piglets, moderate to severe interstitial pneumonia was observed as a major microscopic finding along with lymphoid depletion in tonsils and lymph nodes, and thymic atrophy (Senthilkumar et al. 2017).

7.10 Swine Influenza

The type A influenza virus infection that causes swine flu, which is an acute respiratory illness and highly contagious. Swine influenza virus (SIV) is an orthomyxovirus that belongs to influenza A group with hemagglutinating antigen H1 and neuraminidase antigen N1 (H1N1). Recently, new subtypes of SIV have been reported (H2N3, H3N2, and H1N2). It is primarily a disease of the upper respiratory tract. However, pneumonia may occur due to drainage of copious exudate from the bronchi. Secondary pneumonia due to *Pasteurella multocida* occurs in some cases. The replication of pseudorabies virus, *Haemophilus parasuis*, *Actinobacillus pleuropneumoniae*, and *Mycoplasma hyopneumoniae* may be favored by the typical type A virus infection with weak virulence, which may complicate the outbreaks. In swine, rapid and substantial production of tumor necrosis factor (TNF), IL-1, and interferon-alpha (IFN-α) in the lungs are highly correlated with acute influenza (van Reeth et al. 1999). The lack of NF-kB activation may be the cause of the PRRSV infection's weak or subclinical respiratory involvement.

7.11 Other Diseases

Suppurative bronchopneumonia with multiple abscesses in lungs was found in a 5-month-old swine, which was found associated with Gram-positive bacilli and *Proteus* spp. (Sethi et al. 2017).

7.12 Small Animals

Adenovirus types 1 and 2, parainfluenza virus, feline calicivirus, and canine distemper virus all induce lesions in the distal airways and increase the risk of subsequent bacterial invasion of the lungs. The first report of bacterial pneumonia in dogs co-infected with canine distemper or canine infectious respiratory disease (CIRD) pathogens was described by Batey and Smits (1976). Gram-negative *Escherichia coli* and *Pasteurella* spp. are the most frequently isolated bacteria, followed by Gram-positive cocci *Streptococcus* spp. and *Staphylococcus* spp. (Thayer and Robinson 1984; Jameson et al. 1995; Angus et al. 1997). In the USA, *E. coli* which caused lethal hemorrhagic pneumonia in dogs (Breitschwerdt et al. 2005). A virulence factor known as cytotoxic necrotizing factor-1 (CNF-1), which is widely known in people with extraintestinal pathogenic *E. coli* (ExPEC) infections and present in the extraintestinal *E. coli* strain that was identified in these instances (Breitschwerdt et al. 2005). Other Gram-negative aerobic bacteria are *Pseudomonas* spp., *Klebsiella* spp., *Enterobacter* spp., and *Bordetella bronchiseptica*. The canine infectious respiratory disease (CIRD) complex is mostly caused by the bacterial pathogens *Bordetella bronchiseptica*, *Mycoplasma* spp., and *Streptococcus equi* sp. *zooepidemicus (Str. zooepidemicus)*. Additionally, these have only been seen in canines with pneumonia, especially when the canines are housed in environments with high infection pressure (Radhakrishnan et al. 2007; Zeugswetter et al. 2007; Priestnall and Erles 2011). Pneumonia may develop from parasitic invasion of the bronchi by *Filaroides*, *Aelurostrongylus*, or *Paragonimus* spp. (Dharanesha et al. 2019). It is uncommon to see *Toxoplasma gondii* or *Pneumocystis jirovecii* involved in protozoan infections and tuberculous pneumonia. Dogs more frequently affected than cats. There are more cases of mycotic granulomatous pneumonia in dogs than cats. Cryptococcal pneumonia in cats has been documented, which causes bronchitis and bronchoalveolar pneumonia in the cranial ventral regions of lungs (Bryson 1993).

Canine distemper is a highly contagious disease caused by *Morbillivirus* and replicates initially in the respiratory epithelium and alveolar macrophages before spreading to the bronchial lymph nodes. Main lesions in lungs are purulent bronchopneumonia with infiltration of neutrophils in bronchi and alveoli. Sometimes multinucleated giant cells are found in bronchial and alveolar lumen. The most recent novel CIRD virus, the canine pneumovirus (CnPnV), was first identified in dogs suffering from respiratory illness in two American animal shelters in 2010. The symptoms of CIRD might range from a dry cough and nasal discharge to bronchopneumonia.

Atypical bacteria like *Nocardia asteroides* and *Mycobacteria* spp. have been documented to produce isolated episodes of bacterial pneumonia (Irwin et al. 2000; Leissinger et al. 2015). Severe secondary bacterial pneumonia has been reported in conjunction with adenoviral infections (Damian et al. 2005; Chvala et al. 2007). *Bordetella bronchiseptica* is capable of causing respiratory disease without initiating viral infection and is a primary respiratory pathogen in dogs (Bemis et al. 1977). Simultaneous infections with *B. bronchiseptica* and other pathogens such as canine adenovirus type 2 (CAV-2), canine respiratory coronavirus (CRCoV), canine parainfluenza virus (CPIV), canine herpesvirus (CHV), and *Mycoplasma* spp. are common (Wagener et al. 1984; Schulz et al. 2014). Puppies younger than a year old have been reported to suffer with severe *B. bronchiseptica* infection that results in bronchopneumonia (Radhakrishnan et al. 2007).

In dogs with CIRD, bacterial pneumonia, and non-infectious respiratory disorders, *Mycoplasma* spp. have been isolated from the lower respiratory tract (Chalker et al. 2004; Zeugswetter et al. 2007). *Mycoplasma* spp. infections in dogs typically have a benign course, although an epidemic outbreak of *M. cynos* infection caused fatal bronchopneumonia in puppies (Zeugswetter et al. 2007). Canine parainfluenza-2 is associated with kennel cough syndrome and bronchopneumonia is one of the manifestations along with other clinical signs.

7.13 Immunity to Pneumonia

Local sensor cells initially identify the invaders, initiating cell-intrinsic defensive responses that neutralize the pathogen. Then, chemoattractants are secreted to activate rapid response cells like neutrophils and release first-order cytokines. Natural killer (NK) cells, innate lymphoid cells (ILCs), innate-like lymphocytes, and tissue-resident memory (TRM) T-cells are distinct tissue-resident lymphocytes that react with cytokines of the first order. These lymphocytes transform first-order cytokine signals into second-order cytokines that recruit and activate effector cells that initiate pathogen elimination and tissue repair. Effector mechanisms that may be able to control the infection, inhibit the triggering of additional immune responses, and restrict the inflammatory damage.

As the specific sensors and effector mechanisms differ but the fundamental layered response is applicable to both type 1 immune responses and type 2 immune responses, it is possible to observe an evolving pattern of immune regulation common to a wide range of pathogens (Reynolds 1997). The characteristics of the pathogen and the host, such as amount of the inoculum, characteristics of its surface, its virulence, and the capacity of alveolar macrophages to eliminate the ingested pathogens, affect the outcome of infection (Toews 1994). Two categories can be used to categorize the host response in pneumonia: those that quantify the degree of microbial invasion and those that shed light on the host's cellular reactions.

The number of organisms in the lung represents the balance between the multiplication of the organism and its clearance by the host. The respiratory tract has potential to fight against infections without damaging the lung tissue or compromising the pulmonary physiology. The imminent exposures and severity of infections have put huge selective pressures on pulmonary adaptation to infection. Resident respiratory tract defenses, such as the mucociliary escalator and alveolar macrophages, are capable of eliminating the less dangerous microorganisms in small numbers. However, innate immunity must be activated in order to eliminate the pathogenic or abundant microorganisms.

The main host defensive mechanism in the majority of acute pneumonia cases is innate immunity. However, specialized immunity, including cell-mediated and antibody-mediated mechanisms, are necessary for defense against some species, including mycobacteria and endemic fungi. Pulmonary immunity stimulates a complex network of pro- and anti-inflammatory messenger chemicals to coordinate responses against microorganisms in the lungs. The best studied messenger molecules are the cytokines. Cytokines have a key role in the initial response to a pathogen, including the influx of immune cells to the site of infection, activation of recruited or local cells for phagocytosis of the pathogen, and lung repair during the resolution of acute injury. Numerous cytokines have pleiotropic effects and may be involved in a variety of innate immune response components.

Nuclear factor-kappa-B (NF-κB), a transcription factor, controls the activation of several genes, including those that govern the body's inflammatory and immunological responses. It regulates genes responsible for both innate and adaptive immune responses. It balances the early innate immune responses against microorganisms in the lungs by acting as a molecular fulcrum (Quinton and Mizgerd 2011). Additionally, it shields cells from some impulses that would otherwise make them self-destruct. A protective immuno-inflammatory response to *Pseudomonas aeruginosa* in mice requires NF-kB signaling (Chen et al. 2008).

Animal studies showed that NF-κB signaling disruptions, especially NF-κB RelA mutations (Quinton et al. 2007), intracellular signaling pathways that stimulate NF-κB (Skerrett et al. 2004), or receptor complexes activating these pathways (Jones et al. 2005), can compromise host defenses and predispose the lungs to infections. Conversely, animal models in which NF-κB activity is exaggerated reveal that this transcriptional activity is sufficient to induce or exacerbate lung injury (Mizgerd 2008).

The myeloid differentiation primary response 88 (MyD88), a protein that functions as an adapter, connects proteins that receive signals from the outside of the cell with proteins that convey information inside the cell. The activation of immunological pathways downstream of TLRs and the IL-1 receptor depends on signaling through MyD88. The MyD88 adaptor protein promotes signaling molecules that activate nuclear factor-kappa-B in response to signals from these receptors. According to reports, MyD88 plays a protective role in preventing the growth of fungi such as *Candida albicans*, *Aspergillus fumigatus*, *Cryptococcus neoformans*, and *Paracoccidioides brasiliensis* (Villamon et al. 2004; Biondo et al. 2005; Bretz et al. 2008). For effective alveolar epithelial cell (AEC) and alveolar macrophage (AM) cytokine responses to pneumocystis or pneumocystis cell wall components, MyD88-dependent signaling is necessary (Bello-Irizarry et al. 2012). Mice with a MyD88 deficiency are more vulnerable to bacterial infections, especially Gram-negative infection (Skerrett et al. 2004). MyD88 signaling is necessary for host defense during pneumonia in both hematopoietic and non-hematopoietic cells, according to research using mouse bone marrow chimeras (Hajjar et al. 2005), but it might depend on the specific pathogen. During active *Pneumocystis carinii* pneumonia (PcP) in CD4-depleted mice, Pneumocystis infection must be suppressed by MyD88 signaling in hematopoietic cells. The MyD88 signaling in the hematopoietic compartment was required for control of *Legionella pneumophila* (Archer et al. 2010). The expression of MyD88 in hematopoietic and resident cells aids in the suppression of *Klebsiella pneumoniae* infection. *Pseudomonas aeruginosa* growth was significantly controlled by locally present non-hematopoietic cells (Hajjar et al. 2005; van Lieshout et al. 2012).

7.14 Innate Immunity

Innate immunity has a primary role in lung antimicrobial defenses. Lung adaptive immunity is driven by the innate immune system, which also interacts with the apoptotic pathway and signaling pathways brought on by mechanical stretch. The diversity of innate immune responses may account for the variation in patient reactions to bacterial, fungal, and viral infections of the lungs. Phagocytes (neutrophils and macrophages), dendritic cells (DCs), T-cells, natural killer T (NKT) cells, and epithelial cells lining the alveolar surface and conducting airways are the main components of innate immunity against respiratory infections. The first responders to invading pathogens are the airway epithelial cells. They provide barrier function and a vast array of receptors, act as innate sensors to secrete antimicrobial compounds as first-order cytokines, and serve as effectors of antimicrobial defense. Innate immune responses in the lungs have a critical function for airway epithelial cells, according to recent studies (Voynow et al. 1998). By using a various mechanisms, the airway epithelium controls the development of microorganisms in the conducting airways. The fluid, mucus, and particles are moved, trapped, and expelled from the lungs by the ciliated epithelial cells. Defensins, cathelicidins, lactotransferrin, hypothiocyanite, hypoiodous acid, anionic antimicrobial peptides, and lipocalins are examples of antibacterial compounds. Opsonins include immunoglobulins (Igs), complement proteins, surfactant proteins A and D, and pentraxins. The majority of the above factors are immunomodulatory and aid in tissue healing (Parker and Prince 2011). Innate defenses failed as a result of pathogen resistance to antibacterial compounds and opsonins, lack of synthesis, degradation, or decreased function.

Low quantities of CD14 and TLRs are expressed by airway epithelial cells, which use TLR-dependent processes to detect bacteria in mucociliary fluid. Epithelium-derived cytokines are also important in driving innate inflammatory responses in the airspaces. RANTES (regulated on activation, normal T-cell expressed and secreted), granulocyte-macrophage colony-stimulating factor, transforming growth factor, and other pro-inflammatory cytokines are produced by airway epithelial cells (Diamond et al. 2000). Airway epithelial cells also recognize unmethylated bacterial DNA by membrane TLR-9, leading to NF-κB activation and production of IL-6, IL-8, and β2-defensin in the airways (Platz et al. 2004). Distal airway epithelium also has a role in lipopolysaccharide (LPS) recognition. Respiratory epithelial cells have complex defenses against viral infection, including recognition by TLRs, RIG-I (retinoic acid-inducible gene I), MDA-5 (melanoma differentiation-associated protein-5), and NLRP3 (NLR family pyrin domain containing 3). These defenses activate type I interferons and trigger a variety of antiviral responses (Vareille et al. 2011; Saminathan et al. 2019). NK T-cells offer defense against phospho-antigens and glycolipid antigens produced by numerous respiratory bacterial infections, such as *Streptococcus pneumoniae*; whereas, epithelial cells and DCs control the inflammatory responses in the lungs during infection (Eddens and Kolls 2012). The primary phagocytic cells of the innate immune system in the lungs are alveolar macrophages, which account for around 95% of the airspace leukocytes, followed by lymphocytes (1–4%) and neutrophils (1%). The first identification and development of cytokine signals that coordinate the initial steps of host defense are mediated by alveolar macrophages. Both innate and adaptive immune responses require macrophages. The type of cytokines that macrophages are exposed determines whether these cells are activated by classical (Th1) or alternative (Th2) pathways. Specifically, when activated by IFN-γ or by LPS, classically activated (M1) macrophages promote inflammation by secreting tumor necrosis factor-alpha (TNF-α), IL-12, and chemokines. They also have significant bactericidal activity by going through an oxidative burst and producing nitric oxide from arginine. After being exposed to cytokines like IL-4, IL-10, or IL-13, alternately activated (M2) macrophages arise, express arginase I, and stimulate tissue repair and restoration by secreting IL-10, transforming growth factor-beta (TGF-β), and IL-6 (Van Dyken and Locksley 2013); furthermore, they generate polyamines and proline, which promote collagen formation and cell proliferation, respectively. All forms of inhaled particles that enter the alveolar gaps are ingested by alveolar macrophages, which are voracious phagocytic. Adaptive immune responses are triggered by the presentation of microbial antigens to responding lymphocytes by alveolar macrophages, which also transport them to local lymph nodes and the interstitium. Activated monocytes and lymphocytes are attracted to inflammatory areas in the lungs by CC chemokines like MCP-1 and RANTES, which are produced by alveolar macrophages. In order to maintain alveolar homeostasis, macrophages in the lungs recycle surfactant, phagocytose particulates including bacteria, produce reactive oxygen and nitrogen species, and secrete cytokines and proteases. However, the range of these functions depends on the monocyte subpopulation from which they were derived, the recruitment strategy used, and the stimuli present in the lung microenvironment (Alber et al. 2012). Macrophages also regulate the dose of antigen to prevent the inappropriate development of tolerance and provide a small dose of antigen to T helper (Th) cells (Chauhan and Rana 2010). Alveolar macrophages are thought to be distinct from other histiocytes in the lungs, such as intravascular, interstitial and DCs, which exhibit significant functional heterogeneity. Resident alveolar macrophages in mice are quiescent, with low major histocompatibility complex (MHC) II expression, weak antigen-presenting function, and low production of inflammatory cytokines. The influx of monocytes that results from an inflammatory stimulation produces exudative macrophages and monocyte-derived DCs in the lung tissue. These cells are efficient at presenting antigens, activating T-cells, producing nitric oxide and TNF, and inducing lung tissue damage (Tighe et al. 2011).

Using the processes of phagocytosis and neutrophil extracellular trap (NET) creation, neutrophils are antimicrobial effector cells. By creating bactericidal substances such as reactive oxygen species, antimicrobial proteins, and proteolytic enzymes, they engulf bacteria and kill them (elastase and cathepsins). Antibacterial proteins found in chromatin networks known as extracellular traps enable the engulfing and elimination of extracellular bacteria (Balamayooran et al. 2010). They can also produce a number of soluble mediators, including cytokines often attributed to $CD4^+$ T-cells during adaptive immune responses, and they have affector roles (Yamada et al. 2011). Similar to neutrophils, the migration of inflammatory macrophages boosts the lung's ability to mount phagocytic host defenses. It also creates new opportunities for immunostimulatory signals, and other innate leukocytes such NK cells, NKT cells, and $\gamma\delta$ T-cells to further regulate the responses. Neutrophils and inflammatory macrophages are among the influx of phagocytes that aid in the destruction of germs, but many of their antimicrobial components can also aggravate tissue damage. The leading candidates for non-hematopoietic cells with innate immune functions against respiratory infections are epithelial cells, supported by studies in murine models, in which epithelial cells have interrupted NF-kB signaling (Poynter et al. 2003; Quinton et al. 2007). Hepatocytes regulate plasma proteins during pneumonia to control the spread of bacteria from the diseased lungs, which are the examples of cells with innate immune functions found outside of the affected lungs (Quinton et al. 2007). To support endocrine innate immunological processes, the liver mobilizes immunomodulatory chemicals to the lungs, which secrete them into the blood. The acute phase response, which is characterized by quick changes in blood plasma components, was originally identified in pneumonia patients (Tillett and Francis 1930). Lung innate immunity depends heavily on the soluble components of alveolar and airway fluids. Lysozyme, lactoferrin, immunoglobulin A (IgA), immunoglobulin G (IgG), and defensins, are antimicrobial peptides secreted from leukocytes and respiratory epithelial cells, which are the components of the airway aqueous fluids in the conducting airways (Becker et al. 2000; Lehrer 2004). Smaller particles, including bacterial and viral particles, are transported to the alveolar surface where they interact with soluble elements of the fluid, including alveolar macrophages, IgG, complement, surfactant, and proteins associated with surfactant. The IgG immunoglobulin is the most prevalent in alveolar fluid and serves as additional microbial opsonins in addition to complement proteins and surfactant-associated proteins. Surfactant protein A (SP-A) and D (SP-D), in particular, are collectin family members that encourage alveolar macrophages to phagocytose particles. When LPS interacts with lipopolysaccharide-binding proteins (LBP) in alveolar fluids and the CD14/TLR4 complex on alveolar macrophages, alveolar surfactant lipids SP-A and SP-D bind with LPS to limit its biological effects (Borron et al. 2000; Sano et al. 2000). High levels of LBP and soluble CD14 (sCD14) are present in alveolar fluid, and they play a crucial role in the detection of LPS by alveolar macrophages and other cells in the alveolar environment (Martin et al. 1992). When inflammation develops, concentrations of LBP and sCD14 significantly increase, amplifying the effects of LPS in lung fluid, while concentrations of SP-A and SP-D decline (Skerrett et al. 2007; Adamo et al. 2004). Compared to mature alveolar macrophages, blood monocytes and freshly recruited macrophages exhibit much higher membrane CD14. Alveolar macrophages engulf bacteria that have been opsonized by IgG, complement, SP-A, or SP-D in the airspaces. Toll-like receptors (TLRs) in the phagosomal membranes help to differentiate between the numerous microbial products that enter the cells (Medzhitov et al. 1998).

Signals produced by membrane-bound and cytosolic pattern-recognition receptors are essential for innate immunity (PRRs). The most prevalent PRRs are TLRs and RLRs like RIG-I, MDA-5, and NOD-like receptors, which are retinoic acid-inducible gene-I (RIG-I)-like receptors (NLRs) (Kawai and Akira 2010). A complex network of intracellular signaling pathways is activated by the interaction of viral pathogen-associated molecular proteins (PAMPs) with the PRRs, which in turn causes transcription of numerous cytokine genes to induce an antiviral state in the host (Platanias 2005). The first PRRs to be discovered was the TLRs. TLRs are mostly expressed in immunological tissues like the spleen and leukocytes as well as in tissues exposed to the outside environment including the lungs and digestive system (Singh et al. 2003). TLRs can detect microbial compounds because they are present on the ciliated epithelium of conducting airways and the cells of alveolar walls. When PRRs are active, airway epithelial cells release more antimicrobial defensins and are stimulated to create CXC and CC chemokines, which recruit neutrophils into the airway lumen (Becker et al. 2000). TLRs can sense distinct PAMPs derived from pathogens. One of the mechanisms for controlling bacterial proliferation at the site of infection and reducing bacterial spread is TLR-mediated innate immune responses. The multiple TLRs activate antimicrobial pathways, which destroy bacteria (Opitz et al. 2010). Two different TLR signaling pathways are activated by the engagement of particular adaptor proteins: a MyD88-dependent system involving TLR1, 2, 4, 5, 6, 7, 8, and 10 and a TIR-domain-containing adapter-inducing IFN-β (TRIF)-dependent pathway comprising TLR3 and 4 (Kawai and Akira 2011). The activation of transcription factors like NF-kB, mitogen-activated protein kinases, activator protein 1 (AP-1), and IFN regulatory factor 3 (IRF-3) leads to an upregulation of pro-inflammatory cytokines and chemokines as well as adhesion molecules crucial for phagocyte recruitment and activation. These events are involved in antibacterial defenses and are induced by TLRs. Additionally, TLR signaling promotes DC maturation and IL-12 and TGF-β production. TGF-β and IL-6 can promote the differentiation of Th0 cells into Th17 cells, but IL-12 alone can promote the differentiation of Th0 cells into Th1 cells to produce efficient adaptive immune responses (Balamayooran et al. 2010). Acute stressors enhance many aspects of the innate immune response. In a rat model, stress induces release of heat shock protein 72 from cells, which acts similarly to a damage-associated molecular pattern (DAMP) to enhance production of nitric oxide from macrophages (Fleshner 2013).

7.15 Adaptive Immunity

7.15.1 Humoral Immunity

The host's defense against bacterial pathogens depends on the humoral immune response. Through stimulation of resident antigen-specific memory B-cells, lungs have the ability to respond quickly to some pathogens. Lungs have the ability to create both systemic and local antibody responses on their own following exposure to a novel pathogen. Invading pathogens are eliminated as a result of the creation of antigen-specific IgG and IgA, which also reduces subsequent respiratory epithelium colonization. The local (mucosal) response is crucial in preventing the pathogenic germs from colonizing the upper respiratory tract. In the lower respiratory tract, the IgG is crucial (Prince et al. 1985), because it has opsonizing and complement-activating characteristics, which help phagocytic cells to get rid of the invading bacteria. The IgG2 antibodies are produced in response to polysaccharide antigens; whereas, the IgG1 subclass primarily reacts to protein antigens (Siber et al. 1980). The upper respiratory tract is primarily made up of IgA with lesser amounts of IgG than the lower respiratory tract. The IgA1 is found predominantly in serum. In contrast, IgA2 appears to be crucial for mucosal immunity, as it makes up about half of the IgA in secretions.

Antibodies, i.e., IgA (in respiratory system), exert their protective effect through three mechanisms (Mazanec et al. 1993; Chauhan 1998). First, they inhibit the binding of organisms to mucosal surfaces and serve as an immunologic barrier. Second, they may be effective in neutralizing intracellular pathogens as suggested by their movement from the basilar to apical region of epithelial cells. Finally, pathogens bound to IgA may be taken up by airway macrophages through the phagocytic process. Alveolar macrophages and other antigen-presenting cells are responsible for capturing particulate antigens in the alveolar space. These cells then move through lymphatics to local lymph nodes, where the initial immune response takes place. After developing in lymph nodes, antigen-specific B-cells move back to the lungs, where they differentiate and grow to become either plasma cells or memory B-cells (Curtis and Kaltreider 1989).

Mucosa-associated lymphoid tissue (MALT), a specialized lymphoid tissue directly below the mucosal surface, can provide mucosal immunity, indicating that IgA-secreting plasma cells are formed locally and IgA can easily diffuse back into the airspaces. There is a specialized defense mechanism in animals developed at the interface between mucosal surface and the external environment, which functions to maintain the integrity of the internal environment. This defense mechanism operates independently of the immune system and is designated as MALT (Chauhan 1998). Most animal species have mucosal/submucosal lymphoid tissues in the upper airways where the nose is located; while in mice, bronchus-associated lymphoid tissue (BALT) is readily demonstrable in the lower respiratory tract (McKenzie et al. 2004). After influenza infection, strong protective primary pulmonary B- and T-cell responses were seen in mice lacking secondary lymphoid tissues (Moyron-Quiroz et al. 2004), which supports the concept of inducible BALT. In submucosal tissues, this response was linked to the induction of B-cell follicles centered on follicular DCs. Hence, collection of antigen-presenting cells, B-cells and T-cells in the BALT may only be readily identified during times of antigenic challenge. Once antibody-producing B-cells are formed in secondary lymphoid tissue or MALT, they must traffic back to the original point of entry of the pathogen. When the host is exposed to a potential pathogens, the immune system either responds quickly by activating resident memory B-cells, if the host has previously been exposed to germs, or slowly by inducing both systemic immunity and local mucosal immunity, if the host has never encountered the pathogen. In the first few months of life, maternal antibodies are thought to be crucial in defending against respiratory pathogens.

7.16 Cell-Mediated Immunity

Because of their diversity, specificity, and memory, cell-mediated adaptive immune responses are crucial in the fight against viruses, mycobacteria and fungi as well as other groups of lung pathogens. It depends on the intricate interaction of numerous soluble elements and various cell types. The T-cells, NK cells, and DCs sequentially interact with one another in pairwise interactions. Immature myeloid DCs transport antigens from the lungs to local lymph nodes and responsible for initiating the primary adaptive responses. In healthy lungs, iDCs reside in airway epithelium, alveolar septae and around pulmonary vessels (Holt et al. 1994), but are rare within alveoli. Naive CD4 T-cells must be activated by antigen presentation by mature DCs in order to produce effector responses and strong immunologic memory. Inflamed tissues attract NK cells and DCs, which interact in a contact and tumor necrosis factor-dependent fashion to initiate the immune response polarization. Memory T-cells can migrate directly to infected tissues, where they can be activated without accelerating the secondary immune responses. Previous pulmonary infections or immune responses increase number of lungs DCs and populate the lungs with clones of memory B-cells and T-cells that are promptly available to respond to infections.

The following two DCs phenotypes are crucial for lung host defenses: (i) plasmacytoid DCs (pDCs) express TLR9 and TLR7, enabling them to respond to bacterial DNA and viruses with the production of IFN-α, and (ii) myeloid DCs (mDCs) express TLR1, TLR2, TLR3, and TLR4 allowing them to be activated by LPS, mycopeptides, and viral RNA. In addition to bridging innate and adaptive immunity in the lungs, DCs can also trigger different CD4+ T-cell responses against infectious pathogens, depending on the situation. Additionally, important immuno-regulatory functions that link innate and adaptive responses are performed by NK and NKT cells. The function of NK cells is to lyse the cells with decreased MHC class I expression (missing self). NK cells are essential for protection against cytopathic viruses because they can cause decreased expression to avoid CD8+ T-cells attack (Biron et al. 1999). Defense against *Cryptococcus neoformans* and *Aspergillus fumigatus* is contributed by NK cells (Murphy et al. 1993; Morrison et al. 2003). Invariant NKT (iNKT) cells share properties of both T-cells and NK cells, and recognize antigens presented by the CD1d molecule. Limited T-cell receptors are expressed by the iNKT cells. These cells produce IFN-γ, which are capable of being activated by innate cytokines and antigen-driven pathways, and participate in a number of bacterial infections in the lungs. There are three main types of cell-mediated effector immunity, which can be divided into type 1, type 2, and type 3, based on the growing knowledge about the various effector T-cells and innate lymphoid cells (ILC) lineages.

Type-1 immunity consists of T-bet⁺ IFN-γ producing group 1 ILCs (ILC1 and NK cells), CD8+ cytotoxic T-cells (Tc1), and CD4+ Th1 cells, which are involved in defense against intracellular pathogens, as viruses, some bacteria, and protozoan pathogens through activation of mononuclear phagocytes. Additionally, IL-2, tumor necrosis factor-α, and granulocyte/macrophage colony-stimulating factor (GM-CSF) are produced by these cells. The CD4+ T-cells are a major T-cell subset playing a central role in immune system function. These are necessary for the host to develop long-lasting immunity against infections and for efficient bacterial clearance in the lungs. T-helper (Th) 1 and Th2 cells are two separate populations of CD4+ T-cells, which are distinguished primarily by the effector cytokines they produce but also by differential patterns of expression of cell surface components and transcription factors. IFN-γ and lymphotoxin-alpha (LT-α) are produced by Th1 cells as their signature cytokines (Romagnani 1991). Moreover, Th1 cells are able to produce the antibodies of the IgG2a isotype by B-lymphocytes in mice (Mosmann et al. 1986). Recently, it was discovered that IL-23 and IL-27 showed Th1-polarizing function (Brombacher et al. 2003). Activation of signal transducer and activator of transcription (STAT) 1 by IFN-γ and of STAT 4 by IL-12 is critical for the induction of T-bet, which is considered the hallmark transcription factor for Th1 cells (Farrar et al. 2002). Because alveolar macrophages need exogenous interferons to activate STAT1-dependent effector pathways in response to bacterial or viral products, these responses are essential in the lungs (Punturieri et al. 2004). Chemokine receptors expressed by Th1 cells enable migration of Th1 cells to inflammatory areas. Microbial proteins are processed and presented during intracellular persistence, which initiates T-cell activation. Mononuclear phagocytes (MPs) are activated by Th1, Tc1, and group 1 ILCs, which secrete IFN-γ and TNF, and transforming them into potent effector cells. T-cytotoxic 1 (Tc1)-phenotyped CD8+ T-cells appear to be protective; while, non-Tc1 cells appear to contribute to immunopathology (Chen and Kolls 2013). Due to high specific cytolytic potential of Tc1 cells against infected cells and their capacity to produce IFN-γ and TNF, Tc1 cells are more crucial than Th1 cells for the defense against viruses.

Type-2 immunity comprised of GATA-3⁺ ILC2s, Tc2 cells, and Th2 cells producing IL-4, IL-5, IL-9, IL-10, and IL-13, which induce mast cells, basophils, and eosinophils activation and also IgE and IgG4 antibody production. The primary functions of type 2 immunity are defense against helminth and allergy. In mice, switching of B-cells to produce IgG1 and IgE requires both IL-4 and IL-13 (Mosmann et al. 1986). While IL-13 and IL-4 have some similar roles, IL-13 is a key inducer of airway hyperresponsiveness, goblet cell metaplasia, and mucus hypersecretion in the lungs. The IL-5 is a key mediator of eosinophilopoiesis and eosinophils activation, and plays an important role in the differentiation, activation, and survival of eosinophils in mice (Mosmann et al. 1986). The IL-33 is a regulator of IL-4 and IL-13 and induced by influenza virus in murine lungs (Le Goffic et al. 2011). It influences type 2 ILCs to increase the production of IL-13 and cause airway hyperreactivity (Chang et al. 2011). In fungal infections, the Th2 lineage effector cells are considered to be harmful because they suppress the protective Th1 cell responses (Romani 2004). Because much of the lungs damaged in viral infections can be mediated by the type-1 response, such downregulation may preserve lung integrity, but type 2 responses favors fibrosis (Jakubzick et al. 2004). The IFN-γ inhibits the Th2 cell development, and IL-10 prevents the Th1 cells from producing cytokines.

A third type of immunity, which protects against extracellular bacteria and fungi has recently been discovered. It is mediated by retinoic acid-related orphan receptor γt+ ILC3s, Tc17 cells, and Th17 cells that produce the cytokines IL-17 (IL-17A and IL-17F). These cytokines activate MPs, recruit neutrophils, and trigger epithelial antimicrobial responses. The IL-17-producing CD4+ T-cell population, distinct from Th1 and Th2, was first demonstrated in a mouse model (Infante-Duarte et al. 2000). The IL-17 targets either immune or non-immune cell types and is also key cytokine for the recruitment, activation and migration of neutrophils. Additionally, IL-22 and IL-26 are produced by Th17 cells (Annunziato et al. 2012). The IL-22 has many roles in tissue repair (Akdis et al. 2012) and promotes epithelial cell homeostasis and antimicrobial defense (Rutz et al. 2013). It induces antimicrobial peptide production by epithelial cells (Ye et al. 2001). The susceptibility of IL-17-deficient mice to bacteria and fungi, such as *Candida albicans*, *Staphylococcus aureus*, and *Klebsiella pneumoniae*, has been demonstrated in animal models of infection (Annunziato et al. 2012). The IL-17RA knockout mice was used as *K. pneumoniae* model, which demonstrated decreased pulmonary G-CSF production, neutrophil recruitment, and granulopoiesis, resulting in higher bacterial burden in the lungs and increased systemic dissemination to the spleen (Ye et al. 2001). During *Pneumocystis murina* infection, the IL-17 pathway may provide protection (Rudner et al. 2007). Rhesus macaques infected with the simian immunodeficiency virus (SIV) have CD8+ T-cells that produce IL-17 and IL-22.

The CD4+ T-cells can also develop into regulatory T-cells (Treg), which are cells that control or dampen ongoing effector T-cell responses (Fu et al. 2004; Zheng et al. 2004). The FOXP3 transcription factor regulates a specific CD25+ CD4 T-cell fraction that predominantly mediates the Treg response (Kronenberg and Rudensky 2005). Although IL-10 and TGF-β are not necessary for the effector mechanism of CD4+CD25+ regulatory T-cells, may involve apoptosis of the target, but other T-cell subsets with suppressive properties act through these cytokines. Treg cells play a crucial role in maintaining and reestablishing a homeostatic environment, in addition to reducing excessive inflammation. In respiratory syncytial virus (RSV) infection models, Treg cells limit immunopathology by influencing the trafficking and effector function of virus-specific CD8+ T-cells in the lungs and draining lymph nodes (Fulton et al. 2010). Suppression of inflammatory responses by Treg cells can be both beneficial and deleterious in host defense. These cells are essential for modulating the tolerance to inhaled antigen in the lungs (Chang et al. 2011).

The T follicular helper (Tfh) cells, a new CD4+ T-cell subset that aids in the generation of antigen-specific antibodies, have recently been discovered in the germinal center (Zheng et al. 2004). The IL-21, a cytokine produced by Tfh, is known to facilitate the pathogenic inflammation during pneumovirus infection in mice (Spolski et al. 2012). The precise function of Tfh in this model is still being investigated. The γδ T-cells represent a small subset of T-cells that have a T-cell receptor composed of one γ chain and one δ chain unlike conventional T-cells having a TCR made up of α and β chains. The δ T-cells are common in the gut and other mucosa including the airways but these are rare in blood and lymphoid tissues (D'Souza et al. 1997). During the *Klebsiella* infection in mice, the γδ T-cells are a major source of IFN-γ, TNF-α, and IL-17 (Chen et al. 2011) and mice lacking γδ T-cells showed increased bacterial spread and decreased survival (Moore et al. 2000). In the *Streptococcus pneumoniae* infection, γδ T-cells are a crucial cellular source of TNF-α (Nakasone et al. 2007). The IL-17 is produced by γδ T-cells in influenza-infected mice and seems to contribute to pathogenic inflammation (Crowe et al. 2009). A counterpart of Th cells known as suppressor T-cells also exists, which suppresses the immune response (Chauhan and Rana 2010).

The actions of the innate and adaptive arms are strictly sequential or unidirectional. Humoral immunity also affects cell-mediated responses by activating and inhibiting the Fc receptors that are present on all leukocytes in different combinations. T-cells contribute to *Nocardia* lung infection in a non-redundant way in murine models (King et al. 1999) and are needed to prevent dissemination of *Klebsiella*. Gene-targeted mice lacking T-cells exhibit exaggerated inflammation in response to variety of pathogens.

Murine lymphocytes differ in their dependence on specific adhesion receptors for recruitment to the lungs for instance CD8+ T-cells and Th1 CD4+ cells strongly depend on endothelial selectins, whereas γδ T-cells do not (Curtis et al. 2002; Clark et al. 2004). Lungs that have recovered from infections have large numbers of immune cells that can accelerate subsequent local immune responses. After antigenic stimulation, the B-cells and functioning DCs are persists for months (Julia et al. 2002). Viral pneumonias in mice induce persistence of large numbers of specific T-cell clones among which CD8+ T-cells remaining longer than CD4+ T-cells. These CD8+ clones do not multiply in the lungs but instead exhibit particular antiviral activity and large amounts of receptors that are frequently linked to acute activation (Woodland 2003), hence called as "persistently activated T-cells." According to studies on T-cell clonal deletion and heterologous immunity, each patient's response to respiratory viruses may vary because of the cumulative effect of their infection history on their own adaptive immune responses (Welsh et al. 2004). An effective early immune response in the lungs is critical for a successful elimination of bacteria as they often breach host defense leading to rapid their multiplication in the lungs and dissemination to distant organs.

7.17 Immunodeficiency in Animals

All the living beings have evolved by developing complex defense mechanisms to protect them from several varieties of foreign agents. Hence, the development and intactness of the immune system is important for survival of the organisms. Any defect in development or maintenance of the immune system leads to immunodeficiency and makes the animal prone to many types of infections. The immunodeficiency can be categorized into two classes:

7.17.1 Congenital Immunodeficiency

It is observed rarely in animals. There is defect in basic cellular components during development. These defects may occur during the differentiation and maturation of the bone marrow elements derived from stem cells. These can be recognized early in life by appearance of recurrent infections, increased susceptibility to pathogens, occurrence of systemic disease after vaccination with attenuated vaccines, and poor response to treatment. Further, various types of congenital deficiencies are:

7.17.1.1 Combined Immunodeficiency Syndrome

It occurs due to inherited gene defect. The stem cells are absent or are unable to differentiate into T- and B-lymphocytes. It is characterized by recurrent infections since birth, agammaglobulinemia, and absence of T- and B-lymphocytes. It has been reported in Arabian foals. Death occurs due to recurrent infections such as *Pneumocystis carinii* and adenovirus infections. A similar syndrome characterized by hypoplasia in the thymus, spleen, and lymph nodes has been reported in dogs.

7.17.1.2 Defects in T- and B-Lymphocytes

Thymic hypoplasia in pups leads to defective T-cell function. These pups have increased susceptibility to various infections. In dogs, selective IgA deficiency has been recorded, which is characterized by recurrent respiratory infections. It occurs due to maturation arrest from B-cell to IgA-secreting plasma cells. Recurrent respiratory infections in Arabian horses have been recorded due to selective IgM deficiency. The foals are reported to be infected with *Klebsiella pneumoniae* or *Rhodococcus equi* (Joshi and Chauhan 2012). Increased susceptibility to pyogenic infections and broncho-pneumonia is reported in Danish red cattle with IgG deficiency. During 4–6 months of age, transient hypogammaglobulinemia can be observed in the newborn. The maternal immunoglobulins are catabolized slowly and the antibody level falls below the normal range. This condition has been reported in foals, dogs, and lambs. During this period the animals are prone to various opportunistic pathogen infections.

Partial maturational defects in T- and B-cells are characterized by recurrent infections. Ataxia-telangiectasia is a disorder associated with IgG deficiency. In this also there is recurrence of infections.

7.17.1.3 Deficiency of Complement

Congenital deficiency of complement is rarely seen in animals. Because complement does not mediate opsonization, chemotaxis, and phagocytosis in the absence or deficiency of C3, bacterial infections are more likely to occur.

7.17.2 Acquired Immunodeficiency

Animals can acquire immunosuppression due to diseases, drugs, deficiency of nutrients, neoplasms, and environmental factors. Bovine viral diarrhea virus (BVDV) causes reduction of CD4+, CD8+ T-cells, B-cells, and neutrophils in cattle. The RSV infection in lambs makes them prone to secondary bacterial infection by *Pasteurella multocida*. Bluetongue infection in sheep makes them prone to secondary bacterial infection by *Pasteurella multocida* (Saminathan et al. 2020). Canine distemper virus activates the T-suppressor cells and causes immunosuppression (Chauhan 1998).

7.18 Immunomodulation

Increased resistance of microbes to antibiotics has led to a growing concern towards immunomodulation, which aims to improve the immune system to control the infections. Immunomodulators manipulate the immune system. It comprises of immunostimulation and immunosuppression. Immunostimulation has been a matter of choice in order to increase the host's resistance to diseases. Immunomodulatory compounds can also reverse immunosuppression caused by stress, viruses, or environmental pollution. Among various types of immunomodulatory molecules, certain physiological products act as immunomodulatory molecules such as neuroendocrine hormones, cytokines, thymic hormones, and glucocorticoids. The products of immune system are also capable of transmitting information to neurons known as immunotransmitters that regulate the course of immune response. In animals, acute stress may enhance the immune response, while chronic stress may suppress the immune system mediated by immunotransmitters. Thymic hormones (thymosin α_1, thymulin, thymic humoral factor, etc.) act on T-cell subsets and help to maintain the immune function. Cytokines including interferons, interleukins, growth factors, chemokines, etc. act as intercellular messengers and regulate the immune system. Cytokines may interact in various ways and may enhance or suppress their own production. Cortisol and corticosterone are naturally occurring glucocorticoids and are known to have immunosuppressive and anti-inflammatory effects (Chauhan 2001).

7.19 Evasion Strategies of Microbes

The pathogens have co-evolved with their hosts over millions of years. The viruses have developed mechanisms to evade from the host immune responses, eventhough the hosts have evolved and strengthened the strong components of their immune systems.

7.20 Evasion from Innate Immune Responses

7.20.1 Interference with the Physical Barrier

Pathogens are coated by surfactant proteins A and D on lung epithelial surfaces, making them more amenable to phagocytosis by neutrophils and macrophages. Therefore, the pathogens would benefit if the epithelium were damaged. The BHV-1 invades the upper respiratory tract epithelium, producing cilia and goblet cell loss as well as epithelial erosions that may progress into necrosis of the epithelium and surrounding lymphoid tissues (Schuh et al. 1992). These circumstances encourage the migration and colonization of the lower respiratory system by commensal bacterial pathogens such as *Mannheimia haemolytica* in the nasopharynx of healthy animals. In order to circumvent host defenses and to increase pathogenicity, *Bordetella bronchiseptica* has a number of strategies. Fimbriae and the production of hemagglutinins and adhesins enable the bacteria to adhere to ciliated epithelium and the production of exotoxins suppresses local immunity and contributes to the loss of ciliary function (Keil and Fenwick 1998).

7.20.2 Interference with Phagocytosis by Predisposing Factors and Pathogens

Inhibition of phagocytosis, oxidative burst, and antibody-dependent cell-mediated cytotoxicity by glucocorticoid treatment have been reported in bovine neutrophils (Paape et al. 1981; Roth and Kaeberle 1981). Pathogens have evolved strategies to combat the phagocytes as they are important in the induction of innate and adaptive immunity (Coombes et al. 2004). Alveolar macrophage activity is suppressed by non-cytopathic BVDV. Infection reduces the expression of receptors for immunoglobulin and complement, interferes with fusion of phagosomes to lysosomes, reduces bactericidal activity, reduces the secretion of TNF-α, IL-1β, IL-6 and neutrophil chemoattractants and increases the secretion of prostaglandin E2. However, it has no impact or stimulatory effect on the production of type I interferons and IL-12 (Welsh et al. 1995; Liu et al. 1999). Likewise, alveolar macrophage function has been primarily suppressed by BPIV-3 and BHV-1 by decreasing the phagocytosis and oxidative burst (Slauson et al. 1987; Dyer et al. 1994). Studies on influenza-infected mice revealed that the influenza virus caused type I interferons production, which interfered the production of chemokine C-C motif ligand 2 (CCL2) that reduces the recruitment of macrophages to the lungs and increases the risk of *Streptococcus pneumoniae* colonization (Nakamura et al. 2011). Leukotoxin (LKT), an exotoxin that *Mannheimia haemolytica* produces, which is cytotoxic to neutrophils, macrophages, and all other leukocytes (Berggren et al. 1981). It binds to β2-integrins, which are leukocyte-specific integrins (Jeyaseelan et al. 2000). Viral infections sensitize neutrophils to the damaging effects of *M. haemolytica* LKT. The IL-1β and other cytokines are produced by BHV-1-infected bovine mononuclear cells, and these cytokines increase the expression of CD18 (LFA-1) on neutrophils. Since CD18 is the receptor for M. haemolytica LKT, this increases the binding of this toxin and exacerbates the cytotoxic effect on bovine neutrophils (Leite et al. 2005). The LKT targets phagocytes and other leukocytes by using CD18 as its receptor (Deshpande et al. 2002; Dassanayake et al. 2007). It suggested that *M. haemolytica* LKT-deletion mutant strain does not cause the severe lung lesions as that of wild type strain (Tatum et al. 1998; Highlander et al. 2000). Ruminant neutrophils and macrophages undergo apoptotic or oncotic death when exposed to the *M. haemolytica* LKT (Singh et al. 2011).

Haemophilus somni is able to compromise the phagocytic ability of neutrophils results in evasion of the phagocytic killing by inducing apoptosis of phagocytic cells (Yang et al. 1998). *H. somni* has the ability to prevent neutrophils and alveolar macrophages from undergoing an oxidative burst, and immunoglobulin-binding protein A can prevent phagocytosis and cause cytotoxicity in bovine monocytes (Hoshinoo et al. 2009).

Bacteria possess polysaccharide capsules, which have antiphagocytic properties. *Pasteurella multocida* acapsular mutants were easily ingested by macrophages, but in a mouse model, the wild-type bacteria were found to be significantly resistant to phagocytosis (Boyce and Adler 2000; Priya et al. 2017). *Mycoplasma dispar* polysaccharide capsule hinders the activation of alveolar macrophages and production of the pro-inflammatory cytokines IL-1β and TNF-α (Almeida et al. 1992). *B. bronchiseptica* can enter into the non-phagocytic cells and this ability provides the defense from the host immune system (Keil and Fenwick 1998).

7.20.3 Effects of Predisposing Factors and Pathogens on the Production of Innate Defense Molecules

Corticosteroids impair the LPS-inducible tracheal antimicrobial peptide expression in cattle (Mitchell et al. 2007). Elevated levels of corticosteroids can be seen in animals, which are stressed by transportation, by exposure to cold, and by disruption of social groups (Hickey et al. 2003). Virus infections can lead to failure of expression of innate defense factors. A significant risk factor for bacterial pneumonia in feedlot cattle is non-cytopathic BVDV (Ridpath 2010). Bovine tracheal epithelial cells infected with the virus lose the ability to express lactotransferrin and tracheal antimicrobial peptide in response to LPS (Al-Haddawi et al. 2007). The PRRSV has effectively developed an infectious strategy to bypass the early warning mechanisms of innate immune system. Antiviral and inflammatory cytokines, in particular

IFN-α/β, IL-1, and TNF, are not generated in PRRSV infection (van Reeth et al. 1999). Weak activation of NK cells and an essential regulator of immunological mobilization is the NF-kB (Christman et al. 2000).

Some pathogens directly circumvent these barriers by resisting the action of antimicrobial agents or by promoting their eradication. *Aspergillus fumigatus* protease cleaves a number of complement proteins and thereby preventing the complement activation (Behnsen et al. 2010). Several Gram-positive infections alters the peptidoglycan acetylation patterns in their cell walls as a defense mechanism against lysozyme breakdown (Davis and Weiser 2011).

7.20.4 Effects on Receptors on the Surface of Airway Epithelial Cells and Cell Signal Transduction

Bacterial adhesins bind to host cell receptors and altered expression of these receptors affects colonization of pathogens in the lungs. According to an in vitro study, BHV-1 encouraged the adherence of *M. haemolytica* to airway epithelial cells (Czuprynski 2009). The viral pathogens have evolved to escape the recognition and effector mechanisms like alteration of the immune-inflammatory response to bacterial infections of lungs. Viral infections modify the type I interferon-induced signaling through the RIG-I, MDA-5, and TLR3 pathways (Ballinger and Standiford 2010; Saminathan et al. 2019). Viral infections are known to modulate NF-κB signaling pathway. Viral interference with the host response may exacerbate the immuno-inflammatory reaction to bacterial infection as seen in case of influenza virus. It causes the immune-suppressive substances like glucocorticoids, IL-10, or TGF-β to increase the risk of bacterial infections (Jamieson et al. 2010). Numerous intrinsic regulators are used by pulmonary bacteria or pathogens to modify the TLR signaling in different ways, and this may be influenced by the pathogen's virulence strategy in the host. TLR signaling can be regulated to either provoke or downregulate immune effects (O'Neill 2008). Bacterial effectors directly cause overactivation of signaling molecules or transcription factors (Fontana et al. 2011). Positive host regulators, including the triggering receptors expressed on myeloid cell 1 (TREM-1), which indirectly increases the TLR-mediated inflammation (O'Neill 2008). Pseudomonas aeruginosa uses hyper inflammation-mediated strategies such as the type III secretion system for its survival and growth as observed in a murine pneumonia model (Faure et al. 2014). This includes the promotion of IL-18 production, which exacerbates acute lung inflammation and attenuates the IL-17 production and IL-17-driven antimicrobial peptide production (Faure et al. 2014). During *S. pneumoniae* pneumonia in mice, the receptor for advanced glycation end products (RAGE), a TLR amplifier with a structure similar to TREM-1, is upregulated in the lungs. This increases the pulmonary inflammatory response, which reduces the bacterial clearance and increases the bacterial dissemination (van Zoelen et al. 2009). By directly suppressing the expression or activity of TLRs or TLR signaling molecules via negative regulators, avoiding the TLR recognition, or promoting the production of anti-inflammatory cytokines, bacteria can reduce host TLR signaling. Some negative regulators prevent TLR signaling molecules from functioning, impairing host defense and subsequent downstream signal transduction. During Gram-negative bacteria-induced pneumonia, signals from CD44 have been demonstrated to weaken a number of host defense mechanisms (van der Windt et al. 2010) by inducing the expression of negative regulators such as A20 and interleukin-1 receptor-associated kinase (IRAK)-M. Both *Streptococcus pneumoniae* and *Klebsiella* take the advantage of host IRAK-M, a regulator that prevents IRAKs from functioning, in order to avoid pulmonary immune reactions (Hoogerwerf et al. 2012). Several pulmonary bacteria, including *Chlamydophila pneumoniae*, *Burkholderia pseudomallei*, and *Legionella pneumophila*, have peculiar lipid A moieties in their LPS. Tetra-acylated LPS structure is expressed by *Francisella tularensis* and *Yersinia pestis* during infection to avoid being detected by the host TLR4. Numerous host defense events, such as the induction of autophagy are significantly impacted by failure to activate TRIF and promote TLR4 signaling (Jabir et al. 2014), neutrophil recruitment, and expression of inducible nitric oxide synthase (Baral and Utaisincharoen 2012). $TLR2^{-/-}$ mice have defective lactoferrin production following bacterial challenge (Wu et al. 2011).

7.20.5 Interference with Intracellular Killing

In the bovine respiratory illness complex, PI-3 induces signal transduction disruption and inhibition of oxygen-dependent bactericidal activities of alveolar macrophages, which results in immunosuppression and subsequent bacterial infection (BRDC) (Dyer et al. 1994). To avoid intracellular death, *H. somni* prevents alveolar macrophages and neutrophils from producing superoxide anion (Howard et al. 2004). The neutrophil respiratory burst is inhibited by *Mycobacterium bovis* either during or after protein kinase C activation.

7.20.6 Interference with IFN System

The expression of IFN-α and IFN-β is dysregulated by a number of bovine respiratory viruses. Infected cell polypeptide 0 (ICP0) and ICP27, two viral proteins that are encoded by the BHV-1, prevent the stimulation of IFN-β gene expression (da Silva et al. 2012). The BHV-1 inhibits IFN-β-dependent transcription (Henderson et al. 2005). Increased virulence of BRSV is correlated with non-structural protein blockade of type-I IFN induction (Valarcher et al. 2003). In vitro or in vivo type-1 IFN expression is not induced by PRRSV infection, and there is no intracellular antiviral action (Albina et al. 1998).

7.21 Evasion of Adaptive Immune Response

7.21.1 Infection of Leukocytes and Suppression of Proliferation

Before differentiating into effector cells that can eradicate the infection, the B- and T-lymphocytes undergo clonal proliferation (Janeway et al. 2005). Numerous infections actively attack immune system cells and interfere with their ability to proliferate in order to inhibit the immune system.

7.21.2 Suppression of Proliferation of Leukocytes

BHV-1 infection of lymphocytes contributes to immunosuppression, which could be caused by more than one mechanism including suppression of proliferation of leukocytes (Carter et al. 1989). The BHV-1-induced the reduction of peripheral blood mononuclear cells (PBMCs) proliferative responses to antigen or IL-2 was confirmed by in vitro investigation (Hutchings et al. 1990). *Mycobacterium bovis* induces the death of lymphocytes by apoptosis in vitro (Vanden Bush and Rosenbusch 2002). Leukotoxin in the *Mannheimia haemolytica* culture supernatant suppresses lymphocyte blastogenesis in response to mitogens at sub-lytic doses (Majury and Shewen 1991a; Czuprynski and Ortiz-Carranza 1992). Compared to T-lymphocytes, B-lymphocytes seem to be more vulnerable to the inhibitory effects. Exogenous IL-1 or IL-2 addition reduces the inhibitory effect of leukotoxin (Majury and Shewen 1991b).

7.21.3 Infection of Cells of the Immune System

When calves are experimentally co-infected with BRSV and New York-1 (NY-1) BVDV develop more severe respiratory tract disease compared to calves infected with either virus alone.. The percentage of CD8+ lymphocytes and CD4+ lymphocytes in the thymus and Peyer's patches was lower in co-infected calves (Brodersen and Kelling 1999).

7.21.4 Induction of Humoral and Cellular Immune Tolerance

It has been reported that the leukotoxin released by *M. haemolytica* suppresses the production of class II molecules on macrophages obtained from bovine monocytes (Hughes et al. 1994). Leukotoxin affects the constitutive expression, but not IFN-δ-induced expression of class II molecules.

7.21.5 Inhibition of Antibody Activity

Lack of immunoglobulins acquired through colostrum is linked to a higher occurrence of respiratory illnesses and may be caused by insufficient quantities of protective antibodies in colostrum (Virtala et al. 1999). On bovine monocyte-derived macrophages, leukotoxin produced by *M. haemolytica* inhibits the production of class II molecules (Hughes et al. 1994). *M. haemolytica* secretes a protease that cleaves IgG1 (Gioia et al. 2006). The bacterial pathogens causing bovine respiratory disease (BRD) have several mechanisms to limit antibody-mediated immunity. For *H. somni* and several other bovine respiratory infections, biofilm formation is described (Olson et al. 2002). Immunoglobulin-binding proteins, such as IgG2-binding proteins, are secreted by *H. somni* and are linked to serum resistance because they bind to IgG2 in a non-antigen-specific manner, thus preventing the binding of particular antibodies to the organism (Siddaramppa and Inzana 2004).

7.21.6 Interference with Cytotoxic T-Lymphocyte Response

The self-MHC class I molecules on the cell surface present intracellular viral antigens that are recognized by the cytotoxic T-lymphocytes (CTLs) (Zinkernagel and Doherty 1974). In order to avoid being recognized by CTLs, certain viruses, including BHV-1, have developed ways to interfere at different points along the pathways of antigen processing and presentation (Hewitt 2003). The reduction of CTL has been reported in calves infected with BHV-1 (Joshi and Chauhan 2012). The pathogens have developed a number of immune evasion/immunosuppressive tactics. The strategies developed by one pathogen may not only help that pathogen, but also the others, resulting in exacerbation of the disease.

7.22 Conclusion

Pneumonia is caused by a bacterial and viral infections of the lungs, but the course of the infection is determined by physiological mechanisms integrating the responses across several cell types and the immune system. Pneumonia continues to be a significant cause of illness, mortality, and financial losses to animal husbandry despite improved understanding of the etiology and immune responses involved, the availability and use of numerous respiratory pathogen vaccinations, and new antimicrobial medications. Evolution in microbes to evade host defenses has not only led to failure of the immune system to combat infections but has also led to the emergence of antibiotic resistance and vaccination failure. The immune system is unable to completely protect against this disease complex due to the complicated etiology and myriad immune evasion mechanisms established by the microorganisms. These immune evasion mechanisms contribute to the failure of currently available vaccines and inability to completely protect animals against the bacteria and viruses. Good management, appropriate building design that ensures enough ventilation, minimizing various stress factors, and successful vaccination against the main respiratory pathogens can help in preventing the disease. Disease prevention does not rely on curing all the failed respiratory defenses. To get rid of infection and stop sickness, restoring a few defenses, especially those that pathogens would be unable to get over, may be sufficient. In order to provide instantaneous protection, effective therapeutics should be developed. The strategies of combined host-targeted immunotherapies and cytokine therapies may proved to be helpful to fight against infectious diseases as there has been an emergence of antibiotic resistance. Further, vaccines should be prepared keeping in view the evolved pathogen.

References

Adamo R, Sokol S, Soong G, Gomez MI, Prince A (2004) Pseudomonas aeruginosa flagella activate airway epithelial cells through asialoGM1 and toll-like receptor 2 as well as toll-like receptor 5. Am J Respir Cell Mol Biol 30:627–634

Akdis M, Palomares O, van de Veen W, van Spunter M, Akdis CA (2012) TH17 and TH22 cells: a confusion of antimicrobial response with tissue inflammation versus protection. J Allergy Clin Immunol 129:1438–1449

Alber A, Howie SE, Wallace WA, Hirani N (2012) The role of macrophages in healing the wounded lung. Int J Exp Pathol 93:243–251

Albina E, Carrat C, Charley B (1998) Interferon-alpha response to swine arterivirus (PoAV), the porcine reproductive and respiratory syndrome virus. J Interferon Cytokine Res 18:485–490

Al-Haddawi M, Mitchel GB, Clark ME, Wood RD, Caswell JL (2007) Impairment of innate immune responses of airway epithelium by infection with bovine viral diarrhea virus. Vet Immunol Immunopathol 116:153–162

Almeida RA, Wannemuehler MJ, Rosenbusch RF (1992) Interaction of mycoplasma dispar with bovine alveolar macrophages. Infect Immun 60:2914–2919

Ames TR (1993) The epidemiology of BRSV infection. Vet Med 88:881–885

Angus JC, Jang SS, Hirsh DC (1997) Microbiological study of transtracheal aspirates from dogs with suspected lower respiratory tract disease: 264 cases (1989-1995). J Am Vet Med Assoc 210:55–58

Annunziato F, Cosmi L, Liotta F, Maggi E, Romagnani S (2012) Defining the human T helper 17 cell phenotype. Trends Immunol 33:505–512

Archer KA, Ader F, Kobayashi KS, Flavell RA, Roy CR (2010) Cooperation between multiple microbial pattern recognition systems is important for host protection against the intracellular pathogen legionella pneumophila. Infect Immun 78:2477–2487

Asrani RK, Batta MK, Joshi VB, Katoch RC, Sharma M, Sambyal DS, Singh SP, Nagal KB (1996) Comparative pathology of naturally occurring chlamydial pneumonia among domestic animals in Himachal Pradesh. Indian Vet J 73:623–627

Balamayooran T, Balamayooran G, Jeyaseelan S (2010) Toll-like receptors and NOD-like receptors in pulmonary antibacterial immunity. Innate Immun 16:201–210

Ballinger MN, Standiford TJ (2010) Post influenza bacterial pneumonia: host defenses gone awry. J Interferon Cytokine Res 30:643–652

Baral P, Utaisincharoen P (2012) Involvement of signal regulatory protein alpha, a negative regulator of toll-like receptor signaling, in impairing the MyD88-independent pathway and intracellular killing of Burkholderia pseudomallei-infected mouse macrophages. Infect Immun 80:4223–4231

Baron J, Bin-Tarif A, Herbert R, Frost L, Taylor G, Baron MD (2014) Early changes in cytokine expression in peste des petits ruminants disease. Vet Res 45:22

Batey RG, Smits AF (1976) The isolation of Bordetella bronchiseptica from an outbreak of canine pneumonia. Aust Vet J 52:184–186

Becker MN, Diamond G, Verghese MW, Randell SH (2000) CD14-dependent lipopolysaccharide-induced beta-defensin-2 expression in human tracheobronchial epithelium. J Biol Chem 275: 29731–29736

Behnsen J, Lessing F, Schindler S, Wartenberg D, Jacobsen ID, Thoen M, Zipfel PF, Brakhage AA (2010) Secreted Aspergillus fumigatus protease Alp1 degrades human complement proteins C3, C4, and C5. Infect Immun 78:3585–3594

Bello-Irizarry SN, Wang J, Olsen K, Gigliotti F, Wright TW (2012) The alveolar epithelial cell chemokine response to Pneumocystis requires adaptor molecule MyD88 and interleukin-1 receptor but not toll-like receptor 2 or 4. Infect Immun 80:3912–3920

Bemis DA, Greisen HA, Appel MJ (1977) Pathogenesis of canine bordetellosis. J Infect Dis 135: 753–762

Berggren KA, Baluyut CS, Simonson RR, Bemrick WJ, Maheswaran SK (1981) Cytotoxic effects of Pasteurella haemolytica on bovine neutrophils. Am J Vet Res 42:1383–1388

Biondo C, Midiri A, Messina L, Tomasello F, Garufi G, Catania MR, Bombaci M, Beninati C, Teti G, Mancuso G (2005) MyD88 and TLR2, but not TLR4, are required for host defense against Cryptococcus neoformans. Eur J Immunol 35:870–878

Biron CA, Nguyen KB, Pien GC, Cousens LP, Salazar-Mather TP (1999) Natural killer cells in antiviral defense: function and regulation by innate cytokines. Annu Rev. Immunol 17:189–220

Borron P, McIntosh JC, Korfhagen TR, Whitsett JA, Taylor J, Wright JR (2000) Surfactant-associated protein A inhibits LPS-induced cytokine and nitric oxide production in vivo. Am J Phys Lung Cell Mol Phys 278:L840–L847

Boyce JD, Adler B (2000) The capsule is a virulence determinant in the pathogenesis of Pasteurella multocida M1401 (B: 2). Infect Immun 68:3463–3468

Breitschwerdt EB, Brown TT, De Buysscher EV, Andersen BR, Thrall DE, Hager E, Ananaba G, Degen MA, Ward MD (1987) Rhinitis, pneumonia, and defective neutrophil function in the Doberman pinscher. Am J Vet Res 48:1054–1062

Breitschwerdt EB, DebRoy C, Mexas AM, Brown TT, Remick AK (2005) Isolation of necrotoxigenic Escherichia coli from a dog with hemorrhagic pneumonia. J Am Vet Med Assoc 226:2016–2019

Bretz C, Gersuk G, Knoblaugh S, Chaudhary N, Randolph-Habecker J, Hackman RC, Staab J, Marr KA (2008) MyD88 signaling contributes to early pulmonary responses to Aspergillus fumigatus. Infect Immun 76:952–958

Brodersen BW, Kelling CL (1999) Alteration of leukocyte population in calves concurrently infected with bovine respiratory syncytial virus and bovine viral diarrhea virus infections. Viral Immunol 12:323–334

Broderson JR, Lindsey JR, Crawford JE (1976) The role of environmental ammonia in respiratory mycoplasmosis of rats. Am J Pathol 85:115–130

Brombacher F, Kastelein RA, Alber G (2003) Novel IL-12 family members shed light on the orchestration of Th1 responses. Trends Immunol 24:207–212

Bryson E (1993) Necropsy findings associated with BRSV pneumonia. Vet Med 88:894–899

Carter JJ, Weinberg AD, Pollard A, Reeves R, Magnuson JA, Magnuson NS (1989) Inhibition of T-lymphocyte mitogenic responses and effects on cell functions by bovine herpesvirus 1. J Virol 63:1525–1530

Caswell JL, Hewson J, Slavic E, DeLay J, Bateman K (2012) Laboratory and postmortem diagnosis of bovine respiratory disease. Vet Clin Food Anim Pract 28:419–441

Cerquetella M, Laus F, Paggi E, Zuccari T, Spaterna A, Tesei B (2013) Bronchial vegetal foreign bodies in the dog-localization in 47 cases. J Vet Med Sci 75:959–962

Chalker VJ, Owen WM, Paterson C, Barker E, Brooks H, Rycroft AN, Brownlie J (2004) Mycoplasmas associated with canine infectious respiratory disease. Microbiology 150:3491–3497

Chang YJ, Kim HY, Albacker LA, Baumgarth N, McKenzie AN, Smith DE, DeKruyff RH, Umetsu DT (2011) Innate lymphoid cells mediate influenza-induced airway hyper-reactivity independently of adaptive immunity. Nat Immunol 12:631–638

Chauhan RS (1998) An introduction to immunopathology. G.B. Pant University of Agriculture & Technology, Pantnagar, pp 5, 29, 52–57

Chauhan RS (2001) Immunomodulation: basic concepts. In: Chauhan RS, Singh GK, Agrawal DK (eds) Advances in immunology and immunopathology. SIIP, Pantnagar, pp 1–3

Chauhan RS, Rana JMS (2010) Recent advances in immunobiotechnology. In: Basic concepts in immunology in immunopathology. IBT, Patwadangar, p 32

Chen K, Kolls JK (2013) T cell–mediated host immune defenses in the lung. Annu Rev. Immunol 31:605–633

Chen SM, Cheng DS, Williams BJ, Sherrill TP, Han W, Chont M, Saint-Jean L, Christman JW, Sadikot RT, Yull FE, Blackwell TS (2008) The nuclear factor kappa-B pathway in airway epithelium regulates neutrophil recruitment and host defence following Pseudomonas aeruginosa infection. Clin Exp Immunol 153:420–428

Chen K, McAleer JP, Lin Y, Paterson DL, Zheng M, Alcorn JF, Weaver CT, Kolls JK (2011) Th17 cells mediate clade-specific, sero type-independent mucosal immunity. Immunity 35:997–1009

Christman JW, Sadikot RT, Blackwell TS (2000) The role of nuclear factor–kB in pulmonary diseases. Chest 117:1482–1487

Chvala S, Benetka V, Mostl K, Zeugswetter F, Spergser J, Weissenbock H (2007) Simultaneous canine distemper virus, canine adenovirus type 2, and Mycoplasma cynos infection in a dog with pneumonia. Vet Pathol 44:508–512

Clark JG, Mandac-Dy JB, Dixon AE, Madtes DK, Burkhart KM, Harlan JM, Bullard DC (2004) Trafficking of Th1 cells to lung: a role for selectins and a P-selectin glycoprotein-1-independent ligand. Am J Respir Cell Mol Biol 30:220–227

Confer AW (2009) Update on bacterial pathogenesis in BRD. Anim Health Res Rev 10:145

Confer AW, Clinkenbeard KD, Murphy GL (1995) Pathogenesis and virulence of Pasteurella haemolytica in cattle: an analysis of current knowledge and future approaches. In: Donachie W, Lainson FA, Hodgson JC (eds) Haemophilus, actinobacillus and pasteurella. Plenum Press, London, p 51

Coombes BK, Valdez Y, Finlay BB (2004) Evasive maneuvers by secreted bacterial proteins to avoid innate immune responses. Curr Biol 14:R856–R867

Crowe CR, Chen K, Pociask DA, Alcorn JF, Krivich C, Enelow RI, Ross TM, Witztum JL, Kolls JK (2009) Critical role of IL-17RA in immunopathology of influenza infection. J Immunol 183:5301–5310

Curtis JL, Kaltreider HB (1989) Characterization of bronchoalveolar lymphocytes during a specific antibody-forming cell response in the lungs of mice. Am Rev. Respir Dis 139:393–400

Curtis JL, Sonstein J, Craig RA, Todt JC, Knibbs RN, Polak T, Bullard DC, Stoolman LM (2002) Subset-specific reductions in lung lymphocyte accumulation in endothelial selectin-deficient mice. J Immunol 169:2570–2579

Czuprynski CJ (2009) Host response to bovine respiratory pathogens. Anim Health Res Rev 10:141

Czuprynski CJ, Ortiz-Carranza O (1992) Pasteurella haemolytica leukotoxin inhibits mitogen-induced bovine peripheral blood mononuclear cell proliferation in vitro. Microb Pathog 12:459–463

D'Souza CD, Cooper AM, Frank AA, Mazzaccaro RJ, Bloom BR, Orme IM (1997) An anti-inflammatory role for T lymphocytes in acquired immunity to Mycobacterium tuberculosis. J Immunol 158:1217–1221

da Silva LF, Sinani D, Jones C (2012) ICP27 protein encoded by bovine herpesvirus type 1 (bICP27) interferes with promoter activity of the bovine genes encoding beta interferon 1 (IFN-beta1) and IFN-beta3. Virus Res 169:162–168

Dabo SM, Taylor JD, Confer AW (2007) Pasteurella multocida and bovine respiratory disease. Anim Health Res Rev 8:129

Damian M, Morales E, Salas G, Trigo FJ (2005) Immunohistochemical detection of antigens of distemper, adenovirus and parainfluenza viruses in domestic dogs with pneumonia. J Comp Pathol 133:289–293

Dassanayake RP, Maheswaran SK, Srikumaran S (2007) Monomeric expression of bovine β_2-integrin subunits reveals their role in Mannheimia haemolytica leukotoxin-induced biological effects. Infect Immun 75:5004–5010

Davis KM, Weiser JN (2011) Modifications to the peptidoglycan backbone help bacteria to establish infection. Infect Immun 79:562–570

Deshpande MS, Ambagala TC, Ambagala APN, Kehrli ME, Srikumaran S (2002) Bovine CD18 is necessary and sufficient to mediate Mannheimia (Pasteurella) haemolytica leukotoxin-induced cytolysis. Infect Immun 70:5058–5068

Dharanesha NK, Saminathan M, Mamta P, Ramesh KR, Ananda KJ, Giridhar P, Byregowda SM (2019) Parasitic pneumonia caused by Paragonimus spp. in a wild Royal Bengal Tiger, Mysuru, South India. J Parasit Dis 43:528–533

Diamond G, Legarda D, Ryan LK (2000) The innate immune response of the respiratory epithelium. Immunol Rev 173:27–38

Dyer RM, Majumdar S, Douglas SD, Korchak HM (1994) Bovine parainfluenza-3 virus selectively depletes a calcium-independent, phospholipid-dependent protein kinase C and inhibits superoxide anion generation in bovine alveolar macrophages. J Immunol 153:1171–1179

Eddens T, Kolls JK (2012) Host defenses against bacterial lower respiratory tract infection. Curr Opin Immunol 24:424–430

Farrar JD, Asnagli H, Murphy KM (2002) T helper subset development: roles of instruction, selection, and transcription. J Clin Investig 109:431–435

Faure E, Mear JB, Faure K, Normand S, Couturier-Maillard A, Grandjean T, Balloy V, Ryffel B, Dessein R, Chignard M, Uyttenhove C (2014) Pseudomonas aeruginosa type-3 secretion system dampens host defense by exploiting the NLRC4-coupled inflammasome. Am J Respir Crit Care Med 189:799–811

Fleshner M (2013) Stress-evoked sterile inflammation, danger associated molecular patterns (DAMPs), microbial associated molecular patterns (MAMPs) and the inflammasome. Brain Behav Immun 27:1–7

Fontana MF, Banga S, Barry KC, Shen X, Tan Y, Luo ZQ, Vance RE (2011) Secreted bacterial effectors that inhibit host protein synthesis are critical for induction of the innate immune response to virulent Legionella pneumophila. PLoS Pathog 7:e1001289

Frank GH, Nelson SL, Briggs RE (1989) Infection of the middle nasal meatus of calves with Pasteurella haemolytica serotype 1. Am J Vet Res 50:1297–1301

Fu S, Zhang N, Yopp AC, Chen D, Mao M, Chen D, Zhang H, Ding Y (2004) TGF-β induces Foxp3+ T-regulatory cells from CD4+ CD25− precursors. Am J Transplant 4:1614–1627

Fulton RB, Meyerholz DK, Varga SM (2010) Foxp3+ CD4 regulatory T-cells limit pulmonary immunopathology by modulating the CD8 T-cell response during respiratory syncytial virus infection. J Immunol 185:2382–2392

Galav V, Sharma SK, Agarwal M, Tiwari RK, Kumar B (2017) Pattern of lung lesions in Escherichia coli and Klebsiella spp. associated caprine pneumonia. In: International conference on emerging horizons in diagnosis of animal and poultry diseases towards sustainable production in asian countries held on 9–11 November 2017 at Bengaluru

Gioia J, Qin X, Jiang H, Clinkenbeard K, Lo R, Liu Y, Fox GE, Yerrapragada S, McLeod MP, McNeill TZ, Hemphill L (2006) The genome sequence of Mannheimia haemolytica A1: insights into virulence, natural competence, and Pasteurellaceae phylogeny. J Bacteriol 188:7257–7266

Gogoi K, Rajkhowa TK, Singh YD, Ravindran R, Arya RS, Hauhnar L (2017) Epidemiology of porcine respiratory and reproductive syndrome (PRRS) outbreak in India. Indian J Vet Pathol 41:31–37

Hajjar AM, Harowicz H, Liggitt HD, Fink PJ, Wilson CB, Skerrett SJ (2005) An essential role for non-bone marrow-derived cells in control of Pseudomonas aeruginosa pneumonia. Am J Respir Cell Mol Biol 33:470–475

Henderson G, Zhang Y, Jones C (2005) The bovine herpesvirus 1 gene encoding infected cell protein 0 (bicp0) can inhibit interferon-dependent transcription in the absence of other viral genes. J Gen Virol 86:2697–2702

Hewitt EW (2003) The MHC class I antigen presentation pathway: strategies for viral immune evasion. Immunology 110:163–169

Hickey MC, Drennan M, Earley B (2003) The effect of abrupt weaning of suckler calves on the plasma concentrations of cortisol, catecholamines, leukocytes, acute-phase proteins and in vitro interferon-gamma production. J Anim Sci 81:2847–2855

Highland MA, Herndon DR, Bender SC, Hansen L, Gerlach RF, Beckmen KB (2018) Mycoplasma ovipneumoniae in wildlife species beyond subfamily Caprinae. Emerg Infect Dis 24:2384

Highlander SK, Fedorova ND, Dusek DM, Panciera R, Alvarez LE, Rinehairt C (2000) Inactivation of Pasteurella (Mannheimia) haemolytica leukotoxin causes partial attenuation of virulence in a calf challenge model. Infect Immun 68:3916–3922

Holt PG, Haining S, Nelson DJ, Sedgwick JD (1994) Origin and steady-state turnover of class II MHC-bearing dendritic cells in the epithelium of the conducting airways. J Immunol 153:256–261

Hoogerwerf JJ, van der Windt GJ, Blok DC, Hoogendijk AJ, De Vos AF, van't Veer C, Florquin S, Kobayashi KS, Flavell RA, van der Poll T (2012) Interleukin-1 receptor-associated kinase M-deficient mice demonstrate an improved host defense during gram-negative pneumonia. Mol Med 18:1067–1075

Hoshinoo K, Sasaki K, Tanaka A, Corbeil LB, Tagawa Y (2009) Virulence attributes of Histophilus somni with a deletion mutation in the ibpA gene. Microb Pathog 46:273–282

Howard MD, Boone JH, Buechner-Maxwell V, Schurig GG, Inzana TJ (2004) Inhibition of bovine macrophage and polymorphonuclear leukocyte superanion production by Haemophilus somnus. Microb Pathog 37:263–271

Hughes HP, Campos M, Mcdougall L, Beskorwayne TK, Potter AA, Babiuk LA (1994) Regulation of major histocompatibility complex class II expression by Pasteurella haemolytica leukotoxin. Infect Immun 62:1609–1615

Hutchings DL, Campos M, Qualtiere L, Babiuk LA (1990) Inhibition of antigen-induced and interleukin-2-induced proliferation of bovine peripheral blood leukocytes by inactivated bovine herpes virus 1. J Virol 64:4146–4151

Infante-Duarte C, Horton HF, Byrne MC, Kamradt T (2000) Microbial lipopeptides induce the production of IL-17 in Th cells. J Immunol 165:6107–6115

Irwin PJ, Whithear K, Lavelle RB, Parry BW (2000) Acute bronchopneumonia associated with Mycobacterium fortuitum infection in a dog. Aust Vet J 78:254–257

Jabir MS, Ritchie ND, Li D, Bayes HK, Tourlomousis P, Puleston D, Lupton A, Hopkins L, Simon AK, Bryant C, Evans TJ (2014) Caspase-1 cleavage of the TLR adaptor TRIF inhibits autophagy and beta-interferon production during Pseudomonas aeruginosa infection. Cell Host Microbe 15:214–227

Jain SK, Rajya BS, Mohanty GC, Paliwal OP, Mehrotra ML, Shah RL (1975) Pathology of chlamydial abortions in ovine and caprine. Curr Sci 44:209–210

Jakubzick C, Kunkel SL, Puri RK, Hogaboam CM (2004) Therapeutic targeting of IL-4- and IL-13-responsive cells in pulmonary fibrosis. Immunol Res 30:339–349

Jameson PH, King LA, Lappin MR, Jones RL (1995) Comparison of clinical signs, diagnostic findings, organisms isolated, and clinical outcome in dogs with bacterial pneumonia: 93 cases (1986-1991). J Am Vet Med Assoc 206:206–209

Jamieson AM, Yu S, Annicelli CH, Medzhitov R (2010) Influenza virus-induced glucocorticoids compromise innate host defense against a secondary bacterial infection. Cell Host Microbe 7:103–114

Janeway CA, Travers P, Walport M, Shlomchik MJ (2005) Immuno biology: the immune system in health and disease, 5th edn. Garland Science Publishing, New York

Jeyaseelan S, Hsuan SL, Kannan MS, Walcheck B, Wang JF, Kehrli ME, Lally ET, Sieck GC, Maheswaran SK (2000) Lymphocyte function-associated antigen 1 is a receptor for Pasteurella haemolytica leukotoxin in bovine leukocytes. Infect Immun 68:72–79

Johnson LR, Johnson EG, Vernau W, Kass PH, Byrne BA (2016) Bronchoscopy, imaging, and concurrent diseases in dogs with bronchiectasis: (2003-2014). J Vet Intern Med 30:247–254

Jones MR, Simms BT, Lupa MM, Kogan MS, Mizgerd JP (2005) Lung NF-kappa B activation and neutrophil recruitment require IL-1 and TNF receptor signaling during pneumococcal pneumonia. J Immunol 175:7530–7535

Joshi A, Chauhan RS (2012) Immunological techniques: interpretations, validation and safety measures. Kapish Prakashan, Gurgaon, Haryana, pp 35, 39

Julia V, Hessel EM, Malherbe L, Glaichenhaus N, O'Garra A, Coffman RL (2002) A restricted subset of dendritic cells captures airborne antigens and remains able to activate specific T-cells long after antigen exposure. Immunity 16:271–283

Kaminen PS, Viitanen SJ, Lappalainen AK, Kipar A, Rajamaki MM, Laitinen-Vapaavuori OM (2014) Management of a congenital tracheoesophageal fistula in a young Spanish water dog. BMC Vet Res 10:16

Kanemoto H, Morikawa R, Chambers JK, Kasahara K, Hanafusa Y, Uchida K, Ohno K, Nakayama H (2015) Common variable immune deficiency in a Pomeranian with Pneumocystis carinii pneumonia. J Vet Med Sci 77:715–719

Kawai T, Akira S (2010) The role of pattern-recognition receptors in innate immunity: update on toll-like receptors. Nat Immunol 11:373–384

Kawai T, Akira S (2011) Toll-like receptors and their crosstalk with other innate receptors in infection and immunity. Immunity 34:637–650

Keil DJ, Fenwick B (1998) Role of Bordetella bronchiseptica in infectious tracheobronchitis in dogs. J Am Vet Med Assoc 212:200–207

Kharole MV (1973) Studies on pathology of pneumonitis caused by chlamydial agent in sheep and goats. Thesis, PhD Haryana Agriculture University, Hisar India

King DP, Hyde DM, Jackson KA, Novosad DM, Ellis TN, Putney L, Stovall MY, Van Winkle LS, Beaman BL, Ferrick DA (1999) Cutting edge: protective response to pulmonary injury requires T lymphocytes. J Immunol 162:5033–5036

Kollannur JD, Syam R, Chauhan RS (2014) Epidemiological studies on infectious bovine rhinotracheitis (IBR) in different parts of India. Int J Livestock Res 4:21–27

Kronenberg M, Rudensky A (2005) Regulation of immunity by self-reactive T-cells. Nature 435:598–604

Lather D, Narang G, Sinha AK, Jangir BL, Sharma M (2017) Pathobiological studies on Mycobacterium bovis associated granulomatous pneumonia in an adult cow. In: International conference on emerging horizons in diagnosis of animal and poultry diseases towards sustainable production in Asian countries held on 9–11 November 2017 at Bengaluru

Le Goffic R, Arshad MI, Rauch M, L'Helgoualc'h A, Delmas B, Piquet-Pellorce C, Samson M (2011) Infection with influenza virus induces IL-33 in murine lungs. Am J Respir Cell Mol Biol 45:1125–1132

Lehrer RI (2004) Primate defensins. Nat Rev. Microbiol 2:727–738

Leissinger MK, Garber JB, Fowlkes N, Grooters AM, Royal AB, Gaunt SD (2015) Mycobacterium fortuitum lipoid pneumonia in a dog. Vet Pathol 52:356–359

Leite F, Atapattu D, Kuckleburg C, Schultz R, Czuprynski CJ (2005) Incubation of bovine PMNs with conditioned medium from BHV-1 infected peripheral blood mononuclear cells increases their susceptibility to Mannheimia haemolytica leukotoxin. Vet Immunol Immunopathol 103:187–193

Li Y, Wang X, Bo K, Wang X, Tang B, Yang B, Jiang W, Jiang P (2007) Emergence of a highly pathogenic porcine reproductive and respiratory syndrome virus in the Mid–Eastern region of China. J Vet Sci 174:577–584

Liu L, Lehmkuhl HD, Kaeberle ML (1999) Synergistic effects of bovine respiratory syncytial virus and non-cytopathic bovine viral diarrhea virus infection on selected bovine alveolar macrophage functions. Can J Vet Res 63:41–48

Lopez A (2007) Respiratory system. In: McGavin MD, Zachari JF (eds) Pathologic basis of veterinary disease, 5th edn. Mosby, St. Louis, MO, p 463

Majury AL, Shewen PE (1991a) The effect of Pasteurella haemolytica A1 leukotoxic culture supernate on the in vitro proliferative response of bovine lymphocytes. Vet Immunol Immunopathol 29:41–56

Majury AL, Shewen PE (1991b) Preliminary investigation of the mechanism of inhibition of bovine lymphocyte proliferation by Pasteurella haemolytica A1 leukotoxin. Vet Immunol Immunopathol 29:57–68

Martin TR, Mathison JC, Tobias PS, Leturcq DJ, Moriarty AM, Maunder RJ, Ulevitch RJ (1992) Lipopolysaccharide binding protein enhances the responsiveness of alveolar macrophages to bacterial lipopolysaccharide: implications for cytokine production in normal and injured lungs. J Clin Investig 90:2209–2219

Matsui H, Verghese MW, Kesimer M, Schwab UE, Randell SH, Sheehan JK, Grubb BR, Boucher RC (2005) Reduced three-dimensional motility in dehydrated airway mucus prevents neutrophil capture and killing bacteria on airway epithelial surfaces. J Immunol 175:1090–1099

Mazanec MB, Nedrud JG, Kaetzel CS, Lamm ME (1993) A three-tiered view of the role of IgA in mucosal defense. Immunol Today 14:430–435

McKenzie BS, Brady JL, Lew AM (2004) Mucosal immunity: overcoming the barrier for induction of proximal responses. Immunol Res 30:35–71

McNeil HJ, Shewen PE, Lo RY, Conlon JA, Miller MW (2002) Mannheimia haemolytica serotype 1 and Pasteurella trehalosi serotype 10 culture supernatants contain fibrinogen binding proteins. Vet Immunol Immunopathol 90:107–110

Medzhitov R, Preston-Hurlburt P, Kopp E, Stadlen A, Chen C, Ghosh S, Janeway CA Jr (1998) MyD88 is an adaptor protein in the hToll/IL-1 receptor family signaling pathways. Mol Cell 2: 253–258

Mitchell GB, Al-Haddawi MH, Clark ME, Beveridge JD, Caswell JL (2007) Effect of corticosteroids and neuropeptides on the expression of defensins in bovine tracheal epithelial cells. Infect Immun 75:1325–1334

Mizgerd JP (2008) Acute lower respiratory tract infection. N Engl J Med 358:716–727

Moore TA, Moore BB, Newstead MW, Standiford TJ (2000) γδ-T-cells are critical for survival and early proinflammatory cytokine gene expression during murine klebsiella pneumonia. J Immunol 165:2643–2650

Morrison BE, Park SJ, Mooney JM, Mehrad B (2003) Chemokine-mediated recruitment of NK cells is a critical host defense mechanism in invasive aspergillosis. J Clin Investig 112:1862–1870

Mosmann TR, Cherwinski H, Bond MW, Giedlin MA, Coffman RL (1986) Two types of murine helper T-cell clone. I. Definition according to profiles of lymphokine activities and secreted proteins. J Immunol 175:5–14

Moyron-Quiroz JE, Rangel-Moreno J, Kusser K, Hartson L, Sprague F, Goodrich S, Woodland DL, Lund FE, Randall TD (2004) Role of inducible bronchus associated lymphoid tissue (iBALT) in respiratory immunity. Nat Med 10:927–934

Murphy JW, Hidore MR, Wong SC (1993) Direct interactions of human lymphocytes with the yeast-like organism, Cryptococcus neoformans. J Clin Investig 91:1553–1566

Nakamura S, Davis KM, Weiser JN (2011) Synergistic stimulation of type I interferons during influenza virus coinfection promotes Streptococcus pneumoniae colonization in mice. J Clin Investig 121:3657–3665

Nakasone C, Yamamoto N, Nakamatsu M, Kinjo T, Miyagi K, Uezu K, Nakamura K, Higa F, Ishikawa H, O'Brien RL, Ikuta K (2007) Accumulation of γ/δ T-cells in the lungs and their roles in neutrophil-mediated host defense against pneumococcal infection. Microbes Infect 9:251–258

Nandi S, Kumar M, Manohar M, Chauhan RS (2009) Bovine herpes virus infections in cattle. Anim Health Res Rev 10:85–98

O'Neill LA (2008) When signaling pathways collide: positive and negative regulation of toll-like receptor signal transduction. Immunity 29:12–20

Olson ME, Ceri H, Morck DW, Buret AG, Read RR (2002) Biofilm bacteria: formation and comparative susceptibility to antibiotics. Can J Vet Res 66:86–92

Opitz B, van Laak V, Eitel J, Suttorp N (2010) Innate immune recognition in infectious and noninfectious diseases of the lung. Am J Respir Crit Care Med 181:1294–1309

Paape MJ, Gwazdauskas FC, Guidry AJ, Weinland BT (1981) Concentrations of corticosteroids, leukocytes, and immunoglobulins in blood and milk after administration of ACTH to lactating dairy cattle: effects on phagocytosis of Staphylococcus aureus by polymorphonuclear leukocytes. Am J Vet Res 42:2081–2087

Parker D, Prince A (2011) Innate immunity in the respiratory epithelium. Am J Respir Cell Mol Biol 45:189–201

Peltola VT, McCullers JA (2004) Respiratory viruses predisposing to bacterial infections: role of neuraminidase. Pediatr Infect Dis J 23:S87–S97

Platanias LC (2005) Mechanisms of type-I- and type-II-interferon-mediated signalling. Nat Rev Immunol 5:375–386

Platz J, Beisswenger C, Dalpke A, Koczulla R, Pinkenburg O, Vogelmeier C, Bals R (2004) Microbial DNA induces a host defense reaction of human respiratory epithelial cells. J Immunol 173:1219–1223

Poynter ME, Irvin CG, Janssen-Heininger YM (2003) A prominent role for airway epithelial NF-kappa B activation in lipopolysaccharide induced airway inflammation. J Immunol 170:6257–6265

Priestnall S, Erles K (2011) Streptococcus zooepidemicus: an emerging canine pathogen. Vet J 188:142–148

Prince GA, Horswood RL, Chanock RM (1985) Quantitative aspects of passive immunity to respiratory syncytial virus infection in infant cotton rats. J Virol 55:517–520

Priya GB, Nagaleekar VK, Milton AAP, Saminathan M, Kumar A, Sahoo AR, Wani SA, Kumar A, Gupta SK, Sahoo AP, Tiwari AK, Agarwal RK, Gandham RK (2017) Genome wide host gene expression analysis in mice experimentally infected with Pasteurella multocida. PLoS One 12:e0179420

Punturieri A, Alviani RS, Polak T, Copper P, Sonstein J, Curtis JL (2004) Specific engagement of TLR4 or TLR3 does not lead to IFN-β- mediated innate signal amplification and STAT1 phosphorylation in resident murine alveolar macrophages. J Immunol 173:1033–1042

Purohit VD, Paul Gupta RK (1980) Indian journal of comparative microbiology. Immunol Infect Dis 4:142

Quinton LJ, Mizgerd JP (2011) NF-kB and STAT3 signaling hubs for lung innate immunity. Cell Tissue Res 343:153–165

Quinton LJ, Jones MR, Simms BT, Kogan MS, Robson BE, Skerrett SJ, Mizgerd JP (2007) Functions and regulation of NF-kappa β RelA during pneumococcal pneumonia. J Immunol 178:1896–1903

Radhakrishnan A, Drobatz KJ, Culp WT, King LG (2007) Community acquired infectious pneumonia in puppies: 65 cases (1993-2002). J Am Vet Med Assoc 230:1493–1497

Rajkhowa TK, Mohan Rao GJ, Gogoi A, Hauhnar L (2016) Indian porcine reproductive and respiratory syndrome virus bears discontinuous deletion of 30 amino acids in nonstructural protein 2. Virus Dis 27:287–293

Reynolds HY (1997) Integrated host defense against infections. In: Crystal RG, West JB, Weibel ER, Barnes PJ (eds) The lung: scientific foundations, vol 2, 2nd edn. Lippincott-Raven, Philadelphia PA, pp 2353–2365

Rice JA, Carrasco-Medina L, Hodgins DC, Shewen PE (2007) Mannheimia haemolytica and bovine respiratory disease. Anim Health Res Rev 8:117

Ridpath JF (2010) The contribution of infections with bovine viral diarrhea viruses to bovine respiratory disease. Vet Clin N Am Food Anim Pract 26:335–348

Romagnani S (1991) Human TH1 and TH2 subsets: doubt no more. Immunol Today 12:256–257

Romani L (2004) Immunity to fungal infections. Nat Rev. Immunol 4:1–23

Rossow KD (1998) Porcine reproductive and respiratory syndrome. Vet Pathol 35:1–20

Roth JA, Kaeberle ML (1981) Effects of in vivo dexamethasone administration on in vitro bovine polymorphonuclear leukocyte function. Infect Immun 33:434–441

Rudner XL, Happel KI, Young EA, Shellito JE (2007) Interleukin-23 (IL-23)-IL-17 cytokine axis in murine Pneumocystis carinii infection. Infect Immun 75:3055–3061

Rutz S, Eidenschenk C, Ouyang W (2013) IL-22, not simply a Th17 cytokine. Immunol Rev 252:116–132

Saminathan M, Singh KP, Rajasekar R, Malik YPS, Dhama K (2019) Role of type I interferons in the pathogenesis of bluetongue virus in mice and ruminants. J Exp Biol Agric Sci 7:513–520

Saminathan M, Singh KP, Khorajiya JH, Dinesh M, Vineetha S, Maity M, Rahman ATF, Misri J, Malik YS, Gupta VK, Singh RK, Dhama K (2020) An updated review on Bluetongue virus: epidemiology, pathobiology, and advances in diagnosis and control with special reference to India. Vet Q 40:258–321

Sanders A, Crystal RG (1997) Consequences to the lung of specific deficiencies in host defense. In: Crystal RG, West JB, Weibel ER, Barnes PJ (eds) The lung: scientific foundations, vol 2, 2nd edn. Lippincott-Raven, Philadelphia PA, pp 2367–2379

Sano H, Chiba H, Iwaki D, Sohma H, Voelker DR, Kuroki Y (2000) Surfactant proteins A and D bind CD14 by different mechanisms. J Biol Chem 275:22442–22451

Schneider-Schaulies S, Niewiesk S, Schneider-Schaulies J, ter Meulen V (2001) Measles virus induced immunosuppression: targets and effector mechanisms. Curr Mol Med 1:163–181

Schuh JC, Bielefeldt-Ohmann H, Babiuk LA, Doige CE (1992) Bovine herpesvirus-1-induced pharyngeal tonsil lesions in neonatal and weanling calves. J Comp Pathol 106:243–253

Schulz BS, Kurz S, Weber K, Balzer HJ, Hartmann K (2014) Detection of respiratory viruses and Bordetella bronchiseptica in dogs with acute respiratory tract infections. Vet J 201:365–369

Senthilkumar D, Rajukumar K, Sen A, Kumar M, Shrivastava D, Kalaiyarasu S, Gautam S, Singh F, Kulkarni DD, Singh VP (2017) Pathogenic characterization of porcine reproductive and respiratory syndrome virus of Indian origin in experimentally infected piglets. In: international conference on emerging horizons in diagnosis of animal and poultry diseases towards sustainable production in Asian countries held on 9–11 November 2017 at Bengaluru

Sethi M, Das T, Tomar N, Vamadevan B, Saikumar G (2017) Pathological and bacteriological investigation of severe suppurative bronchopneumonia in swine. In: International conference on emerging horizons in diagnosis of animal and poultry diseases towards sustainable production in asian countries held on 9–11 November 2017 at Bengaluru

Shaila MS, Purushothaman V, Bhavasar D, Venugopal K, Venkatesan RA (1989) Peste des petits ruminants of sheep in India. Vet Rec 125:602–602

Shaila MS, Peter AB, Varalakshmi P, Apte M, Rajendran MP, Anbumani SP (1996) Peste des petits ruminants in Tamilnadu goats. Indian Vet J 73:587–588

Shivashankar BP, Chandranaik BM, Shivaraj, Manjunatha V, Shankar BP, Venkatesha MD, Byregowda SM (2017) Outbreak of porcine reproductive and respiratory syndrome (PRRS) in an organised piggery farm in Karnataka. In: International conference on emerging horizons in diagnosis of animal and poultry diseases towards sustainable production in asian countries held on 9–11 November 2017 at Bengaluru

Siber GR, Schur PH, Aisenberg AC, Weitzman SA, Schiffman G (1980) Correlation between serum IgG-2 concentrations and the antibody response to bacterial polysaccharide antigens. N Engl J Med 303:178–182

Siddaramppa S, Inzana TJ (2004) Haemophilus somnus virulence factors and resistance to host immunity. Anim Health Res Rev 5:79–93

Singh BP, Chauhan RS, Singhal LK (2003) Toll Like Receptors (TLRs) and their role in innate immunity. Curr Sci 85:1156–1164

Singh K, Ritchey JW, Confer AW (2011) Mannheimia haemolytica: bacterial-host interactions in bovine pneumonia. Vet Pathol 48:338–348

Skerrett SJ, Liggitt HD, Hajjar AM, Wilson CB (2004) Cutting edge: myeloid differentiation factor 88 is essential for pulmonary host defense against Pseudomonas aeruginosa but not Staphylococcus aureus. J Immunol 172:3377–3381

Skerrett SJ, Wilson CB, Liggitt HD, Hajjar AM (2007) Redundant toll-like receptor signaling in the pulmonary host response to Pseudomonas aeruginosa. Am J Physiol Lung Cell Mol Physiol 292:L312–L322

Slauson DO, Lay JC, Castleman WL, Neilsen NR (1987) Alveolar macrophage phagocytic kinetics following pulmonary Parainfluenza-3 virus infection. J Leukoc Biol 41:412–420

Spolski R, Wang L, Wan CK, Bonville CA, Domachowske JB, Kim HP, Yu Z, Leonard WJ (2012) IL-21 promotes the pathologic immune response to pneumovirus infection. J Immunol 188:1924–1932

Srikumaran S, Kelling CL, Ambagala A (2007) Immune evasion by pathogens of bovine respiratory disease complex. Anim Health Res Rev 8:215

Tatum FM, Briggs RE, Sreevatsan SS, Zehr ES, Ling Hsuan S, Whiteley LO, Ames TR, Maheswaran SK (1998) Construction of an isogenic leukotoxin deletion mutant of Pasteurella haemolytica serotype 1: characterization and virulence. Microb Pathog 24:37–46

Thayer G, Robinson S (1984) Bacterial bronchopneumonia in the dog-a review of 42 cases. J Am Anim Hosp Assoc 20:731–735

Tighe RM, Liang J, Liu N, Jung Y, Jiang D, Gunn MD, Noble PW (2011) Recruited exudative macrophages selectively produce CXCL10 after noninfectious lung injury. Am J Respir Cell Mol Biol 45:781–788

Tillett WS, Francis T (1930) Serological reactions in pneumonia with non-protein somatic fraction of pneumococcus. J Exp Med 52:561–571

Toews GB (1994) Pulmonary clearance of infectious agents. In: Pennington JE (ed) Respiratory infections—diagnosis and management, 3rd edn. Raven Press, New York NY, pp 43–53

Tong GZ, Zhou YJ, Hao XF, Tian ZJ, An TQ, Qui HJ (2007) Highly pathogenic porcine reproductive and respiratory syndrome, China. Emerg Infect Dis 13:1434–1436

Trowald-Wigh G, Ekman S, Hansson K, Hedhammar A, Hard af Segerstad C. (2000) Clinical, radiological and pathological features of 12 Irish setters with canine leucocyte adhesion deficiency. J Small Anim Pract 41:211–217

Valarcher JF, Furze J, Wyld S, Cook R, Conzelmann KK, Taylor G (2003) Role of alpha/beta interferons in the attenuation and immunogenicity of recombinant bovine respiratory syncytial viruses lacking NS proteins. J Virol 77:8426–8439

van der Windt GJ, Florquin S, de Vos AF, van't Veer C, Queiroz KC, Liang J, Jiang D, Noble PW, van der Poll T (2010) CD44 deficiency is associated with increased bacterial clearance but enhanced lung inflammation during gram-negative pneumonia. Am J Pathol 177:2483–2494

Van Dyken SJ, Locksley RM (2013) Interleukin-4– and interleukin- 13–mediated alternatively activated macrophages: roles in homeostasis and disease. Annu Rev. Immunol 31:317–343

van Lieshout MH, Blok DC, Wieland CW, de Vos AF, van't Veer C, van der Poll T (2012) Differential roles of MyD88 and TRIF in hematopoietic and resident cells during murine gram-negative pneumonia. J Infect Dis 206:1415–1423

van Reeth K, Labarque G, Nauwynck H, Pensaert M (1999) Differential production of proinflammatory cytokines in the pig lung during different respiratory virus infections: correlations with pathogenicity. Res Vet Sci 67:47–52

van Zoelen MA, Schouten M, de Vos AF, Florquin S, Meijers JC, Nawroth PP, Bierhaus A, van der Poll T (2009) The receptor for advanced glycation end products impairs host defense in pneumococcal pneumonia. J Immunol 182:4349–4356

Vanden Bush TJ, Rosenbusch RF (2002) Mycoplasma bovis induces apoptosis of bovine lymphocytes. FEMS Immunol Med Microbiol 32:97–103

Vareille M, Kieninger E, Edwards MR, Regamey N (2011) The airway epithelium: soldier in the fight against respiratory viruses. Clin Microbiol Rev 24:210–229

Vegad JL, Katiyar AK (2015) Contagious bovine pleuropneumonia. In: A textbook of veterinary special pathology, 1st edn. CBS publishers & distributors, p 447

Villamon E, Gozalbo D, Roig P, Murciano C, O'Connor JE, Fradelizi D, Gil ML (2004) Myeloid differentiation factor 88 (MyD88) is required for murine resistance to Candida albicans and is critically involved in Candida-induced production of cytokines. Eur Cytokine Netw 15:263–271

Virtala AM, Grohn YT, Mechor GD, Erb HN (1999) The effect of maternally derived immunoglobulin G on the risk of respiratory disease in heifers during the first 3 months of life. Prev Vet Med 39:25–37

Viuff B, Tjornehoj K, Larsen LE, Røntved CM, Uttenthal Å, Rønsholt L, Alexandersen S (2002) Replication and clearance of respiratory syncytial virus: apoptosis is an important pathway of virus clearance after experimental infection with bovine respiratory syncytial virus. Am J Pathol 161:2195–2207

Vogelweid CM, Zapien KA, Honigford MJ, Li L, Li H, Marshall H (2011) Effects of a 28-day cage-change interval on intracage ammonia levels, nasal histology, and perceived welfare of CD1 mice. J Am Assoc Lab Anim Sci 50:868–878

Voynow JA, Selby DM, Rose MC (1998) Mucin gene expression (MUC1, MUC2, and MUC5/5 AC) in nasal epithelial cells of cystic fibrosis, allergic rhinitis, and normal individuals. Lung 176:345–354

Wagener JS, Sobonya R, Minnich L, Taussig LM (1984) Role of canine parainfluenza virus and Bordetella bronchiseptica in kennel cough. Am J Vet Res 45:1862–1866

Wani SA, Sahu AR, Saxena S, Rajak KK, Saminathan M, Sahoo AP, Kanchan S, Pandey A, Mishra B, Muthuchelvan D, Tiwari AK, Mishra BP, Singh RK, Gandham RK (2018) Expression kinetics of ISG15, IRF3, IFNγ, IL10, IL2 and IL4 genes vis-a-vis virus shedding, tissue tropism and antibody dynamics in PPRV vaccinated, challenged, infected sheep and goats. Microb Pathog 117:206–218

Welsh MD, Adair BM, Foster JC (1995) Effect of BVD virus infection on alveolar macrophage functions. Vet Immunol Immunopathol 46:195–210

Welsh RM, Selin LK, Szomolanyi-Tsuda E (2004) Immunological memory to viral infections. Annu Rev. Immunol 22:711–743

Woodland DL (2003) Cell-mediated immunity to respiratory virus infections. Curr Opin Immunol 15:430–435

Wu Q, Jiang D, Minor MN, Martin RJ, Chu HW (2011) In vivo function of airway epithelial TLR2 in host defense against bacterial infection. Am J Phys Heart Circ Phys 300:L579–L586

Yamada M, Gomez JC, Chugh PE, Lowell CA, Dinauer MC, Dittmer DP, Doerschuk CM (2011) Interferon-γ production by neutrophils during bacterial pneumonia in mice. Am J Respir Crit Care Med 183:1391–1401

Yang YF, Sylte MJ, Czuprynski CJ (1998) Apoptosis: a possible tactic of Haemophilus somnus for evasion of killing by bovine neutrophils? Microb Pathog 24:351–359

Yates WD (1982) A review of infectious bovine rhinotracheitis, shipping fever pneumonia and viral-bacterial synergism in respiratory disease of cattle. Can J Comp Med 46:225–263

Ye P, Rodriguez FH, Kanaly S, Stocking KL, Schurr J, Scwarzenberger P, Oliver P, Huang W, Zhang P, Zhang J, Shellito JE (2001) Requirement of interleukin 17 receptor signaling for lung CXC chemokine and granulocyte colony-stimulatory factor expression, neutrophil recruitment, and host defense. J Exp Med 194:519–527

Zeugswetter F, Weissenbock H, Shibly S, Hassan J, Spergser J (2007) Lethal bronchopneumonia caused by Mycoplasma cynos in a litter of golden retriever puppies. Vet Rec 161:626–627

Zheng SG, Wang JH, Gray JD, Soucier H, Horwitz DA (2004) Natural and induced CD4+CD25+ cells educate CD4+CD25− cells to develop suppressive activity: the role of IL-2, TGF-β, and IL-10. J Immunol 172:5213–5221

Zinkernagel RM, Doherty PC (1974) Restriction of in vitro T-cell-mediated cytotoxicity in lymphocytic choriomeningitis within a syngeneic or semiallogeneic system. Nature 248:701–702

Immunopathology of the Liver in Animals 8

Key Points

1. The liver is the largest gland and accessory organ to the digestive tract with pivotal role in metabolism, biotransformation of xenobiotics, and their release into the bile.
2. The liver contributes about 20–50% of the lymph flow in thoracic duct and is the largest lymph producer in the body.
3. About ~25% of the total blood volume of the heart is received by the liver, and in addition, it receives blood from the portal vein.
4. The liver acts as one of the important lymphoid organs with specialized cells such as resident macrophages (Kupffer cells), sinusoidal endothelial cells (SECs), hepatic stellate cells (HSCs), dendritic cells, lymphocytes, NKT cells, and NK cells.
5. Kupffer cells are resident (fixed) macrophages of the liver and secrete a variety of cytokines and growth factors that contribute to the inflammatory and repair responses.
6. Toll-like receptor 4 is constitutively expressed on hepatocytes, SECs and HSCs, which activates the immune system.
7. The liver is an immunologically highly tolerogenic organ.
8. Balance between pro-inflammatory and anti-inflammatory responses determines the final result of intrahepatic immune responses.
9. Hepatocytes are infected, either by hepatotropic viruses, parasites, bacterium, fungal agents, protozoa, and toxic agents results in activation of complex immune responses by stimulation of diverse immunological cells found in the liver.
10. Autoimmune hepatitis (AIH) is a complex pathogenic process, caused by toxins, drugs, metabolites, commensal and pathogenic organisms, and microbial products resulting in abnormal immune responses that disrupt the tolerance and cause chronic portal inflammation.

11. Infectious diseases affecting the liver are infectious canine hepatitis, Wesselsbron disease, Rift Valley fever, leptospirosis, trematodes, etc.

8.1 Introduction

The liver is a friable, brownish-red, and largest gland in the animal body. The liver is considered as an accessory organ to the digestive tract (Crispe 2009). It represents ~3%, ~2%, and ~1% of the total body weight among fully grown carnivores, omnivores, and herbivores, respectively. The liver is the pivotal organ of metabolism with high level of vascularization, which allows complete access to the cells of the liver to the blood stream (Böttcher et al. 2011). The liver plays a major role for the processing of dietary lipids, carbohydrates, amino acids and vitamins, synthesis of plasma proteins, detoxification, and biliary excretion of endogenous waste and xenobiotic compounds.

The hepatic parenchyma is exposed to various metabolic and tissue-remodeling activities along with continuous encounter of microbial products, which results in sustained and regulated inflammation. These processes of inflammation occur in a very regulated manner and executed in the liver to eliminate the hepatotropic pathogens, cells of malignancy, and toxic products from metabolic activity (Robinson et al. 2016). This may pave the way to the development of chronic pathological inflammation and disruption of tissue homeostasis, leading to fibrosis of the liver, cirrhosis, and hepatic failure (Robinson et al. 2016). In the liver, inflammatory processes of homeostatic control regulate the hemodynamic changes, movement of leukocytes toward tissues and production of inflammatory mediators (Robinson et al. 2016). This regulated homeostatic inflammatory response is crucial to resolve inflammation and safeguard the tissues and organs homeostasis; however, when it gets dysregulated, pathological changes occurs (Robinson et al. 2016).

8.2 Anatomy of the Liver

The liver is covered by a smooth capsular surface, and the hepatic parenchyma has friable reddish-brown tissue that is partitioned into lobes. Liver lobes vary in number and shape among domestic mammals. In the case of monogastric animals, the liver lies in the central cranial area of the abdomen; whereas, among ruminants and to a lesser extent in equines, the location is right side of the cranial abdomen.

8.3 Histology of the Liver

The arrangement of hepatocytes will be either acini or lobules, which is species-specific. The hepatic lobule is hexagonal in shape with the arrangement of hepatocytes as cords radiating from terminal hepatic venule in the center known as "central vein." In pigs, capsule of the liver forms septa, which divides the parenchyma into lobular perimeters; while, in most mammals, hepatic lobules are less obvious, because the connective tissue is more limited to the portal tracts. The portal triad (portal tract) is a well-formed structure consisting of at least one each branch of the bile duct, hepatic artery and portal vein, and surrounded by connective tissue majorly made up of type I collagen.

Liver sinusoids differ from vascular structures of other areas by lacking a characteristic basement membrane and are supported by a discontinuous or loose extracellular matrix (ECM). The hepatic sinusoids have an average diameter of 10 μm, but they can expand up to 30 μm. Periportal sinusoids are tortuous than those in the centrilobular region. Specialized endothelial cells line the hepatic sinusoids and these are fenestrated having 100 nm diameter sieve-like pores. Sinusoids are set apart from the adjacent hepatocytes by an extracellular space, called the space of Disse, which has reticulin fibers, hepatic stellate cells and nerves. Under light microscopy, the space of Disse is not distinct except when there is fluid retention due to impediment to venous outflow.

8.4 The Bile Duct System and Gallbladder

The system of bile ducts is a branching outflow, where bile ultimately enters the anterior duodenum. The gallbladder acts as a bile storage diverticulum in most species except in horse and rat. The gallbladder in cat occasionally is bipartite or divided. The bile duct connects with the pancreatic duct before emptying into the duodenum. The lining of the bile ducts is by cuboidal to low columnar epithelium.

8.5 Cells of the Liver

Hepatocytes constitute the most prominent cell type in the liver, around 90% (average ~70–80%) of the bio-weight. Non-parenchymal cells are bile duct epithelium, sinusoidal endothelium, hepatic stellate cells, and Kupffer cells. Hepatocytes are the type of polygonal epithelial cells and are arranged in anastomosing plates of single cell thick, set apart by hepatic sinusoids. Hepatocytes play a central role in metabolism, biotransformation of xenobiotics, and their release into the bile, because of which, the liver is exposed to a number of toxin-related damage and nutritionally based insults.

Hepatic stellate cells (HSC) also called as Ito cells, lipocytes, or fat-storing cells. These cells reside within the space of Disse. Their key functions are (1) storage of retinoids and vitamin A including their homeostasis; (2) maintenance of sinusoidal ECM; (3) synthesis of growth factors, like hepatocyte growth factor and cytokines; and (4) regulating the diameter of sinusoids by contraction of cellular processes. The activation of HSC has been associated with hepatic fibrosis.

Kupffer cells are resident (fixed) macrophages of the liver, bound to the inner wall of sinusoids and are in direct contact with the blood. Kupffer cells secrete a variety of cytokines and growth factors that contribute to modulate inflammatory and repair responses.

8.6 Blood Supply and Bile Flow

About ~25% of the total output of the heart is received by the liver and in addition, it also receives blood from the portal vein. The portal vein drains from the pancreas, spleen, stomach, and intestine provides ~50% of the oxygen supply and 70–80% of the total hepatic afferent blood flow. Admixture of portal and arterial blood takes place in the low-pressure areas like hepatic sinusoids. Blood exits the liver through the hepatic vein and enters through the posterior vena cava. Blood flow is from the portal area towards the central vein of each lobule, while bile flow is from the central vein to the portal area.

8.7 Immunopathology of the Liver

A diverse populations of hepatic immune cells make the liver as a complex immunological organ (Nemeth et al. 2009). As a part of innate immune system, liver acts as one of the important lymphoid organs. The liver capillary system is lined by specialized cells (non-parenchymal) such as sinusoidal endothelial cells (SECs), HSCs, intravascular resident macrophages (Kupffer cells) and dendritic cells, and parenchymal cells of the liver (hepatocytes and cholangiocytes). These parenchymal cells act as primary sensors and triggers immune responses (Table 8.1). Kupffer cells, DCs, and SECs are the important antigen-presenting cells of the liver (Crispe 2009). Identification of different cell types in the liver can be done by immunohistochemistry using chromogen or fluorescent-tagged antibodies.

Hepatocytes are infected, either by hepatotropic viruses, parasites, and intracellular bacterium, which results in the activation of complex local immune responses by stimulation of diverse immunological cells that are found in the non-parenchymal fractions like SECs, Kupffer cells, HSCs, trafficking monocytes, DCs, natural killer (NK) cells, NKT (natural killer T lymphocytes) cells, and varied types of $CD4^+$ and $CD8^+$ T lymphocytes.

Danger-sensing receptors like Toll-like receptors (TLRs) especially TLR4 is constitutively expressed on hepatocytes, SECs and HSCs, which activates the immune system (Matsumura et al. 2000). These cells oversee antigen presentation, acute-phase protein production, complement factors, and chemokines and cytokines production. Therefore, these cells are key players in initiating and shaping the immune responses in liver (Heymann and Tacke 2016). There is continuous exposure of liver to non-self-proteins and bacterial endotoxins derived from diet or gut microbiota, which would normally trigger immune responses (Racanelli and Rehermann 2006). Liver tolerance mechanisms allow viruses and parasites to persist in the liver chronically (Knolle and Thimme 2014). Injury to the liver due to viruses,

8.7 Immunopathology of the Liver

Table 8.1 Antibodies for the demonstration of cells of the liver

Type of cells	Antibodies
Hepatocytes	CK8 and 18
Bile canaliculi	Polyclonal CEA
Bile duct epithelium	AE1/AE3, CK7 and 19
Endothelial cells	Factor VIII, CD31, and CD34
Monocytes	ED1
Kupffer cells	CD68, ED2, and SRA-E5
Myofibroblasts, smooth muscle cells, and activated hepatic stellate cells	α-SMA
Dendritic cells	OX-6 and NLDC-145
Oval cells	CK20 and α-fetoprotein (AFP)
Apoptosis	Bcl-2, caspase 3 and 8
Proliferative markers	Ki67 and PCNA

References: Davenport et al. (2001), Kashiwagi et al. (2001), Malhotra et al. (2004), Geller et al. (2008)

AE1/AE3 two clones of anti-cytokeratin monoclonal antibodies, *α-SMA* α-smooth muscle actin, *Bcl-2* B-cell lymphoma 2, *CD31 and 34* cluster differentiation 31 and 34, *CEA* carcinoembryonic antigen, *CK* cytokeratin, *ED1* rat homologue of human CD68, *Factor VIII* blood-clotting factor/antihemophilic factor, *F4/80* rat anti-mouse macrophage monoclonal antibody, *Ki-67* nuclear protein associated with proliferation, *NLDC-145* rat anti-mouse dendritic cell monoclonal antibody, *OX-6* MHC Class II Ia antibody, *PCNA* proliferating cell nuclear antigen, *SRA-E5* mouse monoclonal anti-macrophage antibody for scavenger receptor A

drugs, alcohol, and metabolic or cholestatic diseases results in hepatitis, which progresses to chronic liver disease and fibrosis (Heymann and Tacke 2016).

Specific macrophages located in the sinusoidal lumen is called as Kupffer cells. These cells migrate along the sinusoidal spaces and reach the areas of injury. They are derived from blood-borne monocytes. They are proficient phagocytic cells and function without stimulating inflammation, but they are less efficient as antigen presenters. Kupffer cells on activation, secrete TNF-α and nitric oxide, which cause peripheral vasodilation in generalized inflammatory responses during exposure of bacterial toxins. Other cytokines such as IL-1 and IL-6 drive the acute-phase responses and some features of the hepatic immune and regenerative responses. Kupffer cells are more likely to secrete IL-10, which suppresses the activation of macrophages and cytokine secretion. Kupffer cells induced cytokine responses are believed to be crucial for adaptive immune responses or tolerance development.

The liver has organ-specific distribution of lymphocytes, NKT cells and NK cells. Cells of specific immune system like $CD8^+$ T cells are more in number in comparison with peripheral blood. Most of the intrahepatic lymphocyte population is involved in innate immunity instead of acquired immunity.

NK cells of the liver make about ~40% of hepatic lymphocytes, and they are functionally and phenotypically distinct from normal blood NK cells. Intrahepatic

NK cells are vital for defense against external antigens from the gut, infections, metastatic tumors, modulation of hepatic fibrosis, and hepatocellular carcinoma. The NKT cells of the liver reside within the space of Disse. The liver also has the largest population of γδ T cells in the body. This diversity of immune cells is associated with immunologic homeostasis, and put forward that the liver can be appraised as lymphoid organ.

Dendritic cells are crucial for triggering and controlling immunological responses in the liver. They are found within the portal tract and are observed to be functionally less matured in comparison to the DCs of the bone marrow and spleen.

Mast cells are plentiful in the liver, especially in dogs. They are seen in perivenous location. In the liver, mast cell degranulation cause contraction of spiral smooth muscles, which in turn restricts outflow of blood from the canine liver. This is the pathophysiological feature of shock seen in dogs.

Liver contributes 20–50% of the lymph flow in thoracic duct and is the largest lymph producer of the body. Lymph from the liver is high in levels of protein and high cells count consisting of lymphocytes and macrophages. In ovine, the lymphocytic circulation is more through the liver than any typical lymphoid tissues.

8.8 Types and Patterns of Cell Death in the Liver

Cell death results from the irreversible damage to the cells. The necrosis (oncotic necrosis) and apoptosis are the two predominant types of cell death that occur in the liver.

8.9 Necrosis

Initially, necrosis is morphologically observed as cellular swelling, followed by loss of integrity of plasma membrane, formation of large blebs, and lysis of cells. The ATP depletion and subsequent failure to maintain the membrane stability lead to necrosis. Influx of calcium results in disruption of both organelle and plasma membranes, which includes release of catalytic enzymes from lysosomes.

Oncosis is commonly considered as severe injury to the integrity of the cell membrane, leading to enzymes leakage and inflammation. Sequelae events of secondary inflammation due to release of cellular contents cause elevation of the serum enzymes, which are useful to detect hepatic necrosis. But, these events can also occur following apoptosis of hepatocytes, mainly because of the exceeded capacity for phagocytic removal of apoptotic cells and severe insult, which supervene into necrosis.

In post-necrotic stages, disintegrating hepatocytes are seen along with infiltrating neutrophils and/or macrophages. A variety of insults can lead to either necrosis or apoptosis of hepatocytes, which include hypoxia, hepatotoxic chemicals, reactive oxygen metabolites, bacterial toxins, viral infections, and inflammation (Table 8.2).

8.9 Necrosis

Table 8.2 Common hepatotoxic agents of domestic animals and birds

Category	Hepatotoxic agents
Viral agents	Infectious canine hepatitis (*Canine adenovirus* 1) (Figs. 8.1, 8.2, and 8.3)
	Wesselsbron disease (*Flavivirus*)
	Rift Valley fever (*Phlebovirus*)
	Equine serum hepatitis: Theiler's disease (Theiler's disease-associated virus (TDAV)) (*Flavivirus*)
	Infectious bovine rhinotracheitis virus (*Bovine herpesvirus* 1)
	Abortigenic equine herpesvirus (*Equine herpesvirus* 1)
	Canine herpesvirus (*Canine herpesvirus* 1)
	Feline viral rhinotracheitis virus (*Feline herpesvirus* 1)
	Pseudorabies virus (*Sui herpesvirus* 1)
	PCV 2-associated disease (*Porcine circovirus* 2)
	Avian leukosis/big liver disease/lymphoid leukosis: leukosis/sarcoma group of avian retroviruses (Fig. 8.4 and Fig. 8.5)
	Marek's disease: genus *Mardivirus* and family *Herpesviridae* (Fig. 8.6 and Fig. 8.7)
	Highly pathogenic *influenza* A virus H5N1
	Feline calicivirus
	GB-virus-like virus (*Pegivirus*)
	Hepatitis E virus (HEV) genotypes 3 and 4
Bacterial agents	Actinobacillosis (*Actinobacillus equuli*, *A. suis*)
	Yersiniosis (*Yersinia pseudotuberculosis*)
	Tularemia (*Francisella tularensis*)
	Mannheimia (*Pasteurella*) *haemolytica*
	Histophilus somni
	Campylobacteriosis (*Campylobacter fetus*)
	Salmonellosis
	Nocardiosis (*Nocardia asteroids*)
	Necrobacillosis: *Fusobacterium necrophorum* (Figs. 8.8 and 8.9)
	Necrotic hepatitis-black disease (*Clostridium novyi*; type B strain)
Fungal agents	Histoplasmosis (*Histoplasma capsulatum*)
	Cryptococcus spp.
	Coccidioidomycosis (*Coccidioides immitis*)
	Sporotrichosis (*Sporothrix schenckii*)
	Aspergillus spp.
	Prototheca spp.
Trematodes	Fasciolosis: *Fasciola hepatica*, *F. gigantica*, *Fascioloides magna* (Fig. 8.10)
	Dicrocoeliosis (*Dicrocoelium dendriticum*)
	Schistosomiasis (*Heterobilharzia americana*)
	Opisthorchiidae (*Clonorchis sinensis* and *Opisthorchis felineus*)
	Pseudamphistomum truncatum
Cestodes	Cysticercosis in rat: larval stage *Cysticercus tenuicollis*
	Stilesia hepatica
	Hydatid cysts (*Echinococcus multilocularis*, *E. granulosus*)

(continued)

Table 8.2 (continued)

Category	Hepatotoxic agents
	Thysanosoma actinioides
Nematodes	*Strongylus vulgaris*
	Stephanurus dentatus
	Ascaris suum
	Capillaria hepatica
Pentastomids	*Linguatula serrata*
Protozoa	Toxoplasma
	Neospora
	Leishmania
	Hepatozoon canis
	Cytauxzoon felis
	Equine protozoal myeloencephalitis: *Sarcocystis neurona*
	Hepatic coccidiosis in rabbit: *Eimeria stiedae*
Toxic agents	Adverse drug reactions that induced liver injury
	Antibiotics (trimethoprim-sulfonamide)
	Anticonvulsants (zonisamide, primidone, phenytoin, and phenobarbital)
	*Anti*anxiety agent (diazepam)
	Anthelmintic (mebendazole and thiacetarsamide)
	Anti-arrhythmic (amiodarone)
	Anabolic steroid (stanozolol, mibolerone)
	Antidiabetics (glipizide)
	Anticancer drugs (megestrol acetate, methotrexate)
	Antifungals (ketoconazole, griseofulvin)
	Anesthetic agents (methoxyflurane, halothane)
	Photodynamic therapy agent (aluminum phthalocyanine tetrasulfonate)
	Nonsteroidal anti-inflammatory drugs (Carprofen)
	Vaccine (inadvertent subcutaneous injection of intranasal *Bordetella bronchiseptica/Canine parainfluenza*)
	Plants that induced hepatic injury
	Cycadales: methylazoxymethanol (Cycas)
	Solanaceae: Atractyloside (*Cestrum diurnum* and *C. aurantiacum*)
	Myoporaceae: ngaione (*Myoporum acuminatum* and *M. tetrandum*)
	Ulmaceae: trematoxin (*Trema tomentosa, Trema micrantha*)
	Pyrrolizidine alkaloids (*Senecio, Crotalaria, Heliotropium, Cynoglossum, Amsinckia, Echium,* and *Trichodesma*)
	Lantana camara: lantadene A, lantadene C, and icterogenin (Fig. 8.11)
	Heavy metal: copper
	Toxic algae: Cyanobacteria-blue-green algae (*Anabaena, Aphanizomenon, Microcystis,* and *Nodularia*)
	Fungal toxins
	Aflatoxin (*Aspergillus flavus, A. parasiticus,* and *Penicillium puberulum*)
	Fumonisin B1 (*Fusarium verticillioides* and *F. proliferatum*)
	Phomopsin (*Diaporthe toxica*)

(continued)

Table 8.2 (continued)

Category	Hepatotoxic agents
	Facial eczema: Sporidesmin (*Pithomyces chartarum*)
	Larval poisoning
	Sawfly larva (*Lophyrotoma interrupta*, *Arge pullata*, and *Perreyia flavipes*)

8.10 Apoptosis

Apoptosis is a type of programmed cell death, where cells disintegrate without much leakage of cellular contents or inflammation. The main features of apoptosis are maintaining the plasma membrane integrity; proteolytic cleavage of intracellular cytoskeletal proteins; condensation of chromatin and its marginalization; nuclear fragmentation; formation of plasma membrane blebs; and final cell fragmentation into smaller components called apoptotic bodies with intact plasma membrane. These bodies are readily phagocytosed by Kupffer cells or neighboring hepatocytes. The balance between mitosis and apoptosis maintains the liver mass.

Extrinsic apoptotic pathway is via death receptors, a family of cell surface receptors. Death receptors are tumor necrosis factor-α (TNF-α) receptor, Fas, death receptor 4 (DR4), and DR5. Important ligand molecules in the liver are TNF-α, Fas ligand (FasL), and TNF-related apoptosis-inducing ligand (TRAIL). When death receptors bind with their ligand, multiprotein complex, the death-inducing signaling complex (DISC) are formed. Changes in conformation in this complex lead to activation of caspase 8, main mediator of apoptosis, and downstream activation of effector caspases (caspases 3, 6, and 7).

The intrinsic apoptotic pathway involves mitochondrial membrane damage with release of proapoptotic factors. Key activators of this pathway are DNA damage, oxidative stress, toxins, lipid peroxidation, endoplasmic reticulum (ER) stress, like accumulation of unfolded proteins, ultraviolet radiation, and growth factors deprivation. Mitochondrial permeability is altered either by direct mitochondrial membrane damage or more generally by transient mitochondrial permeability (TMP) regulated by bax and other proapoptotic proteins of the Bcl-2 family. Altered permeability causes liberation of the cytochrome C from mitochondrion, which forms an apoptosomal complex in the cytoplasm activating an initiator caspase 9 that executes downstream cell fragmentation events. Further, mitochondrial outer membrane permeabilization (MOMP) can be triggered by multiprotein channels within the membranes of mitochondria, causing the release of proapoptotic factors.

Several ligands (TNF-α, Fas ligand, and TRAIL) are expressed on Kupffer cells and resident macrophages, which lead to increased apoptosis among hepatocytes. Likewise, profibrotic cytokines and type 1 collagen are released by HSCs following the engulfment of apoptotic bodies. Exaggerated apoptosis is presently seen as a driver of inflammation and fibrosis of the liver.

8.11 Autoimmune Hepatitis (AIH)

Autoimmune hepatitis (AIH), also known as autoimmune liver disease, is characterized by intracellular antigen-specific serum antibodies, chronic portal inflammation due to unexplained origin (Peters 2002). However, little is understood about the origin and regulators of autoimmune disorders in the liver (Kita et al. 2001). Actin, chromatin, CYP450 (2D6, 2C9, 2A6, and 1A2), glucuronyltransferase (UGT1A), and UGA repressor tRNA-related protein have all been identified as targets of autoantibodies (Wies et al. 2000; Manns and Strassburg 2001). Pathologically, autoimmune hepatitis is more frequently characterized by chronic active hepatitis with infiltration of mononuclear cells, especially plasma cells, and piecemeal necrosis, and distinct liver cell rosetting. Liver pathology is not a diagnostic. Activated CD4 (predominant) and CD8 T cells are among the additional cellular infiltrates found in the portal regions. Additionally, there is proof of T-cell cytotoxicity and class I upregulation on hepatocytes (Löhr et al. 1994; Tanaka et al. 1997).

The liver is a highly tolerogenic organ. Pathogenesis of AIH is complex and caused by environmental stimuli (toxins, drugs, metabolites, commensal and pathogenic organisms, microbial products including DNA, different antigens, and associated haptens) and misaligned immune processes that disrupt tolerance and cause clinical signs of the illness (Assis 2020). The liver is continually exposed to environmental stimuli through the portal vein. The liver prevents pathological inflammatory responses due to its diverse molecules and functional vascular firewall (Balmer et al. 2014). Liver showed local tolerance and potent systemic immune tolerance during transplantation (Calne et al. 1969; Crispe 2014).

Mechanisms responsible for tolerance is stunning and exhaustion. Immunosuppressive substances inactivate reactive T cells during stunning, while excessive and prolonged antigenic stimulation causes malfunction of T cells during fatigue. In addition to preventing unwanted inflammation, this robust tolerogenic immunological environment can also make it easier for infections to persist, which can cause persistent dysregulated inflammation and chronic viral hepatitis, which can result in autoimmunity (Liberal et al. 2013).

During AIH, loss of tolerance can develop due to a combination of genetic predisposition, environmental stimuli, and an imbalance in immunological regulatory mechanisms. This is true even if there are robust peripheral and central tolerogenic pathways. As a result of the loss of tolerance, numerous T-cell subsets and B cells play a significant role in inflicting cytotoxic T cell-mediated hepatocellular damage (Doherty 2016).

8.12 Key Inflammatory Pathways in the Development of AIH

The formation of T helper 1 (Th1), Th2, and Th17 pathogenic pathways can result from the introduction of self-antigens to naive T cells in the presence of co-stimulation, and the relative predominance of key stimulatory cytokines can favor one pathway over another (Table 8.3). Cytokines can polarize the adaptive

Table 8.3 Important inflammatory mechanisms in the onset of autoimmune hepatitis

Phenotype	Key stimuli	Cytokines secreted	Effects on pathogenesis of AIH
Th1	IL-12	IFN-γ, IL-2, MIF, and IL-1β	• CD8+ effector T-cell identification of self-antigen on hepatocytes and cytotoxic damage caused by MHC class I and II • Activation of NK cell
Th2	IL-4	IL-4, IL-10, IL-13, and IL-21	• CD4$^+$ Th cell • B cell differentiation to plasma cells • Complement activation and antibody-mediated cytotoxicity • NK recognition of Fc on hepatocytes
Th17	TGF-β IL-1β IL-6	IL-17, IL-22, IL-23, and TNF-α	• Secretion of IL-6 by hepatocytes • Th17 effector T-cell-mediated liver cell damage

immune responses in favor of autoantigens, which are produced as a result of local innate immune reactions (Assis 2020).

8.13 Immunopathology of Infectious Diseases Affecting the Liver

8.13.1 Infectious Canine Hepatitis

A prevalent illness in dogs known as infectious canine hepatitis (ICH) or Rubarth's disease, which is caused by canine adenovirus type 1 (CAV-1). The CAV-1 is a double-stranded DNA virus that is non-enveloped and icosahedral symmetry. The CAV-1 infects wolves, coyotes, skunks, bears, and even causes foxes to develop encephalitis (Sykes 2014). This is the only virus having a primary liver tropism (Sellon 2005). Severe hepatic necrosis caused by CAV-1 is accompanied by ocular and renal abnormalities. Following oronasal contact, the virus spreads to nearby lymph nodes before localizing in the tonsils and spreading into the thoracic duct. The primary targets of viral replication are hepatic parenchymal cells and vascular endothelial cells, and damage resulting in centrilobular to panlobular hepatic necrosis can range from self-limiting to deadly. The majority of affected dogs are younger than 1 year old and unvaccinated. Dogs with severe disease may become morbidly ill and pass away within hours of the disease onset and with few warning clinical indications.

Fever, inappetence, diffuse hemorrhages, stomach pain, vomiting, diarrhea, and less frequently dyspnea are some of the clinical symptoms. Due to the buildup of circulating immune complexes, corneal opacity (blue eye) and interstitial nephritis may appear 1–3 weeks after the clinical recovery (Carmichael 1965; Wright 1976). Animals who survive may suffer from chronic liver inflammation and fibrosis, which is probably caused by self-renewing hepatic inflammation rather than a persistent infection (Chouinard et al. 1998).

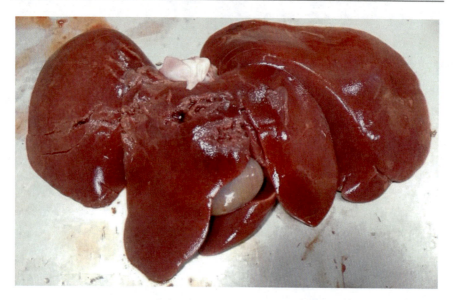

Fig. 8.1 The liver of a dog infected with infectious canine hepatitis: markedly enlarged, congested and friable liver. Focal areas contained hemorrhages and pale tan-yellow foci of necrosis

Blood-tinged ascites or hemoabdomen, enlarged, congested, mottled liver (Fig. 8.1), mild splenomegaly, enlarged, congested and edematous lymph nodes, and fibrin deposition on the surface of the abdominal viscera are the gross pathologic features in dogs affected with ICH. Markedly thickened and edematous gallbladder wall is seen. Hepatocellular necrosis, particularly centrilobular (periacinar) zonal necrosis, and intranuclear viral inclusion bodies within Kupffer cells and hepatocytes (Fig. 8.2) are the most characteristic histologic findings (Thompson et al. 2010). Lymph nodes showed lymphoid depletion (Fig. 8.3). In dogs with persistent liver damage, fibrosis may be seen. There may also be focal neutrophils and mononuclear cells accumulations, and fibrosis results in interstitial nephritis (Caudell et al. 2005).

The condition known as "corneal oedema" or "blue eye" is characterized by diffused corneal clouding that develops suddenly or usually over a short period of time and is accompanied by anterior uveitis. It is brought on by either a naturally occurring CAV-1 infection or by receiving a live modified CAV-1 vaccine. This kerato-uveitis is a type III hypersensitivity manifestation that is characterized by immune complex development as a result of virus release, particularly from the infected corneal endothelial cells, which results in corneal endothelium damage and edema. Most of the cases never reach a conclusion. It seems that the Afghan hound breed is particularly vulnerable. Vaccination with CAV-2 did not cause endogenous ocular disease, a temporally correlated increase in neutralizing antibody titers and corneal edema. Although, it often takes place between 14 and 21 days after infection (dpi), it can happen as early as 7 dpi. Fluorescent techniques can identify

8.13 Immunopathology of Infectious Diseases Affecting the Liver

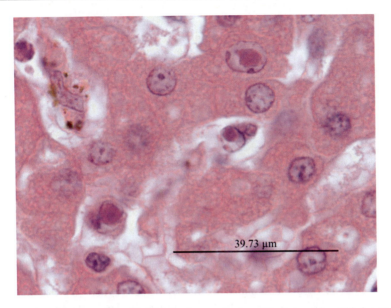

Fig. 8.2 The liver of a dog infected with infectious canine hepatitis: large eosinophilic intranuclear inclusions in the hepatocytes and degenerative changes are evident. H&E ×1000

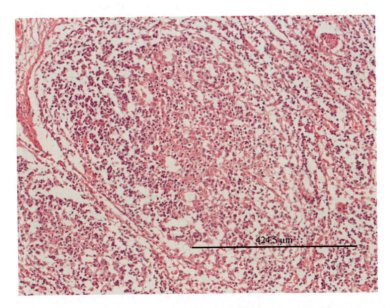

Fig. 8.3 The lymph node of a dog infected with infectious canine hepatitis: the lymph node showed marked lymphocytic depletion in the cortex. H&E ×100

viral antigen in these eyes, but not in the corneal structures. The iris, ciliary apparatus, and corneal propria exhibit inflammatory edema, and the filtration angle and iris both contain a large number of inflammatory cells. There is evidence that the ocular lesion is a hypersensitive reaction to circulating immune complex deposition with complement fixation and chemotaxis of inflammatory cells because the infiltrates are primarily plasma cells.

8.14 Wesselsbron Disease

Wesselsbron virus (WSLV), a neglected flavivirus spread by mosquitoes and widespread on the African continent. In the Wesselsbron area of South Africa, the WSLV was originally discovered in the liver and brain of a dead lamb in 1955 (Weiss et al. 1956). Numerous domesticated animals, including cattle, camels, horses, sheep, and goats are infected with the WSLV (Blackburn and Swanepoel 1980; Swanepoel 1988; Mushi et al. 1998). The virus causes a self-limiting disease in humans and teratogenic to small and large ruminants (Oymans et al. 2020). High neonatal mortality rates and congenital malformations of the central nervous system in ovine fetus namely, hydrops amnii and abortion in ewe are linked with the WSLV (Jupp and Kemp 1998). Humans are also susceptible to clinical and inapparent infection and causes non-fatal influenza-like illness (McIntosh 1986). Various *Aedes* mosquitoes especially *Aedes caballus juppi* are the vectors (Jupp and Kemp 1998; Weyer et al. 2013). The virus causes outbreaks of abortion and perinatal mortality in sheep. Adults were susceptible to infection and exhibited few clinical symptoms, but they could have a biphasic febrile reaction. Hepatitis and jaundice are further clinical manifestations. Although the reservoir host is unknown, Senegal virus isolation has been recently made from black rats (Diagne et al. 2017).

Lambs died within 12 h of birth typically have extensive petechiae and gastrointestinal bleeding as their primary pathologies. Longer-lived lambs had jaundice and an enlarged, friable, orange-yellow liver. Bile in the gallbladder can thicken and turn dark under certain conditions; hemolysis is less likely to be the cause than gallbladder hemorrhages. Lymph nodes are constantly swollen, clogged, and edematous. The most distinctive histopathologic changes are found in the liver and occasional foci of necrosis with apoptosis and proliferation of sinusoidal lining cells were noticed. Accumulation of mononuclear cells and macrophages were noticed in the portal stroma and sinusoidal spaces. Hepatocyte nuclei occasionally have eosinophilic irregular inclusions that are not accompanied by nuclear chromatin margination usually seen with typical viral inclusions, and the significance of these inclusions are unknown. Necrotic, acidophilic and degenerating hepatocytes can show Wesselsbron viral antigen, but inclusions very rarely seen. Animals with jaundice may have severe canalicular cholestasis. In the least severe cases, hepatocellular proliferation is visible. In lymph nodes and spleen, lymphoid follicles had severe lymphocyte necrosis and lymphoblast activation.

8.15 Rift Valley Fever

Rift Valley fever (RVF) is a newly discovered zoonotic virus that is spread by mosquitoes and causes high rates of illness and mortality in both human and animal populations (Fawzy and Helmy 2019). The RVF is caused by RVF virus (RVFV), which is a single-stranded ambi-sense RNA virus that belongs to the genus *Phlebovirus*, family *Phenuiviridae*, and the order *Bunyavirales* (Gerrard and Nichol 2007; Pepin et al. 2010; Moutailler et al. 2011). In Kenya's Rift Valley province, where the name was given, the RVF disease was discovered in sheep for the first time in 1931. The RVFV can be spread to people by drinking unpasteurized milk, coming into close contact with contaminated animal blood, breathing aerosol, or bitten by an infected mosquito. *Aedes*, *Culex*, *Anopheles*, and *Mansonia* mosquito genera are capable of transmitting the virus and serving as a vector (Diallo et al. 2008; Bird et al. 2009). *Culex* and *Aedes* are the RVF virus vectors, which are classified into amplifying and maintenance vectors, respectively (Pepin et al. 2010). Sheep, lamb, goats, cattle, buffalo, some wild animals, and mice are the most vulnerable host to RVF infection (Pepin et al. 2010). Human sickness can range from a simple cold to more serious conditions like hemorrhagic fever, encephalitis, renal failure, retinitis, and miscarriage (Baudin et al. 2016; Hassan et al. 2017). The age of animal significantly influences and young animals are susceptible to the severe type of RVF infection (WHO 2018). The abortion rate in pregnant ewes may approach up to 100%, and the mortality rates for lambs and adult sheep were 90% and 20–60%, respectively (Gerdes 2002; Budasha et al. 2018). The most important clinical manifestation of RVF infection in pregnant animals is an abortion storm. Due to the direct impact of virus on the fetus, infected animals may abort at any point of the gestation period, and the abortion rate can reach up to 100% (Pepin et al. 2010).

As the disease develops, juvenile animals experience fever, anorexia, and eventually death. In contrast, adult animals have fever, weakness, bloody diarrhea, and vomiting as the disease progresses from an apparent form to an acute form (Busquets et al. 2010). Necrotizing hepatitis, necrosis of the spleen, renal tubular damage, and lesions in other organs, including the lymph nodes, lungs, heart, adrenal glands, gall bladder, skin, and digestive system, were highly prevalent in infected sheep (Coetzer 1977; Odendaal et al. 2019). Within the liver, necrotic foci are more or less evenly distributed. In lambs, these foci can combine to produce diffuse necrotic lesions.

Using immunohistochemistry (IHC), the cellular tropism of RVFV was investigated in experimentally and spontaneously infected newborn lambs. Extensive hepatocyte necrosis and a gradual rise in viral antigen in the liver were observed (Van der Lugt et al. 1996). It was consistent that the primary distinguishing lesion of RVF cases in adult sheep was liver necrosis (Odendaal et al. 2019). Innate and adaptive immune systems of Infected animals can help to limit the RVFV infection (Bird et al. 2009; do Valle et al. 2010). It is reported that interferon (IFN)-alpha within 12 h of release provides defence against RVFV infection and the affected animals did not get the illness (Morrill et al. 1990). However, the RVFV non-structural (NS) protein prevents the secretion of IFN-α and IFN-β, allowing for early replication and viremia (Bouloy et al. 2001; Ikegami et al. 2009a, b).

After an infection, anti-RVFV antibodies might be seen 4 to 8 days later (Paweska et al. 2005a, b; Williams et al. 2011). It is thought that neutralizing antibodies are essential for the defense of diseased animals (Morrill et al. 1990; Pepin et al. 2010). Serum from goats infected with RVFV showed elevated levels of IFN-γ, IL-12, and other pro-inflammatory cytokines (TNF-α, IL-6, and IL-1β), but not IFN-α, one of the most effective antiviral cytokines. It is reported that innate immunity through the IL-12 to IFN-γ circuit offered early protection against RVFV despite the lack of IFN-γ because neutralizing antibodies were only identified after viremia had ceased (Nfon et al. 2012).

However, research has shown that IFN-α plays a role in the elimination of RVFV (Morrill et al. 1990). Additionally, the virus has evolved strategies to prevent IFN-γ production or response in cells infected with RVFV by using the NS protein (Bouloy et al. 2001; Ikegami et al. 2009a, b; McElroy and Nichol 2012). This would open up a window for the occurrence of high viremia, which typically happens within 24 h following infection. However, IL-12 and IFN-γ peaked around 2–4 dpi, indicating that goats had a functional innate immune response to RVFV. According to earlier results in sheep, innate immunity was probably responsible for this early protection because RVFV was eliminated from blood many days before neutralizing antibodies were found (Busquets et al. 2010).

It is known that IL-12 causes NK cells from cows and sheep to release IFN-γ (Elhmouzi-Younes et al. 2010), which in turn activates NK cells for better cytotoxicity (Biron and Brossay 2001). The release of IFN-γ by NK cells, macrophages, and DCs could have been aided by the IL-12 (Ansari et al. 2002). Human monocyte-derived macrophages infected with wild-type RVFV showed productive infection and suppression of innate immune responses due to decreased production of TNF-α, IFN-α, and IFN-β (McElroy and Nichol 2012). RVF is characterized by obvious focal hepatic necrosis and cholestasis, which is not as prominent as it is in Wesselsbron disease. Liver lesions in the Wesselsbron disease consist of smaller, randomly distributed foci of hepatocellular necrosis, more active reaction by the sinusoidal lining cells, and more obvious cholestasis (Maxie 2016).

8.16 Lymphoid Leukosis in Poultry

Lymphoid leukosis (LL) is a neoplastic disease of poultry caused by avian leukosis virus (ALC), which belongs to the genus *Alpharetrovirus* and the family *Retroviridae*. The disease is characterized by B-cell lymphoma, which occurs in approximately 16 weeks of age and/or older chickens. Subclinical infection of LL decreases several important performance traits, including egg production. Chickens are the natural hosts for the ALC and the virus is shed by the birds into the yolk results in vertical or congenital infection. Horizontal infection mainly occurs after hatching, especially when the chicks are exposed to faeces of congenitally infected chicks or birds and through contaminated vaccines. Neoplastic disease is more frequent during congenital infection than horizontal infection.

Four types of avian leukosis virus infections are reported in adult birds namely, no viremia and no antibody (V-A-); no viremia and with antibody (V-A+); viremia and with antibody (V+A+); and viremia and no antibody (V+A-). Birds from an infection-free flock and genetically-resistant birds from a susceptible flock belong to the V-A- category. Genetically susceptible birds in an infected flock belong to the one of the three categories of V-A+, V+A+, and V+A-. Out of these, most common category is V-A+. The minority category, usually 10% is V+A-. Most of the V+A- category birds transmit the virus relatively high proportion to their progeny. Lymphoid leukosis causes the clonal malignancy of the bursal-dependent lymphoid system. Lymphoid leukosis tumours are composed of mainly B lymphocytes and have IgM on their surfaces. During LL, no antitumor immune responses have been reported; however, antibodies are readily induced after infection, except when tolerance occurs. Most important gross lesions are diffuse or nodular lymphoid tumours frequently in the liver (Fig. 8.4), spleen and bursa, and occasionally in the kidneys, gonads and mesentery. Lesions in the bursa have been considered virtually pathognomonic. Microscopically, the tumour cells are uniform, large lymphoblasts and mitotic figures are frequent (Fig. 8.5).

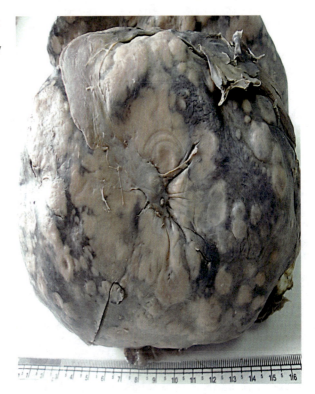

Fig. 8.4 Avian leukosis (big liver disease or lymphoid leukosis) in chicken: a greatly enlarged liver (17-cm length and approximately 1-kg weight) with diffuse grey nodular tumor foci

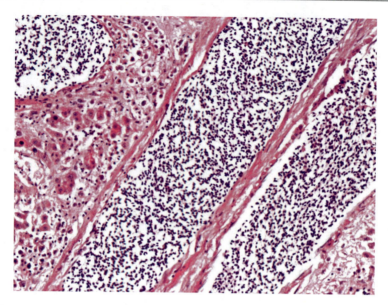

Fig. 8.5 Avian leukosis (big liver disease or lymphoid leukosis) in chicken: a greatly enlarged liver (17-cm length and approximately 1-kg weight) with diffuse grey nodular tumor foci

8.17 Marek's Disease in Poultry

Marek's disease (MD) is a highly contagious viral disease of poultry characterized by T-cell lymphomas and enlargement of peripheral nerves, caused by Marek's disease virus (MDV), belongs to the genus Mardivirus, within the subfamily *Alphaherpesvirinae* and family *Herpesviridae*. The *Gallid alphaherpesvirus 2* (MDV serotype 1) is further divided into various pathotypes, namely mild (m), virulent (v), very virulent (vv), and very virulent plus (vv+). Chickens are the most important natural host for MD. The MDV is a highly cell-associated herpesvirus. The MD is one of the most ubiquitous diseases among various avian virus infections identified in the chicken flocks of worldwide. Marek's disease is highly contagious and readily transmitted among chickens.

Currently, four phases of Marek's disease infection are recognized by in vivo. This includes the early cytolytic infection (productive-restrictive); latent infection; second phase of cytolytic, productive-restrictive infection coincident with permanent immunosuppression; and proliferative phase, involving non-productively infected lymphoid cells that may or may not progress to the point of lymphoma formation. Productive infection may occur transiently in B lymphocytes within a few days after infection with virulent MDV strain and characterized by antigen production, which leads to the cell death. In case of restrictive-productive infection, only few virions are produced. In case of productive infection, enveloped virions are produced in the feather follicle epithelium. Latent infection of activated T cells is responsible for the

8.17 Marek's Disease in Poultry

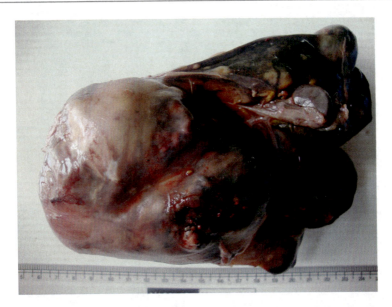

Fig. 8.6 A liver with Marek's disease in turkey: an enlarged liver (19 cm in length and approximately 600 g in weight) with grey nodular tumor foci. The tumor is soft, smooth, and glistening

long-term carrier state. During latent infection, no antigens were expressed, but the MDV can be recovered from the lymphocytes by co-cultivation with susceptible cells in tissue cultures. In case of proliferative phase, some T lymphocytes are latently infected with oncogenic MDV strains, which undergo neoplastic transformation. These transformed cells escape from the immune system of the host and proliferate to form characteristic lymphoid neoplasms.

Most consistent gross lesions in affected birds are enlarged peripheral nerves, particularly brachial, vagus and sciatic nerves, which become enlarged and lose their striations. Diffuse or nodular lymphoid tumors may be seen in various organs, particularly spleen, liver (Fig. 8.6), heart, gonads, kidneys, lungs, proventriculus and muscle. Enlarged feather follicles are commonly noticed during skin leucosis in broilers, which was evident after defeathering during processing and are suitable for condemnation. In case of MD, the bursa is only rarely affected with tumorous and more frequently undergoes atrophy. In case of LL, the bursa is more frequently affected with tumorous condition. Histopathologically, the tumours consist of a mixed population of pleomorphic small, medium, and large lymphoid cells with plasma cells, large anaplastic lymphoblast cells, cancerous cells, and reactive inflammatory cells (Fig. 8.7). When the bursa is involved, the cancerous cells typically appear in interfollicular areas.

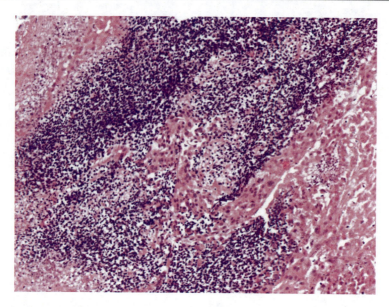

Fig. 8.7 A liver with Marek's disease in turkey: diffused areas of mixed population of small, medium, and large lymphoid cells with anaplastic lymphoblast cells. H&E ×100

8.18 Leptospirosis

Infection with a Gram-negative, slender, spiral, and motile bacteria of the genus *Leptospira* causes the zoonotic disease leptospirosis (Levett et al. 2006). Leptospirosis is a significant zoonotic disease for both humans and animals worldwide. Leptospirosis can be transmitted by when damaged skin or mucous membranes come into contact with water or soil that has been contaminated with the urine of reservoir animals, particularly rats. Gram-negative LPS has a higher endotoxic potential than leptospiral LPS, which may be due to the peculiar characteristics of its lipid A component (Que-Gewirth et al. 2004). According to mutagenesis data, only four virulence factors have been identified in leptospires: proteins Loa22 (Ristow et al. 2007), heme oxygenase (Murray et al. 2008), FliY (flagellar motor switch protein) (Liao et al. 2009), and LPS (Murray et al. 2010). *Leptospira interrogans*, one of two species, can infect animals and cause sickness. There are more than 200 serovars and more than 23 pathogenic serogroups that are antigenically diverse, which complicates the taxonomy of these organisms. In terms of the species affected, the organs involved, and the severity of the illness, each serovar can vary.

Leptospires enter the body through the skin or mucous membranes, if the natural defenses of the skin are damaged. Because the organism is excreted in urine, contaminated soil, water, and bedding are frequently the sources of infection. Transplacental infections can affect fetuses, which are frequently terminated as abortion. Depending on the serovar causing the infection, the red blood cells, kidneys, liver, and other tissues may be affected. Liver is often involved in acute, severe leptospirosis of all domestic species because various serovars cause intravascular hemolytic anemia leading to ischemic injury and centrilobular areas. Further, using silver-staining technique, it is possible to demonstrate a lot of organisms in the liver, although the direct effects of leptospiral toxins on hepatocytes are less well understood.

When animals are infected with serovars that cause hemolysis, gross manifestations include icterus. Depending on the progression of the infection and the serovars involved, hepatic hemorrhage and ascites may develop. Acute infection may occasionally result in focal necrosis and/or centrilobular necrosis. Hepatocyte dissociation is a frequent, non-specific change found in the liver of sick dogs. The affected hepatocytes showed shrunken and hyperbasophilic nuclei, while their cytoplasm becomes eosinophilic and granular. There are frequently visible bile casts in canaliculi. Hemosiderin concentrations in Kupffer cells may be high. *Leptospira grippotyphosa* infection in dogs has been linked to the development of chronic-active hepatitis, but it is unclear that *Leptospira* are responsible for the pathophysiology of many cases of spontaneous chronic hepatitis.

The first line of defense for the host is the innate immune system, which is essential for the early detection and elimination of leptospires. One of the most important effector mechanisms during the first few hours following infection is activation of the alternative pathway of the complement system (Meri et al. 2005).

Pathogenic *Leptospira* species can survive, and are more resistant to the activity of complement system, especially if they are virulent (Barbosa et al. 2009). The term "virulent" refers to phenotypic traits through which pathological alterations may be produced in the host; whereas, the term "pathogenic" refers to genotypic qualities of leptospires that may or may not be manifested. Leptospires are extracellular pathogens; thus the production of antibodies and activation of the classical pathway of complement system are essential for the acquired immune responses. The majority of the specific antibodies produced in leptospirosis are directed against the LPS. Therefore, passive vaccination with polyclonal or monoclonal anti-LPS antibodies can provide immunity against leptospirosis (Jost et al. 1986). It became clear from numerous experimental models that *Leptospira* can only be effectively phagocytosed by neutrophils and macrophages when they are opsonized by specific IgG (Wang et al. 1984). For humans, dogs, pigs, guinea pigs, and hamsters to be protected against leptospirosis, these antibodies must be able to agglutinate leptospires and activate the traditional pathway of humoral-mediated immunity in addition to opsonization. However, little is known about the function of cell-mediated immunity. Development of cellular immune responses has been linked to leptospirosis defense in cattle. Vaccination of cattle with a killed *L. borgpetersenii* preparation results in INF-γ production and proliferation of both CD4+ ab and WC1+ cd T cells following peripheral blood mononuclear cell (PBMC) stimulation with Leptospira (Naiman et al. 2002).

When stimulated with *Leptospira* in humans, PBMC from healthy donors or patients who have recovered from leptospirosis showed an increase in both ab and cd T lymphocytes (Tuero et al. 2010). But more cd T cells have been found in the peripheral blood of those with acute leptospirosis (Klimpel et al. 2003). Therefore, it would appear that the leptospiral immune responses involve both ab and cd T cells. Interestingly, although pathogenic Leptospira is not considered as typical intracellular pathogen, it was reported that L. interrogans may be able to escape from the phagolysossome to the cytosol of a human macrophage cell line (THP-1) (Li et al. 2010). Therefore, Leptospiral peptides might interact with MHC class I molecules and then be presented to CD8+ T cells. Indeed, CD8+ T lymphocytes specific to peptides derived from leptospiral immunoglobulin-like (Lig) A protein were identified in human patients (Guo et al. 2010).

8.19 Fusobacterium necrophorum

Fusobacterium necrophorum causes hepatic abscesses, foot rot, necrotic laryngitis, and lip-leg ulceration in cattle, and sporadic abortion in sheep, which are of significant concern to the cattle and sheep industry. *F. necrophorum* is a normal and opportunistic inhabitant of the respiratory, alimentary, and genital tract of animals and humans, but it can be pathogenic for many species under certain conditions. *F. necrophorum* is a Gram-negative anaerobic, non-spore-forming, and non-motile pleomorphic bacterium present worldwide. Two subspecies of *F. necrophorum* subsp. *necrophorum* (biotype A) and *F. necrophorum* subsp. *funduliforme* (biotype B) have been identified, which differ biochemically, morphologically, and biologically. *F. necrophorum* subsp. *necrophorum* is more virulent and isolated more frequently from infections than subsp. *funduliforme*.

F. necrophorum causes necrotic condition known as necrobacillosis as either specific or non-specific infections in various animals. Ruminants are highly susceptible to hepatic abscesses and foot abscesses, but carnivores are resistant. The pathogenic mechanism of *F. necrophorum* is complex and not well defined. *F. necrophorum* inhabits the rumen and enters the portal circulation and liver. After the entrance of the bacterium or its toxins into the circulation, it can cause sepsis, resulting in hepatic abscesses. It is often associated with ruminal acidosis and rumenitis complex in grain-fed cattle. Grossly, hepatic abscesses in cattle are pale yellow and spherical with irregular outlines of multiple abscesses surrounding an intense zone of hyperemia. Abscesses are usually 1–3 cm in diameter (Fig. 8.8). Histopathologically, the liver showed coagulative necrosis of hepatocytes with central zone of bacterial colonies and surrounding zone of inflammation (Fig. 8.9). Foot rot is the major cause of lameness in dairy and beef cattle. Infected placenta showed purulent exudate on the chorionic surface, necrosis of cotyledons and intercotyledonary areas, edema, and hemorrhage. The skin of the fetus may show severe multifocal dermatitis. Several virulence factors such as endotoxin, leukotoxin, hemagglutinin, hemolysin, adhesin, and proteases etc. have been implicated in the pathogenesis. Among these, the major virulent factor appears to be leukotoxin, which is a secreted protein of high molecular weight and acts specifically on leukocytes of ruminants. *F. necrophorum* is a human pathogen, and the human strains are different from the animal strains.

8.19 Fusobacterium necrophorum

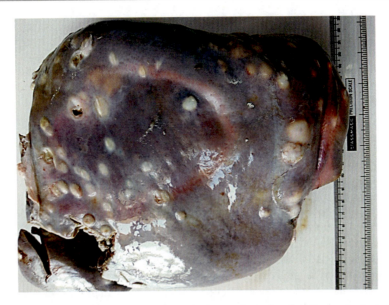

Fig. 8.8 Liver abscesses in cattle (*Fusobacterium necrophorum*): pale yellow and spherical with irregular outlines of multiple abscesses surrounding intense zone of hyperemia. Abscesses are usually 1–3 cm in diameter

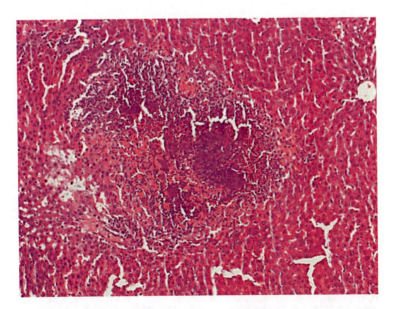

Fig. 8.9 Liver abscesses in cattle (*Fusobacterium necrophorum*): coagulative necrosis of hepatocytes with central zone of bacterial colonies and surrounding zone of inflammation. H&E ×200

8.20 Tematodes

Members of the three main families of trematodes namely, *Dicrocoeliidae*, *Opisthorchidae*, and *Fasciolidae*, cause the majority of the parasitic liver damage. The most important infection among these is fasciolosis. It is mostly caused by the liver fluke *Fasciola hepatica* and affects sheep and cattle. Around the world, hepatic fascioliasis can be found in places where the climate is favorable for the survival of aquatic snails, which act as intermediate hosts for the parasites. These places are often low marshy environments. Adult *Fasciola hepatica* parasites live in the biliary system, which are leaf-shaped. Their eggs pass through the bile from the digestive tract to the feces. Then, in the intermediate host snail, miracidium develops (genus *Lymnaea*). Cercariae come out from the snail encyst and settle on vegetation, where they grow into infectious metacercariae. The ruminant host consumes metacercariae, which then pass through the wall of the duodenum to reach the peritoneal cavity and then the liver. Before settling inside the bile ducts, they move within the liver. Hemorrhagic tracts in the necrotic liver parenchyma are produced when immature flukes migrate across the liver. These tracts are grossly visible and are initially dark red during acute infection, they eventually become paler than the adjacent parenchyma (Fig. 8.10). Fibrosis is a common form of repair. These migrations can cause a number of unfavorable sequelae, such as acute peritonitis, hepatic abscesses, and death of the host due to acute, widespread hepatic necrosis produced by a significant infiltration of immature flukes. Bacillary hemoglobinuria or infectious necrotic

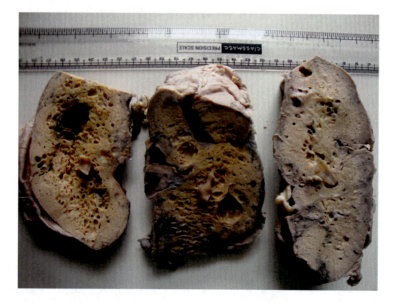

Fig. 8.10 Fasciolosis in cattle (*Fasciola hepatica*): the liver became enlarged, thickened Glisson's capsule and parenchymal destruction due to formation of numerous migratory tracts/tunnels caused by *F. hepatica*

8.20 Trematodes

hepatitis is caused by the growth of *Clostridium haemolyticum* or *Clostridium novyi* spores in necrotic tissues, respectively.

The larger extrahepatic and intrahepatic bile ducts are home to mature flukes that cause cholangitis. Chronic cholangitis and bile duct obstruction cause the ectasia of ducts, stenosis, and development of periductular fibrosis, which thicken the walls and causes the ducts to become more noticeable. Mineralization may occur, producing the classic "pipestem" appearance to the affected bile ducts. Because of a combination of abnormal bile, cellular debris, and iron-porphyrin pigment excreted by the flukes, the bile duct contents are frequently dark brown and viscous. Cholestasis results from the ducts being blocked.

Animals suffering from chronic fasciolosis frequently have poor body condition. *Fasciola gigantica* and *Fascioloides magna* are important causes of liver fluke disease of ruminants in some areas of the world. North America is home to *Fascioloides magna*, while the regions of Africa and its neighbors are the most common locations for *Fasciola gigantica*. In India, *Fasciola gigantica* and *Fasciola hepatica* adults frequently found in the bile ducts. In contrast, adult *Fascioloides magna*, whose normal hosts are elk and white-tailed deer, reside in the hepatic parenchyma in aberrant hosts, such as cattle and sheep. Immature *Fascioloides magna* flukes in cattle travel through the liver and causes significant tissue damage, whereas adults are encased in cysts filled with a dark fluid and are protected by fibrous connective tissue. The flukes continuously migrate through the liver of sheep and goats, resulting in severe injury and eventual death.

The bile ducts may also be home to other trematodes, such as *Eurytrema pancreaticum* and *E. coelomaticum* in ruminants; *Opisthorchis tenuicollis* in pigs, dogs, and cats; *Opisthorchis felineus* in dogs and cats; *Dicrocoelium dendriticum* in horses, ruminants, pigs, and carnivores; and *Pseudamphistomum truncatum*, *Metorchis conjunctus*, *Metorchis albidus*, *Parametorchis complexus*, *Concinnum (Eurytrema) procyonis*, and *Platynosomum fastosum* in dogs and cats. All have the ability to cause alterations that are comparable to those caused by *Fasciola hepatica*, although they are typically much milder. Additionally, they can infrequently block the bile ducts. Fluke infections, most frequently *Opisthorchiidae* and *Platynosomum fastosum*, can infect cats and less frequently dogs to suffer from severe chronic cholangitis. Microscopically, concentric fibrosis, drastically thickened larger intrahepatic bile ducts, which are typically dilated and frequently with papillary projections of the biliary epithelium into the lumen. The ducts frequently have mild to moderate inflammatory infiltrations of neutrophils and macrophages, while the portal tracts have an infiltrate of neutrophils, lymphocytes, and plasma cells. Eosinophils are rarely found. Adult flukes or their ova are frequently difficult to find in infected animals. *Heterobilharzia americana*, a schistosome that generally infects raccoons, can also infect dogs. When infected raccoons travel over water, their ova shed into the water and release miracidia from their feces, which infect intermediate host snails. Dogs become infected with the disease when cercariae, which are released from the intermediate host snail, pierce their skin. When adult schistosome ova lodge in affected tissues, trigger an inflammatory response, results in development of granulomatous lesions of the liver, pancreas, intestines, and mesentery. *Heterobilharzia americana* has recently been demonstrated to cause hepatic granulomas in horses; however in all cases the infection was asymptomatic.

Fasciola hepatica and *F. gigantica* can migrate to the liver passing through the peritoneal cavity after oral entry into the final host, such as buffaloes, cattle and small ruminants (Ashrafi et al. 2014). Clinically affected animals showed a reduction in the growth rate, development and productivity, and in severe cases of fasciolosis may lead to death. In extreme circumstances, fasciolosis may also result in death (Kuchai et al. 2011). Fasciolosis causes liver fibrosis, cirrhosis, cancer, and significant economic losses (Spithill and Dalton 1998; Machicado et al. 2016).

An infection with the liver fluke results in dominant Th2/T-regulatory type immune responses (Fu et al. 2016), and it is well known for modulating the host immune responses through a number of mechanisms, such as the alternate activation of macrophages and the production of immunosuppressive cytokines (Flynn and Mulcahy 2008), increased stimulation of regulatory T cells (Walsh et al. 2009), and the modulation of differentiation and function of dendritic cells (Hamilton et al. 2009; Rodríguez et al. 2015). However, the immune response to *F. gigantica* infection is a mix of Th1/Th2 response, with a Th2-biased pattern predominating (Molina 2005; Chantree et al. 2013).

Fasciola hepatica infection in lambs can induce a dominant Th2-biased immune responses along with suppression of Th1/Th17 responses (Fu et al. 2016), and can negatively impact Th1 responses to bystander infections, such as during coinfection with *Mycobacterium tuberculosis* (Flynn et al. 2007). Buffaloes can exhibit a combination of Th1 and Th2 cytokine expression pattern in response to *F. gigantica* infection (Changklungmoa et al. 2016). The development of a local immune response in the liver of large ruminants infected with *F. gigantica* is indicated by the infiltration of T and B lymphocytes, plasma cells, eosinophils, and mast cells in hepatic lesions. This reaction was most likely brought on by the increased antigen load that the developing flukes were releasing. In addition, the continuous immune responses might be explained by tissue damage and the subsequent production of autoantigens. In bovine and bubaline *F. gigantica* infection, the T lymphocytes may aid and assist in selecting the particular antibody responses, in producing cell-mediated responses, and recruit and activate macrophages and granulocytes. The T-cell responses in the liver of large ruminants displayed various patterns. While the quantity of T cells in buffaloes gradually increased, it started to decline in cattle after 3 weeks. This shows that there was increasing host responsiveness to the antigenic products released by flukes and to the stimulus induced by necrotic tissues in the liver in buffaloes; whereas, in cattle the T cell responses may be depressed to a certain extent after 3 weeks. Proliferative responses of lymphocytes from sheep infected with *F. hepatica* to concanavalin A were reduced after 4 weeks of infection (Zimmerman et al. 1983). *Fasciola gigantica* may have either inhibited the proliferation of T lymphocytes or suppressed the local cellular response to a certain degree in cattle to facilitate their migration through the hepatic parenchyma. As leucocyte infiltration was hampered in sheep with fasciolosis, there may be a decrease of the local inflammatory and immunological responses in the infected liver to permit their migration across the hepatic parenchyma (Chauvin and Boulard 1996). The rapid migration of *F. hepatica* in goats was thought of as a possible mechanism of immune evasion by the parasite (Martinez-Moreno et al. 1999).

Fasciola hepatica employs a variety of ways to alter the host immune responses, rendering it ineffective to kill the parasites (Molina-Hernández et al. 2015). The stimulation of T regulatory cells (Foxp3), a strategy shared by other helminths, which promotes parasite survival and modulates tissue damage (McNeilly et al. 2013). The majority of helminth parasite infections result in a potent type-2 immune responses with early production of IL-4 over IFN-γ, which is thought to play a dominating role in the protective immunity of the host and associated with a reduction in both worm burden and disease severity (Moreau and Chauvin 2010). In previous studies, it has been reported that F. hepatica is able to downregulate the Th1 immune responses and upregulate the Th2 responses at early stages of infection in sheep, mice, and chronic stages in cattle (Pacheco et al. 2017; Chung et al. 2012; Ingale et al. 2008). Regulatory cytokines and cells that modify and/or decrease inflammatory responses mediate this imbalance toward a Th2 immune profile. The induction of a regulatory environment by the expression of cytokines such as IL-10 and TGF-β has been shown as a common strategy used by parasites and microorganisms to extend their survival (Curotto de Lafaille and Lafaille 2008). The expression of Foxp3 T cells are elevated as a outcome of this regulatory environment. Particularly, it has been demonstrated that Foxp3 T lymphocytes play a decisive role in *F. hepatica* infection, contributing to the parasite survival throughout the migratory stages (Escamilla et al. 2016). In addition, F. hepatica develops other mechanisms to evade the host's immune response in early stages in sheep where larvae can induce apoptosis of peritoneal leukocytes, allowing the migration of larvae through the peritoneum (Escamilla et al. 2017).

In both vaccinated and non-immunized sheep, upregulation of Foxp3 along with overexpression of IL-10 and TGF-β indicates that *F. hepatica* induces a modulation of the host response during the initial stages of infection to facilitate the survival of parasites during these crucial phases of the disease (Pacheco et al. 2018). However, while cytokine qPCR analysis showed elevated levels of IL-10, IL-12, IL-13, IL-23, and TGF-β in comparison to uninfected animals at 18 days post-infection, this suggested that the immune response is muted and has not yet been skewed towards a Th2-type response that is linked to chronic disease (Ruiz-Campillo et al. 2017). The most severe liver damage and cirrhosis were seen in goats with numerous hepatic calcareous granulomas. These goats also had a striking infiltrate of CD3+ T lymphocytes and lambda IgG+ plasma cells that replaced large areas of the hepatic parenchyma, where there was a clear hypertrophy of the smooth endoplasmic reticulum of hepatocytes. These results were primarily seen in the goats that received multiple infective doses (Pérez et al. 2002). These studies provide the first evidence to suggest that the induction of an early type-1 immune response in natural host sheep may be responsible for the resistance to liver fluke infection (Pleasance et al. 2011).

8.21 Cysticercus fasciolaris

The adult tapeworm (Cestoda), *Taenia taeniaeformis* occurs in the small intestines of the definitive host, cat and related carnivores all over the world. In intermediate host rat and mice, the prevalence of this parasite, ranges from 4.3% to 67.7%. The infected definitive host excretes thousands of eggs daily (average 12,000 partially developed eggs, called as oncospheres) into the host feces from the proglottids of the adult parasite. The intermediate host, rodents and less frequently lagomorphs become infected through contaminated environment, feed, and water containing viable oncospheres. Common intermediate host species are laboratory, urban, and wild rodents such as rats (*Rattus norvegicus* and *R. rattus*) and mice (*Mus musculus*).

The metacestode or bladder worm or larval stage, *Cysticercus fasciolaris* also known as *Strobilocercus fasciolaris*, *Hydatigera fasciolaris* and *Taenia crassicolis* develops in the liver of the infected rodents. Occasionally, the cysts also develop in the abdominal wall and kidneys, filled with purulent exudate without larvae. Under experimental conditions, one-month old mice infected with low numbers of *T. taeniaeformis* eggs (200-500) developed 11 to 250 metacestodes in the liver. The *T. taeniaeformis* eggs lose their membrane in the stomach or intestine of intermediate host, soon after being ingested and release the larvae, which pass through the intestinal wall. Larvae then migrate via the hepatic portal system and reach the liver. Laboratory rodents that have been experimentally infected with *C. fasciolaris* have a prepatent period of 34-80 days (41.1 ± 5.9); at the end of this period, the ingested larvae become fully developed and infectious. The *T. taeniaeformis* life cycle is completed when the definitive host cats consume infected intermediate host rodents or any other intermediate host containing larval stage in their liver.

The parasite is of zoonotic significance and human beings can act as accidental intermediate host. Adult parasites and metacestodes have been detected in intestines and liver of people from Czech Republic, Argentina, Denmark, Sri Lanka, and Taiwan. Infection of the rat liver by *C. fasciolaris* may cause fibrosarcomas. The cat tape worm *T. taeniaeformis* produce cysts with fibrous tissue capsule around in the intermediate host rat liver with marked infiltration of inflammatory cells especially mononuclear cells and eosinophils (Fig. 8.11a-d).

8.22 Lantana camara toxicity

Lantana camara is the species of tropical flowering plant within the family Verbenaceae (verbena family). Hepatotoxicity is caused by leaves and unripened fruits of lantana. The hepatotoxic compounds are pentacyclic triterpenoids called as Lantadenes. The allelochemicals (compounds that participate in the defense of plants against microbial attack, herbivore predation, and competition with other plants) have been identified from lantana are phenolic compounds and most common phytotoxins are methylcoumarin, umbelliferone and salicylic acid. Recent studies

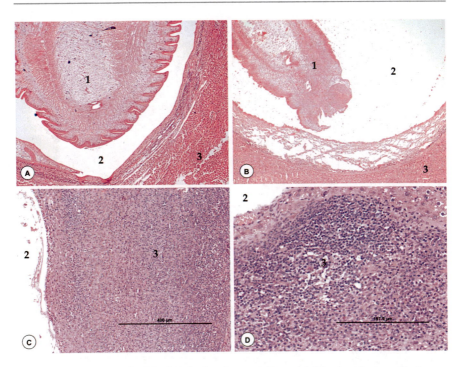

Fig. 8.11 *Cysticercus fasciolaris* infection in a rat liver. (**a**) The larval stage *Cysticercus fasciolaris* (1) in the cystic cavity (2) of liver (3). H&E ×40. (**b**) The mature larval stage *C. fasciolaris* showed oral suckers (1) in the cystic cavity (2) of liver (3). H&E ×40. (**c**) Liver showed *C. fasciolaris* cyst (2) and marked infiltration of inflammatory cells, especially mononuclear cells and few eosinophils (3). H&E ×100. (**d**) Higher magnification of Fig. (**c**). H&E ×200

revealed that most potent allelochemicals of phenolic groups present in *L. camara* are Lantadene A and B.

Lantana camara poisoning in cattle, sheep, buffalo, and guinea pigs caused obstructive jaundice, photosensitization, and increased activity of serum glutamic oxaloacetic transaminase (SGOT) or aspartate transaminase (AST) enzyme. Liver and kidneys are the most affected organs during lantana poisoning especially Lantadene A. Feeding of *L. camara* dried leaves to sheep as a single dose of 10 gram per kg body weight for two consecutive days caused jaundice and photosensitivity. Histopathologically, swollen hepatocytes, necrosis, diffuse macro and micro cytoplasmic vacuoles with displacement of the nuclei to the periphery of affected hepatocytes (fatty change), and congestion of hepatic artery in periportal areas with reduced glycogen content were noticed (Fig. 8.12). The activities of enzymes like esterase, succinate dehydrogenase (SDH), and glutamate dehydrogenase (GDH) were reduced. There was rise in the concentration of bilirubin and phylloerythrin in the serum of affected animals. The activities of enzymes like sorbitol dehydrogenase, arginase and SGOT were increased in serum. There was also reduced clearance of bromosulphate. However, feeding of *L. camara* dried leaves to sheep as a divided

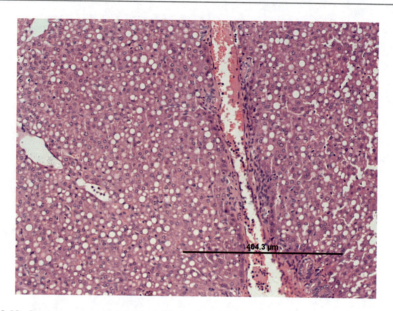

Fig. 8.12 *Lantana camara* toxicity in the liver of a guinea pig: the liver showed diffuse macro and micro cytoplasmic vacuoles in hepatocytes with displacement of the nuclei to the periphery of affected hepatocytes (fatty change) with congestion of hepatic artery. H&E × 100

dose for five consecutive days instead of two days results in slight histopathological changes with no release of enzymes into serum and no retention of bilirubin or phylloerythrin.

Major clinical manifestations in *L. camara* poisoning are photosensitization (excessive sensitivity of skin to sunlight), anorexia, sluggish, dehydration, jaundice, and yellow discolouration of visible mucous membranes, white portion of eye, skin and muzzle. Reddening and inflammation of non-pigmented areas of skin, and swelling of ears and eyelids with discharge from eyes were noticed. In chronic cases, ulcer may develop and bacterial invasion may lead to sloughing of skin surface. Diarrhoea with foul smell and black colour faeces were noticed. Death may occur within 2 days in severely poisoned cattle and 1 to 3 weeks in less severely affected cattle.

8.23 Conclusion

The liver is the largest organ in the body, and has several special immunological characteristics, such as the capability to induce adaptive immune responses, innate immunity, immune tolerance, and suppression of over-reactive autoimmunity, and in the fetal liver, it causes hematopoiesis. Therefore, it has been suggested that the liver is "an immunological organ." Although the liver conducts numerous crucial immune-related actions, its fundamental functions are not typically thought of as immunological. There is evidence to support the idea that hepatocytes, non-parenchymal cells, and liver immune cells must interact in a complicated way for immunological tolerance to be mediated by the liver. The balance between pro-inflammatory and anti-inflammatory T-cell populations and the functional variety of dendritic cells and macrophages determine the final result of intrahepatic immune responses. Therefore, maintaining hepatic immunological homeostasis is crucial for the body to produce the proper immune responses.

References

Ansari AA, Mayne AE, Sundstrom JB, Bostik P, Grimm B, Altman JD, Villinger F (2002) Administration of recombinant rhesus interleukin-12 during acute simian immunodeficiency virus (SIV) infection leads to decreased viral loads associated with prolonged survival in SIVmac251-infected rhesus macaques. J Virol 76(4):1731–1743

Ashrafi K, Bargues MD, O'Neill S, Mas-Coma S (2014) Fascioliasis: a worldwide parasitic disease of importance in travel medicine. Travel Med Infect Dis 12:636–649

Assis DN (2020) Immunopathogenesis of autoimmune hepatitis. Clin Liver Dis 15(3):129

Balmer ML, Slack E, De Gottardi A, Lawson MA, Hapfelmeier S, Miele L, Grieco A, Van Vlierberghe H, Fahrner R, Patuto N, Bernsmeier C (2014) The liver may act as a firewall mediating mutualism between the host and its gut commensal microbiota. Sci Transl Med 6(237):237–237

Barbosa AS, Abreu PA, Vasconcellos SA, Morais ZM, Gonçales AP, Silva AS, Daha MR, Isaac L (2009) Immune evasion of Leptospira species by acquisition of human complement regulator C4BP. Infect Immun 77(3):1137–1143

Baudin M, Jumaa AM, Jomma HJ, Karsany MS, Bucht G, Näslund J, Ahlm C, Evander M, Mohamed N (2016) Association of Rift Valley fever virus infection with miscarriage in Sudanese women: a cross-sectional study. Lancet Glob Health 4(11):e864–e871

Bird BH, Ksiazek TG, Nichol ST, MacLachlan NJ (2009) Rift Valley fever virus. J Am Vet Med Assoc 234(7):883–893

Biron CA, Brossay L (2001) NK cells and NKT cells in innate defense against viral infections. Curr Opin Immunol 13(4):458–464

Blackburn NK, Swanepoel R (1980) An investigation of flavivirus infections of cattle in Zimbabwe Rhodesia with particular reference to Wesselsbron virus. Epidemiol Infect 85(1):1–33

Böttcher JP, Knolle PA, Stabenow D (2011) Mechanisms balancing tolerance and immunity in the liver. Dig Dis 29(4):384–390

Bouloy M, Janzen C, Vialat P, Khun H, Pavlovic J, Huerre M, Haller O (2001) Genetic evidence for an interferon-antagonistic function of Rift Valley fever virus nonstructural protein NSs. J Virol 75(3):1371–1377

Budasha NH, Gonzalez JP, Sebhatu TT, Arnold E (2018) Rift Valley fever seroprevalence and abortion frequency among livestock of Kisoro district, South Western Uganda (2016): a prerequisite for zoonotic infection. BMC Vet Res 14(1):1–7

Busquets N, Xavier F, Martín-Folgar R, Lorenzo G, Galindo-Cardiel I, Del Val BP, Rivas R, Iglesias J, Rodríguez F, Solanes D, Domingo M (2010) Experimental infection of young adult European breed sheep with Rift Valley fever virus field isolates. Vector Borne Zoonotic Dis 10(7):689–696

Calne RY, White HJ, Binns RM, Herbertson BM, Millard PR, Pena J, Salaman JR, Samuel JR, Davis DR (1969) Immunosuppressive effects of the orthotopically transplanted porcine liver. Transplant Proc 1(1):321–324

Carmichael LE (1965) The pathogenesis of ocular lesions of infectious canine hepatitis: II. Experimental ocular hypersensitivity produced by the virus. Pathol Vet 2(4):344–359

Caudell D, Confer AW, Fulton RW et al (2005) Diagnosis of infectious canine hepatitis virus (CAV-1) infection in puppies with encephalopathy. J Vet Diagn Investig 17:58–61

Changklungmoa N, Phoinok N, Yencham C, Sobhon P, Kueakhai P (2016) Vaccine potential of recombinant cathepsinL1G against *Fasciola gigantica* in mice. Vet Parasitol 226:124–131

Chantree P, Phatsara M, Meemon K, Chaichanasak P, Changklungmoa N, Kueakhai P et al (2013) Vaccine potential of recombinant cathepsin B against Fasciola gigantica. Exp Parasitol 135(1): 102–109

Chauvin A, Boulard C (1996) Local immune response to experimental Fasciola hepatica infection in sheep. Parasite 3:209–215

Chouinard L, Martineau D, Forget C et al (1998) Use of polymerase chain reaction and immunohistochemistry for detection of canine adenovirus type 1 in formalin-fixed, paraffin-embedded liver of dogs with chronic hepatitis or cirrhosis. J Vet Diagn 10:320–325

Chung JY, Bae YA, Yun DH, Yang HJ, Kong Y (2012) Experimental murine fascioliasis derives early immune suppression with increased levels of TGFβ and IL-4. Korean J Parasitol 50:301–308

Coetzer JA (1977) The pathology of Rift Valley fever. I. Lesions occurring in natural cases in new-born lambs. Onderstepoort J Vet Res. 44(4):205–211

Crispe IN (2009) The liver as a lymphoid organ. Annu Rev. Immunol 27:147–163

Crispe IN (2014) Immune tolerance in liver disease. Hepatology 60(6):2109–2117

Curotto de Lafaille MA, Lafaille JJ (2008) Natural and adaptive FoxP3+ regulatory cells: more of the same or a division of labor? Immunity 29:114–126

Davenport M, Gonde C, Redkar R, Koukoulis G, Tredger M, Mieli-Vergani G, Portmann B, Howard ER (2001) Immunohistochemistry of the liver and biliary tree in extrahepatic biliary atresia. J Pediatr Surg 36(7):1017–1025

Diagne MM, Faye M, Faye O, Sow A, Balique F, Sembène M, Granjon L, Handschumacher P, Faye O, Diallo M, Sall AA (2017) Emergence of Wesselsbron virus among black rat and humans in eastern Senegal in 2013. One Health 3:23–28

Diallo D, Ba Y, Dia I, Lassana K, Diallo M (2008) Use of insecticide-treated cattle to control Rift Valley fever and West Nile virus vectors in Senegal. Bull Soc Pathol Exot 101(5):410–417

do Valle TZ, Billecocq A, Guillemot L, Alberts R, Gommet C, Geffers R, Calabrese K, Schughart K, Bouloy M, Montagutelli X, Panthier JJ (2010) A new mouse model reveals a critical role for host innate immunity in resistance to Rift Valley fever. J Immunol 185(10): 6146–6156

Doherty DG (2016) Immunity, tolerance and autoimmunity in the liver: a comprehensive review. J Autoimmun 66:60–75

Elhmouzi-Younes J, Boysen P, Pende D, Storset AK, Le Vern Y, Laurent F, Drouet F (2010) Ovine CD16+/CD14- blood lymphocytes present all the major characteristics of natural killer cells. Vet Res 41(1):1

Escamilla A, Zafra R, Pérez J, McNeilly TN, Pacheco IL, Bufoni L, MartínezMoreno FJ, Molina-Hernández V, Martínez-Moreno A (2016) Distribution of Foxp3+T cells in the liver and hepatic lymph nodes of goats and sheep experimentally infected with *Fasciola hepática*. Vet Parasitol 230:14–19

Escamilla A, Pérez-Caballero R, Zafra R, Bautista MJ, Pacheco IL, Ruiz MT, Martínez-Cruz MS, Martínez-Moreno A, Molina-Hernández V, Pérez J (2017) Apoptosis of peritoneal leucocytes during early stages of *Fasciola hepatica* infection in sheep. Vet Parasitol 238:49–53

Fawzy M, Helmy YA (2019) The One Health approach is necessary for the control of Rift Valley fever infections in Egypt: a comprehensive review. Viruses 11(2):139

Flynn R, Mulcahy G (2008) The roles of IL-10 and TGF-beta in controlling IL-4 and IFN-gamma production during experimental *Fasciola hepatica* infection. Int J Parasitol 38:1673–1680

Flynn RJ, Mannion C, Golden O, Hacariz O, Mulcahy G (2007) Experimental *Fasciola hepatica* infection alters responses to tests used for diagnosis of bovine tuberculosis. Infect Immun 75: 1373–1381

Fu Y, Chryssafidis AL, Browne JA, O'Sullivan J, McGettigan PA, Mulcahy G (2016) Transcriptomic study on ovine immune responses to *Fasciola hepatica* infection. PLoS Negl Trop Dis 10:e0005015

Geller SA, Dhall D, Alsabeh R (2008) Application of immunohistochemistry to liver and gastrointestinal neoplasms: liver, stomach, colon, and pancreas. Arch Pathol Lab Med 132(3):490–499

Gerdes GH (2002) Rift valley fever. Vet Clin North Am Food Anim Pract 18(3):549–555

Gerrard SR, Nichol ST (2007) Synthesis, proteolytic processing and complex formation of N-terminally nested precursor proteins of the Rift Valley fever virus glycoproteins. Virology 357(2):124–133

Guo YJ, Wang KY, Sun SH (2010) Identification of an HLA-A* 0201-restricted CD8+ T-cell epitope encoded within Leptospiral immunoglobulin-like protein A. Microbes Infect 12(5): 364–373

Hamilton C, Dowling D, Loscher C, Morphew R, Brophy P, O'Neill S (2009) Fasciola hepatica tegumental antigen suppresses dendritic cell maturation and function. Infect Immun 6:2488–2498

Hassan OA, Affognon H, Rocklöv J, Mburu P, Sang R, Ahlm C, Evander M (2017) The One Health approach to identify knowledge, attitudes and practices that affect community involvement in the control of Rift Valley fever outbreaks. PLoS Negl Trop Dis 11(2):e0005383

Heymann F, Tacke F (2016) Immunology in the liver—from homeostasis to disease. Nat Rev Gastroenterol Hepatol 13(2):88

Ikegami T, Narayanan K, Won S, Kamitani W, Peters CJ, Makino S (2009a) Dual functions of Rift Valley fever virus NSs protein: inhibition of host mRNA transcription and post-transcriptional downregulation of protein kinase PKR. Ann N Y Acad Sci 1171(1):E75

Ikegami T, Narayanan K, Won S, Kamitani W, Peters CJ, Makino S (2009b) Rift Valley fever virus NSs protein promotes post-transcriptional downregulation of protein kinase PKR and inhibits eIF2α phosphorylation. PLoS Pathog 5(2):e1000287

Ingale SL, Singh P, Raina OK, Mehra UR, Verma AK, Gupta SC, Mulik SV (2008) Interferon-gamma and interleukin-4 expression during *Fasciola gigantica* primary infection in crossbred bovine calves as determined by real–time PCR. Vet Parasitol 152:158–161

Jost BH, Adler B, Vinh T, Faine S (1986) A monoclonal antibody reacting with a determinant on leptospiral lipopolysaccharide protects Guinea pigs against leptospirosis. J Med Microbiol 22(3):269–275

Jupp PG, Kemp A (1998) Studies on an outbreak of Wesselsbron virus in the Free State Province, South Africa. J Am Mosq Control Assoc 14(1):40–45

Kashiwagi R, Kaidoh T, Inoué T (2001) Immunohistochemical study of dendritic cells and kupffer cells in griseofulvin-induced protoporhyric mice. Yonago Acta Med 44(1):7–16

Kita H, Van De Water J, Gershwin ME, Mackay IR (2001) The lymphoid liver: considerations on pathways to autoimmune injury. Gastroenterology 120(6):1485–1501

Klimpel GR, Matthias MA, Vinetz JM (2003) Leptospira interrogans activation of human peripheral blood mononuclear cells: preferential expansion of TCRγδ+ T cells vs TCRαβ+ T cells. J Immunol 171(3):1447–1455

Knolle PA, Thimme R (2014) Hepatic immune regulation and its involvement in viral hepatitis infection. Gastroenterology 146(5):1193–1207

Kuchai JA, Chishti MZ, Zaki MM, Rasool SAM, Ahmad J, Tak H (2011) Some epidemiological aspects of fascioliasis among cattle of Ladakh. Global Vet 7:342–346

Levett PN, Morey RE, Galloway RL, Steigerwalt AG (2006) Leptospira broomii sp. nov., isolated from humans with leptospirosis. Int J Syst Evol Microbiol 56(3):671–673

Li S, Ojcius DM, Liao S, Li L, Xue F, Dong H, Yan J (2010) Replication or death: distinct fates of pathogenic Leptospira strain Lai within macrophages of human or mouse origin. Innate Immun 16(2):80–92

Liao S, Sun A, Ojcius DM, Wu S, Zhao J, Yan J (2009) Inactivation of the fliY gene encoding a flagellar motor switch protein attenuates mobility and virulence of Leptospira interrogans strain Lai. BMC Microbiol 9(1):1–10

Liberal R, Grant CR, Mieli-Vergani G, Vergani D (2013) Autoimmune hepatitis: a comprehensive review. J Autoimmun 41:126–139

Löhr HF, Schlaak JF, Gerken G, Fleischer B, Dienes HP, zum Büschenfelde KHM (1994) Phenotypical analysis and cytokine release of liver-infiltrating and peripheral blood T lymphocytes from patients with chronic hepatitis of different etiology. Liver 14(3):161–166

Machicado C, Machicado JD, Maco V, Terashima A, Marcos LA (2016) Association of Fasciola hepatica infection with liver fibrosis, cirrhosis, and cancer: a systematic review. PLoS Negl Trop Dis 10:e0004962

Malhotra V, Sakhuja P, Gondal R (2004) Immunohistochemistry in liver diseases. J Gastroenterol Hepatol 19:S364–S369

Manns MP, Strassburg CP (2001) Autoimmune hepatitis: clinical challenges. Gastroenterology 120(6):1502–1517

Martinez-Moreno A, Jimenez-Luque V, Moreno T, Redondo ES, de las Mulas JM, Perez J (1999) Liver pathology and immune response in experimental Fasciola hepatica infections of goats. Vet Parasitol 82:19–33

Matsumura T, Ito A, Takii T, Hayashi H, Onozaki K (2000) Endotoxin and cytokine regulation of toll-like receptor (TLR) 2 and TLR4 gene expression in murine liver and hepatocytes. J Interf Cytokine Res 20(10):915–919

Maxie MG (2016) Jubb, Kennedy & Palmer's pathology of domestic animals-E-book, vol 2. Elsevier Health Sciences

McElroy AK, Nichol ST (2012) Rift Valley fever virus inhibits a pro-inflammatory response in experimentally infected human monocyte derived macrophages and a pro-inflammatory cytokine response may be associated with patient survival during natural infection. Virology 422(1):6–12

McIntosh BM (1986) Mosquito-borne virus diseases of man in southern Africa. S Afr Med J 70(4):69–72

McNeilly TN, Rocchi M, Bartley Y, Brown JK, Frew D, Longhi C, McLean L, McIntyre J, Nisbet AJ, Wattegedera S, Huntley JF, Matthews JB (2013) Suppression of ovine lymphocyte activation by Teladorsagia circumcincta larval excretory–secretory products. Vet Res 44:70

Meri T, Murgia R, Stefanel P, Meri S, Cinco M (2005) Regulation of complement activation at the C3-level by serum resistant leptospires. Microb Pathog 39(4):139–147

Molina EC (2005) Serum interferon-gamma and interleukins-6 and -8 during infection with Fasciola gigantica in cattle and buffaloes. J Vet Sci 6:135–139

Molina-Hernández V, Mulcahy G, Pérez J, Martínez-Moreno A, Donnelly S, O'Neill SM, Dalton JP, Cwiklinski K (2015) Fasciola hepatica vaccine: we may not be there yet but we're on the right road. Vet Parasitol 208:101–111

Moreau E, Chauvin A (2010) Immunity against helminths: interactions with the host and the intercurrent infections. J Biomed Biotechnol 2010:428–593

Morrill JC, Jennings GB, Johnson AJ, Cosgriff TM, Gibbs PH, Peters CJ (1990) Pathogenesis of Rift Valley fever in rhesus monkeys: role of interferon response. Arch Virol 110(3–4):195–212

Moutailler S, Roche B, Thiberge JM, Caro V, Rougeon F, Failloux AB (2011) Host alternation is necessary to maintain the genome stability of rift valley fever virus. PLoS Negl Trop Dis 5(5):e1156

Murray GL, Ellis KM, Lo M, Adler B (2008) Leptospira interrogans requires a functional heme oxygenase to scavenge iron from hemoglobin. Microbes Infect 10(7):791–797

Murray GL, Srikram A, Henry R, Hartskeerl RA, Sermswan RW, Adler B (2010) Mutations affecting Leptospira interrogans lipopolysaccharide attenuate virulence. Mol Microbiol 78(3):701–709

Mushi EZ, Binta MG, Raborokgwe M (1998) Wesselsbron disease virus associated with abortions in goats in Botswana. J Vet Diagn Investig 10(2):191–191

Naiman BM, Blumerman S, Alt D, Bolin CA, Brown R, Zuerner R, Baldwin CL (2002) Evaluation of type 1 immune response in naïve and vaccinated animals following challenge with Leptospira borgpetersenii serovar Hardjo: involvement of WC1+ γδ and CD4 T cells. Infect Immun 70(11): 6147–6157

Nemeth E, Baird AW, O'Farrelly C (2009) Microanatomy of the liver immune system. Semin Immunopathol 31(3):333–343

Nfon CK, Marszal P, Zhang S, Weingartl HM (2012) Innate immune response to Rift Valley fever virus in goats. PLoS Negl Trop Dis 6(4):e1623

Odendaal L, Clift SJ, Fosgate GT, Davis AS (2019) Lesions and cellular tropism of natural Rift Valley fever virus infection in adult sheep. Vet Pathol 56(1):61–77

Oymans J, van Keulen L, Wichgers Schreur PJ, Kortekaas J (2020) Early pathogenesis of wesselsbron disease in pregnant ewes. Pathogens 9(5):373

Pacheco IL, Abril N, Morales-Prieto N, Bautista MJ, Zafra R, Escamilla A, Ruiz MT, Martínez-Moreno A, Pérez J (2017) Th1/Th2 balance in the liver and hepatic lymph nodes of vaccinated and unvaccinated sheep during acute stages of infection with Fasciola hepatica. Vet Parasitol 238:61–65

Pacheco IL, Abril N, Zafra R, Molina-Hernández V, Morales-Prieto N, Bautista MJ, Ruiz-Campillo MT, Pérez-Caballero R, Martínez-Moreno A, Pérez J (2018) *Fasciola hepatica* induces Foxp3 T cell, proinflammatory and regulatory cytokine overexpression in liver from infected sheep during early stages of infection. Vet Res 49(1):1–10

Paweska JT, Burt FJ, Swanepoel R (2005a) Validation of IgG-sandwich and IgM-capture ELISA for the detection of antibody to Rift Valley fever virus in humans. J Virol Methods 124(1–2): 173–181

Paweska JT, Mortimer E, Leman PA, Swanepoel R (2005b) An inhibition enzyme-linked immunosorbent assay for the detection of antibody to Rift Valley fever virus in humans, domestic and wild ruminants. J Virol Methods 127(1):10–18

Pepin M, Bouloy M, Bird BH, Kemp A, Paweska J (2010) Rift Valley fever virus (*Bunyaviridae*: *Phlebovirus*): an update on pathogenesis, molecular epidemiology, vectors, diagnostics and prevention. Vet Res 41(6):61

Pérez J, Ortega J, Moreno T, Morrondo P, López-Sández C, Martínez-Moreno, A. (2002) Pathological and immunohistochemical study of the liver and hepatic lymph nodes of sheep chronically reinfected with *Fasciola hepatica*, with or without triclabendazole treatment. J Comp Pathol 127(1):30–36

Peters MG (2002) Animal models of autoimmune liver disease. Immunol Cell Biol 80(1):113–116

Pleasance J, Wiedosari E, Raadsma HW, Meeusen E, Piedrafita D (2011) Resistance to liver fluke infection in the natural sheep host is correlated with a type-1 cytokine response. Parasite Immunol 33(9):495–505

Que-Gewirth NL, Ribeiro AA, Kalb SR, Cotter RJ, Bulach DM, Adler B, Saint Girons I, Werts C, Raetz CR (2004) A methylated phosphate group and four amide-linked acyl chains in *Leptospira interrogans* lipid A: the membrane anchor of an unusual lipopolysaccharide that activates TLR2. J Biol Chem 279(24):25420–25429

Racanelli V, Rehermann B (2006) The liver as an immunological organ. Hepatology 43(S1):S54–S62

Ristow P, Bourhy P, McBride FWDC, Figueira CP, Huerre M, Ave P, Girons IS, Ko AI, Picardeau M (2007) The OmpA-like protein Loa22 is essential for leptospiral virulence. PLoS Pathog 3(7): e97

Robinson MW, Harmon C, O'Farrelly C (2016) Liver immunology and its role in inflammation and homeostasis. Cell Mol Immunol 13(3):267–276

Rodríguez E, Noya V, Cervi L, Chiribao ML, Brossard N, Chiale C et al (2015) Glycans from Fasciola hepatica modulate the host immune response and TLR-induced maturation of dendritic cells. PLoS Negl Trop Dis 9(12):e0004234

Ruiz-Campillo MT, Hernandez VM, Escamilla A, Stevenson M, Perez J, Martinez-Moreno A, Donnelly S, Dalton JP, Cwiklinski K (2017) Immune signatures of pathogenesis in the peritoneal compartment during early infection of sheep with Fasciola hepatica. Sci Rep 7(1):1–14

Sellon RK (2005) Canine viral diseases. In: Ettinger SJ, Feldman EC (eds) Textbook of veterinary internal medicine (ed 6). Elsevier, St Louis, pp 646–652

Spithill TW, Dalton JP (1998) Progress in development of liver fluke vaccines. Parasitol Today 14:224–228

Swanepoel R (1988) Wesselsbron virus disease. In the arboviruses: epidemiology and ecology, vol 5. CRC Press, Boca Raton, FL, pp 31–57

Sykes JE (2014) Infectious canine hepatitis. Canine Feline Infect Dis:182

Tanaka A, Iwabuchi S, Takatori M, Ohno A, Yamada H, Hashimoto N, Ikeda Y, Kato T, Nishioka K, Iino S, Yamamoto K (1997) Clonotypic analysis of T cells in patients with autoimmune and viral hepatitis. Hepatology 25(5):1070–1076

Thompson H, O'Keeffe AM, Lewis JC, Stocker LR, Laurenson MK, Philbey AW (2010) Infectious canine hepatitis in red foxes (*Vulpes vulpes*) in the United Kingdom. Vet Rec 166(4):111–114

Tuero I, Vinetz JM, Klimpel GR (2010) Lack of demonstrable memory T cell responses in humans who have spontaneously recovered from leptospirosis in the Peruvian Amazon. J Infect Dis 201(3):420–427

Van der Lugt JJ, Smit MME, Coetzer JA (1996) 1996. Distribution of viral antigen in tissues of new-born lambs infected with Rift Valley fever virus. Onderstepoort J Vet Res 63(4):341–347

Walsh KP, Brady MT, Finlay CM, Boon L, Mills KH (2009) Infection with a helminth parasite attenuates autoimmunity through TGF-beta-mediated suppression of Th17 and Th1 responses. J Immunol 183:1577–1586

Wang B, Sullivan J, Sullivan GW, Mandell GL (1984) Interaction of leptospires with human polymorphonuclear neutrophils. Infect Immun 44:459–464

Weiss KE, Haig DA, Alexander RA (1956) Wesselsbron virus—A virus not previously described, associated with abortion in domesticated animals. Onderstepoort J Vet Res 27:183–195

Weyer J, Thomas J, Leman PA, Grobbelaar AA, Kemp A, Paweska JT (2013) Human cases of Wesselsbron disease, South Africa 2010–2011. Vector Borne Zoonotic Dis 13(5):330–336

WHO (2018) Rift Valley fever. Available online: http://www.Who.Int/news-room/fact-sheets/detail/riftvalley-fever. Accessed 19 Feb 2018

Wies I, Brunner S, Henninger J, Herkel J, Kanzler S, zum Büschenfelde KHM, Lohse AW (2000) Identification of target antigen for SLA/LP autoantibodies in autoimmune hepatitis. Lancet 355(9214):1510–1515

Williams R, Ellis CE, Smith SJ, Potgieter CA, Wallace D, Mareledwane VE, Majiwa PAO (2011) Validation of an IgM antibody capture ELISA based on a recombinant nucleoprotein for identification of domestic ruminants infected with Rift Valley fever virus. J Virol Methods 177(2):140–146

Wright NG (1976) Canine adenovirus: its role in renal and ocular disease: a review. J Small Anim Pract 17(1):25–33

Zimmerman GL, Kerkvliet NI, Brauner JA, Cerro JE (1983) Modulation of host immune responses by Fasciola hepatica: responses by peripheral lymphocytes to mitogens during liver fluke infections of sheep. J Parasitol 69:473–477

Immunopathology of Diarrhea in Animals

Key Points

1. Enteritis is defined as an inflammation of the intestine.
2. Diarrhea is defined as an increase in the frequency of feces output and decrease in the consistency.
3. Diarrhea has been a most consistent feature of enteritis and gastrointestinal infection.
4. Diarrhea is caused by bacterial, viral, and parasitic in origin.
5. Persistent diarrhea is defined as the passage of watery feces more than three times a day over a period of 2 weeks and resulting into loss of weight.
6. Chronic diarrhea is defined as the passage of loose stool or feces for a period of more than 3 to 4 weeks resulting in consistent loss of weight.
7. Increased frequency of defecation, often decreased volume, and presence of mucus and fresh blood in feces are suggestive of large bowel diarrhea and commonly associated with parasitic infection.
8. Bacterial pathogens cause diarrhea are *Escherichia coli* (EPEC, ETEC, EHEC, EAEC, and EIEC), *Shigella, Salmonella, Clostridium*, etc.
9. Rotavirus and coronavirus are the most commonly identified viral causes of diarrhea of neonatal food animals.
10. Protozoal pathogens cause diarrhea are amoebiasis, giardiasis, cryptosporidium, balantidiasis, etc.
11. Diagnosis of diarrhea is based on the symptoms, fecal examination, molecular techniques for demonstration of microbial pathogens, and endoscopy.
12. Hydration and nutrition play major role from the recovery of diarrhea.

9.1 Introduction

Enteritis is defined as an inflammation of the intestine and affects wide age groups and is characterized by dull and depressed appearance, abdominal pain, weight loss, and characteristically diarrhea. Diarrhea has been a most consistent finding and feature of enteritis. Diarrhea is defined as increase in the frequency of feces output and a decrease in the consistency (Mullhaupt 2002). The World Health Organization (WHO) has defined diarrhea as the passage of loose feces frequently more than three to four times a day and may lead to severe dehydration and in many cases leads to death. Diarrhea is a condition affecting both humans and animals. Globally, billions of peoples are found to be affected with diarrhea and most badly driven is the developing country where people die of diarrhea. Thus, crucial management of diarrhea is necessary as excess loss of water and electrolyte may lead to death. Diarrhea is mainly seen as a manifestation of gastrointestinal infection which may be bacterial, viral, and parasitic in origin. Diarrhea is spread through ingestion of contaminated food and water and poor hygienic conditions. Worst struck are the young and immunocompromised animals. Studies reveal that the prime sources for origin of diarrhea is the small intestines followed by the large intestines and accessory digestive organs. Disease and infections affecting the large intestines causes diarrhea due to disturbances in water conservation, whereas, in the small intestines, it is osmotic or secretary (Bhutta et al. 2004).

Diarrhea results when there is alteration of normal physiologic process. Balance between secretion and absorption of the electrolytes is a dynamic process, and any imbalance results into diarrhea, as the rectum is filled with low-viscosity watery contents, which induces an involuntary fecal reflex making it onerous for the subject even with normal sphincter function to prevent leaking of rectal contents (Spiller 2006; Whyte and Jenkins 2012). Frequency and movement of bowel are both important as it may sometime reveal the type of diarrhea or the origin, as small and frequent stools indicate left colon or rectal disease, whereas, immense quantity of stools indicates small bowel or right colon disease.

Globally, the most important trigger for persistent diarrhea (PD) is an acute diarrheal episode caused by an enteric infection. Poor intestinal repair is regarded as a key component of the abnormal mucosal morphology. However, the factors underlying this ineffective repair process and continuing injury are poorly understood. The result of this mucosal derangement is poor absorption of luminal nutrients and increased permeability of the bowel to abnormal dietary or microbial antigens. Alterations of intestinal permeability in early childhood may reflect changes in intestinal mucosal maturation and may be affected by concomitant enteric infections.

There are multiple causes for diarrhea, and the following classification provides a useful framework for approaching diarrhea: (1) diarrhea secondary to altered mucosal transport or secretory dysfunction, (2) osmotic diarrhea, (3) diarrhea secondary to malabsorption, (4) exudative diarrhea, and (5) diarrhea secondary to altered bowel motility. Besides the information mentioned above, there are various mediators involved in the diarrhea: they are broadly categorized into two types: intracellular and extracellular mediators. The intracellular mediators encompass cyclic adenosine monophosphate (c-AMP), cyclic guanosine monophosphate (c-GMP), calmodulin, calcium, and phospholipids, and extracellular mediators are hormones, neurotransmitter, prostaglandins, and enterotoxins (Ooms and Degryse 1986).

9.2 Etiology

A variety of factors are responsible for the onset of diarrhea in animals, which include bacterial *Clostridium perfringens* (Fig. 9.1) (Enteroaggregative *Escherichia coli* (EAEC or EAggEC), enteropathogenic *Escherichia coli* (EPEC) (Fig. 9.2), *Campylobacter* spp. (Prince Milton et al. 2017), *Salmonella Enteritidis*, *Shigella* spp., *Clostridium difficile*, *Arcobacter butzleri*, and *Klebsiella* spp.), viral (rotavirus, coronavirus, bovine virus diarrhea, parvovirus (Fig. 9.3), peste des petits ruminants virus, bovine enteric calicivirus, and bovine astrovirus), and protozoan (*Giardia lamblia*, *Blastocystis hominis*, *Cryptosporidium* spp., *Entamoeba histolytica*, *Cyclospora cayetanensis*, and *Enterocytozoon bieneusi* (*Microsporidium* spp.)) pathogens (Table 9.1). The presence of parasite like *Toxocara canis* (Fig. 9.4) or protozoan may further cause bloody or tarry color feces in animals predisposing them to severe anemic condition, nutritional deficiency. Important diarrhea-causing viral agents are rotavirus, coronavirus, bovine viral diarrhea, human astrovirus, *Enteroviruses*, and

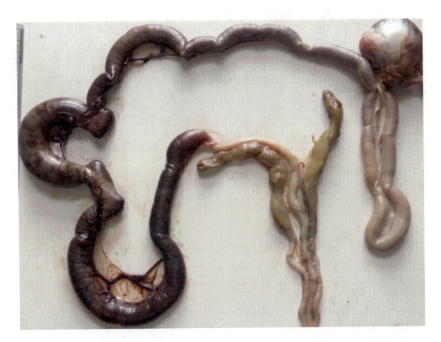

Fig. 9.1 Necrotic enteritis in chicken caused by *Clostridium perfringens*: gross lesions are primarily found in the jejunum and ileum, showed ballooning, severe congestion, hemorrhages, and necrosis with foul-smelling, brownish content

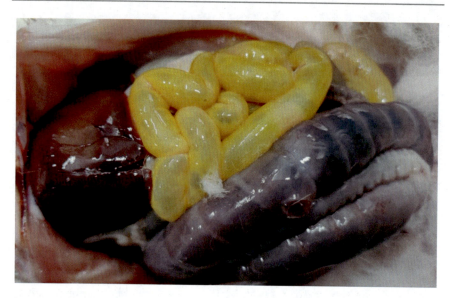

Fig. 9.2 Enterotyphlitis in guinea pig due to colibacillosis: the small intestine is dilated, flaccid, and filled with translucent yellow fluid and gas. The caecum showed flaccid, severe congestion, hemorrhages, and necrosis

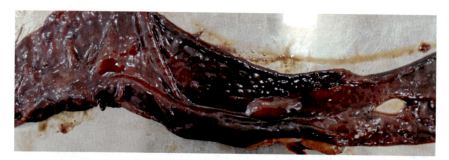

Fig. 9.3 Hemorrhagic enteritis in a dog due to canine parvovirus: the small intestinal mucosa showed thickening, reddish discoloration with hemorrhagic intestinal contents and diffusely wrinkled intestinal wall

Picornaviruses, and particularly associated with HIV infection. Nutritional deficiency including micronutrient deficiencies contribute toward poor intestinal repair. Key micronutrient is zinc, and studies over zinc supplements during diarrhea indicate a significant reduction in the duration and severity of diarrheal illnesses (Bhutta et al. 2007; Aggarwal et al. 2007), indicating that zinc deficiency significantly contributes to the prolongation of mucosal injury. Some of the inflammatory conditions such as Crohn's disease and ulcerative colitis, poor hygiene of the young ones, contamination of the drinking water with feces, sudden change in the diet, consuming food products which have high-fat and high-sugar content, presence of artificial sweetener in food, and lactose intolerance cause diarrhea. The use of

9.2 Etiology

Table 9.1 Most important infectious and noninfectious causes of diarrhea in ruminants

Etiology	Host	Disease	Susceptibility age	Organ affected
Enterotoxigenic *E. coli*	Calves	Neonatal diarrhea Colibacillosis	During the first week of life	Distal small intestine, cecum, and colon
Enteropathogenic *E coli*	Calves and lambs			
Salmonella enterica serovar Typhimurium and *Salmonella enterica* serotype Dublin	Calves	Salmonellosis	6 days of age or older. Sometimes 2–12 weeks old also affected	Small intestine
Clostridium perfringens types A, B, C, and E	Calves and lambs	Fatal hemorrhagic abomasitis and enteritis, enterotoxaemia (pulpy kidney)	Lambs: Less than 21 days of age Calves: Less than 10 days of age	Small and large intestine
Campylobacter jejuni	Calves and lambs	Enteritis	–	Small intestine
Yersinia enterocolitica	Calves and lambs	Enteritis	–	Distal small intestine (ileum)
Mycobacterium paratuberculosis	Adult cattle	Johne's disease/ paratuberculosis	Over 1 to 2 years	Terminal ileum and colon
Rotavirus Groups A and B	Calves and lambs	Enteritis	Within 24 h of birth	Small intestine
Coronavirus	Calves	Enteritis	Over 5 days of age	Small and large intestine
Bovine virus diarrhea	Calves	Calf diarrhea	All ages (before 3 months of age)	Small intestine
Peste des petits ruminants	Sheep and goats	Fibrinohemorrhagic enteritis	All ages	Small and large intestine
Infectious bovine rhinotracheitis	Calves	Calf diarrhea	All ages	Small and large intestine
Bovine torovirus (Breda virus)	Calves	Enteritis	Up to 4 months of age	Caudal portion of the small intestine (mid-jejunum through ileum)
Bovine enteric calicivirus	Calves	Enteritis	–	Small intestine
Bovine astrovirus	Calves	Enteritis	–	Small intestine
Bovine parvovirus; genus: *Bocavirus*	Calves	Enteritis	Between 5 and 21 days of age	Small intestine

(continued)

Table 9.1 (continued)

Etiology	Host	Disease	Susceptibility age	Organ affected
Coccidiosis	Calves and lambs	Hemorrhagic enteritis	3 weeks of age and older	Small and large intestine
Cryptosporidium parvum	Calves and lambs	Cryptosporidiosis	Less than 6 weeks of age	Distal small intestine and colon
Giardia duodenalis	Young calves and lambs	Chronic mucoid diarrhea	As early as 4 days of age	Proximal small intestine (duodenum)
Strongyloides papillosus	Calves	Enteritis	Up to 6 months of age	Small intestine

Noninfectious causes of diarrhea

More quantities of milk, inappropriately formulated milk replacers, lush green feed, oral administration of antimicrobials such as neomycin or tetracycline, ruminal drinking, acidosis (grain overload), cobalt or selenium deficiency, and copper deficiency or toxicity

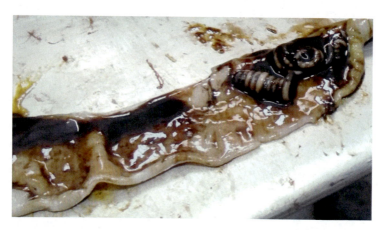

Fig. 9.4 Enteritis in dogs caused by *Toxocara canis*: the small intestine contained adult worms of *T. canis* with edema, erosions, and dark-brown (tarry)-colored contents

antibiotics over a period of time may lead to diarrhea. Also stress and tumorous condition may also cause diarrhea.

9.3 Classification of Diarrhea

Diarrhea is classified into various types depending upon the severity of occurrence and the time period for which the individual has been affected. It is based upon signs and dehydration and is classified as acute watery diarrhea, dysentery, and chronic or persistent diarrhea leading to malnutrition and malabsorption.

9.3 Classification of Diarrhea

9.3.1 Acute Diarrhea

It is defined as occurrence of loose or watery stool for less than 2 weeks frequently three or more times a day. It is the leading cause of death in the low- and middle-income countries and accounts for high death rates in children and animals and is ranked as seventh most cause of mortality in the developing countries.

9.3.2 Persistent Diarrhea (PD)

It is defined as the passage of watery feces more than three times a day over a period of 2 weeks and resulting into either no gain or loss in weight. The PD identified in children as a substantial diarrhea-related morbidity and accounts for between 36% and 54% of all diarrhea-related deaths (Bhutta et al. 2004). Persistent diarrhea is associated with the episode of occurrence of acute diarrhea and is also related or is a consequence of nutritional deficiency especially the micronutrients. Zinc is the main micronutrient, which is known to prevent diarrhea (Bhutta et al. 2004). Studies have revealed that deficiency of micronutrients may cause poor intestinal repair. In a study, based upon meta-analysis of zinc, it was found that supplement of zinc in diarrheal illness help in prevention (Bhutta et al. 2007). However, the mechanism of zinc in prevention of diarrhea is still not completely known, but studies suggested that deficiency of zinc contribute to prolongation of mucosal injury and delayed intestinal repair mechanism. Diarrheal disorders mainly resolve within the first week of illness; however, a smaller proportion of diarrheal illness may fail to resolve and persist for more than 2 weeks. Many infants and toddlers in developing countries may have frequent recurrent episodes of diarrhea, resulting in nutritional deficiencies and predisposing them to PD. Noting the close relationship between diarrheal disorders and malnutrition, persistent diarrhea is widely recognized as a nutritional disorder, and optimal nutritional rehabilitation is needed for its management (Bhutta et al. 2004).

9.3.3 Chronic Diarrhea

It is defined as passage of loose stool or feces for a period of more than 3 to 4 weeks resulting in consistent loss of weight.

9.3.4 Small Bowel Diarrhea

Disorders of the small intestine are either malabsorptive or secretory in nature, but most disorders of the small intestinal mucosa result in both excess secretion and failure of absorption. Diarrhea of small bowel is more often noninflammatory. Postprandial diarrhea, bloating, malodorous flatus, pale stools which leave oil slick, and difficult to flush are indication of malabsorption. A normal appetite besides gradual weight loss might also suggest malabsorption. Any improvement of diarrhea after fasting suggests an osmotic component of the symptoms. Pain is a common symptom of small bowel diseases including celiac disease. The pain may be focal or diffuse; it is often associated with meals (Murray and Rubio-Tapia 2012). Delay in intestinal transport result in bowel stasis and further help in bacterial colonization and growth leading to mucosal injury—a phenomenon commonly associated with anaerobic bacteria. The underlying mechanism responsible for this is bile salt deconjugation, in which bile acids are converted into secondary bile acid forms, which are highly damaging to the mucosa. This results in diarrhea due to fat malabsorption and increased colonic secretion. Diarrhea is also induced from water and sodium secretion and glucose malabsorption leading to breach in the continuity of the epithelium of the intestine.

9.3.5 Large Bowel Diarrhea

There is increased frequency of defecation, often decreased volume and the presence of mucus and fresh blood in feces are suggestive of large bowel diarrhea (Table 9.2). Large bowel diarrhea is commonly manifested during parasitic infestation.

Table 9.2 Differentiating features for small and large bowel diarrhea

Characteristics	Small bowel diarrhea	Large bowel diarrhea
Frequency of defecation	Normal to slightly increased	Very frequent
Fecal volume	Large quantity of bulky or watery feces	Small quantities often
Fecal mucus	Usually absent	Often present
Fecal blood	Melena (dark black)	Hematochezia (red and fresh)
Tenesmus	Absent	Often present
Urgency	Absent	Often present
Dyschezia	Absent	Often present
Vomiting	May be present	Infrequently present
Weight loss	Often present	Infrequently present
Steatorrhea	May be present	Absent
Undigested food	May be present	Absent
Color	Color variations occur, e.g., creamy brown, green orange, or clay	Color variations rare; may be hemorrhagic
Gas	Sometimes	Absent
Smell of stool	Very foul	Foul
Nature of stool	Soupy and greasy	Mucinous/jelly like

9.3.6 Osmotic Diarrhea

It occurs when the osmotically active substances increase in the gut, fluid passes passively down the osmotic gradient, and this overwhelms the intestine absorptive capacity resulting into diarrhea. Osmotic diarrhea results from the ingestion of solutes, mucosal damage, malabsorption, and motility disorders. Certain laxatives such as lactulose or maldigestion of certain food substances such as milk are common causes of osmotic diarrhea. This type of diarrhea ceases with fasting.

9.3.7 Secretory Diarrhea

It is also known as diarrhea secondary to altered mucosal transport. Such diarrhea may occur when the mucosa secretes excess amount of fluid, which may be due to bacteria, toxins, and other infectious diseases. Secretary diarrhea may occur due to excessive secretion of certain hormones, viz., vasoactive intestinal peptide (VIP) and gastrin produced by pancreatic tumors and calcitonin produced by medullary cancer of the thyroid, and can also stimulate excessive mucosal secretion leading to diarrhea. Secretary diarrhea occur independent of the dietary intake, and there is no significant stool osmotic gap. Stool osmotic gap is calculated using following formula: $290 - 2 \times$ (stool Na + stool K). Here, 290 mOsm/kg is the presumed stool osmolality and measured concentration of sodium (Na^+) and potassium (K^+) cations in stool. A normal stool osmotic gap is between 50 and 100 mOsm/kg, which depends on the concentration of other solutes such as magnesium salts and sugar. Decreased stool osmotic gap indicates secretory diarrhea, in which the digestive tract is hyperpermeable and losing electrolytes. The reason is secreted sodium and potassium ions make up a greater percentage of stool osmolality in secretory diarrhea. More stool osmotic gap suggests osmotic diarrhea, in which the digestive tract is unable to absorb solutes from the chyme, either due to the digestive tract is hypopermeable (because of inflammation) or nonabsorbable compounds (Epsom salt). The reason is unabsorbed carbohydrates responsible for the stool osmolality.

Diarrhea results when either decreased absorption or increased secretion occurs. Classic secretory diarrhea is caused most commonly by toxins produced by various bacterial pathogens such as *Staphylococcus* spp., *Escherichia coli*, and *Vibrio cholerae*. Experimental evidence suggested that elevated levels of cyclic AMP can stimulate net anion secretion, thus causing diarrhea. Such diarrhea does not stop upon fasting as they are diet independent (Woods 1990).

9.3.8 Exudative Diarrhea

Diseases associated with large amount of inflammatory exudates like, blood, pus, and proteinaceous material can produce diarrhea. These cause increased stool volume and frequency. Such type of diarrhea can be seen in invasive enteric infections such as *Shigella, Salmonella*, or *Campylobacter* and inflammatory bowel diseases (Woods 1990; Prince Milton et al. 2017).

9.4 Pathogenesis of Diarrhea

9.4.1 Bacterial Pathogens of Diarrhea

Bacterial diarrhea is a major health problem and causes mortality in a very high number if untreated. Worst hit are the infants, young animals, and developing countries that suffer from malnutrition (Gracey 1986). Occurrence of bacterial diarrhea has increased over the past few years because of antimicrobial resistance and shown a wide range of 4–33% occurrence (Harries 1976). Pathogenesis of diarrhea due to bacterial agents is classified into two types: (i) bacterial mucosal interaction and (ii) induction of intestinal fluid loss by enterotoxin. Interaction between bacteria and mucosa involves adherence to epithelial cell villi, adherence to enterocytes (classical example is EPEC), and mucosal invasion (commonly shown by *Shigella* spp. and *Salmonella* spp.) (Bockemühl 1980; Cantey 1985). Another way of classifying diarrhea-causing bacterial pathogens is on the basis of their colonization in the bowel, mainly invasive and noninvasive. Invasive pathogens include *Shigella* and *Salmonella*, which affect the large intestine. Noninvasive includes *V. cholerae* and *E. coli*, which affects the small intestine (Harries 1976).

9.5 *Escherichia coli*

The most important cause of the bacterial diarrhea is Gram-negative *Coccobacilli* that belong to the *Enterobacteriaceae* family (Fig. 9.2). There are five pathogenic types responsible for diarrhea specifically enterotoxigenic *E. coli* (ETEC) and enteropathogenic *E. coli* (EPEC), which causes noninflammatory type of diarrhea; enterohemorrhagic *E. coli* (EHEC); enteroinvasive *E. coli* (EIEC); and enteroadherent *E. coli* (EAEC), later named as enteroaggregative (Vial et al. 1988) that cause inflammatory diarrhea (Holland 1990; Hart et al. 1993). These are generally termed as diarrheagenic *E. coli* (DEC) and differ over the virulence mechanism, colonization sites, and clinical symptoms. *E. coli* synthesizes various fimbriae that enables the organism to colonize in the intestinal tract in different species. However, it has been mentioned that diarrheagenic strains of *E. coli* exhibit only one type of fimbrial antigen, but it has been found that ETEC express multiple fimbrial antigen, which includes K88 and 987P antigen. Fimbriae helps the organism in overcoming the physiological barrier, ETEC attachment, and rapid proliferation (Milton et al. 2019).

9.6 Enteropathogenic *E. coli* (EPEC)

They have a usual three-dimensional microcolonies arrangement and therefore produce a localized adherence pattern (Scaletsky et al. 1984; Nataro and Kaper 1998). EPEC causes diarrhea and produces attaching and effacing lesions. EPEC strain is sub-classified into typical EPEC and atypical EPEC (Trabulsi et al. 2002; Kaper et al. 2004). Typical EPEC is known to possess a virulence plasmid and causes infectious diarrhea (Nataro and Kaper 1998; Trabulsi et al. 2002). The hallmark of both typical and atypical EPEC is the ability to produce attaching and effacing lesions. EPEC causes disruption of the microvilli through vesiculation; the process is known as attaching and effacement. EPEC is the causal organism for summer and neonatal diarrhea (Milton et al. 2019).

9.7 Enterotoxigenic *E. coli* (ETEC)

It produces mainly two types of toxins, namely, heat labile toxin (LT) and heat stable toxin (ST). It is the main cause of diarrhea in neonates in developing countries. ETEC strain activates the enterotoxins and produces a secretory diarrhea (Čobeljić et al. 1996; Henderson et al. 2004). *E. coli* produces diarrhea by attaching to the intestinal mucosa and producing effect through either heat labile or heat stable or both the toxins. This pathotype is the cause of economic burden to the farmers and causes huge farm and industry losses. The LT toxin consist of A and B subunits. The B subunit consists of five identical monomer structures and arranged in a pentameric ring-shaped manner. The A subunit is linked with the B subunit by A2 helical domain. The B subunit binds with the cell surface receptors and promotes toxin internalization and causes cleavage of A1 domain from A2 domain. A1 domain stimulates G protein and activates adenylate cyclase leading to increased intracellular c-AMP. This in turn activates protein kinase A and causes phosphorylation of the ion channels resulting in increased release of chloride ions and decreased uptake of sodium ions, thus producing a secretory diarrhea (Spangler 1992). The ST toxin activates guanylate cyclase C in the intestinal cells and produces cGMP, which induces osmotic deregulation and secretes chloride ions and water from the intestinal epithelium.

9.8 Enterohemorrhagic *E. coli* (EHEC)

It is a common inhabitant of the gastrointestinal tract in variety of animals. The EHEC is also designated as Shigella toxic *E. coli* (STEC). Cattle are the most common reservoir host but is also found in feces of other animals (Borges et al. 2012; Martins et al. 2013, 2015; Beraldo et al. 2014; Maluta et al. 2014), including birds (Gioia-Di Chiacchio et al. 2016) and fishes (Ribeiro et al. 2016). The EHEC can be found in soil, manure, and water; thus it is a serious matter of concern. In a report from Lascowski et al. (2013), EHEC/STEC has been isolated from drinking water, which shows the extent of EHEC transmission. Lascowski et al. (2012) has reported the presence O157:H7 from hides of cattle in Brazil. Such reports indicate the zoonotic importance of EHEC strains. EHEC attaches at the intestinal mucosa and produces verocytotoxins VT1 and VT2. These toxins damage the colonic enterocytes and vascular endothelial cells resulting in hemorrhagic urinary syndrome.

9.9 Enteroadherent or Enteroaggregative E. coli (EAEC)

The EAEC is the major cause of diarrhea in children. The EAEC causes damage to the colonic villi that results in shortening (Hart et al. 1993). In watery diarrhea with or without blood, often mucus is present along with abdominal pain and vomiting (Hebbelstrup Jensen et al. 2014). Recent research findings confirmed that EAEC is diarrheagenic *E. coli*, which produces aggregative adherence (AA) in the cultured epithelial cells but lack main genetic markers that are present in other DEC (Tânia et al. 2016).

9.10 Enteroinvasive E. coli (EIEC)

There has been discussion among researchers about this particular type of *E. coli* because of similarity in disease symptoms as that of *Shigella* spp. It is summarized that EIEC strain is in intermediate stage and are precursor of the fully mature *Shigella* strain (Pupo et al. 1997; Bando et al. 1998; Rolland et al. 1998; Martinez et al. 1999; Lan et al. 2004). The EIEC penetrates the colonic enterocytes and replicates therein. The M cells in the intestinal mucosa are the targets of *E. coli*, invade deeper tissues, and cause dysentery (Sansonetti and Phalipon 1999; Parsot 2005). The EIEC invades the intestinal epithelial cells by endocytosis (Sansonetti et al. 1982; Levine 1987), causing its destruction. Also, it shows high adaptability, uses iron capture system for metabolic needs, requires less energy, and facilitates infectious process (Dall'Agnol and Martinez 1999; Andrade et al. 2000).

9.10.1 Shigella

They are a group of Gram-negative, and facultative intracellular pathogens. *Shigella* was recognized as the etiologic agent of bacillary dysentery or shigellosis in the year 1890. Biochemical characteristics (e.g., ability to ferment D-mannitol) and antigenic properties form the basis for classification into subgroups and serotypes of *Shigella* (Gomez and Cleary 1997). Feco-oral route is the most common route of transmission and others being ingestion and contact with inanimate objects. As few as ten *S. dysenteriae* bacilli can cause clinical disease; possible reason for such low dose of infectivity could be virulent *Shigellae* are able to withstand the low pH (2–2.5) of gastric juice (Phalipon and Sansonetti 2007). The virulence trait is encoded on a large plasmid, which is in turn responsible for cytotoxicity. *Shigellae* that lose the virulence plasmid are no longer pathogenic. *Escherichia coli* O157:H7 that harbor this plasmid clinically behave as *Shigella* bacteria (Friedrich et al. 2002).

Virulent *Shigella* strains produce disease after invading the intestinal mucosa. Shiga toxin is an AB_5 toxin, i.e., made up of one A subunit and five B subunits. The A subunit provides the enzymatic activity as it permanently inactivates the ribosome of the host cells and the B subunits bind to the host cells at a surface receptor, globotriaosylceramide (Gb3). This initiates an uptake mechanism by the host cells, and eventually toxins gain access to the cytoplasm. *Shigella* infects by invading the epithelial cells, multiplies, and destroys them. The early step in invasion is the invasion of the microfold cells (M cells). The function of the healthy M cells is to transport the antigen and present to the macrophages, but during infection, M cells transport the bacterial antigen, thereby evading the immune mechanisms. When the macrophages are exposed to *Shigella* organisms, it undergoes apoptosis and releases the proinflammatory cytokine interleukin 1 (IL-1). The process begins with *S. dysenteriae* protein, called IpaB protein, which activates the programmed cell death in macrophages and converts pro-IL-1 into the active form of IL-1. By lysing the macrophage, *S. dysenteriae* has access to the epithelial cells. A type III secretion system (T3SS) of the pathogen penetrates the host cell membrane and is an important virulence factor for cell entry. Then, *S. dysenteriae* spreads across the epithelium. The spread of the bacteria is a chain event, and actin plays a role in the spread of bacteria. The bacterium moves from cell to cell without exposing into the lumen, thus evading from the immune system. A potent inflammatory response is responsible for the characteristic dysentery. The host cell and bacterial cell are both negatively charged in nature, which causes them to repel. Thus, the fimbriae contain adhesions on their tips to contradict this repulsion (Siciliani 2017). It is part of the genus *Shigella*, which can cause the acute intestinal illness, known as shigellosis. It is characterized by watery diarrhea at first, followed by the classic dysenteric stool, which is little in volume and grossly bloody (Edwards 1999; Siciliani 2017). Lesions consist of mucosal edema, erythema, ulceration, and focal mucosal hemorrhage involving the rectosigmoid junction. Microscopic lesions are epithelial cell necrosis, goblet cell depletion, infiltration of polymorphic and mononuclear cells, and crypt abscess formation (Phalipon and Sansonetti 2007).

9.10.2 *Salmonella*

It is a Gram-negative bacterium with more than 1800 serovars. Some of the serotypes are host limited (*S. gallinarum, S. pullorum,* and *S. typhimurium*), but some has a wide range of host and may even infect humans. Salmonellosis is manifested with diverse clinical signs including enteric fever, enterocolitis, abdominal pain, vomiting, and diarrhea along with blood and mucus (Rubin and Weinstein 1977). *Salmonella* is among the global causes of diarrhea; the species commonly associated with diarrhea is *S. enterica* (McWhorter-Murlin and Hickman-Brenner 1994; Milton et al. 2018).

Salmonella is a common disease affecting poultry birds. The affected poultry appears symptomless and thus acts as carrier for others. The pathogen may enter the eggs either through contamination with the feces and cracks on the shell, and transovarian transmission from adult to chick is also reported. The increase in incidences of *Salmonella* in the poultry sector has the witness of salmonellosis in humans because of the hike in demand for eggs and its products. Humans are generally infected by consumption of contaminated food products and partially cooked meat and egg products (Milton et al. 2018).

The organism enters the body through ingestion and colonizes in the intestine. Studies revealed that Peyer's patches are the most common site, and also the villus epithelium is most preferred as compare to the crypts epithelium. However, noninvasive *Salmonella typhimurium* mutants are avirulent because of their inability to enter and destroy M cells of ileal Peyer's patches (Penheiter et al. 1997). The pathogen invades the mucosa through ruffling by binding with the receptor of the epithelial cells. As the mucosal barrier is invaded, the organisms multiply and release the pro-inflammatory cytokines, which induce acute inflammation and cause ulceration, inhibition of protein synthesis, and release of prostaglandins. This sends impulse for the activation of adenyl cyclase and increases the production of c-AMP. Increase in the cyclic AMP causes secretion of fluid in the intestine resulting into diarrhea (Finlay et al. 1992).

9.10.3 *Clostridium*

Clostridium difficile (CD) is an established human and animal pathogen that primarily causes gastroenteritis (Milton et al. 2017). It is transmitted through the feco-oral route. It is a Gram-positive, anaerobic, spore-bearing bacillus and present as a common inhabitant in contaminated environments. Clostridium pathogen produces two types of toxins, toxin A and B, and generates severe inflammation of the colonic mucosa, which is manifested as profound diarrhea along with abdominal pain (Brown and Wilson 2018). Clostridium pathogenesis is manifested in three phases: (1) microbial suppression, (2) collateral damage, and (3) a wide range of vulnerability (Yacyshyn 2016). Evidently, it is the most important nosocomial pathogen responsible for diarrhea and generally affects individuals associated with antibiotics (Milton et al. 2015; Segar et al. 2017). Clostridium is responsible for antibiotic-associated diarrhea and colitis, as the intestinal microflora is altered due to antibiotics providing conducive environment for the proliferation of pathogenic bacteria (Brown and Wilson 2018; Kumar and Uma 2019). In recent years, the reports of *Clostridium difficile*-associated diarrhea (CDAD) have increased due to the indiscriminate use of antibiotics, which has resulted in emergence of BI/NAP1/027. *C. difficile* is a pathogen of zoonotic importance and is a potent source of diarrhea in food animals (Songer 2004; Rodriguez-Palacios et al. 2006). *C. difficile* also has been identified in the meat products (Rodriguez-Palacios et al. 2009) and in products intended for pet consumption (Weese et al. 2005; Hensgens et al. 2012). Clostridium organisms form spores, which are heat resistant and can survive high temperatures and adverse environment. Common heat-resistant ribotypes of clostridia are RT027 and RT078 (Rodriguez-Palacios and LeJeune 2011; Deng et al. 2015). *C. perfringens* causes severe necrosis in the small intestine (primarily jejunum). Necrosis is segmental, involving varying degrees of hemorrhage and intramural gas (Fig. 9.1).

9.11 Viral Pathogens of Diarrhea

Rotaviruses and coronaviruses are the most commonly identified viral causes of diarrhea of neonatal food animals (Chauhan and Singh 1993a, b). These viruses have also been associated with diarrhea in adult food animals, but the disease incidence is less in adults when compared to neonates. However, both clinically and subclinically, infected adults shed the viruses and provide sources of infection for others, and mostly to the young ones (Esper et al. 2010).

9.11.1 Rotavirus

Rotavirus is ubiquitous in nature and causes diarrhea by eminently disrupting the absorptive area in the intestine (Chauhan 1991; Chauhan and Singh 1992a, b; 1993a, b). It is the leading cause of diarrhea worldwide both in humans and animals (Graham et al. 1984; Chauhan and Singh 1993a, b; 1994, 1996). Rotavirus belongs to the family *Reoviridae* and mainly has its effect on the mature villi of the intestine. Virus consists of 11 segments (Chauhan and Singh 1993a, b), 6 structural and non-structural proteins (NSP), each having a unique genome except NSP5 and NSP6 (Ramig 2004). Serologically, the virus is classified into groups, namely, groups A to E, and groups A to C are found to infect humans and the rest affect animal species (Chauhan and Singh 1994, 1996).

Rotavirus survives wide range of pH and buffering action of the milk in the gut. Rotavirus significantly affects intensively reared calves (Chauhan 1991; Chauhan and Singh 1992a, b; 1993a, b; Rathi et al. 2007). Rotavirus diarrhea can be due to several mechanisms, namely, malabsorption, enteric nervous system (ENS) stimulation via viral toxins, and villus ischemia (Conner and Ramig 1997). The virus increases the depth of the crypts and decreases the enzyme including sodium pump ($Na^+K^-ATPase$) (Graham et al. 1984).

Enterocytes in the intestine is divided into (1) enterocytes and (2) the crypt cells. Villus enterocytes are the mature non-proliferating cells. Replication of the virus in these mature cells suggests the expression of favorable factor required for efficient replication and subsequent infection. Rotavirus infection results in the vacuolization of the enterocytes, villus blunting, and crypts hyperplasia. Disruption of the villi causes malabsorption, ionic imbalance by depleting the major ions (sodium, chloride, and bicarbonate) (Chauhan and Singh 1992a, b; 1993a, b), and passage of undigested bolus. The undigested food particle being osmotically active causes osmotic diarrhea (Graham and Estes 1988). Viral NSP4 in many researches has been revealed for inducing diarrhea (Ball et al. 1996; Estes and Morris 1999; Zhang et al. 2000). The NSP4 enterotoxin mediates diarrheagenic changes and causes disruption of tight junction leading to paracellular permeability. The NSP4 on the crypt cells causes increase in calcium ions. Increased calcium causes secretion in crypts mediated through the activation of chloride ions resulting in secretory diarrhea.

Rotavirus diarrhea is related to age-dependent protease expression. Viral infectivity requires protease cleavage of VP4 protein (Greenberg et al. 1994). Proteolytic cleavage induces conformational changes in the structure of RNA virus and produces additional attachment sites on surface for interaction with series of co-receptors (Brunet et al. 2000; Ruiz et al. 2000; Crawford et al. 2006; Greenberg and Estes 2009). Replication of the virus depends upon the concentration of calcium ions in the cells, and the absence of proper calcium levels results in the stoppage of viral morphogenesis (Poruchynsky et al. 1991). The NSP4 causes release of calcium from the endoplasmic reticulum. Increased level of calcium induces numerous cellular mechanisms including disruption of microvilli cytoskeleton, decreased expression of enzymes, general inhibition of the sodium solute co-transport system, and necrosis.

Diarrhea is initiated when the virus infects the enterocytes mediated via interaction of series of sialic acid containing and non-sialylated receptor molecules (Chauhan et al. 2008). Various studies have led to distinguishing fact about the virus; even virus with the same morphological characteristic had been identified in the samples from diarrheic pigs, calves, lambs, and humans (Chauhan and Singh 1994, 1996). These are referred to as atypical rotavirus, pararotavirus or group C rotaviruses, antigenically distinct rotaviruses, rotavirus-like viruses or group B rotaviruses, and novel rotaviruses (Esper et al. 2010). Other experimental studies have also identified the different groups of rotaviruses (Chauhan 1991; Chauhan and Singh 1992a, b, c; 1993a, b; Dhama et al. 2009).

The extensive havoc played by rotavirus leads to the development of vaccines to safeguard the humans from diarrhea. The initiative started with the Jennerian approach to vaccinate the children against rotavirus, which commonly infects animals (Greenberg and Estes 2009). Research studies in gnotobiotic calves revealed that vaccination with attenuated bovine rotavirus in calves safeguarded them against bovine rotaviruses (Vesikari 2008). Subsequently, other vaccines produced were more efficient and effective, which included RIT4237, RotaShield (Vesikari 2008), simian rotavirus vaccine (RRV) (Joensuu et al. 1997), and Rotovac. The newest being Rotosiil, which is being considered as revolutionary as it is a thermostable vaccine and yielded good results in the trials (Desai et al. 2018).

9.11.2 Bovine Viral Diarrhea (BVD)

The BVD in cattle causes sub-acute benign infection, fatal mucosal disease, and peracute fatal diarrhea (Brownlie 1990). Venereal route of infection is of utmost important as it can transfer disease vertically to fetus. BVD virus triggers another disease called mucosal disease (MD), which is mainly responsible for diarrhea in cattle. It is associate with severe erosions in the intestinal mucosa. Several studies reported that both MD and BVD are serologically similar. Researchers have concluded etiology for the mucosal disease that only persistently viremic animals succumb to mucosal disease (Liess et al. 1974). Secondly persistently viremic animals had only the non-cytopathogenic virus, whereas those that died of mucosal disease were infected with both biotypes, namely, non-cytopathogenic and cytopathogenic (Brownlie et al. 1984). Cytopathogenic biotype of the BVD virus localizes in germinal centers and gut lymphoid tissue of Peyer's patches before spreading to the gastrointestinal epithelium (Liebler-Tenori et al. 1997; Liebler-Tenorio et al. 2000). Cytopathogenic biotype causes monocyte activation and differentiation and inhibits antigen presentation to the T cells leading to uncontrolled viraemia and weakening of the defense mechanism against virus (Lee et al. 2009). Studies reveal that affected young calves develop respiratory disorders, whereas the older calves develop enteric diseases (Bachofen et al. 2010; Lanyon et al. 2014).

9.11.3 Coronavirus

Coronaviruses are associated with diarrhea in animals and humans (Pedersen et al. 2008; Esper et al. 2010). Human coronavirus is responsible for enteric diseases. Rousset et al. (1984) found coronavirus-like particles by electron microscopy in stool samples of children with diarrhea and infants with necrotizing enterocolitis. New coronaviruses have been reported in affected patients with the evidence of gastrointestinal involvement (Esper et al. 2005, 2006; Vabret et al. 2006). However, large studies on coronaviruses in humans are lacking (Esper et al. 2010).

Other viruses that have been implicated in diarrhea of young farm animals include togavirus (bovine viral diarrhea virus), parvovirus (Fig. 9.3), calicivirus, adenoviruses, Breda viruses and astroviruses. Researchers have demonstrated a higher proportion of children with gastroenteritis with antibody responses to coronaviruses (Gerna et al. 1984). During the SARS-CoV outbreak in 2002–2003, enteric involvement was reported in 38–70% of patients and detected frequently in stool samples collected from infected individuals. Recently, Vabret et al. (2006) identified HCoV-HKU1 from stools in pediatric patients, whose respiratory samples were screened positive for HCoV-HKU123.

9.11.4 Norovirus

Noroviruses are the leading cause of acute gastroenteritis in the developed countries, one of them being the United States (Wikswo et al. 2015). Human noroviruses are now being considered as the major cause of diarrhea and gastroenteritis across the globe. Though sporadic occurrences have been rectified, globally they are the leading cause of diarrhea in parts where rotavirus vaccination is implemented.

Noroviruses are food-borne disease in nature (Koo et al. 2010; Becker-Dreps et al. 2014).

A diarrheal epidemiological study of norovirus has revealed that noroviruses are responsible for nearly 20% of all cases of acute gastroenteritis (Ahmed et al. 2014). Recent advances in research have led to understanding the pathogenesis of norovirus. The pathogenicity of the virus is due to the exploitation of the balance between commensal bacteria and the immune system. Virus infects the immune cells of the gastric mucosa, and the transportation of the virus through the lumen is via M cells in the small intestine. Human noroviruses are most common in immunocompromised patients where they lead to life-threatening dehydration (Bok and Green 2012; Green 2014).

9.12 Diarrhea due to Intestinal Parasites

Diarrhea caused by intestinal parasites are broadly classified into two types either acute or chronic diarrhea. Acute diarrhea is commonly seen in amoebiasis, giardiasis, balantidiasis, etc., and chronic diarrhea is caused by trichuriasis, *Toxocara canis* (Fig. 9.4), and strongyloidiasis. Parasitic diarrhea is also classified based upon the site where they produce major effects such as the small intestine in the case of giardia, strongyloides, and capillaria, and the large intestine in entamoeba, balantidina, and trichuris (Marsden and Schultz 1969).

9.12.1 Giardia

Infection with *Giardia lamblia* could lead to osmotic diarrhea associated with malabsorption and maldigestion along with signs of intestinal hypermotility (Ebrahim 1990). Giardia produces diarrhea without penetrating the epithelia (Buret et al. 2002; Müller and Von Allmen 2005; Gaseon 2006). Close contact of the sucking end of the trophozoite damages the microvilli of enterocytes (Ebrahim 1990). Trophozoites do not produce or release enterotoxin but causes reduction in the absorptive surface area (Scott et al. 2000). In most cases, it is believed to be self-limiting. In humans, it is commonly associated with the deficiency of secretory IgA (Ebrahim 1990). In vivo and in vitro studies reveal that giardia causes malabsorption of glucose, sodium, and water. Findings suggests that toxic products released from the parasite damages the intestinal barrier and activates T lymphocytes, which causes retraction of the brush border leading to diarrhea (Buret et al. 2002; Müller and Von Allmen 2005; Gaseon 2006). Researchers have revealed that giardia prevents nitric oxide formation (Eckmann et al. 2000) by consuming arginine, the substrate commonly needed by the enterocytes and thus predisposes the enterocytes to giardia-induced apoptosis.

9.12.2 Cryptosporidium

The protozoa *Cryptosporidium* enters into the host cells by attaching to its target host cells i.e., epithelial cells of the intestine, forms the parasitophorus vacuoles and rest of its life cycle reside in it (O'Hara and Chen 2011; Certad et al. 2017). Attachment of the parasite to the target cells is mediated via two proteins, namely, mucin-like glycoprotein and thrombospondin-related adhesive protein (Leitch and Qing 2011). *Cryptosporidium* infection causes release of pro-inflammatory cytokines and chemokines and results in increased epithelial permeability and impaired intestinal absorption and secretion (Di Genova and Tonelli 2016). Further, it causes disruption of tight junction, loss of barrier function, host cell actin polymerization, remodeling of the cytoskeleton, and increased rate of cell death. This alteration in the absorption and increased secretion accelerates the intestinal transit. Research findings have revealed that *Cryptosporidium* activates nuclear factor kappa B (NF-κB) in the infected biliary epithelial cells, which inhibits apoptosis, provides protection to parasite, and promotes propagation of the parasite in the infected cells (Chen et al. 2001; Schmid-Hempel 2008). Researchers have reported that *Cryptosporidium* escapes the host immune system by residing in the parasitophorus vacuoles. The parasite infects both man and animals and causes nutrient malabsorption (Huang et al. 2003; Hunter et al. 2004).

9.12.3 Trichuris

Trichuriosis is the most common infection in tropics. The intensity of infection determines the symptoms, whether diarrhea or dysentery. Infection with over 20,000 eggs per gram of feces is classified as severe diarrhea or dysentery. *Trichuris* causes necrosis of the cells with inflammation and infiltration of cells. Diarrhea is due to impaired water absorption and damage of colon (Marsden and Schultz 1969).

9.12.4 Strongyloides

It penetrates the intestinal mucosa and damages the mucosa. It causes ulcerative enteritis along with marked inflammatory response, which is responsible for diarrhea (Marsden and Schultz 1969).

9.12.5 Traveler's Diarrhea (TD)

TD is defined as the passage of three or more unformed stools per day associated with enteric symptoms and occurring in a traveler after arrival. TD is caused by bacterial, viral, or protozoal pathogens. Feco-oral route is the most common route of transmission of TD. Etiologies for TD are similar to those causing acute diarrhea in young ones. Norovirus and rotavirus are identified as the most common viral etiologies of TD. Protozoa *Giardia duodenalis* and *Entamoeba histolytica* are the main pathogens (Giddings et al. 2016).

9.13 Chemical Mediators Influencing the Intestinal Motility

9.13.1 Serotonin

Approximately 95% of the serotonin in the body is located in the gut. Reports suggested the role of serotonin in functional GI disorders. Researchers have claimed there may be a role for circulating serotonin in determining predominant bowel function. Serotonin is increased during diarrhea and celiac disease, while it is decreased in constipation. Studies have revealed its role in small intestinal motility, inhibition of gastric juices, and colonic contractions (Hendrix et al. 1957; Misiewicz et al. 1966). Increased sigmoid colonic motility was reported in patients with irritable bowel syndrome (IBS) (Houghton et al. 2007). However, involvement of 5-hydroxytryptamine (5-HT) in IBS remains unclear. The experiment data showed a possible relationship between endogenous concentrations of 5-HT and sigmoid colonic motility. There were significant correlations of sigmoid colonic motor activity index with platelet-depleted plasma 5-HT concentration in IBS patients and healthy volunteers. Serotonin is released diffusely into the lamina propria, and its action is rapidly terminated by reuptake by nerve terminals, enterocytes, and vascular endothelial cells (Camilleri 2009).

9.13.2 Prostaglandins

Prostaglandins (PGs) showed mucosa protective effects. PGs also affect intestinal physiology, contribute toward diarrhea, and influence inflammatory reactions. In the context of exogenous prostaglandins, diarrhea is often the most obvious consequence of the oral ingestion of prostaglandins (Horton et al. 1968; Misiewicz et al. 1969; Karim and Filshie 1970). Two underlying mechanism involves the following: (1) they act on smooth muscles—largely contraction of longitudinal muscles by E and F prostaglandins, contraction of circular muscles by F prostaglandins, and relaxation of circular muscles by E prostaglandins contribute to diarrhea and associated abdominal cramps; (2) intestinal secretory properties of prostaglandins; and (3) prostaglandins affect intestinal transport by inhibiting Na^+/K^+-adenosine triphosphatase (ATPase) activity (Sharon et al. 1984; Hawkey and Rampton 1985). In humans, it has been found that prostaglandin E stimulates secretion of chloride, sodium, potassium, and water in vivo (Matuchansky and Bernier 1973; Matuchansky et al. 1976; Modigliani et al. 1979) and in laboratory animals (Pierce et al. 1971). In vitro studies on prostaglandin E showed that it stimulates chloride secretion and reduces sodium absorption (Bukhave and Rask-Madsen 1980). Studies revealed that stimulation of adenylate cyclase and accumulation of cAMP by prostaglandins are central events in the stimulation of intestinal secretion.

9.13.3 Claudin

Claudin-2 is a structural component of tight junction (TJ) strands and forms cation channels. However, the functional consequence on epithelial barrier function depends on the background of all other claudins in the TJ. In the small and large intestine, claudin-2 expression allows a better passage of sodium and water by formation of paracellular channels being permeable to these. Claudin-2 seems to contribute to TJ strand discontinuities, although it cannot be the only determinator of this phenomenon. Therefore, claudin-2 distinctively upregulated in most inflammatory and infectious diseases of the intestine is rather a contributor or even only an indicator than the reason for an increased macromolecule passage through the intestinal wall, although claudin-2 itself contributes to diarrhea in many intestinal diseases via a leak flux mechanism. Tsai et al. (2017) showed that diarrhea is critical to pathogen clearance, and diarrhea development requires claudin-2 upregulation that increases tight junction permeability to Na + and water.

The intestinal barrier is often compromised during enteric infection. In the case of invasive and toxigenic organisms, this typically involves direct epithelial damage. In contrast, noninvasive, attaching, and effacing (A/E) pathogens, such as human and mouse pathogens, namely, enteropathogenic *E. coli* and *Citrobacter rodentium*, respectively, use type III secretion system to inject proteins into the host cells. These effector proteins promote cytoskeletal reorganization and increase intestinal permeability (Guttman et al. 2006).

However, neither the mechanisms that underlie these permeability increases nor their significance to pathogenesis are well understood. Claudin-2 is a well-established mediator of pore pathway permeability, and claudin-2 upregulation drives the increased pore pathway permeability within 2 days of infection. Analyses of mucosal cytokines during infection showed that only IL-22 was significantly increased by 2 days of infection. However, IL-22 has not been reported to regulate claudin-2 transcription. Cytokines that have been linked to claudin-2 upregulation were increased only at later times (IL-6, TNF, IL-17A) or were unchanged (IL-13). Despite many advantages, presence of numerous cell types and potential for complex intercellular signaling limits the utility of in vivo models to determine whether IL-22 signalling is directly related to intestinal epithelia (Tsai et al. 2017).

Expression of claudin-2 is changed under different pathologic conditions, such as cancer, infectious diseases, and inflammation (Günzel and Fromm 2012). In inflammatory bowel diseases (IBDs), increased claudin-2 is associated with decreased and/or redistribution of sealing TJ proteins including claudin-1, -3, -4, -5, and/or -8. These changes in conjunction with the induction of epithelial apoptosis led to barrier dysfunction and increased ion and water permeability, which in turn results in leak-flux diarrhea (Amasheh et al. 2009; Prasad et al. 2005; Zeissig et al. 2007). Claudin-2 impairs barrier function in several intestinal diseases presenting with inflammation and/or diarrhea. These barrier defects often include an increased claudin-2 expression, which occurs in IBDs, namely, Crohn's disease and ulcerative colitis, infectious diseases including human immunodeficiency virus (HIV) infection, and gluten-sensitive enteropathy (Heller et al. 2005; Zeissig et al. 2007; Oshima et al. 2008; Schumann et al. 2012; Epple and Zeitz 2012).

Furthermore, claudin-2 is not only the TJ protein dysregulated in intestinal diseases, and changes in barrier-strengthening and other channel-forming TJ proteins must also be considered in the overall picture of barrier modification processes. Increased claudin-2 expression is a predominant feature. This upregulation is an early and functionally important alteration in the inflamed mucosa of Crohn's disease patients, while TJ proteins with sealing properties, including claudins-3, -4, -5, and -8 and occludin, are downregulated and redistributed off the TJ domain (Prasad et al. 2005; Zeissig et al. 2007; Das et al. 2012).

9.13.4 Nutrition and Diarrhea

Nutrition plays a very important role in the development of diarrhea (Scrimshaw et al. 1968). The nutritional state alters the host immune responses to infection; vice versa infectious illness alters nutritional state. Reports of the Committee on International Nutrition Programs have focused on improved case management, including oral rehydration therapy and appropriate nutritional therapy. In humans, breastfeeding of the child is the vital phenomenon, which provides the nutrients to prevent diarrhea. Protective mechanism of the human milk is the attribute of the immunological properties and the high nutritive value (Scrimshaw et al. 1968). Recurrent diarrheal cases may become circular, and increase in frequency results in a parallel and progressive deterioration in host nutritional status proceeds to overt protein energy malnutrition unless treated (Keusch and Scrimshaw 1986).

Many studies have revealed that probiotics are effective in treating diarrhea. Synbiotic (combination of probiotic and prebiotic) is also effective in preventing diarrhea (Nomoto 2005; Yan and Polk 2006; Guarino et al. 2009; Whelan and Schneider 2011). The mechanism through which probiotics acts include (1) the release of bacteriocins from the lumen, restricting the growth and pathogenicity of nonhomologous pathogens. Probiotics also generate lactic acid, short-chain fatty acids, and hydrogen peroxide, which lower the pH and contribute to a hostile environment for pathogenic species. *Saccharomyces boulardii* (probiotic) produces proteases, which degrade toxins produced by pathogens such as *Clostridium difficile*, *Vibrio cholera*, or pathogenic *Escherichia coli* (Castagliuolo et al. 1999). Probiotics have useful nutritional or clinical activity. Enzyme ß-galactosidase produced by lactobacilli is useful in preventing diarrhea (de Vrese et al. 2001). (2) Probiotic agents bind directly to invasive species and disrupt their ability to interact with or bind to endothelial receptors in the intestinal mucosa. Probiotic *Lactobacillus* spp. upregulate the production of mucins from goblet cells and protective trefoil factor defensins. In addition, probiotics influence the proteins that control the tight junctions between enterocytes and reduce the potential for the absorption of harmful macromolecules (Hill et al. 2014). (3) Recognizing the microbe-associated molecular patterns (MAMPs) that are found more frequently on the surface of microbial species from a wide range of molecules (Lebeer et al. 2010; Mandal and Sahi 2017).

9.13 Chemical Mediators Influencing the Intestinal Motility

Table 9.3 Effect of probiotics on cytokine production

Probiotic bacteria	Route	Form	Species	Assessment	Effect on cytokines
Lactobacillus casei	Oral	Dry	Human	Serum interferon-γ	Increased cytokine production
Lactobacillus rhamnosus GG (LGG)	Oral	Live	Human	TNF-α in patients with food allergy	Decreased fecal TNF-α
Lactobacillus spp., Bifidobacterium spp., and streptococcus spp.	Oral	Live	Rodent	Mitogen-induced IL-6, IL-12, IFN-γ, and TNF-α production by intestinal lymphoid cells	Lactobacillus casei and L. acidophilus: Enhanced IL-6 and IL-12 L. Acidophilus: Enhanced IFN-γ and nitric oxide production
Bacillus subtilis natto	–	–	Calf	Stimulation of overall CMI response by helping in absorption of antigens from dead microbes	Elevation in the level of vital immune factors such as interferons, etc.; increased macrophage, lymphocyte, and NK cells activity; upregulation of oxidative burst and degranulation of heterophils.
Lactococcus lactis BFE920	–	–	Olive flounder (fish)	Stimulation of host innate immunity	Increased production of IL-12 and IFN-γ

Probiotics also influence the adaptive immune responses, stimulate the immunoglobulin production, and modulate the development and activity of T lymphocytes (Table 9.3). The potential of probiotics to influence a series of interactions through the activation of cellular immune responses can be effective in responses to acute infection within the gastrointestinal tract (Lebeer et al. 2010).

Other than the probiotics, low-lactose diet formulation has also been studied and followed for the prevention and management of diarrhea. Low-lactose diet should be provided to the young ones, who have encountered diarrhea to ensure an efficient recovery. Lactose malabsorption is seen in diarrhea-affected individuals; therefore the presence of lactose in diet predisposes to osmotic diarrhea (Sethi et al. 2018). The use of low-lactose diet is emphasized by both the WHO and the Indian Academy of Pediatrics in nutritional management of persistent diarrhea (Bhatnagar et al. 2007). Thus it is good to use a low-lactose formula instead of eliminating lactose completely in the management of diarrhea. These formulations need to be based on our understanding of the gut absorptive capacity and the critical nutrients required for repair and should consist of an appropriate balance of macronutrients and micronutrients. Past dietary approaches have promoted soy formulations and elemental diets; superiority to other diets or combinations is not validated in facility settings in developing countries.

9.14 Immunity

Immunity in neonates is mainly through the immunoglobulins received from the colostrum (Table 9.4). Among the immunoglobulins, IgG is most important that confers the immunity and provide protection against enteric infections. Selman (1973) reported that in sows, as the lactation proceeds, the amount of IgA increases and thus confers local immunity in the gut. The IgM gets absorbed in the crypt epithelium and provides protection against enteropathogens. Immunity in neonates completely depends upon the antibodies acquired via colostrum, and thus neonates deprived of colostrum fall an easy prey to systemic and gastric infections.

Immunity of the intestine is mainly conferred due to the presence of gut-associated lymphoid tissue (GALT). The hallmark of organized GALT is the presence of lymphoid follicles. Lymphoid follicles are the site where effector T cells are present in concentration. The GALT comprises of Peyer's patches, mesenteric lymph nodes, and intestinal cryptopatches. The GALT plays the vital role in balancing the brief line between tolerance and inflammation. The embryonic development of the GALT (Peyer's patches, mesenteric lymph node, and B cells of lamina propria) depends upon the interaction between lymphotoxin beta (β). Lymphotoxin alpha (α) and β regulates the development of intestinal lymphoid organs (Koboziev et al. 2010; Jung et al. 2010).

Peyer's patches are the highly specialized lymphoid follicles present in the small intestine. It consists of B- and T-cell areas, and follicular dendritic cells covered by follicular-associated epithelium (FAE). The FAE differs from the villus mucosa as there is weak mucus production, less expression of digestive enzymes, and the brush

Table 9.4 Colostral and milk immunoglobulin levels in domestic animals

Species	Fluid	Immunoglobulin (mg/dL)				
		IgA	IgM	IgG	IgG3	IgG6
Horse	Colostrum	500–1500	100–350	1500–5000	500–2500	50–150
	Milk	50–100	5–10	20–50	5–20	0
Cow	Colostrum	100–700	300–1300	2400–8000	–	–
	Milk	10–50	10–20	50–750	–	–
Ewe	Colostrum	100–700	400–1200	4000–6000	–	–
	Milk	5–12	0–7	60–100	–	–
Sow	Colostrum	950–1050	250–320	3000–7000	–	–
Bitch	Colostrum	500–2200	14–57	120–300	–	–
	Milk	110–620	10–54	1–3	–	–
Queen	Colostrum	150–340	47–58	4400–3250	–	–
	Milk	240–620	0	100–440	–	–

border glycocalyx has different pattern. Peyer's patches consist of M cells (specialized epithelial cell). The M cells are present in the follicular-associated epithelium of Peyer's patches and has high capacity of transcytosis of microorganism and serves as antigen-presenting system. The cellular composition of the FAE can be modulated by the presence of pathogen in the gut. The FAE exhibit an increased expression of claudin-3 and occluding, thereby reducing the opening of tight junction. The M cells surpass the luminal antigen directly to the Peyer's patches bypassing the intestinal epithelial cells. Other lymphoid organs include intestinal cryptopatches and isolated lymphoid follicles. Lymphoid follicles also consist of B- and T-cell areas, germinal center, and M cells; therefore, they are regarded as inductive site for mucosal immune responses (Spahn and Kucharzik 2004).

The GALT provides antigen priming, activation, polarization, and expansion, which then release the Th1 or Th17 or both of the effector cells. Effector cells enter the systemic circulation through lymphatics and help to destroy the pathogens. Experimental studies have laid emphasis over M cells for the prime site of T-cell production in the gut. Production of the T cells in the intestine is a complex process and involves distinct adhesion and signaling steps, (1) localization of the T cells to the endothelial surface, (2) rolling along the endothelial cell surface, and (3) activation and adhesion of lymphocytes to the endothelium. This causes extravasation of the T cells in the mesenteric lymph node and Peyer's patches. When CD4 cell enters the intestine, they encounter the enteric antigens presented along with the MHC class II, and this association initiates cell activation and results in more vigorous response of the effector T cells. Increased production of proinflammatory cytokines and reactive oxygen and nitrogen metabolites causes activation of leucocytes and induces gut inflammation (Koboziev et al. 2010).

9.15 Diagnosis

Prior to treatment and medication, knowledge about the origin of diarrhea (whether the large or small intestine) is necessary for effective control of diarrhea and its consequences. In the case of diarrhea from small bowel, there is weight loss with an increased volume of stool, no straining, and normal to slight increase in frequency of bowel movement. Blood is generally absent; however, digested blood may give black or tarry color to feces. In the case of diarrhea from the large intestine, weight loss is uncommon with normal or increased or decreased volume of stool and straining, and the frequency of bowel movement is increased. Fresh blood can be seen along with mucus in feces.

Stool testing should be performed under standard protocol for the presence of pathogens such as *Salmonella*, *Shigella*, *Campylobacter*, *Yersinia*, *C. difficile*, and STEC. The STEC O157 should be assessed by culture, and non-O157 STEC should be detected by Shiga toxin or genomic assays (Prince Milton et al. 2017). Blood samples should be taken from affected individuals with signs of septicemia or enteric fever, immunocompromised animals or humans as they are at high-risk, and peoples who traveled to endemic areas or had contact with affected persons. Bloody feces are not the common manifestation in the case of *Clostridial* infection. In the case of *Yersinia enterocolitica*, persistent abdominal pain is noticed, which mimics appendicitis. In peoples with large volume of watery stools, recent exposure to salty or brackish waters, consumption of raw or undercooked shellfish, and travel to endemic regions within 3 days prior to the onset of diarrhea should be subsequently suspected for vibriosis.

A differential diagnosis is recommended in immunocompromised people with diarrhea, especially those with moderate and severe primary or secondary immune deficiencies. The stool specimens should be evaluated by culture, viral studies, and examination for parasites. People with acquired immune deficiency syndrome (AIDS) with persistent diarrhea should undergo additional testing for other organisms including *Cryptosporidium, Cyclospora, Microsporidia, Mycobacterium avium* complex, etc. Travelers with diarrhea lasting 14 days or longer should be evaluated for intestinal parasitic infections. Testing for *C. difficile* should be performed in travelers treated with antimicrobial agents within the preceding 8–12 weeks. In addition, gastrointestinal tract disease including IBD and postinfectious irritable bowel syndrome (IBS) should be considered for evaluation (Shane et al. 2017).

The optimal specimen for laboratory diagnosis is a diarrheal stool sample or a rectal swab. Molecular techniques generally are more sensitive and less dependent than culture on the quality of specimen. For identification of viral and protozoal agents and *C. difficile* toxin, fresh stool is preferred. Serologic tests are recommended for diagnosis and to rule out any discrepancy (Carey-Ann and Carroll 2013; Yoldaş et al. 2016).

Endoscopy or proctoscopic examination should be considered in people with persistent diarrhea, unexplained diarrhea, certain underlying conditions, people with acute diarrhea, clinical colitis, and proctitis (Schiller et al. 2017). Duodenal aspirate may be considered in people for diagnosis of *Giardia, Strongyloides, Cystoisospora,* and *Microsporidia* infection. Clinical and laboratory re-evaluation may be indicated in people who do not respond to an initial course of therapy and should be considered for noninfectious conditions including lactose intolerance. Noninfectious conditions, including IBD and IBS, should be considered as underlying etiologies in people with symptoms lasting for 14 or more days with unidentified etiologies.

A broader set of bacterial, viral, and parasitic agents should be considered regardless of the presence of fever, bloody or mucoid stools, and other markers of more severe illness in the context of a possible outbreak of diarrheal illness. Suitable example is outbreak of diarrhea in many peoples who shared a common meal or a sudden rise in diarrheal cases. Selection of agents for testing should be based on a combination of host and epidemiologic risk factors and ideally in coordination with public health authorities. Specimens from peoples who are involved in an outbreak of enteric disease should be tested for enteric pathogens as per the public health department guidance. Testing may be considered for *C. difficile* in people with more than 2 years of age who have a history of diarrhea following antimicrobial use and in people with healthcare-associated diarrhea. Testing for *C. difficile* may be

9.15.1 Prevention and Prophylaxis

Major contributors toward restoration of health in diarrhea are hydration and nutrition. Oral rehydration is one of the best remedies for curing or preventing diarrhea and death due to diarrhea, as it restores the hydration in the body and maintains the electrolyte balance (Whyte and Jenkins 2012). Nutritional management plays key role to manage diarrhea. The WHO and United Nations Children's Fund (UNICEF) recommend feeding along with oral rehydration solution (ORS) and zinc supplementation in the management of diarrhea. The ORS does not actually stop the diarrhea, which often continues, but the absorption of water and solutes will exceed the secretion and ensures hydration (Whyte and Jenkins 2012). The optimal diet in the management of diarrhea is a matter of ongoing debate. Lactose malabsorption is one of the causes associated with diarrhea, which occurs as a result of secondary deficiency of lactase during diarrhea. This is one of the primary reasons for avoiding lactose during diarrhea (Sethi et al. 2018). Lactose avoidance is one of the strategies that had gained importance over time in diarrhea management. The osmotic effects of undigested lactose draw fluid into the intestinal lumen causing loose stools. Thus, low lactose plays an important role in effective management of diarrhea. An acronym most commonly used by Jog (2016) for diarrheal management is zinc ORS diet immunization antibiotics and adjuvants and cleanliness (ZODIAC). This management deals with administration of the vital minerals, electrolytes, and salt lost during diarrhea in the right amount. Zinc is an important component in the intestinal villi. Supplementation of zinc for 14 days reduces the duration and severity of diarrhea. Excessive dehydration during diarrhea results in the death of the affected individual. The ORS restores the electrolytes and salt lost during diarrhea, resulting in the restoration of the health of individuals.

Other preventive practices for the control of diarrhea encompasses (1) the impact of food and water hygiene, as most of the cases of diarrhea have a history of ingestion of contaminated food and water. Proper management of food and water hygiene reduces the risk of traveler's diarrhea. However, there is a little evidence of such incidences. (2) Vaccination, as there are few vaccines available against diarrhea. The whole cell-based vaccine against cholera pathogen has been used in the cases of diarrhea induced by ETEC pathogens because of homogeneity with the heat labile toxin of the pathogen and also provided some amount of protection against traveler's diarrhea (Peltola et al. 1991). The efficacy of the vaccine on diarrhea has revealed only 28% of protection. (3) Probiotics are recommended for the prevention of diarrhea, but there are several challenges with usage of probiotic products, which include diversity of probiotic strains, adequate quality control, optimal dose and duration of therapy, and specific storage requirement. A positive result for the use of probiotics against diarrhea has been shown (Guarino et al. 2009). (4) Antibiotic chemoprophylaxis can provide up to 90% protection. Fluoroquinolones are effective prophylactic agents.

Researchers have found a relation between diarrhea and zinc and copper status in a metabolic study and concluded that the balance of these minerals was strongly negative during the diarrheic phase due to malabsorption and maldigestion. However, during recovery the zinc balance increases and become positive, but copper remains negative. Net retention of these minerals is required for the normal growth, which gets hampered due to increased fecal output or decreased uptake during diarrhea. It was found that serum copper levels were significantly lower in diarrhea. On the basis of this study, treatment regimens for diarrhea should contain supplemental amounts of copper and zinc, but the positive results of these minerals on diarrhea is yet to be demonstrated.

9.15.2 Public Health

The present scenario of shift in the food habit had led to an increased demand of animal food products and animal-based food products, which makes the animal as a potent source of transmission of pathogens to humans, and these pathogens have a zoonotic potential (Archer and Young 1988; Holland 1990). Diarrheic and asymptomatic animals act as reservoir and sources of infection for others. Cases of hemorrhagic urinary syndrome and hemorrhagic colitis in humans are mainly due to the contamination of food products with EHEC from dairy animals. Undercooked meat and consumption of raw meat and milk have acted as a potential source of transmission of diseases such as O157:H7 (Mohammad et al. 1986; Orskov et al. 1987; Dorn 1988). Rotavirus that belongs to serogroup beta has been identified in humans, which is zoonotic importance. Young children and travelers are usually affected and water serves as the common mode of transmission (Navin and Juranek 1984; D'Antonio et al. 1985).

The new and resistant strains of the pathogenic organisms have resulted from the administration of antibiotics as growth promoter in farm animals, which are now a potent source of zoonoses. Management protocols designed for facility settings in developing countries need to be widely disseminated and used. Efforts should be made to devise agreed-on and appropriate diagnostic algorithms that reflect contemporary management strategies, i.e., the place of parenteral nutrition, place of specific therapies, and the place/timing of intestinal transplantation. As noted, early and unhygienic introduction of other than mother's milk and poorly managed recurrent acute diarrheal episodes are important predisposing factors for PD and should be prevented if possible. Thus, promotion of exclusive breastfeeding for at least 6 months, avoidance of formula feeding, timely and adequate weaning, and hygienic nutritious foods can help to prevent episodes of post infectious PD (Bhutta et al. 2004).

The WHO has developed a comprehensive strategy on strengthening food-borne disease surveillance. The most virulent food-borne pathogens that cause food-borne diseases are *Campylobacter*, *Escherichia coli*, *Salmonella*, *Shigella* species, and

Trichinella (Prince Milton et al. 2017). One of the initiatives to strengthen the surveillance systems for food-borne disease was the Global Foodborne Infections Network (GFN), establishment in January 2000. The GFN consists of institutions and individuals working in human health, veterinary, and food-related disciplines. In the area of food-borne diseases, the WHO also is involved in (1) outbreak investigations and responses, (2) pre-harvest control strategies, (3) burden of foodborne disease illness, and (4) antimicrobial resistance due to nonhuman antimicrobial usage.

Compared to other species of *Shigella*, *S. dysenteriae* is less of a global health risk. It is most commonly isolated in sub-Saharan Africa and South Asia. Moreover, 56% of *S. dysenteriae* infections are associated with global travel. The countries that pose the highest risk for contraction of shigellosis are Africa, Central America, South America, and Asia in descending order. Oral antibiotics, either singly or in combination, have not been proven useful, but antimicrobial therapy is required for *Clostridium difficile* enterocolitis, cryptosporidial enteritis, and giardiasis. The role of antibiotics in the treatment of associated systemic infections that are seen in almost 30 to 40% of the children with PD is poorly appreciated.

The government is also contributing much in this regard to prevent the occurrence of diarrhea. In March 2016, Rotavac vaccine was included in universal immunization program (UIP). Under clinical trials, the vaccine has shown reduction in rotavirus diarrhea by 56%, but there is limit in the availability of the vaccine. Also, the major drawbacks of vaccine are maintenance of the cold chain, which if altered renders the vaccine ineffective. This drawback is overruled by the production of a heat-stable rotavirus vaccine. ROTASIIL, a product from Serum Institute of India, is the world's first thermostable vaccine. The vaccine is administered to infants orally in a three-course dose at ages of 6, 10, and 14 weeks. Rotasiil consist of bovine-human reassortant rotavirus against the most common rotavirus serotypes (G1, G2, G3, G4, and G9) developed by the National Institute of Health (NIH). Bovine rotavirus pentavalent vaccine (BRV-PV) consists of G1, G2, G3, G4, and G9 serotypes, and G1, G2, G3, G9, and G12 serotypes were responsible for about 90% of severe rotavirus gastroenteritis (SRVGE), indicating that the vaccine can induce broad protection. This finding is important for potential use of the vaccine globally. The BRV-PV developed in India was found efficacious and safe in Indian infants. The BRV-PV can be cost-effective and heat-stable option in the global strategy for the prevention of diarrhea and does not interfere with the immune responses of other vaccines (Kulkarni et al. 2017; Desai et al. 2018).

9.16 Conclusion

Diarrhea though preventable and treatable through safe drinking and adequate hygiene still pertains to be one of the leading causes of illness and death in developing countries, where the diarrheic episodes are frequent. Young ones may spend more than 15% of their days with diarrhea. About 80% of deaths occur due to diarrhea. The main causes of death in diarrhea are from dehydration and undernutrition (due to increased nutrient requirement and reduced ability to absorb nutrients). Diarrheal disease represents an economic burden for the developing countries as worldwide millions of humans and animals die off due to diarrhea. Also, the changing trends in food web, more demand of the animal product, and consumption of raw or undercooked meat have made the transmission between humans and animals easy resulting in altered and resistant strains of pathogenic organisms. The free use of antibiotics as growth promoters in production of farm animals increases the resistivity of the pathogens.

Continued breastfeeding is universally accepted and recommended during diarrhea. The diarrheic disorder is frequently seen when deprived of colostrum. Firstly, good nutrition is the key for the complete recovery. Therefore, development and assessment of cost-effective enteral multinutrient formulations for the nutritional rehabilitation and therapy for children remain a priority. Secondly, vaccination against deadly pathogens should be practiced in regular intervals. In due course, public awareness through advertisements should be made so as to safeguard the children.

The main drawbacks in fighting against diarrhea are lack of education and resource allotment. Still people in the villages prohibit the optimum diet of the children during diarrhea; thus there is a need of improved outreach program for the management of diarrhea. The mother should be correctly guided to prevent the occurrence of diarrhea in toddlers and infants. The shift in pathogen from animals to human has paved the way for zoonotic occurrences of diarrhea; thus hygienic practices should be followed by peoples those in contact with animals.

References

Aggarwal R, Sentz J, Miller MA (2007) Role of zinc administration in prevention of childhood diarrhea and respiratory illnesses: a meta-analysis. Pediatrics 119(6):1120–1130

Ahmed SM, Hall AJ, Robinson AE, Verhoef L, Premkumar P, Parashar UD, Koopmans M, Lopman BA (2014) Global prevalence of norovirus in cases of gastroenteritis: a systematic review and meta-analysis. Lancet Infect Dis 14:725–730

Amasheh S, Dullat S, Fromm M, Schulzke JD, Buhr HJ, Kroesen AJ (2009) Inflamed pouch mucosa possesses altered tight junctions indicating recurrence of inflammatory bowel disease. Int J Color Dis 24(10):1149

Andrade A, Dall'Agnol M, Newton S, Martinez MB (2000) The iron uptake mechanisms of enteroinvasive Escherichia coli. Braz J Microbiol 31:200–205

Archer DL, Young FE (1988) Contemporary issues: diseases with a food vector. Clin Microbiol Rev 1:377–398

Bachofen C, Braun U, Hilbe M, Ehrensperger F, Stalder H, Peterhans E (2010) Clinical appearance and pathology of cattle persistently infected with bovine viral diarrhoea virus of different genetic subgroups. Vet Microbiol 141(3-4):258–267

Ball JM, Tian P, Zeng CQY, Morris AP, Estes MK (1996) Age-dependent diarrhea induced by a rotaviral nonstructural glycoprotein. Science 272(5258):101–104

Bando SY, Valle GRD, Martinez MB, Trabulsi LR, Moreira-Filho CA (1998) Characterization of enteroinvasive Escherichia coli and Shigella strains by RAPD analysis. FEMS Microbiol Lett 165(1):159–165

References

Becker-Dreps S, Bucardo F, Vilchez S, Zambrana LE, Liu L, Weber DJ, Peña R, Barclay L, Vinjé J, Hudgens MG, Nordgren J, Svensson L, Morgan DR, Espinoza F, Paniagua M (2014) Etiology of childhood diarrhea after rotavirus vaccine introduction: a prospective, population-based study in Nicaragua. Pediatr Infect Dis J 33:1156–1163

Beraldo LG, Borges CA, Maluta RP, Cardozo MV, Rigobelo EC and de Avila F.A. 2014. Detection of Shiga toxigenic (STEC) and enteropathogenic (EPEC) Escherichia coli in dairy buffalo. Vet Microbiol 170(1–2):162-166

Bhatnagar S, Lodha R, Choudhary P, Sachdev HP, Shah N, Narayan S, Wadhwa N, Makhija P, Kunnekel K, Ugra D (2007) IAP guidelines 2006 on hospital based management of severely malnourished children (adapted from the WHO guidelines). Indian Paediatr 44:443–461

Bhutta ZA, Ghishan F, Lindley K, Memon IA, Mittal S, Rhoads JM (2004) Persistent and chronic diarrhea and malabsorption: Working Group report of the second World Congress of Pediatric Gastroenterology, Hepatology, and Nutrition. J Pediatr Gastroenterol Nutr 39:S711–S716

Bhutta ZA, Bird SM, Black RE, Brown KH, Gardner J, Gore S, Hidaat A, Khatun F, Martorell R, Ninh N, Penny M, Rosado J (2007) Therapeutic effects of oral zinc in acute and persistent diarrhea in children in developing countries: pooled analysis of randomized controlled trials. Am J Clin Nutr 2:1516–1522

Bockemühl J (1980) Characteristics and function of enterotoxins of Gram-negative bacteria (author's transl). Immunitat und Infektion 8(2):43–49

Bok K, Green KY (2012) Norovirus gastroenteritis in immunocompromised patients. N Engl J Med 367:2126–2132

Borges CA, Beraldo LG, Maluta RP, Cardozo MV, Guth BEC, Rigobelo EC, de Avila FA (2012) Shiga toxigenic and atypical enteropathogenic Escherichia coli in the feces and carcasses of slaughtered pigs. Foodborne Pathog Dis 9(12):1119–1125

Brown AW, Wilson RB (2018) Clostridium difficile colitis and zoonotic origins—a narrative review. Gastroenterol Rep 6(3):157–166

Brownlie J (1990) The pathogenesis of bovine virus. Revue scientifique et technique (International Office of Epizootics) 9:43–59

Brownlie J, Clarke MC, Howard CJ (1984) Experimental production of fatal mucosal disease in cattle. Vet Rec 114(22):535–536

Brunet JP, Cotte-Laffitte J, Linxe C, Quero AM, Géniteau-Legendre M, Servin A (2000) Rotavirus infection induces an increase in intracellular calcium concentration in human intestinal epithelial cells: role in microvillar actin alteration. J Virol 74(5):2323–2332

Bukhave K, Rask-Madsen J (1980) Saturation kinetics applied to in vitro effects of low prostaglandin E2 and F2α concentrations on ion transport across human jejunal mucosa. Gastroenterology 78(1):32–42

Buret AG, Scott KG, Chin AC (2002) Giardiasis: pathophysiology and pathogenesis. In: Giardia, the cosmopolitan parasite, pp 109–1126

Camilleri M (2009) Serotonin in the gastrointestinal tract. Curr Opin Endocrinol Diabetes Obes 16(1):53

Cantey JR (1985) Infectious diarrhea: pathogenesis and risk factors. Am J Med 78(6):65–75

Carey-Ann BD, Carroll KC (2013) Diagnosis of Clostridium difficile infection: an ongoing conundrum for clinicians and for clinical laboratories. Clin Microbiol Rev 26(3):604–630

Castagliuolo I, Riegler MF, Valenick L, LaMont JT, Pothoulakis C (1999) Saccharomyces boulardii protease inhibits the effects of Clostridium difficile toxins A and B in human colonic mucosa. Infect Immun 67(1):302–307

Certad G, Viscogliosi E, Chabé M, Cacciò SM (2017) Pathogenic mechanisms of Cryptosporidium and Giardia. Trends Parasitol 33(7):561–576

Chauhan RS (1991) Immunopathological studies on rotavirus infection in calves. PhD Thesis, GB Pant University of Agriculture and Technology, Pantnagar, Nainital (UP), pp 140

Chauhan RS, Singh NP (1992a) Assessment of intestinal damage in rotavirus infected calves by D-xylose malabsorption test. Indian J Vet Pathol 16:13–16

Chauhan RS, Singh NP (1992b) Cell-mediated immune response in rotavirus-infected calves: leucocyte migration inhibition assay. J Comp Pathol 107:115–118

Chauhan RS, Singh NP (1992c) Cytopathology induced by rotavirus in fetal rhesus monkey kidney cells (MA104). Indian J Vet Pathol 16:76–78

Chauhan RS, Singh NP (1993a) Rotavirus infection in calves- diagnosis by polyacrylamide gel electrophoresis. Indian J Anim Sci. 63:1–3

Chauhan RS, Singh NP (1993b) Rotavirus infection in calves-electron microscopic studies. Israel J Vet Res 48:110–112

Chauhan RS, Singh NP (1994) Epidemiology of rotavirus infection in calves in India. Kenya Vet J 18:575

Chauhan RS, Singh NP (1996) Epidemiology of rotavirus infection in calves in India. Int J Anim Sci 11:221–223

Chauhan RS, Dhama K, Mahendran M (2008) Pathobiology of rotaviral diarrhea in calves and its diagnosis and control: a review. J Immunol Immunopathol 10:1–13

Chen XM, Levine SA, Splinter PL, Tietz PS, Ganong AL, Jobin C, Gores GJ, Paya CV, LaRusso NF (2001) Cryptosporidium parvum activates nuclear factor κB in biliary epithelia preventing epithelial cell apoptosis. Gastroenterology 120(7):1774–1783

Čobeljić M, Miljković-Selimović B, Paunović-Todosijević D, Veličković Z, Lepšanović Z, Zec N, Savić D, Ilić R, Konstantinović S, Jovanović B, Kostić V (1996) Enteroaggregative Escherichia coli associated with an outbreak of diarrhoea in a neonatal nursery ward. Epidemiol Infect 117(1):11–16

Conner ME, Ramig RF (1997) Viral enteric diseases. Viral pathogenesis. Lippincott-Raven Publishers, Philadelphia, PA, pp 713–743

Crawford SE, Patel DG, Cheng E, Berkova Z, Hyser JM, Ciarlet M, Finegold MJ, Conner ME, Estes MK (2006) Rotavirus viremia and extraintestinal viral infection in the neonatal rat model. J Virol 80(10):4820–4832

D'Antonio RG, WinnR E, TaylorJ P, Gustafson TL, Current WL, Rhodes MM, Gray W Jr, Zajac A (1985) A waterborne outbreak of cryptosporidiosis in normal hosts. Ann Intern Med 103:886–888

Dall'Agnol M, Martinez MB (1999) Uptake of iron from different compounds by enteroinvasive Escherichia coli. Rev Microbiol 30(2):149–152

Das P, Goswami P, Das TK, Nag T, Sreenivas V, Ahuja V, Panda SK, Gupta SD, Makharia GK (2012) Comparative tight junction protein expressions in colonic Crohn's disease, ulcerative colitis, and tuberculosis: a new perspective. Virchows Arch 460(3):261–270

de Vrese M, Stegelmann A, Richter B, Fenselau S, Laue C, Schrezenmeir J (2001) Probiotics compensation for lactase insufficiency. Am J Clin Nutr 73(2):421S–429S

Deng K, Plaza-Garrido A, Torres JA, Paredes-Sabja D (2015) Survival of Clostridium difficile spores at low temperatures. Food Microbiol 46:218–221

Desai S, Rathi N, Kawade A, Venkatramanan P, Kundu R, Lalwani SK, Dubey AP, Rao JV, Narayanappa D, Ghildiyal R, Gogtay NJ (2018) Non-interference of Bovine-Human reassortant pentavalent rotavirus vaccine ROTASIIL® with the immunogenicity of infant vaccines in comparison with a licensed rotavirus vaccine. Vaccine 36(37):5519–5523

Dhama K, Chauhan RS, Mahendran M, Malik SVS (2009) Rotavirus diarrhea in bovines and other domestic animals. Vet Res Commun 33:1–23

Di Genova BM, Tonelli RR (2016) Infection strategies of intestinal parasite pathogens and host cell responses. Front Microbiol 7:256

Dorn CR (1988) Hemorrhagic colitis and hemolytic uremic syndrome caused by Escherichia coli in people consuming undercooked beef and unpasteurized milk. J Am Vet Med Assoc 193:1360–1361

Ebrahim GJ (1990) Diarrhoea due to intestinal parasites. J Trop Pediatr 36(3):98–100

Eckmann L, Laurent F, Langford TD, Hetsko ML, Smith JR, Kagnoff MF, Gillin FD (2000) Nitric oxide production by human intestinal epithelial cells and competition for arginine as potential determinants of host defense against the lumen-dwelling pathogen Giardia lamblia. J Immunol 164(3):1478–1487

Edwards BH (1999) Salmonella and Shigella species. Clin Lab Med 19(3):469–487

Epple HJ, Zeitz M (2012) Intestinal mucosal barrier function in HIV infection. Annals of the New York. Acad Sci 1258:19–24

Esper F, Weibel C, Ferguson D, Landry ML, Kahn JS (2005) Evidence of a novel human coronavirus that is associated with respiratory tract disease in infants and young children. J Infect Dis 191(4):492–498

Esper F, Weibel C, Ferguson D, Landry ML, Kahn JS (2006) Coronavirus HKU1 infection in the United States. Emerg Infect Dis 12(5):775

Esper F, Ou Z, Huang YT (2010) Human coronaviruses are uncommon in patients with gastrointestinal illness. J Clin Virol 48(2):131–133

Estes MK, Morris AP (1999) A viral enterotoxin. In: Mechanisms in the pathogenesis of enteric diseases 2. Springer, Boston, MA, pp 73–82

Finlay BB, Leung KY, Rosenshine I, Portillo FG (1992) Salmonella interactions with the epithelial cell: a model to study the biology of intracellular parasitism. ASM Am Soc Microbiol News 58(9):486–489

Friedrich AW, Bielaszewska M, Zhang WL, Pulz M, Kuczius T, Ammon A, Karch H (2002) Escherichia coli harboring Shiga toxin 2 gene variants: frequency and association with clinical symptoms. J Infect Dis 185(1):74–84

Gaseon J (2006) Epidemiology, etiology and pathophysiology of traveller's diarrhea. Digestion 73: 1102–1108

Gerna G, Passarani N, Battaglia M, Revello MG, Torre D, Cereda PM (1984) Coronaviruses and gastroenteritis: evidence of antigenic relatedness between human enteric coronavirus strains and human coronavirus OC43. Microbiologica 7(4):315–322

Giddings SL, Stevens AM, Leung DT (2016) Traveler's diarrhea. Medical. Clinics 100(2):317–330

Gioia-Di Chiacchio RM, Cunha MPV, Sturn RM, Moreno LZ, Moreno AM, Pereira CBP, Martins FH, Franzolin MR, Piazza RMF, Knöbl T (2016) Shiga toxin-producing Escherichia coli (STEC): zoonotic risks associated with psittacine pet birds in home environments. Vet Microbiol 184:27–30

Gomez HF, Cleary TG (1997) Shigella species. Principles and practice of pediatric infectious diseases. Churchill Livingstone, New York, NY, pp 429–434

Gracey M (1986) Bacterial diarrhea. Clinical. Gastroenterology 15(1):21–37

Graham DY, Estes MK (1988) Viral infections of the intestine. In: Gitnick G (ed) Gastroenterology. Medical Examination Publishing Company, New Hyde Park, NY, pp 566–578

Graham DY, Sackman JW, Estes MK (1984) Pathogenesis of rotavirus-induced diarrhea. Dig Dis Sci 29(11):1028–1035

Green KY (2014) Norovirus infection in immunocompromised hosts. Clin Microbiol Infect 20: 717–723

Greenberg HB, Estes MK (2009) Rotaviruses: from pathogenesis to vaccination. Gastroenterology 136(6):1939–1951

Greenberg HB, Clark HF, Offit PA (1994) Rotavirus pathology and pathophysiology. Curr Top Microbiol Immunol 185:255–283

Guarino A, Vecchio AL, Canani RB (2009) Probiotics as prevention and treatment for diarrhea. Curr Opin Gastroenterol 25(1):18–23

Günzel D, Fromm M (2012) Claudins and other tight junction proteins. Compr Physiol 2(3): 1819–1852

Guttman JA, Li Y, Wickham ME, Deng W, Vogl AW, Finlay BB (2006) Attaching and effacing pathogen-induced tight junction disruption *in vivo*. Cell Microbiol 8:634–645

Harries JT (1976) The problem of bacterial diarrhea. Ciba Found Symp 42:3–25

Hart CA, Batt RM, Saunders JR (1993) Diarrhea caused by E. coli. Ann Trop Paediatr 13(2): 121–131

Hawkey CJ, Rampton DS (1985) Prostaglandins and the gastrointestinal mucosa: are they important in its function, disease, or treatment? Gastroenterology 89(5):1162–1188

Hebbelstrup Jensen B, Olsen KE, Struve C, Krogfelt KA, Petersen AM (2014) Epidemiology and clinical manifestations of enteroaggregative Escherichia coli. Clin Microbiol Rev 27:614–630

Heller F, Florian P, Bojarski C, Richter J, Christ M, Hillenbrand B, Mankertz J, Gitter AH, Bürgel N, Fromm M, Zeitz M (2005) Interleukin-13 is the key effector Th2 cytokine in ulcerative colitis that affects epithelial tight junctions, apoptosis, and cell restitution. Gastroenterology 129(2):550–564

Henderson IR, Navarro-Garcia F, Desvaux M, Fernandez RC, Ala'Aldeen D (2004) Type V protein secretion pathway: the autotransporter story. Microbiol Mol Biol Rev 68(4):692–744

Hendrix TR, Atkinson M, Clifton JA, Ingelfinger FJ (1957) The effect of 5-hydroxytryptamine on intestinal motor function in man. Am J Med 23(6):886–893

Hensgens MP, Keessen EC, Squire MM, Riley TV, Koene MG, de Boer E, Lipman LJ, Kuijper E (2012) Clostridium difficile infection in the community: a zoonotic disease? Clin Microbiol Infect 18(7):635–645

Hill C, Guarner F, Reid G, Gibson GR, Merenstein DJ, Pot B, Morelli L, Canani RB, Flint HJ, Salminen S, Calder PC (2014) Expert consensus document. The international scientific Association for Probiotics and Prebiotics consensus statement on the scope and appropriate use of the term probiotic. Nat Rev Gastroenterol Hepatol 11(8):506–514

Holland RE (1990) Some infectious causes of diarrhea in young farm animals. Clin Microbiol Rev 3(4):345–375

Horton EW, Main IH, Thompson CJ, Wright PM (1968) Effect of orally administered prostaglandin E1 on gastric secretion and gastrointestinal motility in man. Gut 9(6):655

Houghton LA, Atkinson W, Lockhart S, Fell C, Whorwell PJ, Keevil B (2007) Sigmoid-colonic motility in health and irritable bowel syndrome: a role for 5-hydroxytryptamine. Neurogastroenterol Motil 19(9):724–731

Huang K, Akiyoshi DE, Feng X, Tzipori S (2003) Development of patent infection in immunosuppressed C57Bl/6 mice with a single Cryptosporidium meleagridis oocyst. J Parasitol 89(3):620–622

Hunter PR, Hughes S, Woodhouse S, Nicholas R, Syed Q, Chalmers RM, Verlander NQ, Goodacre J (2004) Health sequelae of human cryptosporidiosis in immunocompetent patients. Clin Infect Dis 39(4):504–510

Joensuu J, Koskenniemi E, Pang XL, Vesikari T (1997) Randomised placebo-controlled trial of rhesus-human reassortant rotavirus vaccine for prevention of severe rotavirus gastroenteritis. Lancet 350(9086):1205–1209

Jog P (2016) ZODIAC of diarrhea management. Indian Pediatr 53(7):563–564

Jung C, Hugot JP, Barreau F (2010) Peyer's patches: the immune sensors of the intestine. Int J Inflamm:1–12

Kaper JB, Nataro JP, Mobley HLT (2004) Pathogenic E. coli. Nat Rev Microbiol 2:123–140

Karim SMM, Filshie GM (1970) Therapeutic abortion using prostaglandin F2α. Lancet 295:157–159

Keusch GT, Scrimshaw NS (1986) Selective primary health care. Strategies for control of disease in the developing world. XXIII. Control of infection to reduce the prevalence of infantile and childhood malnutrition. Rev Infect Dis 8:273–287

Koboziev I, Karlsson F, Mathew B (2010) Gut-associated lymphoid tissue T cell trafficking, and chronic intestinal inflammation. Ann N Y Acad Sci 1207(Suppl 1):E86–E93

Koo HL, Ajami N, Atmar RL, DuPont HL (2010) Noroviruses: the principal cause of foodborne disease worldwide. Discov Med 10:61–70

Kulkarni PS, Desai S, Tewari T, Kawade A, Goyal N, Garg BS, Kumar D, Kanungo S, Kamat V, Kang G, Bavdekar A (2017) A randomized phase III clinical trial to assess the efficacy of a bovine-human reassortant pentavalent rotavirus vaccine in Indian infants. Vaccine 35(45):6228–6237

Kumar GSV, Uma BM (2019) Clostridium difficile: a neglected, but emerging pathogen in India. i medpub LTD

Lan R, Alles MC, Donohoe K, Martinez MB, Reeves PR (2004) Molecular evolutionary relationships of enteroinvasive Escherichia coli and shigella spp. Infect Immun 72(9): 5080–5088

Lanyon SR, Hill FI, Reichel MP, Brownlie J (2014) Bovine viral diarrhoea: pathogenesis and diagnosis. Vet J 199(2):201–209

Lascowski KMS, Gonçalves EM, Alvares PP et al (2012) Prevalence and virulence profiles of Shiga toxin-producing Escherichia coli isolated from beef cattle in a Brazilian slaughter house. Zoonoses Public Health 59(1):19–90

Lascowski KMS, Guth BEC, Martins FH, Rocha SPD, Irino K, Pelayo JS (2013) Shiga toxin-producing Escherichia coli in drinking water supplies of north Praná state, Brazil. J Appl Microbiol 114(4):1230–1239

Lebeer S, Vanderleyden J, De Keersmaecker SC (2010) Host interactions of probiotic bacterial surface molecules: comparison with commensals and pathogens. Nat Rev Microbiol 8(3): 171–184

Lee SR, Nanduri B, Pharr GT, Stokes JV, Pinchuk LM (2009) Bovine viral diarrhea virus infection affects the expression of proteins related to professional antigen presentation in bovine monocytes. Biochimica et Biophysica Acta (BBA)-Proteins and Proteomics 1794(1):14–22

Leitch GJ, Qing H (2011) Cryptosporidiosis-an overview. J Biomed Res 25(1):1–16

Levine MM (1987) Escherichia coli that cause diarrhea: enterotoxigenic, enteropathogenic, enteroinvasive, enterohemorrhagic, and enteroadherent. J Infect Dis 155(3):377–389

Liebler-Tenori EM, Greiser-Wilke I, Pohlenz JF (1997) Organ and tissue distribution of the antigen of the cytopathogenic bovine virus diarrhea virus in the early and advanced phase of experimental mucosal disease. Arch Virol 142(8):1613–1634

Liebler-Tenorio EM, Lanwehr A, Greiser-Wilke I, Loehr BI, Pohlenz J (2000) Comparative investigation of tissue alterations and distribution of BVD-viral antigen in cattle with early onset versus late onset mucosal disease. Vet Microbiol 77(1-2):163–174

Liess B, Frey HR, Kittsteiner H, Baumann F, Neumann N (1974) Beobachtungen und Untersuchungen über die "Mucosal disease" des Rindes. Deutsche Tierärztliche Woschenschrift 81:477–500

Maluta RP, Fairbrother JM, Stella AE, Rigobelo EC, Martinez R, de Avila FA (2014) Potentially pathogenic Escherichia coli in healthy, pasture-raised sheep on farms and at the abattoir in Brazil. Vet Microbiol 169(1-2):89–95

Mandal A, Sahi PK (2017) Probiotics for diarrhea in children. J Med Res Innov 1(2):AV5–AV12

Marsden PD, Schultz G (1969) Intestinal parasites. Gastroenterology 57:724–750

Martinez MB, Whittan TS, McGraw EA, Rodrigues J, Trabulsi LR (1999) Clonal relationship among invasive and non-invasive strains of enteroinvasive Escherichia coli serogroups. FEMS Microbiol Lett 172(2):145–151

Martins RP, da Silva MC, Dutra V, Nakazato L, da Silva Leite D (2013) Preliminary virulence genotyping and phylogeny of Escherichia coli from the gut of pigs at slaughtering stage in Brazil. Meat Sci 93(3):437–440

Martins FH, Guth BEC, Piazza RM, Leao SC, Ludovico A, Ludovico MS, Dahbi G, Marzoa J, Mora A, Blanco J, Pelayo JS (2015) Diversity of Shiga toxin-producing Escherichia coli in sheep flocks of Paraná state, southern Brazil. Vet Microbiol 175(1):150–156

Matuchansky C, Bernier JJ (1973) Effect of prostaglandin E1 on glucose, water, and electrolyte absorption in the human jejunum. Gastroenterology 64(6):1111–1118

Matuchansky C, Mary JY, Bernier JJ (1976) Further studies on prostaglandin E1-induced jejunal secretion of water and electrolytes in man, with special reference to the influence of ethacrynic acid, furosemide, and aspirin. Gastroenterology 71(2):274–281

McWhorter-Murlin AC, Hickman-Brenner FW (1994) Identification and serotyping of salmonella and an update of the Kauffmann-white scheme. Centers for Disease Control and Prevention, Atlanta, GA

Milton AAP, Priya GB, Aravind M, Parthasarathy S, Saminathan M, Jeeva K, Agarwal RK (2015) Nosocomial infections and their surveillance in veterinary hospitals. Adv Anim Vet Sci 3(2s):1–24

Milton AA, Agarwal RK, Bhuvana Priya G, Saminathan M, Aravind M, Reddy A, Athira CK, Ramees T, Sharma AK, Kumar A (2017) Prevalence and molecular typing of Clostridium perfringens in captive wildlife in India. Anaerobe 44:55–57

Milton AAP, Agarwal RK, Priya GB, Athira CK, Saminathan M, Reddy A, Aravind M, Kumar A (2018) Occurrence, antimicrobial susceptibility patterns and genotypic relatedness of salmonella spp. isolates from captive wildlife, their caretakers, feed and water in India. Epidemiol Infect 146(12):1543–1549

Milton AAP, Agarwal RK, Priya GB, Aravind M, Athira CK, Rose L, Saminathan M, Sharma AK, Kumar A (2019) Captive wildlife from India as carriers of Shiga toxin-producing, enteropathogenic and enterotoxigenic Escherichia coli. J Vet Med Sci 81(2):321–327

Misiewicz JJ, Waller SL, Eisner M (1966) Motor responses of human gastrointestinal tract to 5-hydroxytryptamine *in vivo* and *in vitro*. Gut 7(3):208

Misiewicz JJ, Waller S, Kiley N, Horton EW (1969) Effect of oral prostaglandin E1 on intestinal transit in man. Lancet 293(7596):648–651

Modigliani R, Matuchansky C, Bernier JJ (1979) Depressed jejunal secretion of water and ions in response to prostaglandin E1 in adult celiac disease. Dig Dis Sci 24(10):763–768

Mohammad A, PeirisJ SM, Wijewanta EA (1986) Serotypes of verocytotoxigenic Escherichia coli isolated from cattle and buffalo calf diarrhoea. FEMS Microbiol Lett 35:261–265

Müller N, Von Allmen N (2005) Recent insights into the mucosal reactions associated with Giardia lamblia infections. Int J Parasitol 35(13):1339–1347

Mullhaupt B (2002) Diarrhea. Praxis(Bern 1994) 91(42):1749–1756

Murray JA, Rubio-Tapia A (2012) Diarrhoea due to small bowel diseases. Best Pract Res Clin Gastroenterol 26(5):581–600

Nataro JP, Kaper JB (1998) Diarrheagenic Escherichia coli. Clin Microbiol Rev 11(1):142–201

Navin TR, Juranek DD (1984) Cryptosporidiosis: clinical. Epidemiologic, and parasitiologic review. J Infect Dis 6:313–327

Nomoto K (2005) Prevention of infections by probiotics. J Biosci Bioeng 100(6):583–592

O'Hara SP, Chen XM (2011) The cell biology of Cryptosporidium infection. Microbes Infect 13(8-9):721–730

Ooms L, Degryse A (1986) Pathogenesis and pharmacology of diarrhea. Vet Res Commun 10(1):355–397

Orskov F, Orskov I, Vilar JA (1987) Cattle as a reservoir of verotoxin-producing Escherichia coli 0157:H7. Lancet 1:276

Oshima T, Miwa H, Joh T (2008) Changes in the expression of claudins in active ulcerative colitis. J Gastroenterol Hepatol 23:S146–S150

Parsot C (2005) Shigella spp. and enteroinvasive Escherichia coli pathogenicity factors. FEMS Microbiol Lett 252(1):11–18

Pedersen NC, Allen CE, Lyons LA (2008) Pathogenesis of feline enteric coronavirus infection. J Feline Med Surg 10(6):529–541

Peltola H, Siitonen A, Kataja M, Kyrönseppa H, Simula I, Mattila L, Cadoz M (1991) Prevention of travellers' diarrhoea by oral B-subunit/whole-cell cholera vaccine. Lancet 338(8778):1285–1289

Penheiter KL, Mathur N, Giles D, Fahlen T, Jones BD (1997) Non-invasive Salmonella typhimurium mutants are avirulent because of an inability to enter and destroy M cells of ileal Peyer's patches. Mol Microbiol 24(4):697–709

Phalipon A, Sansonetti PJ (2007) Shigella's ways of manipulating the host intestinal innate and adaptive immune system: a tool box for survival? Immunol Cell Biol 85(2):119–129

Pierce NF, Carpenter CC, Elliott HL, Greenough WB (1971) Effects of prostaglandins, theophylline, and cholera exotoxin upon transmucosal water and electrolyte movement in the canine jejunum. Gastroenterology 60(1):22–32

Poruchynsky MS, Maass DR, Atkinson PH (1991) Calcium depletion blocks the maturation of rotavirus by altering the oligomerization of virus-encoded proteins in the ER. J Cell Biol 114(4): 651–656

Prasad S, Mingrino R, Kaukinen K, Hayes KL, Powell RM, MacDonald TT, Collins JE (2005) Inflammatory processes have differential effects on claudins 2, 3 and 4 in colonic epithelial cells. Lab Investig 85(9):1139

Prince Milton AA, Agarwal RK, Priya GB, Saminathan M, Aravind M, Reddy A, Athira CK, Anjay, Ramees TP, Dhama K, Sharma AK, Kumar A (2017) Prevalence of Campylobacter jejuni and Campylobacter coli in captive wildlife species of India. Iranian J Vet Res 18(3): 177–182

Pupo GM, Karaolis DK, Lan R, Reeves PR (1997) Evolutionary relationships among pathogenic and nonpathogenic Escherichia coli strains inferred from multilocus enzyme electrophoresis and mdh sequence studies. Infect Immun 65(7):2685–2692

Ramig RF (2004) Pathogenesis of intestinal and systemic rotavirus infection. J Virol 78(19): 10213–10220

Rathi R, Kadian SK, Khurana B, Grover YP, Gulati BR (2007) Evaluation of immune response ton bovine rotavirus following oral and intraperitoneal inoculation in mice. Indian J Exp Biol 45: 212–216

Ribeiro LF, Barbosa MMC, de Rezende Pinto F, Guariz CSL, Maluta RP, Rossi JR, Rossi GAM, Lemos MVF, do Amaral LA. (2016) Shiga toxigenic and enteropathogenic Escherichia coli in water and fish from pay-to-fish ponds. Lett Appl Microbiol 62(3):216–220

Rodriguez-Palacios A, LeJeune JT (2011) Moist-heat resistance, spore aging, and superdormancy in Clostridium difficile. Appl Environ Microbiol 77(9):3085–3091

Rodriguez-Palacios A, Stämpfli HR, Duffield T, Peregrine AS, Trotz-Williams LA, Arroyo LG, Brazier JS, Weese JS (2006) Clostridium difficile PCR ribotypes in calves, Canada. Emerg Infect Dis 12(11):1730

Rodriguez-Palacios A, Reid-Smith RJ, Staempfli HR, Daignault D, Janecko N, Avery BP, Martin H, Thomspon AD, McDonald LC, Limbago B, Weese JS (2009) Possible seasonality of Clostridium difficile in retail meat, Canada. Emerg Infect Dis 15(5):802

Rolland K, Lambert-Zechovsky N, Picard B, Denamur E (1998) Shigella and enteroinvasive Escherichia coli strains are derived from distinct ancestral strains of E. coli. Microbiology 144(9):2667–2672

Rousset S, Moscovici O, Lebon P, Barbet JP, Helardot P, Macé B, Bargy F, Vinh LT, Chany C (1984) Intestinal lesions containing coronavirus-like particles in neonatal necrotizing enterocolitis: an ultrastructural analysis. Pediatrics 73(2):218–224

Rubin RH, Weinstein L (1977) Salmonellosis; microbiologic, pathologic and clinical features (No. 616.927 R896). Stratton Intercontinental Medical Book Corp

Ruiz MC, Cohen J, Michelangeli F (2000) Role of Ca2+ in the replication and pathogenesis of rotavirus and other viral infections. Cell Calcium 28(3):137–149

Sansonetti PJ, Phalipon A (1999) M cells as ports of entry for enteroinvasive pathogens: mechanisms of interaction, consequences for the disease process. Semin Immunol 11(3): 193–203. (Academic Press)

Sansonetti PJ, Kopecko DJ, Formal SB (1982) Involvement of a plasmid in the invasive ability of Shigella flexneri. Infect Immun 35:852–860

Scaletsky IC, Silva ML, Trabulsi LR (1984) Distinctive patterns of adherence of enteropathogenic Escherichia coli to HeLa cells. Infect Immun 45(2):534–536

Schiller LR, Pardi DS, Sellin JH (2017) Chronic diarrhea: diagnosis and management. Clin Gastroenterol Hepatol 15(2):182–193

Schmid-Hempel P (2008) Immune defence, parasite evasion strategies and their relevance for 'macroscopic phenomena' such as virulence. Philos Trans R Soc B Biol Sci 364(1513):85–98

Schumann M, Günzel D, Buergel N, Richter JF, Troeger H, May C, Fromm A, Sorgenfrei D, Daum S, Bojarski C, Heyman M (2012) Cell polarity-determining proteins Par-3 and PP-1 are involved in epithelial tight junction defects in coeliac disease. Gut 61(2):220–228

Scott KE, Logan MR, Klammer GM, Teoh DA, Buret AG (2000) Jejunal brush border microvillous alterations in Giardia muris-infected mice: role of T lymphocytes and interleukin-6. Infect Immun 68(6):3412–3418

Scrimshaw NS, Taylor CE, Gordon JE (1968) Interaction of nutrition and infection. Monograph series No. 57. World Health Organization, Geneva, p 329

Segar L, Easow JM, Srirangaraj S, Hanifah M, Joseph NM, Seetha KS (2017) Prevalence of Clostridium difficile infection among the patients attending a tertiary care teaching hospital. Indian J Pathol Microbiol 60(2):221

Selman IE (1973) The absorption of colostral globulins by newborn calves. Ann Resear Vet 4:213–221

Sethi G, Sankaranarayanan S, Sukhija M (2018) Low lactose in the nutritional management of diarrhea: case reports from India. Clin Epidemiol Global Health 6(4):160–162

Shane AL, Mody RK, Crump JA, Tarr PI, Steiner TS, Kotloff K, Langley JM, Wanke C, Warren CA, Cheng AC, Cantey J (2017) Infectious Diseases Society of America clinical practice guidelines for the diagnosis and management of infectious diarrhea. Clin Infect Dis 65(12):e45–e80

Sharon P, Karmeli F, Rachmilewitz D (1984) Effects of prostaglandins on human intestinal Na-K-ATPase activity. Isr J Med Sci 20:677–680

Siciliani E (2017) Shigella dysenteriae. https://mechpath.com/2017/11/20/shigella-dysenteriae/

Songer JG (2004) The emergence of Clostridium difficile as a pathogen of food animals. Anim Health Res Rev 5(2):321–326

Spahn TW, Kucharzik T (2004) Modulating the intestinal immune system: the role of lymphotoxin and GALT organs. Gut 53:456–465

Spangler BD (1992) Structure and function of cholera toxin and the related Escherichia coli heat-labile enterotoxin. Microbiol Rev 56(4):622–647

Spiller R (2006) Role of motility in chronic diarrhoea. Neurogastroenterol Motil 18(12):1045–1055

Tânia AT, GomesaWaldir P, Elias, Isabel CA, Scaletskya Beatriz EC, Gutha Juliana F, Rodriguesc Roxane MF, Piazzab Luís CS, Ferreirac Marina B, Martinezd. (2016) Diarrhegenic E. coli review. Braz J Microbiol 47S:3–30

Trabulsi LR, Keller R, Gomes TAT (2002) Typical and atypical enteropathogenic Escherichia coli. Emerg Infect Dis 8(5):508

Tsai PY, Zhang B, He WQ, Zha JM, Odenwald MA, Singh G, Tamura A, Shen L, Sailer A, Yeruva S, Kuo WT (2017) IL-22 upregulates epithelial claudin-2 to drive diarrhea and enteric pathogen clearance. Cell Host Microbe 21(6):671–681

Vabret A, Dina J, Gouarin S, Petitjean J, Corbet S, Freymuth F (2006) Detection of the new human coronavirus HKU1: a report of 6 cases. Clin Infect Dis 42(5):634–639

Vesikari T (2008) Rotavirus vaccines. Scandinavian J Infect Dis 40:691–695

Vial PA, Robins-Browne R, Lior H, Prado V, Kaper JB, Nataro JP, Maneval D, Elsayed AED, Levine MM (1988) Characterization of enteroadherent-aggregative Escherichia coli, a putative agent of diarrheal disease. J Infect Dis 158(1):70–79

Weese JS, Rousseau J, Arroyo L (2005) Bacteriological evaluation of commercial canine and feline raw diets. Can Vet J 46(6):513

Whelan K, Schneider SM (2011) Mechanisms, prevention, and management of diarrhea in enteral nutrition. Curr Opin Gastroenterol 27(2):152–159

Whyte LA, Jenkins HR (2012) Pathophysiology of diarrhoea. Paediatr Child Health 22(10):443–447

Wikswo ME, Kambhampati A, Shioda K, Walsh KA, Bowen A, Hall AJ; Centers for Disease Control and Prevention (CDC) (2015) Outbreaks of acute gastroenteritis transmitted by person-to-person contact, environmental contamination, and unknown modes of transmission—United States, 2009–2013. MMWR Surveill Summ 64(12):1–16

Woods TA (1990) Diarrhea in- clinical methods: the history, physical, and laboratory examinations. In: Walker HK, Hall WD, Hurst JW (eds). Butterworths Boston

Yacyshyn B (2016) Advances in Clostridium difficile associated Diarrhea. Digest Dis Week

Yan F, Polk DB (2006) Probiotics as functional food in the treatment of diarrhea. Curr Opin Clin Nutrit Metab Care 9(6):717–721

Yoldaş Ö, Altındiş M, Cufalı D, Aşık G, Keşli R (2016) A diagnostic algorithm for the detection of clostridium difficile-associated diarrhea. Balkan Med J 33(1):80–86

Zeissig S, Bürgel N, Günzel D, Richter J, Mankertz J, Wahnschaffe U, Kroesen AJ, Zeitz M, Fromm M, Schulzke JD (2007) Changes in expression and distribution of claudin 2, 5 and 8 lead to discontinuous tight junctions and barrier dysfunction in active Crohn's disease. Gut 56(1): 61–72

Zhang M, Zeng CQY, Morris AP, Estes MK (2000) A functional NSP4 enterotoxin peptide secreted from rotavirus-infected cells. J Virol 74(24):11663–11670

Immunopathology of Reproductive Disorders of Animals

10

Key Points

1. Immune system of the vaginal mucosa is regularly modulated by physiological events such as menstruation, fertilization, pregnancy, and hormonal changes.
2. Immune cells found in the endometrium as well as endometrial stromal and epithelial cells produce innate uterine immune responses through PRRs.
3. Cervicovaginal mucus and local immune cells serve a crucial function in providing immunity to female reproductive system.
4. Immunity and inflammation are crucial for healthy ovarian and uterine cycles, implantation, placentation, and fetal development, as well as body's defense against microbial infection.
5. Abortion refers to the deliberate ending of a pregnancy with the evacuation of a recognizable-sized fetus before it is viable.
6. Important bacterial infections that cause abortion include brucellosis, listeriosis, campylobacteriosis, leptospirosis, bluetongue, infectious bovine rhinotracheitis, bovine herpesvirus 4, bovine viral diarrhea, etc.
7. Important protozoal infections cause abortion include *Tritrichomonas foetus*, *Toxoplasma gondii*, *Anaplasma marginale*, *Neospora caninum*, etc.

10.1 Introduction

The endometrial lining of the uterus has important role in the normal functioning of the reproductive cycles, implantation, placentation, and supporting the health of fetus up to the parturition. Pathogens cannot enter into the uterus through the vagina because of the mucosal lining and epithelial cells acting as gatekeepers (Hickey et al. 2011). Infections reach the uterus through the vaginal route or through the cervix (Table 10.1). The innate immunity of vagina consists of cellular, chemical, and physical elements (Wira et al. 2005). These elements interact to create a complex microenvironment in the vagina, which regulate the immune responses that are

Table 10.1 Portals of entry into the female reproductive system

Portals of entry	Causes
Ascending infection through the cervix	• At insemination
	• Excessive vaginal contamination
	• Postpartum and retained fetal membranes
Hematogenous	• Localization in maternoplacental interface
• Descending from the ovary via the uterine tube	–
• Direct penetration with foreign body (setae)	
• Transneural with recrudescence of herpesvirus infection	

controlled by sex hormones and a unique microbiome. The immune system of the vaginal mucosa is regularly modulated by physiological events such as menstruation, fertilization, pregnancy, and hormone changes (Wira et al. 2011). The epithelial lining of the vagina also prevents the entry of pathogens into the uterus. In addition to acting as a barrier against pathogens, the stratified squamous epithelium of the vagina also senses the pathogens, which causes immune cells to become activated and secrete immune mediators that trigger inflammation and immunological responses (Kurita 2010). Both humans and animals are susceptible to uterine microbial infections, which are crucial because they can lead to clinical illness, uterine abortion, and infertility (Wira et al. 2005; Jabbour et al. 2009; Sheldon et al. 2009; Mor and Cardenas 2010). While some viruses enter into the uterus through the circulation, and many diseases reach from the genital tract via the cervix. The uterus and endometrium are important because innate and adaptive immunity of uterus and endometrium may detect microbial invasion and fight it off (Wira et al. 2005; Sheldon et al. 2009). Immunity and inflammation are crucial for healthy ovarian and uterine cycles, implantation, placentation, and fetal development, as well as for the body's defense against microbial infection.

Antimicrobial, epithelial barrier, and the complement system are the components of innate immunity that provide protection against pathogens. The discovery of unique cellular pattern recognition receptors that identify chemicals frequently associated with bacteria in the laboratories of Jules Hoffmann and Bruce Beutler led to the expansion of research on innate immunity. In *Drosophila melanogaster*, the Toll protein, which is involved in dorsoventral polarity during embryonic development in the uterus, is necessary for efficient immune responses against fungal infection. The inflammatory response to lipopolysaccharide (LPS), a component of cell wall of Gram-negative bacteria, which acts as an endotoxin in animals, depend on the Toll-like receptor 4 (TLR4), which was functionally significant in mice (Poltorak et al. 1998). The pattern recognition receptors (PRRs) of innate immune system have been shown to be crucial for the detection of microbial infections in the animal uteri through studies employing mice or RNA to target

TLR4. The uterus offers a sterile environment for the growth of the fetus and healthy pregnancy (Cronin et al. 2012; Funkhouser and Bordenstein 2013).

Because, bacteria in the uterine cavity could harm the fetus and induce systemic inflammation and various organ damage, their presence in the uterus is viewed as a risk factor (Martius and Eschenbach 1990). The lower urogenital tract has been the primary source of the germs entering the uterine cavity. The bacteria subsequently enters the uterus through the cervix, crosses the placental barrier, and enters the amniotic fluid and fetus (Goldenberg et al. 2000; Keelan and Payne 2015). Negative pregnancy outcomes have frequently been linked to the detection of bacteria such as *Ureaplasma* and *Fusobacterium* in the uterine cavity was determined by culture-dependent or culture-independent methods (Han et al. 2004, 2009, 2010). The amniotic fluid, uterus, and placenta thought to be sterile however, recently demonstrated to harbor unique microbiomes (Collado et al. 2016; Franasiak and Scott 2017).

10.2 Uterine Function

The nourishment of the blastocyst and embryo, as well as a successful pregnancy, depends on a healthy endometrium. Some pathogenic microorganisms cause difficulties in conception of animals. There is embryo mortality, if uterine infection occurs with these microorganisms after conception (Semambo et al. 1991). Viruses such as bovine viral diarrhea have a similar effect (Mcgowan et al. 1993). The uterus is typically sterile; nevertheless, the presence of microbes or molecules linked to the pathogens seems to elicit an immune response. Immune cells found in the endometrium as well as endometrial stromal and epithelial cells produce the uterine immune responses. The epithelial cells are the first line of defense against microbes in the uterine lumen. The expression of PRRs is crucial for innate immunity in the genital tract to identify the pathogen associated molecular patterns (PAMPs). These PRRs recognize a variety of PAMPs linked to bacteria, viruses, and fungi and are highly conserved across phyla, such as the Toll-like receptor (TLR) family (Akira et al. 2006). Nuclear factor kappa B (NF-κB), transcription factors, and mitogen-activated protein kinase (MAPK) are activated when PAMPs bind to PRRs, causing the release of prostaglandins, cytokines, and chemokines (Ghosh et al. 1998; Li and Verma 2002). Epithelial and stromal cells express TLR4, the innate immune receptor for LPS, which is the key PAMP of the common uterine pathogen *E. coli* (Herath et al. 2006). This concept of endometrial cell expression of PRRs is supported in other species by expression of other TLRs for bacteria and viruses (Schaefer et al. 2004; Hirata et al. 2005; Soboll et al. 2006), while the absence of CD45 expression in bovine cell cultures indicated that they are free of professional immune cells contamination, which gives them an advantage over other species (Herath et al. 2006). The bovine TLR4 signaling pathways are also emerging (Connor et al. 2006). This makes the uterine system of cattle and other mammals as a useful model for explaining the mechanisms of uterine illness (Herath et al. 2006). Pathogen-associated molecules not only cause inflammation in the uterine cells but also have an impact on endocrine function. Prostaglandin F2 (PGF2) and PGE2 are the main hormones released by the endometrium, and *E. coli* or LPS can influence the secretion of these hormones (Herath et al. 2006). Eicosanoids also directly affect uterine immunity, and exogenous PGF2α is a successful therapy for uterine illness (Lewis and Wulster-Radcliffe 2006). Similar to luteinizing hormone, LPS stimulates the progesterone secretion from the mixed populations of luteal cells (including steroidogenic, endothelial, and immune cell types) during in vitro *condition*, but at greater concentrations, LPS kills the cells (Grant et al. 2007).

10.3   Innate Immune Defense of the Uterus

The primary factor in the removal of bacterial contamination of the uterus following parturition is innate immunity (Fig. 10.1). The first innate immune cells to gather at the site of infection are neutrophils, natural killer cells, and macrophages in response to immune mediators produced by affected epithelial cells (Table 10.2). Tumor necrosis factor alpha (TNF-α) is released by neutrophils, which regulates the expression of TLR4 on epithelial cells (Weindl et al. 2007). This involves local cellular defenses to neutralize the pathogens and anatomical and physiological barriers to inhibit bacterial entrance. If the anatomical barriers are breached, immune cells and cells of the endometrium, which are equipped with TLRs, are quick to detect the presence of invasive bacteria. The LPS activation of TLRs initiates the signaling

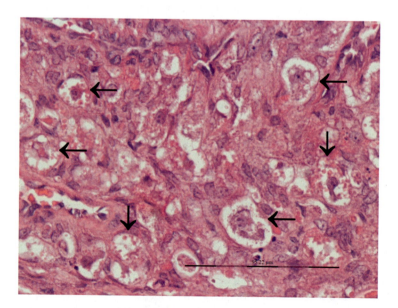

Fig. 10.1 Uterine natural killer (uNK) cells in mouse uterus on day 9 of pregnancy: Infiltration of mature and ruptured uterine natural killer (uNK) cells with the presence of granules in their cytoplasm in the mesometrium of the uterus. H&E x400

10.3 Innate Immune Defense of the Uterus

Table 10.2 Innate and adaptive defenses of the female reproductive system

Immune defenses	Component
Innate defenses	• Vaginal epithelium
	• Cervical barrier
	• Conformation
	• Myometrial tone and contraction
	• Drainage of secretions
	• Neutrophils
	• Macrophages
	• Complement
	• Cytokines
	• Microbial recognition molecules
Adaptive defenses	• Humoral immunity including the common mucosal immune system
	• Cellular immunity

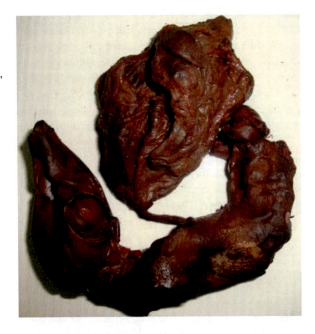

Fig. 10.2 Abortion, mummified fetus, cattle: The fetus died *in utero*; fetal and placental tissues underwent necrosis; fluids were resorbed, dehydrated, and mummified fetus

cascades that lead to the synthesis and production of pro-inflammatory cytokines such as TNF-α, which mobilize the immune cells (Kim et al. 2005).

10.4 Adaptive Immune Defense of the Uterus

10.4.1 Humoral Immunity

Although there are antibody-secreting cells in the bovine uterus, it is unclear, how they contribute to local immunity (Butt et al. 1993). By directly acting on the surface of the bovine uterine mucosa, the specific antibodies are crucial for neutralizing bacterial infections. For instance, it has been observed that cattle received vaccinations against *Campylobacter foetus* subspecies *venerealis* or *Haemophilus somnus* have specific antibodies in their uterine and cervico-vaginal secretions (Butt et al. 1993). An increase in the proportion of specific antibodies to total immunoglobulins in uterine secretions was observed after intrauterine inoculation with *Actinomyces pyogenes* (Watson et al. 1990). It has been demonstrated that immunoglobulin classes are present in the uterine secretions of cows and that they serve as a defense against infections (Dhaliwal et al. 1996). The presence of all other major immunoglobulins in bovine endometrial secretions is regarded as a reflection of an endometrial inflammatory process after bacterial harmness and clinical recovery. By directly lysing the bacteria, acting as opsonins to improve phagocytosis, and activating complement pathways, these immunoglobulins have antibacterial effects (Butler 1983). The type of IgG species produced in the genital tract also depends on the nature of the stimulating antigens. For example, *Tritrichomonas foetus* infection is characterized by a T helper type 2 response, interleukin 4 production, and IgG1 production. When exposed to *Brucella abortus*, the body produces IgG2 and cytotoxic CD8+ T cells as part of the T helper 1 response (Estes and Brown 2002; Oliveira et al. 2002). The IgG opsonizes bacteria to promote phagocytosis, and IgA binds to bacteria to prevent their adherence to mucosal surfaces (Butler 1983). Antigen-antibody complexes also stimulate the classical pathway of complement in the uterine lumen (Butler 1983).

10.4.2 Cell-Mediated Immunity

The cellular form of the immune system plays a very important role in uterine immune defense, but the role of the local humoral immune response is limited (Mestecky et al. 2005). The uterine immune system is significantly modulated by pregnancy, and the number of lymphocytes and macrophages in the uterus varies depending on the stage of gestation (French and Northey 1983; Skopets et al. 1992). To prevent the immunological fetal rejection during the first and second trimesters of pregnancy, the quantity of lymphocytes and macrophages in the bovine uterus is decreased (Vander Wielen and King 1984; Hansen 1997). Macrophages and lymphocytes are found in the inter-caruncular endometrium but not in the caruncular endometrium during mid- and late-stages pregnancy, indicating that the immune response is local and specific to the areas surroundings to fetal tissues or foreign antigens (Gogolin Ewens et al. 1989; Low et al. 1990; Wooding 1992). Lymphocytes and antigen-presenting macrophages were infiltrated into the endometrium of cows, which may be crucial for recognizing and processing of foreign antigens, such as germs that enter the uterus (Leung et al. 2000). Compared to other areas of the endometrium and myometrium, the subepithelial uterine stroma has higher concentrations of T helper cells, B lymphocytes, and antigen-presenting macrophages (Leung et al. 2000).

10.5 Anatomical and Physiological Barriers Against Uterine Infections

A physical barrier that prevents the bacteria from entering the reproductive tract is cervico-vaginal mucus (Bondurant 1999). Within minutes, an infection can travel from the vagina to the cervix and into the uterus (Zervomanolakis et al. 2007). Although the cervical mucus plug inhibits the bacterial growth, it does not entirely block (Hansen et al. 2014). Mucus-trapped bacteria are expelled through the circular and longitudinal muscle layers of uterus (Table 10.2). The cervico-vaginal mucosa also offers defense against many urogenital pathogens. The microbiota play a crucial role in gynecological functions and are an essential component of the female reproductive mucosa. The local immune cells of cervico-vaginal mucosa provides immunity against any pathogen that could affect the female reproductive system.

10.6 Prevalence of Uterine Infections

Prevalence of uterine infections depends on the risk factor associated with the female reproductive tract diseases. There are differences in the prevalence of uterine infections (Konyves et al. 2009; Plontzke et al. 2010). Different classification methods, management strategies, breed characteristics, environmental conditions, nutrition, age, and parity among others, have all been implicated in variations in the prevalence rates (Gautam et al. 2010). In US dairy herds, endometritis was prevalent at a rate of 53% (Gilbert et al. 2005). Endometritis prevalence ranged from 2.6 to 4.5% in Spain (Lopez-Gatius 2003), 23.6% in Japan (Gautam et al. 2010), 47.6% in Korea (Kim and Kang 2003), and 6.25% in Denmark (Bruun et al. 2002). On pasture-based extensive systems, it ranged from 5.6 to 10.9% in Australia (Moss et al. 2002) and from 10 to 38% in Argentina (Madoz et al. 2008; Plontzke et al. 2010). The frequency of uterine infections was 10.1% in the United Kingdom (Azawi 2008).

10.7 Risk Factors Associated with Uterine Infections

There are no known risk factors associated with prepartum or postpartum uterine infections in cows. Various studies have identified some risk factors and they have found that risk factors may vary among different regions or countries due to differences in general management, environment, and herd health conditions (Kim and Kang 2003; Bell and Roberts 2007). Various risk factors related to management and individual cows have been identified. It includes retention of the fetal membranes (Abdelhameed et al. 2009), dystocia, age (Sheldon et al. 2006), parity (Gautam et al. 2009), calving season (Buckley et al. 2010), breed, and nutrition (Bell and Roberts 2007). If we concentrated on nutrition and herd management, the uterine infections could be avoided. The transition period of animal is very important for preventing the uterine infection because in this period the immune status of animal is not being balanced. Additionally, dairy farmers should obtain advice from Nutrition Experts and implement strategies for feeding management of various groups of cows, especially the dry group during the transitional phase. Recently, many antimicrobials and hormonal therapy is used to prevent the uterine infections.

10.8 Abortion

The term "abortion" refers to the deliberate termination of a pregnancy with the expulsion of a recognizable sized fetus before it is viable, which is determined arbitrarily to be 260 days for cattle, 290 days for horses, and 110 days for pigs. Abortion is not always preceded by fetal death. The growing fetus is at great risk at any stage of gestation due to the prolonged gestation in domestic ruminants and horses. A wide range of agents have the ability to harm a fetus by crossing the placenta. Abortions can be either spontaneous or induced, infectious or non-infectious. A significant portion of pregnancy loss in farm animals is caused by infectious abortions. Due to the nature of the placenta (six-layered syndesmochorial placenta) in ruminants, the majority of viral infections do not cross to the fetus. However, some viruses that infect domestic animals can pass through the placenta and infect the fetus, causing disease and/or developmental defects like teratogenesis. Compared to sheep or horses, non-infectious abortions are more common in dairy cattle. Genetic, chromosomal, hormonal, or nutritional factors are the causes of non-infectious spontaneous abortion. Animals that are bred just after puberty or after parturition are likely susceptible to spontaneous abortion. Between the fifth and tenth months of pregnancy, mares appear to be endocrinologically susceptible to abortion. Although, chromosomal abnormalities are known to cause embryonic losses in farm animals, their importance in abortion is unknown. The important features in various diseases associated with abortions along with their immunopathology will be discussed here in detail.

10.9 Etiology of Abortion

Infectious agents are the most frequently identified etiology of abortions in many field outbreaks; however, the cause of every abortion cannot be determined. Various bacterial, viral, protozoan and fungal pathogens, heat stress, toxic agents, nutritional deficiencies, or trauma have been associated with infertility, abortions, congenital anomalies in cattle. Bacterial pathogens like *Escherichia coli*,

Campylobacter foetus subsp. *venerealis*, *Brucella abortus*, *Leptospira interrogans*, *Listeria monocytogenes*, and *Bacillus* spp. are known to cause abortions (Tables 10.3 and 10.4). Viruses from several different families, including *Flaviviridae*, *Bunyaviridae*, *Reoviridae*, and *Parvoviridae*, cause abortion and congenital infections in ruminants (Maclachlan and Osburn 2017). Bovine herpesvirus-1, bovine viral diarrhea virus, epizootic bovine abortion virus, Rift Valley fever virus, Akabane virus, bluetongue virus, epizootic hemorrhagic sickness virus, etc. are important viral causes of abortion (Maclachlan and Osburn 2017). In domestic animals, these viruses cause teratogenic effects on the central nervous system and musculoskeletal abnormalities (Zanella et al. 2012). Fungal causes include *Aspergillus fumigatus*, *Mucor* spp., etc. Important protozoal causes include *Tritrichomonas foetus*, *Toxoplasma gondii*, *Anaplasma marginale*, and *Neospora caninum* (Tables 10.3 and 10.4). Abortions may be idiopathic (occurring without known cause) or the result of metabolic or hormonal abnormalities. High fever from severe maternal illness (due to mastitis or pneumonia), hypoxia (due to anaplasmosis or severe anemia), or endotoxemia may lead to abortion. Autolysis of aborted fetus is one of the criteria for the identification of etiological agent of abortion (Table 10.5).

10.10 Immunopathology of Abortions

The under developed immune system of fetus makes them extremely vulnerable to infection, even with low-virulent organisms transmitted through the placenta. To prevent the fetus from being rejected, immune system is suppressed at the junction of the fetal and maternal placentas. Although the exact mechanism causing this suppression is unclear, it may be caused by soluble serum proteins such as alpha fetoprotein, pregnancy-related protein, and alpha regulatory protein. Because the immune system is suppressed, during this period, any pathogenic agent can reach, multiply and produce lesions at the junction of the maternal and fetal placentas. Opportunistic saprophytic fungi and bacteria with low virulence may result in abortion during these immunologic circumstances. Most of these organisms are quickly eliminated from the body during normal immunological responses by the reticuloendothelial system of an adult cow. Therefore, under immunosuppressive conditions, pregnant animals may frequently be prone to abortions caused by the virulent pathogens.

Toll-like receptors (TLRs), antimicrobial peptides (AMPs), acute-phase proteins, and components of the innate immune system are necessary for the first line of defense in the endometrium of mammals against microorganisms. Pattern-recognition receptors (PRRs) are found on mammalian host cells and have binding molecules particular to pathogens, referred to as pathogen-associated molecular patterns, which are used to detect pathogens (PAMPs). TLRs 1–10 make up the most significant group of such receptors and these receptors are widely encoded in the mammalian genome, and are frequently identified in a variety of immune cells. TLR1, TLR2 and TLR6 recognize bacterial lipids such as lipoteichoic acid. Viral nucleic acids are recognized by TLR3, TLR7, TLR8, and TLR9. TLR4 is able to

Table 10.3 Summary of infectious causes of abortion in cattle

Disease	Age at abortion	Abortion rate	Clinical signs in dam	Fetal/placental gross lesions	Mode of spread	Test samples	Diagnostic tests
Viral							
Infectious bovine rhinotracheitis	Any gestational age; mostly in the second half of gestation	Variable	Abortion storm possible. No clinical signs in aborting cows or some animals showed upper airway disease and pneumonia	Fetus: no lesions and autolyzed. Rarely may have pale foci of hepatic multifocal necrosis. Placenta: edema or no significant gross lesions	Animal to animal contact with aerosol spread	Organ pools including the kidneys, lungs, liver, adrenal, spleen, and placenta	Viral isolation, PCR, fluorescent antibody test, immunohistochemistry, and histopathology
Bovine virus diarrhea	Abortions usually occur in first 4 months (first trimester). Sometimes any time during gestation	Less than 10%	Usually no clinical signs	Abortions and mummification (Fig. 10.2). No obvious gross lesions in the placenta. Variable clinical outcome in calves: none or deformities like cerebellar hypoplasia, hydrocephalus, ocular and myocardial lesions, alopecia, and thymic hypoplasia Live full-term calves infected in utero may have cleared virus or	Calves may become persistently infected prior to birth and may be introduced into the herd by an infected animal	The kidneys, lungs, spleen, brain, eye, pleural fluid, and serum	Viral isolation, PCR, fluorescent antibody test, immunohistochemistry, fetal antibody titer, gross pathology, and histopathology

10.10 Immunopathology of Abortions

Bacterial				persistently infected depending on type of virus or timing of infection		
Leptospirosis (*Leptospira interrogans* serovar *pomona*, *L. hardjo*, *L. borgpetersenii* serovar *hardjo*)	Abortion at third trimester (*L. pomona*) or occurs at any gestational age (other serovars) during acute febrile illness	25–30%	Infertility and abortion storms are possible. No signs or agalactia and mastitis are possible in aborting cows	Fetus usually autolyzed with no gross lesions. Placenta: retained, avascular, atonic yellow-brown cotyledons, brown gelatinous edema between allantois and amnion. Acute fatal disease in young ones with icterus and hemoglobinuria	Water contaminated by wildlife or infected animals	The kidneys, maternal pleural fluid, urine, aqueous humor and fetal fluids	Fluorescent antibody test, PCR, serology, direct examination of cow urine by dark-field microscopy and bacterial isolation
Vibriosis (*Campylobacter fetus* subsp. *venerealis*)	Abortions occurs primarily between 4 and 7 months of gestation	Low, up to 5%, may be up to 20%	Infertility, early embryonic death, irregular moderately prolonged diestrus, metritis, and sporadic abortions. Longer vaginal carrier state	Fetus: fresh, autolyzed, or mummified. Fibrin may be present in serosal cavities, flakes of pus on visceral peritoneum, suppurative pneumonia in fetus. Placenta: semiopaque, thickened with	Venereal transmission. Bulls are the main mode of transmission. Infected cows can reinfect clean bulls. AI equipment may transmit infection	Preputial smegma, vaginal secretions, placenta, fetal abomasal fluid, lungs.	Bacterial isolation, dark-field microscopy, histopathology, fluorescent antibody test, and vaginal mucous agglutination

(continued)

Table 10.3 (continued)

Disease	Age at abortion	Abortion rate	Clinical signs in dam	Fetal/placental gross lesions	Mode of spread	Test samples	Diagnostic tests
			(up to 4 months)	surface exudate, petechiae, localized avascularity, and edema			
Brucellosis (*Brucella abortus*)	Abortions in third trimester. After 5 months	High, up to 90% in susceptible herds	Generally, no signs other than abortion. Chronic infection, retained placenta, and metritis	Fetuses are usually fresh. Fetal bronchopneumonia. Severe placentitis, thickened with surface exudates, retained placenta, and mottled cotyledons	Zoonotic disease	Placenta, fetal abomasal and pleural fluid, lungs, uterus, milk, maternal lymph nodes, maternal serum	Bacterial isolation, serology, histopathology, milk ring test, serum and blood agglutination test, whole milk plate agglutination test
Listeriosis (*Listeria monocytogenes*)	Second or more commonly third trimester (about 7 months)	Low	Cows that abort may die of septicemia near term and metritis	Autolysis, foci of necrosis in liver and other organs. Retained placenta	Most commonly found in poor-quality or spoiled silage	Fetal stomach, liver, placenta, and uterine fluid	Agglutination test
Ureaplasma diversum, *Mycoplasma bovigenitalium*	Any stage of gestation	—	May cause abortion storms in previously uninfected herds	—	Infected animals (especially bulls) introduced into clean	Can be found in reproductive tracts of normal, healthy cows	Bacterial isolation, histopathology

10.10 Immunopathology of Abortions

Opportunistic bacteria (*Salmonella*)	Abortions occur at any stage, but most common in last half of gestation	—	Usually no clinical signs. Sporadic abortions or abortion storms	Primarily placentitis and bronchopneumonia. Fetus autolyzed	herds; poor AI practices	Placenta, fetal abomasal fluid, lungs, liver	Bacterial isolation, histopathology
Parasitic							
Trichomoniasis (*Trichomonas foetus*)	Abortions occurs primarily in the first 5 months of gestation (first trimester)	Moderate, 5–30%	Primarily infertility, early embryonic loss with occasional abortions. Occasional cow with pyometra	Fetuses are autolyzed with no gross lesions. Histologically, fetal giant cell pneumonia. Placenta: edematous, flocculent material and clear, serous fluid in uterine exudate	Venereal transmission. Bulls are the main mode of transmission. Infected cows can reinfect clean bulls. AI equipment may transmit infection	Preputial smegma, cervical mucus, placenta, fetal lungs, and stomach content	Protozoal isolation, direct wet mount examination, histopathology, cervical mucous agglutination test, serology
Neosporosis (*Neospora caninum*)	Abortions occur at 3–8 months of gestation (mean 5.5 months). However, at any stage of gestation	Sporadic or outbreaks common. Repeat abortions from same cows can occur 20–40%.	Abortion storms and mummification are possible. No clinical signs in cows. Animals that abort due to Neospora are at increased risk	Autolyzed mid gestation fetus, widespread histologic inflammatory lesions in fetus including non-suppurative necrotizing	Canines play a role in the transmission and congenital transmission	Major organs, brain, muscle. The brain, primarily	Histopathology, immunohistochemistry, PCR, IFAT, and ELISA for serologic detection

(continued)

Table 10.3 (continued)

Disease	Age at abortion	Abortion rate	Clinical signs in dam	Fetal/placental gross lesions	Mode of spread	Test samples	Diagnostic tests
			of aborting again	encephalitis and myocarditis. No characteristic gross lesions in the placenta			
Miscellaneous diseases							
Mycoses (*Aspergillus* spp., *Absidia* spp.)	Abortion usually occurs in the third trimester. Sometimes, occur at 3–7 months.	6–7% of all abortions encountered	Sporadic abortions. No clinical signs in cows	Fetuses have skin lesions, may be small raised, grey-buff, soft lesions, or diffuse white areas on the skin and resemble ringworm. Fetuses are usually fresh and bronchopneumonia. The placenta may be retained. Necrosis of maternal cotyledon, adherence of necrotic material to chorionic cotyledon causes soft, yellow, cushion-like structure. Small yellow, raised, leathery lesions on intercotyledonary areas		Placental or fetal lesions, fetal abomasal fluid, skin lesions, fetal lungs	Fungal isolation, KOH wet mount, histopathology
Epizootic bovine abortion	Abortion usually in the third trimester Occasionally birth of premature live, weak calves	Abortion storms may occur, usually in heifers and newly introduced cattle. High, 30–40%	No clinical signs in aborting cattle. Herd immunity develops. Incubation period is 3 months after exposure to agent	Fresh fetus with petechiae in the mucosa and thymus, enlarged lymph nodes and spleen, subcutis edema, ascites with fibrin in body cavities, and nodular swollen liver	Tick-transmitted bacterial infection and occurs in dry foothill pastures	Major organs, thymus, lymph node, and the brain	Histopathology, PCR, Steiner silver staining, immunohistochemistry

10.10 Immunopathology of Abortions

Table 10.4 Summary of infectious causes of abortion in ewes

Disease	Age at abortion	Clinical signs in dam	Fetal/placental gross lesions	Mode of spread	Test samples	Diagnostic test	Vaccine
Brucellosis (*Brucella ovis*)	Abortions in the third trimester	Abortion in ewes and epididymitis in rams	Late or stillbirth, weak lambs	Passive venereal transmission, ram to ram	Fetal stomach and placenta	CFT or ELISA	*B. abortus* strain 19 and killed *B. ovis* vaccine or *B. melitensis* Rev. 1 vaccine
Campylobacter fetus or *C. jejuni*	Last 6 weeks of pregnancy	Mainly young ewes affected. Metritis in ewes after abortion	Large necrotic foci in the fetal liver. Stillbirths or weak lambs	Ingestion, high stocking rate, intensive grazing, feeding on the ground	Fetal stomach and liver	Agglutination test	Formalin-inactivated bivalent vaccine
Enzootic abortion of ewes (*Chlamydophila abortus*)	Last 2–3 weeks of pregnancy	No sickness in ewes	Degenerative changes in the placenta, stillbirths, or weak lambs	Ingestion	Fetal cotyledons	ELISA, CFT, PCR	Killed vaccine and live attenuated vaccine
Listeriosis (*Listeria monocytogenes*)	After 3 months of pregnancy	Retained placenta, metritis, and septicemia in some ewes	Fetal autolysis and necrotic foci in liver	Probably ingestion	Fetal stomach	Agglutination and complement fixation test	Killed or live attenuated vaccines
Salmonellosis (*Salmonella abortusovis*)	Last 6 weeks of pregnancy	Metritis after Abortion	–	Probably ingestion and carrier sheep	Fetal stomach	Agglutination test	–
Salmonellosis (*S. dublin*,	Last month of pregnancy	Abortion and metritis	–	Ingestion	Fetal stomach	Agglutination test	–

(continued)

Table 10.4 (continued)

Disease	Age at abortion	Clinical signs in dam	Fetal/placental gross lesions	Mode of spread	Test samples	Diagnostic test	Vaccine
S. montevideo, S. typhimurium							
Toxoplasmosis	Late or stillbirths	Abortion and no illness in ewe	Multiple small necrotic foci in fetal cotyledons. Stillbirths and neonatal mortality	Ingestion	Fetal cotyledons, pleural fluid	Modified agglutination test, ELISA, PCR	Live S48 tachyzoite vaccine in single dose, 3 weeks before mating
Rift Valley fever	Any stage of gestation	Abortion and heavy mortality in young animals	Acidophilic inclusions hepatic cells	Insects	Fetal stomach and spleen	Hemagglutination inhibition, ELISA, fluorescent antibody test	Available in endemic countries
Coxiellosis (Q fever)	Later term and weak lambs	No illness in ewe, neonatal mortality	Fresh fetus and intercotyledonary necrotizing placentitis	Inhalation and ingestion	Fetal stomach and spleen	Fluorescent test, PCR, serology	Vaccine available in Europe
Tick-borne fever	Late, following systemic disease	Fever and abortion	Nonspecific	Ticks	Fetal stomach and spleen	Giemsa smear of blood, PCR, counterimmunoelectrophoresis	–
Border disease	All stages, stillbirth	Infertility in ewes	Hairy shaker lambs	Ingestion	Fetal stomach and spleen	Virus isolation	–

Table 10.5 Assessment of fetal autolysis

Time since death	Changes
12 h	Cloudiness of cornea and blood tinged amnionic fluid
24 h	Fluid in body cavities
36 h	Gelatinous fluid in the subcutis
72 h	Dehydrated eyes
144 h	Dehydrated carcass and no abomasal contents

identify LPS from Gram-negative bacteria. TLR5 can detect flagellin, and TLR9 can detect bacterial DNA. Uterine bacterial infections of bovine induce TLRs to get activated, which in turn triggers signaling cascades that produce proinflammatory cytokines and chemokines, which in turn activate and cause an influx of immune cells into the uterus, especially polymorphonuclear cells (PMNs) from the blood. A healthy, non-pregnant endometrium of cattle expresses TLR1 to TLR10. The TLR2, TLR3, TLR4, TLR6, and TLR9 are expressed in the intercaruncular and caruncular endometrium during before and after parturition. The TLR expression is more in caruncular endometrium than intercaruncular endometrium on 4–6 h postpartum.

Ruminants, horses, and swine have epitheliochorial placentation. Humans and rodents have hemotropic placentae. Ruminants (cattle, sheep, deer, giraffe etc.) have syndesmochorial placentation. Because of the six layers separating the maternal and fetal circulatory systems, maternal immunoglobulins cannot pass through the placenta and enter into the fetal circulation. In ruminant placenta, instead of having a single large area of contact between maternal and foetal vascular system, there are numerous placentomes. The chorioallantois membrane, also referred to as cotyledon, where the fetal side of the placenta develops in a placentome. Caruncle refers to as maternal side of the placenta. Therefore, in ruminants, the development of any immunological responses in the fetus is solely attributable to the fetus and not the dam (Almeria et al. 2011, 2012).

Transplacental transmission of viral infections are dependent upon the complex interactions between maternal and feto-placental immune responses, as well as the stage of fetal development at which the infection occurs. Pregnant cows showed changes in specific leukocyte populations like macrophages, γδT cells, and natural killer cells during different stages of pregnancy (Oliveira and Hansen 2008). In cows, there was no specific changes in the population of CD4, CD8, γδT cell receptors, and CD68 (monocyte marker) in the peripheral blood mononuclear cells (PBMCs) at week 34 of pregnancy. However, preparturient cows showed increased percentage of regulatory T cells (Treg), γδT cells, and CD4+CD25+FOXP3+ cells and decreased percentage of CD68+ cells in PBMCs (Yang et al. 2008). The function of T lymphocytes is downregulated by these cells (Yang et al. 2008), temporary anergy of maternal lymphocytes to conceptus MHC class I antigens (Tafuri et al. 1995), and immunosuppressive proteins like IL-10 and transforming growth factor β1 (TGFβ1) are produced at the maternal-fetal interface (Simpson et al. 2002). According to Bilinski et al. (2008), NK cells have a role in vascular remodeling, γδT cells suppress the immune system by secreting IL10 and TGFβ1

(Nagaeva et al. 2002), and macrophages are responsible for parturition. By suppressing local inflammatory responses, the Th2 cytokine dominance is crucial for the successful implantation of the fetus and maintenance of early pregnancy, but this may cause the pregnant animals unable to control microbial infections. Further, immunolocalization technology showed that increased numbers of CD68+ cells in the endometrial stroma of pregnant cows as early as 54–100 days of gestation and this increase was persisted until 240 days of gestation (Almeria et al. 2011, 2012).

10.11 Brucellosis

The genus *Brucella* contains facultative intracellular Gram-negative coccobacilli, which are the members of the alpha-2 *Proteobacteraceae* family and causes brucellosis. Division of the genus into six classical Brucella species is still widely used for historical and clinical reasons. *Brucella melitensis, Brucella abortus, Brucella suis, Brucella ovis, Brucella canis,* and *Brucella neotomae* are among these species (Osterman and Moriyon 2006). *Brucella* species are distinguished by a strong affinity for specific natural hosts, but they can infect a variety of hosts (Boschiroli et al. 2001). With the exception of *B. ovis* and *B. neotomae*, all other species are capable of infecting humans (Hartigan 1997). Brucellosis is one of the most important zoonotic diseases worldwide, particularly in developing countries, Mediterranean countries, and Central Asia. Fever, anorexia, polyarthritis, meningitis, pneumonia, endocarditis, and other less common clinical manifestations are the clinical signs of human brucellosis (Sauret and Vilissova 2002). Bovine brucellosis outbreaks are linked to abortions during the last trimester of pregnancy (Fig. 10.3), which results in weak newborn calves and infertility in cows and bulls (Enright et al. 1984; Poester et al. 2005; Xavier et al. 2009). Reduced milk production, an increase in the number of somatic cells in the milk, and decreased reproductive efficiency are other clinical signs of infected cows (Meador et al. 1989). Infected bulls may develop systemic signs of infection including fever, anorexia and depression, although infection is often inapparent (Campero et al. 1990). The most severe lesion caused by *B. abortus* in bulls is orchitis, which is frequently accompanied by seminal

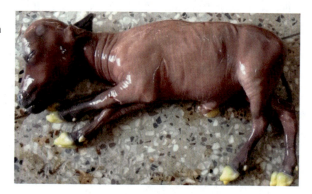

Fig. 10.3 Fetal loss (abortion) with no autolysis in brucellosis: Fetuses are usually fresh with retained placenta and lungs showed bronchopneumonia

vesiculitis and epididymitis (Trichard et al. 1982). Affected bulls may experience permanent infertility as a result of chronic orchitis and fibrosis of the testicular parenchyma (Campero et al. 1990). Under normal circumstances, venereal transmission is not a significant route of infection, but artificial insemination with contaminated semen is a potential source of infection. The most common route of infection in cattle is the gastrointestinal tract (Crawford et al. 1990), from which infection spreads to nearby lymph nodes where *Brucella* replicates intracellularly in phagocytes. Infection can also occur through the skin, conjunctiva, or respiratory mucosa by inhalation (Crawford et al. 1990; Ko and Splitter 2003; Anderson et al. 1986). *Brucella* organisms resist killing by neutrophils and multiply inside of macrophages and other types of phagocytes. Due to elevated levels of erythritol and steroid hormones in the uterus during the third trimester of pregnancy, *B. abortus* is assumed to have a strong affinity for the organ. Erythritol favours bacterial survival because it can be metabolised by *B. abortus* as a source of carbon and energy (Samartino and Enright 1996). Typically, pregnant cows develop a local lymphadenopathy at the infection site that progresses to acute lymphadenitis (Schlafer and Miller 2007). Variable amounts of a foul-smelling, yellow to brownish exudate with fibrin and necrotic debris were noticed in the infected uterus (Xavier et al. 2009). Importantly, the placental lesions are randomly distributed across placentomes, with some normal placentomes and others having severely necrotic and hemorrhagic areas (Xavier et al. 2009). Microscopic changes are also not pathognomonic, but they are more specific than gross changes (Xavier et al. 2009). Histologically, the trophoblastic cells are the primary target cells in the placenta, which are swollen and filled with coccobacilli. Neutrophilic and histiocytic inflammatory infiltrates are typically associated with necrosis, oedema, fibrin deposition, and occasionally vasculitis (Xavier et al. 2009). A severe infiltration of neutrophils, lymphocytes, plasma cells, and a few eosinophils were noticed in the endometrium. The luminal epithelium showed superficial ulcerations or multifocal erosions as a result of the inflammatory response (Meador et al. 1988).

Since innate immunity reduces the initial bacterial load and may influence the development of a protective adaptive immunity, which is crucial for *B. abortus* infection. A system of pattern recognition receptors (PRRs), namely, TLRs, involved in the early recognition of *Brucella* by neutrophils, macrophages, and dendritic cells (DCs) (Campos et al. 2004; Duenas et al. 2004; Weiss et al. 2005). The PAMPs, conserved elements of microorganisms and triggers TLRs. PAMPs from bacteria such as lipoproteins, lipopolysaccharide (LPS), flagellin, and DNA are recognised by TLR2, TLR4, TLR5, and TLR9, respectively. Recognition of PAMPs by TLRs stimulates the recruitment of intracellular TIR domain-containing adaptors, including MyD88, TIRAP, TRIF and TRAM via TIR-TIR interactions to initiate signalling. Upon TLR-mediated recognition of PAMPs, a downstream adaptor protein known as myeloid differentiation factor 88 (MyD88) also participates in macrophage activation. The MyD88 initiates a cascade of events that activates the MAP kinases (MAPKs) namely, ERK, JNK, and p38. The MyD88 is also necessary for the nuclear factor kappa B (NF-κB)-mediated production of pro-inflammatory cytokines by TLRs, which is a crucial step in establishing an immune response to

B. abortus (Weiss et al. 2005). The TIRAP mediates the activation of MyD88-dependent pathway downstream of TLR2 and TLR4. Alternatively, TLR3 and TLR4 may recruit TRIF and activate another pathway (TRIF-dependent pathway) that leads to the activation of transcription factor IRF3 and involves the production of type II IFN, particularly IFN-γ. The TRAM selectively participates in the activation of TRIF-dependent pathway downstream of TLR4, but not TLR3. Therefore, each TLR recruits a specific set of TIR domain-containing adapters, which in turn triggers different transcription factors and controls innate immune responses, leading to the development of antigen-specific acquired immune responses (He 2012). However, *Brucella* LPS is not a strong agonist of TLR4, which favors evasion from the host innate immune responses (Carvalho Neta et al. 2008). Conversely, *Brucella* lipoproteins are TLR2 ligands and exhibit pro-inflammatory effect. Interaction of the *Brucella* with trophoblastic cells results in placental acute inflammatory responses by the trophoblastic cells. *Brucella* elicits pro-inflammatory trophoblastic response, which may play a fundamental role in the pathogenesis of placentitis in bovine brucellosis.

Being an intracellular organism, *Brucella* requires cell-mediated immunity for protection by activating CD4+ and CD8+ T lymphocytes, Th1 cytokines (IFN-γ and TNF-α), activated macrophages, and dendritic cells (DCs). The CD8+ T cells are responsible for predominant protection against *B. abortus* infection. This protection can be produced by the destruction of *Brucella*-infected macrophages and the production of type II IFN particularly IFN-γ. Bacteria are released when macrophages are lysed into the extracellular space, where they can be engulfed by other activated macrophages in a IFN-γ rich microenvironment. These cells have improved anti-*Brucellae* defense mechanisms and able to eliminate the pathogen and inhibit the *Brucella* spread. Moreover, the type II IFN produced by CD8+ T cells induces down-regulation of Th2 cytokines and IL-10. When dendritic cells become active during *B. abortus* infection, T cells are stimulated to produce IFN-γ, which is an important regulatory mechanism. The DCs activation and maturation requires MyD88, whose signalling is required for the development of IFN-γ production by the T-cells, and control of *B. abortus* infection in mice (Copin et al. 2007; Macedo et al. 2008). Importantly, smooth *Brucella* LPS causes DCs to produce IL-12 by activating CD4+ T cells (Billard et al. 2007). Innate immunity against *B. abortus* includes natural killer (NK) cell cytotoxicity (Salmeron et al. 1992). According to Golding et al. (2001), bovine NK cells may act directly through the secretion of cytokine IFN-γ, which enhances the bactericidal activity of macrophages (Oliveira et al. 2002; Wyckoff 2002). Complement system proteins primarily contribute to innate immune responses by opsonizing the extracellular *Brucella* and quickly removing it or by interacting with bacteria that have been neutralized by antibodies (Corbeil et al. 1988). Cell-mediated immunity is crucial for efficient adaptive immune responses, which is promoted by *B. abortus*-specific T-cells activation (Oliveira et al. 1998). T cells first recognize *B. abortus* via co-receptor molecules CD4+ in T helper cells or CD8+ in T cytotoxic cells in order to process and present bacterial antigens to MHC class II or I molecules that are unique to that antigen (Wyckoff 2002).

The CD4+ T cells are stimulated by the IL-12 secreted by infected macrophages (Jones and Winter 1992; Jiang and Baldwin 1993). The IL-12 promotes the development of T helper cell (Th0) differentiation into Th1, the most significant cell type in the host immune response against *B. abortus*. The IL-12 is also involved in adaptive immunity against CD8+ T-cells direct activation. Other cytokines released by active phagocytes include TNF-α and IL-1. The IFN-γ is the primary cytokine produced by Th1 cells, which controls the *Brucella* infection both in vitro and in vivo by activating macrophages (Jones and Winter 1992; Stevens et al. 1992; Jiang and Baldwin 1993; Golding et al. 2001). The CD8+ T cells are also essential for the defense against *B. abortus* (Oliveira et al. 1998; Wyckoff 2002). In fact, CD8+ knockout mice are more susceptible to *Brucella* infection (Oliveira et al. 1998). In addition, CD8+ T-cells secrete IFN-γ and increase the cytotoxic ability of *B. abortus* infected macrophages (Oliveira et al. 2002). In human brucellosis, *B. abortus* increases CD35 and CD11b expression while decreasing the CD62L expression along with IL-8 secretion. This response is compatible for neutrophil activation, which can lead to tissue damage and pathology. This neutrophil activation is also induced by the stimulation of *Brucella* lipoprotein known as lipidated-outer-membrane protein 19 (LOmp19). *Brucella* lipoproteins contain pro-inflammatory properties that may cause tissue injury and inflammation because they can directly activate neutrophils (Zwerdling et al. 2009).

To provide a definitive diagnosis, laboratory techniques such as serological assays or direct diagnostic tests, which include isolation and biochemical characterisation of the organism must be performed (Nielsen and Ewalt 2004). *Brucella* genomic DNA can be detected by using PCR-based methods as an alternative to isolation (Leal-Klevezas et al. 1995; Bricker 2002). Immunohistochemistry is a different approach for direct diagnosis by localizing the *Brucella* antigens in tissue sections (Chauhan and Rana 2010). Despite not being widely used for diagnosis, this method is a very significant tool for studying the pathophysiology of the disease (Lopez et al. 1984; Meador et al. 1986; Santos et al. 1998; Xavier et al. 2009). The milk ring test and the buffered acidified plate antigen test are examples of high-sensitivity screening assays at herd level. These assays are complemented by confirmatory tests like complement fixation or 2-mercaptoethanol reduction. Indirect or competitive ELISA, as well as fluorescence polarization tests, are also utilized as confirming assays (Nielsen 2002). Because strain 19 is a smooth strain, it can be more challenging to arrive a serological diagnosis after immunization. This limitation has been overcome with the RB51 vaccine, a rough strain, which does not interfere the serological assays (Schurig et al. 1991; Cheville et al. 1993; Poester et al. 2006).

10.12 Mycotic Abortion in Cattle and Sheep

Some of the fungi that can infect cattle and cause abortion include *Aspergillus*, *Absidia*, *Mucor*, and *Rhizopus*. Fungal abortion or mycotic placentitis are other names for mycotic abortion, which is caused by several fungus and yeast. About

35 different types of fungi are known to cause abortion, with *Aspergillus fumigatus* being the most frequently diagnosed casual organism. The infection is secondary because the primary lesions are in the lungs, abomasum (ulcers), and intestines. Infection spreads through the bloodstream. Abortion occurs in infected cows during the later half of the gestation period between 6–8 months of pregnancy. The placenta is retained. Macroscopically, the infection first appears in the placentomes, which showed necrotic plaques and the fungus can be demonstrated in these locations. In affected cows, chorion-allantois is leathery and thick. The fetus may show circumscribed greyish plaques on the skin resembling ring worm lesions. Histopathologically, the typical lesions consist of focal infiltration of inflammatory cells with predominating macrophages with widespread necrosis of the placentomes. In the uterine wall, intercaruncular regions showed red patches covered with a thin yellowish-grey pseudomembrane. Hyphae can be visible in the tissues and on the mucosal surface with thrombosis and perivascular necrosis. Throughout the uterine wall, there is degeneration of the circular muscles and hyalinization of the small arteries were noticed. In the affected areas, hemorrhages and hyperemia are frequent.

The effects of infection on pregnancy and foetal development are mediated by pro-inflammatory cytokines (Raghupathy 1997). These cytokines are directly connected to the placenta through the maternal blood, and signaling may be amplified across the placental barrier through the stimulation of inflammation within the placenta (Kwak-Kim et al. 2005). The cytotoxic effects of TNF-α, which is predominantly mediated by TNF receptor 1 (TNFR1) through its intracellular death domain and activate the caspase apoptotic cascade on the placenta. Further, TNF-alpha can cause vascular injury in uterine endothelial cells, placental ischemia, and fetal injury leading to placental and foetal damage (Fortunato et al. 2001).

A preliminary field diagnosis can be made the sporadic nature of the disease with appearance of placental and fetal skin lesions. Abortions usually occur in late pregnancy and the placenta is usually retained. Confirmation of mycotic abortion is made by microscopical and cultural examination. Hyphae may be detected by direct examination of wet preparations of affected cotyledons and abomasal contents. The fungus is isolated from the cotyledons and abomasal contents. Foetal stomach contents provide more useful material for culture and produce a pure growth of causative organisms.

10.13 Listeriosis

Listeriosis, often referred to as silage disease, circling sickness, and meningoencephalitis, is caused by *Listeria monocytogenes*. *L. monocytogenes* may invade, survive and multiply inside the DCs, macrophages, and epithelial cells. It is a facultative intracellular pathogen. It is an infectious and fatal disease of animals, birds, fish, crustaceans and humans, where septicaemia and encephalitis are predominantly observed (Low and Donachie 1997; George 2002; Kahn 2005; OIE 2014). Listeriosis occurs in a sporadic or epidemic form throughout the world (Mitchell 1996; Barbuddhe et al. 2008). Most of the time, infection in animals is subclinical but

10.13 Listeriosis

severe forms can also occur (OIE 2014). The hallmark clinical manifestations of the disease include septicemia, encephalitis, meningitis, meningoencephalitis, rhombencephalitis, abortion, stillbirth, perinatal infections, and gastroenteritis (Brugere-Picoux 2008; Okada et al. 2011; Barbuddhe et al. 2012; Disson and Lecuit 2013; Limmahakhun and Chayakulkeeree 2013; Mateus et al. 2013; OIE 2014). The organism has an intracellular life cycle that can pass directly from cell to cell without release from the cell or exposing to extracellular environment, which involves a cellular mechanism known as paracytophagy, by the way it is escaping from the humoral immune responses (Czuczman et al. 2014). This mechanism shows the potential to cross placental barrier and blood-brain barrier, explaining its pathogenesis and clinical signs (Janakiraman 2008). Inadequate quality control practices during food processing, handling, and packing may result in *L. monocytogenes* contamination, which endangers the health of public (Carpentier and Cerf 2011; Rocourt and Bille 1997; Kaufmann 1988; Oliver et al. 2005). Abortions usually occur during the last trimester of pregnancy. The aborted fetus showed catarrhal gastroenteritis, cardiac vegetations, hemopericardium, anasarca, areas of necrosis, hemorrhage and granulomas in the liver, spleen, lungs, and kidneys.

Listeria possesses unique virulence factors that enable to infect the host while evading the immune system and to cause disease. Major virulence factors of Listeria are actin assembly-inducing protein (ActA), which is responsible for polymerization of host actin; listeriolysin O (LLO), which is a toxin having pore-forming activity; two phospholipases namely, phosphatidylinositol-specific phospholipase C (PlcA) and broad-range phospholipase C (PlcB); group of internalin family proteins namely, internalin A (InlA) and InlB, which play a major role in entry; metalloprotease (Mpl) and hexose-6-phosphate:phosphate antiporter (UhpT), which is a system for uptake of sugars (Dussurget et al. 2004; Schnupf and Portnoy 2007). The UhpT helps bacteria absorb glucose-6-phosphate inside the cells, which enhances the growth and replication. These virulence factors are directly regulated by the transcriptional factor known as positive regulatory factor A (PrfA) (Lecuit 2007). This PrfA is controlled by a thermosensor, and this sensor's 5' UTR can take up several secondary structures depending on the environmental temperature (de las Heras et al. 2011). The PrfA is downregulated at lower temperatures, while, PrfA is expressed optimally at higher temperatures. All virulence genes are expressed maximally at 37 °C compared to lower temperatures. *L. monocytogenes* has the ability to cross the fetoplacental, blood-brain, and intestinal barriers (Johansson et al. 2002). The bacterium gets internalized by phagocytosis within the epithelial cells of host after entering the digestive tract, where it multiplies and causes infection. The harboring and conquering of host cells by *Listeria* involves various stages, such as adhesion, invasion, lysis of vacuoles, multiplication, evasion of the host defense mechanisms, and cell-to-cell transmission. Various bacterial surface proteins and host receptors involved in the initial stage of attachment (Jagadeesan et al. 2010). *Listeria* proteins like adhesion protein (LAP), autolytic amidase (Ami), fibronectin-binding protein (Fbp), d-alanyl carrier protein ligase (DltA), listeria adhesion protein (LapB), internalin J (InlJ), ActA, internalin F (InlF), and recombinase A (RecA) are important for adhesion of Listeria to the host cells (Sabet et al. 2008; Reis et al.

2010). Listeria can infect both phagocytic and non-phagocytic cells. In the case of phagocytic cells like macrophages, phagocytosis mediates bacterial entry; whereas, *Listeria*-invasive proteins mediate entry in non-phagocytic cells (Cossart 2011). Internalins A and B are important invasion proteins (Dramsi et al. 1995). The organism usually killed in phagocytic vacuoles due to the acidic environment. However, *Listeria* employs various ways to counteract this mechanism. The LLO is the main factor contributing to the degeneration of vacuoles (Beauregard et al. 1997; Gedde et al. 2000). The LLO also regulates calcium ions influx into the host cells, which aids in bacterial invasion, activates the NF-kB and MAP kinase pathways, and inhibits the host immune system by suppressing the host cell protein small ubiquitin-like modifier (SUMO)ylation (Ribet et al. 2010). The p60 alters the host immune responses by activation of NK cells results in pro-inflammatory cytokines release (Humann et al. 2007). Flagellin stimulates pro-inflammatory cytokines through TLR5 (Hayashi et al. 2001). The LLO plays a major role in the destruction of vacuoles and downregulate the host immune system through dephosphorylation of H3 and deacetylation of H4 histones of the host cells (Hamon et al. 2007; Hamon and Cossart 2011). The LLO in secreted form can cause fission of the mitochondrial network (Stavru et al. 2011). *Listeria* also has the enzyme superoxide dismutase, which aids in the defense against reactive oxygen species produced by host cells (Archambaud et al. 2006). The immunity against listeria is primarily cell-mediated. Live *L. monocytogenes* have been shown to rapidly stimulate IL-1α, IL-1β, IL-6, and TNF-α mRNAs, in contrast to killed bacteria, which only induce IL-1β mRNA. The bacterial cell wall polymer lipoteichoic acid has been shown to induce the expression of pro-inflammatory cytokines such as IL-1α/β, IL-6, and TNF-α (Vázquez-Boland et al. 2001).

Diagnosis is based on the history, clinical signs, pathological lesions, and pathogen identification. Previous exposure to the disease, feeding habits, grazing pastures, and observation of clinical signs are helpful for presumptive diagnosis. Definitive diagnosis can be made only after isolation and identification of the bacterium (Kahn 2005). Anton's eye test (experimental keratoconjunctivitis test) is used for detecting *Listeria*, where the infected material is instilled on the conjunctiva of an eye of a rabbit that produces kerato-conjunctivitis within 24-36 hours. Immunohistochemical testing is particularly helpful for detecting antigen in lesions with few bacteria in order to diagnose encephalitic listeriosis. Serodiagnostic methods that are useful include the serum agglutination test, complement fixation test, hemagglutination inhibition test, antibody precipitation test, growth inhibition test, and enzyme-linked immunosorbent assay (ELISA) (Capita et al. 2001; OIE 2014).

10.14 Trichomoniasis

The most important *Tritrichomonas* species is *Tritrichomonas foetus*, which is the primary cause of bovine venereal tritrichomonosis, an infection transmitted sexually, and can cause infertility and abortion. *T.ritrichomonas foetus* is a flagellate protozoan parasite and the normal host for *T. foetus* is cattle (*Bos taurus* and

B. indicus). Major routes of transmission are spread from asymptomatic bulls to cows at the time of coitus or by artificial insemination using contaminated semen. Normally in bulls, infection persists for years without clinical signs. The protozoa are frequently found in the preputial cavity and occasionally found in the deeper portions of the urogenital system. The parasites invade and colonize the vagina, uterus and oviduct after infecting the cow. Transient or permanent infertility may occur as a result of endometritis and uterine catarrh. If conception takes place, abortion typically occurs early in pregnancy (6–16 weeks). In a few cases, the fetus is not expelled, but pyometra and intrauterine maceration are seen. In 1998, there was a report of the first human infection by *T. foetus*, which manifested as meningoencephalitis following peripheral blood stem cell transplantation. However, tritrichomonosis cannot be classified as a zoonotic disease, because there is no obvious route of transmission.

The protozoa *Tritrichomonas suis* is closely related to *T. foetus*, can be found in the nasal cavity and digestive system (mostly cecum, colon, small intestine and stomach) of swine. This parasite is thought to be extremely common but non-pathogenic in pigs, or it may only be linked to mild rhinitis symptoms. Acute *T. foetus* infection in bulls is characterized by swelling and inflammation of the preputial tissue, which is sometimes followed by mucopurulent discharge. However, 2 weeks after infection, symptoms disappears, and the carriers typically asymptomatic. However, invasion of deeper tissues may occur and *T. foetus* predominantly found on the mucosal surfaces of the reproductive tract (Rhyan et al. 1995). In vitro experiments have demonstrated that *T. foetus* can attach to bovine vaginal epithelial cells (Corbeil et al. 1989). The parasites have a tendency to adhere to these cells initially by the posterior flagellum and then by the cell body, which was evident by phase-contrast microscopy (Corbeil et al. 1989). In the intestine of cattle, non-pathogenic trichomonad species are found. *T. suis* of pigs is indistinguishable morphologically, serologically and genetically from *T. foetus* (Felleisen et al. 1997).

Light microscopy may identify living organisms by their jerky, rolling motion. The specific details including morphological descriptions required for identification must be observed using phase-contrast dark-field microscopy or electron microscopy. *T. foetus* can be cultivated in vitro using the Diamond's medium. Molecular techniques such as polymerase chain reaction can be used to detect the protozoa (Felleisen et al. 1998; Campero et al. 2003). Transmission of infection occurs by coitus, artificial insemination, and gynecological examination of cows. According to BonDurant (1997), the preputial cavity is the main site of infection in bulls, and there is minimal or no clinical manifestation. In bulls older than 3–4 years, spontaneous recovery rarely occurs, resulting in permanent source of infection in herds. Infection may be transient in bulls younger than 3–4 years old. Chronically infected bulls showed no gross lesions. The initial lesion in infected cows is vaginitis, which can be followed by invasion of the cervix and uterus in pregnant animals. The placentitis results in an early abortion (1–16 weeks), uterine discharge, and pyometra are the sequelae of infection. In some cases, despite infection, pregnancy is not terminated by abortion and a normal, full-term calf is born. Following infection, cows may exhibit irregular oestrous cycles, uterine discharge, pyometra, or early abortion on their herd basis (Fitzgerald 1986; Skirrow and BonDurrant 1988; BonDurant 1997). Cows typically recover from their infection and develop immunity, at least throughout that particular breeding season (Fitzgerald 1986; BonDurant 1997).

Studies on the immune response to *T. foetus* infection in bulls are scarce. Young animals are more resistant to infection due to the microscopic structure of the lining of the penis and foreskin rather than an effective immune response (Rae and Crews 2006). The immunological responses against *T. foetus* can be effectively developed in females. The parasite causes a mild inflammatory reaction associated with the abortion. An immunological system mediates the inflammation, which frequently eliminates the infection. This immune system most likely fails in carrier cows, which maintains the infection in the herd. Bovine females respond to the initial *T. foetus* infection by producing IgG and IgA immunoglobulins locally in the cervicovaginal mucus produced by the uterus. Elimination of infection is probably mediated by specific immunoglobulins, since the organism is an extracellular parasite. Monoclonal antibodies cause agglutination and complement-mediated lysis, which prevents the protozoa from adhering to vaginal epithelial cells and facilitates the phagocytosis of *T. foetus* by monocytes. The combination of specific anti-*T. foetus* antibodies and complement enhances the killing the parasites by polymorphonuclear leukocytes (Rae and Crews 2006).

Bovine immune sera and monoclonal antibodies targeted against *T. foetus* surface epitopes are the main mechanisms of complement-dependent killing of the parasite in vitro (Aydintug et al. 1990, 1993). By colonizing in the female reproductive tract, which serves as a niche where only modest levels of complement are present, *T. foetus* is able to evade from the host immunological defenses. Bovine immunoglobulins can be cleaved by extracellular and membrane-bound cysteine proteinases from *T. foetus*. The *T. foetus* proteinases effectively cleaved the IgG1 and IgG2, which have been shown to kill *T. foetus* in vitro via complement-mediated and independent immune effector mechanisms result in the clearance of the parasite in vivo (De Azevedo and De Souza 1992, 1996; Aydintug et al. 1993; Corbeil 1994; Talbot et al. 1991). However, IgA was either little or not at all proteolyzed in vitro (Talbot et al. 1991). The binding and internalization of antibodies on the surface of parasites are a another potential defense strategy against the immune responses of host. The non-specific binding and exposition of IgG on the surface of *T. foetus*, as shown by Corbeil et al. (1991), may be a key molecular mimicry strategy for the masking of parasite antigens. Additionally, it was proposed that *T. foetus* exhibits antigenic variation as a potentially significant method of immune evasion (Corbeil 1994). The antigenic variation of the protective superficial antigen TF1.17 served as the basis for this hypothesis (BonDurant et al. 1993; Ikeda et al. 1993). In experiments using the appropriate monoclonal antibodies, variations in the expression of TF190 adhesion complex epitopes were also reported. Within a few months of infection, *T. foetus* is often eliminated from the female reproductive system of cattle (Corbeil 1994). Animals that recovered from a *T. foetus* infection exhibits some degree of temporary resistance to re-infection (Skirrow and BonDurant 1990). Since *T. foetus* is mostly found in the lumen of reproductive organs and on the surface of the mucosal tissues of its host in adult cattle, it can be hypothesized that the mucosal immune system is crucial in recognizing and combating a *T. foetus* infection. The surface antigen TF1.17 (Hodgson et al. 1990) has gained significant interest as a possible vaccine candidate for tritrichomonosis in cattle and has undergone extensive studies as a model antigen for the evaluation of the host immune response against *T. foetus*.

The cell-mediated immunological responses induced by *T. foetus* antigens in cattle was studied by Voyich et al. (2001). Cattle can be systemically immunized with *T. foetus* antigen, which can prime antigen-specific T cells and trigger an anamnestic IFN-γ response upon subsequent stimulation with *T. foetus* antigens. Tf190 adhesin vaccination primes CD4+ T cells, which thereafter increase IFN-γ expression in response to antigen challenge. Additionally, vaccination with *T. foetus* antigens primes the T-cell responses in cows that can result in cell-mediated immune responses by activating macrophages.

Based on the clinical history, early abortion symptoms, repeated returns to service, or irregular oestrous cycles, trichomonosis is tentatively diagnosed as a root cause of reproductive failure in a herd. The demonstration of protozoa in placental fluid, the stomach contents of the aborted fetus, uterine washings, pyometra discharge, vaginal mucus, or preputial smegma are confirms the infection. Preputial or vaginal washings or scrapings are the most reliable material for diagnosis in infected herds (Schonmann et al. 1994; Kittel et al. 1998; Parker et al. 1999; Mukhufhi et al. 2003). Where there are insufficient organisms to permit direct detection and precise identification, cultures should be made. *T. foetus* must be cultured because, in the majority of cases, the number of organisms are not large enough to reliably make a diagnosis on direct examination. Several media can be used. The preferred media are commercial culture kits or Diamond's trichomonad medium (Ribeiro 1990; Eaglesome and Garcia 1992; Parker et al. 2003). Clausen's and Oxoid's media are other culture media that could be used (Eaglesome and Garcia 1992). The organisms can be recognized based on their morphological characteristics. The pear-shaped organisms having an undulating membrane that reaches the posterior end of the cell with three anterior and one posterior flagella. Additionally, they have an axostyle that typically extends beyond the posterior end. These features can be revealed using rapid staining procedure or phase-contrast microscopy (Lun and Gajadhar 1999). To identify *T. foetus*, molecular-based methods utilizing PCR technology have been created (Campero et al. 2003; Cobo et al. 2007; Felleisen et al. 1997, 1998; Parker et al. 2001). For the diagnosis of bovine trichomonosis, several immunological tests have been utilized in the past or newly developed (Soto and Parma 1989; Rhyan et al. 1999). However, they are not advised for the *T. foetus* detection in individual animals and have a limited use. Mucus agglutination tests and intradermal diagnostic tests were developed in the 1940s; however their effectiveness is limited by issues with sensitivity and specificity. Other immunological tests based on the antigen-trapping ELISA have been developed (Gault et al. 1995; BonDurant 1997). *T. foetus* organisms can be demonstrated in formalin-fixed tissues utilizing immunohistochemical methods and monoclonal antibodies (Rhyan et al. 1995).

10.15 Neosporosis

Neospora caninum is an apicomplexan protozoan infection that causes significant economic losses in cattle through abortions. Worldwide, *N. caninum* is a significant contributor of abortion and reproductive failure in cattle. The most common route of *N. caninum* infection appears to be transplacental (vertical) transfer of the parasite from mother to fetus, which can lead to abortion or the birth of clinically normal but persistently infected offspring. An important factor in determining the transplacental transfer of parasites to the fetus and subsequent abortion in cattle is the immunological response or immunomodulation seen during pregnancy. Experimental *N. caninum* tachyzoites infection in heifers by intravenous route at 110 days of gestation (Almeria et al. 2011) showed cytokine gene expression at the maternofetal interface. Real-time RT-PCR analysis of infected heifers revealed increased Th1, Th2, and Treg cytokine gene expressions in the maternal (caruncle) and fetal (cotyledon) placentas. The IFN-γ, IL-12p40, IL-6, and IL-10 were elevated in the caruncle; whereas, cotyledon showed upregulated expression of IFN-γ and downregulation of TGF-β. This cytokine production pattern was linked to live transplacentally infected fetuses, suggesting a protective effect for fetus survival; however, it could have a role in the transplacental transmission of parasites. The key to understanding the process of abortion and/or transplacental transmission to the fetus may lie in the immunological control of the parasite in the placenta or by the fetus. Furthermore, it is still unknown that why some infected animals abort and others not.

Cell-mediated immunity is crucial in preventing *N. caninum* proliferation and lowering parasitemia. The Th1 cytokines including IFN-γ and IL-12 are known to play a significant protective immunological response against *N. caninum* in pregnant cattle. The IFN-γ is produced as a result of the Th1 immune response at the maternofetal interface, which is characterized by the infiltrations of CD4+ T cells, γδ-T cells, macrophages, and NK cells. Strong Th1 cytokine responses are incompatible with a successful pregnancy and the survival of the fetus, but they have important consequences for pregnancy in cattle by causing destruction of the placental tissues. Pro-inflammatory Th1 response during pregnancy protects the dam by significantly inhibiting the multiplication of *N. caninum* tachyzoites. The development of protective immune responses against the abortion during a second Neospora exposure in chronically infected cows has been shown. When cattle are first time infected with *N. caninum*, the likelihood of abortion is 3–7 times higher than that of subsequent pregnancies. Neosporosis-affected animals are less likely to abort during subsequent pregnancies. This shows that after infection, a certain levels of protective immunity develops.

When compared to seronegative animals, the *N. caninum*-infected-aborted cows showed upregulated mRNA gene expression of pro-inflammatory Th1 cytokines such as IFN-γ, TNF-α, IL-4, IL-12p40, and Treg cytokine IL-10 in PBMCs and antigen-specific cell proliferation. Chronically infected cattle showed significantly greater levels of IFN-γ are essential for controlling infection and providing protection (Almeria et al. 2011, 2012). Activating host immunological responses, including inflammatory pathways during *N. caninum* infection in cattle causes placental damage and abortion. It is not well known that whether water buffaloes (*Bubalus bubalis*) are susceptible to neosporosis; however, vertical transmission and fetal death have been reported in buffaloes.

Following experimental inoculation with *N. caninum* during late gestation, Canton et al. (2013) reported the phenotypic characterization of immune cells infiltration in the placenta of cattle. Macrophages were primarily seen at 14 days after inoculation. Inflammation was generally mild and mainly characterized by CD3+, CD4+ and γδT-cells; whereas, CD8+ and NK cells were less in number. When pregnant cattle were infected with *N. caninum* during early gestation, the immune cells infiltration were similar to that of late gestation. However, cellular infiltrates were less severe than Neospora infection during first trimester. This may be the reason for milder clinical outcome in animals infected during late gestation. Experimental infection of water buffaloes with Nc-1 strain of *N. caninum* during early gestation results in placentome inflammation characterized by infiltrations of CD3+, CD4+, and γδT cells by immunohistochemistry (Canton et al. 2014). Infiltration of these cellular subsets in buffalo placentomes were similar to that of cattle infected with *N. caninum* during early gestation. However, the lesions were milder and lower number of abortions were reported in buffaloes. The protozoa *N. caninum* causes tissue damage. The TLR-2 expression was elevated in inflammatory peritoneal macrophages and bone marrow-derived DCs after exposure to *N. caninum* soluble antigens, and this upregulation was associated with the maturation of TLR2/MyD88-dependent antigen-presenting cells and secretion of pro-inflammatory cytokines. Recognition of *N. caninum* by TLR2 results in generation of effector immune responses against *N. caninum* (Mineo et al. 2010).

Although, the intracellular nature of *N. caninum* induces host cell-mediated immune (CMI) responses, which is probably crucial to protect the host, this response could also be the cause of placental damage leading to abortion (Almeria et al. 2011; Canton et al. 2013). Cattle experimentally challenged with *N. caninum* on 70 day of gestation showed development of strong CMI responses in dams and foetuses, infiltrations of more numbers of immune cells and increased levels of expression of IFN-γ mRNA in the placenta lead to foetal death and abortion.

10.16 Campylobacteriosis

The most common causes of enteritis in domesticated animals and humans are *Campylobacter* spp., particularly *C. jejuni* and *C. coli*. *Campylobacter fetus* subsp. *venerealis* causes reproductive diseases in sheep and cattle. Many animals shed the *Campylobacter* spp. organism in their feces asymptomatically and spread the bacteria. Poultry, particularly broiler chickens are important source of the bacterium, though they usually do not show clinical signs. Some strains of *C. jejuni*, *C. fetus* subsp. *venerealis*, and *C. fetus* subsp. *fetus* (also known as *C. fetus*) causes infertility and abortions in ruminants. Although other *Campylobacter* species can cause disease, they appear to be of less significance in domesticated animals. These include

C. upsaliensis, C. helveticus, C. lari, and *C. hyointestinalis*. Cattle, sheep and goats have been found infected with *C. foetus* subsp. *foetus*, while *C. foetus* subsp. *venerealis* has been reported in cattle. Consumption of contaminated or undercooked meat (particularly poultry), unpasteurized milk or dairy products, and untreated water are the main routes of transmission in humans. People can also be infected by contact with infected animals or faeces. Human campylobacteriosis can range from mild to severe disease, but the majority of cases are self-limiting. Although complications are uncommon, *C. jejuni* is a major triggering event for Guillain-Barre syndrome (an acute, rapidly progressive, immune-mediated polyneuropathy that occurs in up to 30% of cases).

The incubation period for *Campylobacter* infections is generally short. Signs of enteritis appear within 3 days in gnotobiotic puppies and rapidly in chicks and poults. Cattle, sheep, and goats are susceptible to being ingested by *Campylobacter foetus* subsp. *foetus* by ingestion. Animals can become infected after contact with feces, vaginal discharge, aborted fetus, and fetal membrane. The *Campylobacter fetus* subsp. *fetus* and *C. fetus* subsp. *venerealis* can cause bovine genital campylobacteriosis (BGC) or bovine venereal campylobacteriosis (BVC) and are transmitted venereally in cattle. The BGC or BVC is a venereal disease that affects cattle and is characterized by infertility, early embryonic mortality, and prolonged calving season. Abortions are uncommon but are occasionally seen. Although infected cows occasionally show other systemic symptoms, they may develop a mucopurulent endometritis. *Campylobacter* spp. can also cause abortion in goats. Cattle and sheep can also experience abortions when exposed to *C. jejuni*. Cattle fetuses that have been aborted may suffer peritonitis, moderate fibrinous pleuritis, or bronchopneumonia (Fig. 10.4). The cotyledons may be hemorrhagic and the intercotyledonary areas are edematous; placentitis is often mild. In sheep, the fetus is usually autolyzed after *C. fetus* abortions; occasionally, 1–2 cm orange/yellow necrotic foci can be observed in the liver. Placentitis may be evident with hemorrhagic necrotic cotyledons and edematous or leathery areas between the cotyledons.

In order to protect against antibody-mediated opsonization, the surface layer protein (SLP) of *C. foetus* subsp. *venerealis* undergoes cyclical antigenic variation, which promotes both persistence and systemic infection. Antigenic variation is one of the bacterial mechanisms for evading from the host immune responses and ensuring chronicity of infection. Both antigenic variation and complement resistance provided by SLP indicated their potential importance as virulence factors for this obligately extracellular pathogen (Grogono-Thomas et al. 2003).

Campylobacter has developed strategies in the intestine to avoid the activation of innate immunity. For instance, flagella of *Campylobacter* do not trigger Toll-like receptor 5 (TLR5), the pattern recognition receptor for flagellin (Watson and Galan 2005). Further, TLR9, the CpG dinucleotide receptor, is not efficiently activated. However, it has recently been discovered that mice lacking MyD88, a critical signaling protein downstream of TLRs, are vulnerable to *Campylobacter* infection (Watson et al. 2007), demonstrating the importance of TLR pathways for the defense against diseases. This is supported by the observation that NF-κB-regulated transcription is readily activated in in vitro models (Jones et al. 2003) and necessary for

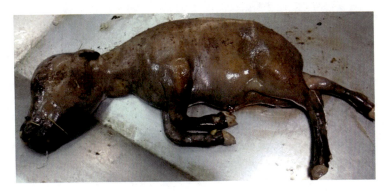

Fig. 10.4 Fetal loss (abortion) with autolysis in campylobacteriosis: The fetus showed autolysis with subcutaneous edema; fibrinous exudates within the body cavities and pneumonia in the fetus

the defense, since NF-κB-gene deleted mice displayed increased susceptibility to infection (Fox et al. 2004). Therefore, even though *Campylobacter* can circumvent the activation of TLR5 and TLR9-mediated innate immunity, innate immune systems are crucial for host defense. Recent studies have demonstrated that the intracellular pattern recognition receptor nucleotide-binding oligomerization domain 1 (NOD1) partly mediates the innate immune responses to *Campylobacter* and the susceptibility to campylobacteriosis is influenced by macrophage activation through the natural resistance-associated macrophage protein gene (Watson et al. 2007). Recently, both viable and killed Campylobacter preparations were shown to induce the maturation of dendritic cells in vitro and the induction of various pro-inflammatory cytokines (Hu et al. 2006), demonstrating that *Campylobacter* induces both innate and specific cell-mediated immune responses. There are also indications that Campylobacter extracts induce the in vitro expansion of γ/δ T cells obtained from healthy controls. The mucosal immune system has been linked to this cell type. These cells respond to non-protein elements in the *Campylobacter* extract. More recently, it was demonstrated that campylobacter infection causes gastroenteritis in NF-κB-deficient mice, which are deficit in the activation of the production of pro-inflammatory cytokines such as tumor necrosis factor alpha, IL-12, IL-1, and IL-6 (Fox et al. 2004). Recently, two novel murine *Campylobacter* models were described, one employing MyD88 gene-deleted mice and the other using IL-10 gene-deleted mice (Mansfield et al. 2007; Watson et al. 2007). The MyD88 gene-deleted mice is a severely immunocompromised model, revealed a role for the gene encoding natural resistance-associated macrophage protein in determining resistance to campylobacteriosis, which suggested that macrophage activation and intracellular survival may contribute to pathology (Watson et al. 2007).

In darkfield or phase contrast preparations, *Campylobacter* spp. showed characteristic darting motility, which can be used to make a presumptive diagnosis. Enteritis can be diagnosed by isolating the causative organism in fresh fecal samples. Nowadays, majority of the laboratories most frequently used diagnostic tool is the polymerase chain reaction (PCR) assay. Gene sequencing targeting 16S rRNA and multi locus sequence typing etc. is also employed for epidemiological typing and identification. Bovine genital campylobacteriosis can be diagnosed by detecting specific IgA in the cervical mucus and these antibodies are present for several months in the infected cows. The vaginal mucus agglutination test (VMAT) and ELISAs are commonly used tests for detecting specific IgA in the cervical mucus. Individual responses in the VMAT are variable hence, a minimum of 10 cows or 10% of the herd should be sampled. Sheath washings taken twice from bulls approximately one week apart can be submitted for culture or immunofluorescent testing. A real-time PCR assay has been developed to differentiate the causative organisms of bovine genital campylobacteriosis, including C. fetus subsp. fetus and C. fetus subsp. venerealis.

10.17 Leptospirosis

Leptospirosis is a significant zooanthroponotic disease that has spread globally and is a re-emerging tropical infectious disease (Xue et al. 2013; Adler and de la Pena Moctezuma 2010). Human and animal leptospirosis is caused by spirochetes of the genus *Leptospira* and manifests as a mild febrile illness to severe multi-organ failure, particularly pulmonary hemorrhage and renal failure (Bharti et al. 2003). The disease is transmitted to humans by contact with contaminated urine from mammalian reservoir hosts such as rodents but also farm, wild, and domestic mammals, either directly or indirectly (Levett 2001). Asymptomatic form of leptospirosis with fever, headache and myalgia that can spontaneously resolve is one of clinical presentations (Bharti et al. 2003). Most of the cases are inapparent infection and associated with host-adapted serovars such as Bratislava in horses and pigs, Canicola in dogs, Hardjo in cattle, and Australis and Pomona in pigs (Ellis et al. 1986; Bernard 1993; Andre-Fontaine 2006; Grooms 2006). Chronically infected cattle with *Leptospira borgpetersenii* serovar Hardjo showed reproductive failure, which lowers animal productivity and continuously endangers the health of animal husbandry workers. The second stage of acute leptospirosis is also known as immunological phase, during which the organism disappears from the bloodstream with appearance of antibodies (Levett 2001). Asymptomatic to serious infections occur in human infections. The classical manifestation of leptospirosisis is an acute biphasic illness. Leptospirosis can occur in a various forms, like mild, flu-like infection, which may not be recognized as leptospirosis, and unusual syndrome or progressive fulminant illness without two distinct phases namely, acute or septicemic phase and anicteric or icteric phase.

Since, the lack of microorganisms at the site of tissue damage, strengthens the hypothesis that the involvement of toxins or toxic substances in the pathogenesis of leptospirosis has long been contemplated (Vinh et al. 1986). Glycoprotein (GLP) extracted from the cell walls of a strain of serovar L. interrogans Copenhageni showed cytotoxic effect against the fibroblasts of mice (L-929). Later research showed that GLP stimulated the peripheral blood monocytes of healthy volunteers to produce the cytokines namely, TNF-α and IL-10 (Diament et al. 2002). Numerous researches have focused on the mechanism by which *Leptospira* activate the immune system, particularly in relation to the role of cytokines (Yang et al. 2000; Marangoni et al. 2004). High levels of TNF-α were found in the macrophage culture supernatant and serum of leptospirosis patients (Estavoyer et al. 1991; Tajiki and Salomao 1996; Marinho et al. 2005, 2006), and they were also related to the severity of the infection. During the late stage of infection with Leptospira interrogans Icterohaemorrhagiae, the quantitative real-time PCR showed higher levels of inflammatory cytokines, IL-4 and IL-10, confirming the role of type 1 cellular immunity (Marinho et al. 2009). It is thought that humoral-mediated reaction is serovar specific, which may result from the naturally acquired immunity. The development of humoral response is related to activation-dependent mechanism of leptospiral LPS through TLR2 activation, via the innate immune system (Werts et al. 2001). Other researchers (Klimpel et al. 2003) proved that Leptospira can activate T-cell proliferation, particularly γ-δ and α-β T cells, which suggests that these cell types may be involved in host defense or the pathogenesis of leptospirosis. However, leptospire adherence to host cell components is a significant step in the infection and pathogenesis. Further, current studies were focused on the outer membrane proteins (OMPs), such as the leptospiral 32-kDa lipoprotein (LipL32), the *Leptospira* immunoglobulin-like domain containing proteins A–C (LigA–C), and the leptospiral endostatin–like proteins A–F (LenA–F) of leptospires (Stevenson et al. 2007). Recombinant *Leptospira* immunoglobulin-like (Lig) proteins have been shown to mediate interactions with fibronectin, fibrinogen, collagen, laminin, tropoelastin, and elastin in vitro proved by various recent investigations (Choy et al. 2007; Lin et al. 2009). During leptospirosis infection, presence of IgM, IgG, IgA, and C3 along the alveolar basement membrane was demonstrated, indicating that the autoimmune process is the cause of severe hemorrhagic complications. In BALB/c mice injected with *Leptospira interrogans* serovar Canicola showed glomerular hypercellularity and a strong immunostaining of both IL-6 and TNF-α (Marinho et al. 2008).

Limiting the renal colonization and bacterial shedding through urine appears to be depend heavily on the development of an antigen-specific Th1 response. Vaccinated animals showed increased CD4+, CD8+, and γδ T-cells proliferation. The NK cells from both infected and vaccinated animals displayed an IFN-γ recall response. Importantly, NK cells immediately react to *L. borgpetersenii* serovar Hardjo infection and offer protective immunity (Zuerner et al. 2011). IFN-γ production and cytotoxic CD8+ T-cell activation are responsible for cell-mediated immunity against *Leptospira*. The IFN-γ plays a crucial role in the clearance of extracellular microorganisms by activating the macrophages and increase the secretion of immunoglobulin G2 (IgG2). Bovine IgG2 and IgG1 antibodies are able to fix complement and bovine IgG2 act as opsonins, and these acts together as important effector molecules for the control of leptospires by potentially increasing the phagocytosis of leptospires. Leptospires are not intracellular pathogens that can survive phagocytosis; however, macrophages activated by IFN-γ may improve the effectiveness of killing (Zuerner et al. 2011). The main defense against leptospirosis is thought to be the humoral immune response. Since, the levels of agglutinating anti-LPS antibodies in patient sera correspond with passive immunity, LPS appears to be the main target for the protective antibody responses. The naive mice are passively protected from leptospirosis by anti-LPS monoclonal antibodies. However, it is not known whether antibodies against other leptospiral antigens in addition to LPS also confer protection (Gopalakrishnan et al. 2016). Protective immunity against leptospirosis is not only limited to humoral immune responses. In order to control a fatal infection, mice need functional TLR2 and TLR4 signaling pathways of innate immunity.

Leptospirosis can sometimes be diagnosed by detecting the antigens or nucleic acids of leptospira in clinical samples such as blood (acute infections), urine, milk, liver, kidneys, and other tissue samples collected at necropsy. There may be intermittent or continuous organism shedding in the urine. Usually, immunofluorescence, immunohistochemical staining, or polymerase chain reaction (PCR) methods are used to detect *Leptospira* in clinical samples. These organisms do not stain well with the Gram stain and cannot be seen under a microscope unless special stains or techniques are used. As an auxiliary method, immunogold-silver staining or silver staining can be helpful. *Leptospira* can also be detected by using darkfield microscopy, but this method is less sensitive and non-specific. Leptospirosis is frequently identified using serology. Paired acute and convalescent samples are preferred from animals, and increased antibody titers are usually seen in acute cases. High titers of antibodies in a single sample raise the suspicion of leptospirosis, but they are not definitive. However, single positive sample from an aborted fetus can be diagnostic. Herd level tests are often used in ruminants. The microscopic agglutination test (MAT) and enzyme-linked immunosorbent assays are the most commonly used serological tests in animals. The MAT evaluates the antibody responses against a specific *Leptospira* serovars (often 5–7 in veterinary assays), and this test is serogroup-specific but not serovar-specific. Since antibodies do not form during the early stages of the biphasic sickness in humans, and early cases must be diagnosed using assays that detect the organism, its antigens, or nucleic acids. *Leptospira* can be detected in human tissue samples, cerebrospinal fluid, blood, and urine. The tests used are similar to those employed in animals, which include immunofluorescence, immunohistochemical staining, PCR, culture, and microscopy. Although the serovar is frequently not identified, it can be useful in the epidemiology of cases and outbreaks and in directing prevention strategies to the most likely source of the infection. Leptospirosis is frequently diagnosed using serology, particularly MAT or ELISA. High titers of antibodies with consistent symptoms is suggestive of an acute disease, but a rising titer is necessary for a definitive diagnosis. Cattle are the maintenance hosts for serovar Hardjo and development of vaccines that provide long-term protective immunity is difficult and induction of high titers of anti-serovar Hardjo antibodies does not appear to be protective. The protective immunity against L. borgpetersenii serovar Hardjo in bovine is cell-mediated. Immunization trials in cattle found that protection against Hardjo serovar conferred by whole-cell inactivated leptospira (bacterin) vaccines, which was correlated with Th1 responses and not with agglutinating antibody titres (Rinehart et al. 2012).

10.18 Bluetongue Virus

Bluetongue (BT) is an infectious, non-contagious disease of domestic (mostly sheep) and wild ruminants that is spread by biting midges of the *Culicoides* spp. Bluetongue virus (BTV) belongs to the member of the *Reoviridae* family and the genus *Orbivirus* (Saminathan et al. 2020a). There have been 28 BTV serotypes identified to date worldwide, and 23 serotypes have been reported from India. Sheep typically showed the most pronounced clinical symptoms, while cattle and goats typically exhibit subclinical or mild symptoms prior to the outbreaks of BTV-1 and BTV-8 in Northern Europe. The World Organization for Animal Health (OIE) has classified BT as a notifiable disease that results in significant socio-economic losses. The severe hemorrhagic syndrome caused by BT includes coronitis, mucosal erosions and ulcerations, fever, edema, hemorrhages, and dyspnea (Saminathan et al. 2016, 2020a). BTV infection caused birth defects such as porencephaly and hydranencephaly as well as abortion and the birth of viremic calves in pregnant animals (MacLachlan and Osburn 2017).

The transplacental transmission (TPT) of BTV causes significant economic losses since it increases the risk of stillbirth, abortion, congenital abnormalities, low birth weight in young ones, decreased milk production, and decreased fertility (Saminathan et al. 2020b; MacLachlan and Osburn 2017). The TPT caused the BTV to overwinter in the *in utero* infected fetuses at the time when *Culicoides* activity was absent during winter (Mayo et al. 2016). Birth of viraemic lambs or calves become persistently infected and act as carriers to introduce the disease in BTV free regions during vector-free seasons (van der Sluijs et al. 2016). The TPT of BTV in ruminants was associated with live attenuated vaccination strains of BTV (BTV-1, -2, -9, -10, -11, -13, and -17) prior to the wild-type BTV-8 outbreak in Europe in 2006 (Maclachlan and Osburn 2017). The development of quasispecies with altered phenotypic characteristics, such as alteration in virulence, tissue tropism, and ability to traverse the placenta, was the result of multiple passages of BTV in susceptible cell lines (Shaw et al. 2013). The TPT of field or wild-type strains of BTV-8 in northern Europe has been reported in various experimental studies (van der Sluijs et al. 2011; Coetzee et al. 2013) and field observations (Zanella et al. 2012) in cows, ewes, and goats. From the reports, it has become apparent that field strains of BTV-1, BTV-2, and BTV-8 crosses the placenta with relative ease at 70–75 days of gestation and caused severe encephalopathy in ewes.

Prior to 2006, TPT of field or wild BTV strains had not been described, but has been reported with modified live or attenuated vaccine virus strains namely, BTV-10, BTV-11, BTV-13, and BTV-17 in cattle (van der Sluijs et al. 2016; MacLachlan and Osburn 2017). The first TPT of wild-type BTV-8 was reported in Western Europe in August 2006. Subsequently, it spread to majority of the northern Europe and caused disease in sheep and cattle (Maclachlan and Osburn 2017). The TPT rate varies depending on the species and gestational stage. The TPT rate was estimated around 10–41.7% in cows and up to 69% in ewes (van der Sluijs et al. 2011). Most significant consequences of TPT are the birth of BTV-positive calves and the spread of BTV in disease-free areas as a result of viral persistence in heifers.

In Sardarkrushinagar, Gujarat state, India, BTV serotype-1 was first detected in goat fetuses that had been aborted and stillborn in 2007 (Chauhan et al. 2014). Before 2007, transplacental infection of BTV serotypes in ruminants has not been reported from India. BTV-1 was isolated from foetuses, which indicated the first evidence of TPT of wild-type BTV-1 from India and attenuated or laboratory adapted BTV-1 strains have never been used in this region. Indian BTV-1 unusually showed new characteristics in its clinical manifestation, more than 50% of pregnant goats were aborted or gave birth to dead kids in the BTV affected farm (Chauhan et al. 2014).

For the first time, Saminathan et al. (2020b) investigated the TPT of Indian BTV-1 (isolated from stillborn and aborted goat fetal spleens) in IFNAR1-blocked pregnant mice at various gestational stages. The mid-stage TPT rate was greater (71.43%) than the early-stage (57.14%) of gestation. Reduced implantation sites, early embryonic deaths, abortion, and necro-hemorrhagic lesions had been reported in the early stage of pregnancy. The IFNAR1-blocked animals developed congenital defects and neurological lesions in foetuses during the mid stage of gestation, including hemorrhages, diffuse cerebral edema, necrotizing encephalitis, and smaller bones. First-time detection of BTV-1 antigen by immunohistochemistry and quantification by real-time qRT-PCR in cells of the mesometrium, decidua of embryos, placenta, uterus, ovary, and brain of fetuses. BTV-inoculated mice underwent seroconversion by 7 and 5 dpi, and reached peak levels 15 dpi and 9 dpi, respectively, in early- and mid-gestation. Early gestation, CD4+ and CD8+ T cells were significantly reduced (increased ratio) on 7 dpi but then increased on 15 dpi. Increased CD8+ T cells (decreased ratio) were seen during mid gestation. Peak viral load was accompanied by an increase in apoptotic cells in PBMCs and tissues. The IFNAR1-blocked mouse model will be ideal for further studies on the mechanisms underlying TPT, overwintering, and vaccine strategies. Even though BTV infection has been present in India since 1964, not much is known about the possible birth defects associated with TPT in ruminants, and distribution of viral antigen in reproductive organs.

The IFN-α and IFN-β, two type I IFNs, are crucial for antiviral innate immune responses against BTV. Only plasmacytoid DCs (pDCs) release a considerable amount of IFN-α/β, despite the fact that both conventional DCs and pDCs significantly increased BTV replication. Numerous in vivo and in vitro models have demonstrated that BTV is a strong inducer of type I IFNs in a variety of cell types from different tissues and host species (Saminathan et al. 2018, 2019). The IFN levels peaked between 8 and 12 hpi, reached maximum levels at 4 hpi, and then fell to undetectable levels at 24 hpi (Saminathan et al. 2018, 2019). The IFN-α/β levels were found in sheep serum at 2 and 6 days after BTV-8 inoculation. Peak IFN levels reduced the BTV titers by 90% in sheep after BTV infection, and it was found that there was a temporal link between IFN activity and viremia (Foster et al. 1991). The NS3 and NS4 proteins of BTV play a vital role in counteracting the antiviral innate immune response of the host by modulating/inhibiting the IFN-Is synthesis signalling pathways. The BTV VP2 and VP5 outer capsid proteins can trigger neutralizing antibodies. Ruminant fetuses infected with BTV develop immunological competence before mid-gestation. Since the VP7 protein is conserved among BTV strains and serotypes, antibodies against VP7 are serogroup-specific. Hence, the serological diagnosis of BTV infection in ruminants frequently involves the identification of antibodies against BTV-VP7 using c-ELISA assay. The BTV-specific neutralizing antibodies provide long-lasting protection to re-infection with homologous serotype of BTV. The neutralizing epitopes of BTV are located in the specific interactive regions of VP2 protein. Development of immune response against BTV involves antigen presenting cells (APCs), such as cDCs and pDCs of skin. Studies have shown that cDCs are essential for the production of cytokines such as IL-12, IL-1β, IFN-γ, and IL-6, which are crucial for the proliferation of BTV-specific CD4+ and CD8+ T-lymphocytes and for protection against BTV. Serotype-specific outer coat protein (VP2) and NS1 protein of BTV are major immunogens for CTLs and play a significant role in inducing CMI responses in sheep, whereas VP5 and NS3 are minor immunogens (Saminathan et al. 2020a).

The BTV-17 infected sheep showed increased CD4/CD8 T-cells ratio (more than 3) in PBMCs due to significantly decreased number of CD8+/MHC class I-restricted T-lymphocytes than CD4+/MHC class II-restricted T-lymphocytes on 7 dpi with panlymphocytopenia. However, CD4/CD8 T cells ratio was decreased (average 0.6) on 14 dpi due to increased number of CD8+ T-lymphocytes in sheep (Ellis et al. 1990). BTV is a strong IFN inducer in wild-type mice (Saminathan et al. 2018, 2019). The IFNAR$^{(-/-)}$ mice have been utilized as a laboratory animal model to study the pathogenicity, virulence, and vaccine testing of BTV. The IFNAR$^{(-/-)}$ mice were vulnerable to numerous BTV serotypes, including BTV-1, -4, and -8, and differential serotype virulence was reported. For the first time, Saminathan et al. (2021) characterized the BTV serotype-1 infection in immunocompetent adult mouse with type I IFNs blockade. Typically, epizootiology, vector distribution, clinical symptoms, and pathological lesions are used to make the field diagnosis of BT. Viral isolation, sandwich ELISA, RNA-polyacrylamide gel electrophoresis, dot immunoperoxidase assay, PCR, and a complement fixation test can be used to detect the BTV antigen. Real-time PCR and RT-PCR are very sensitive and quick diagnostic methods for identifying the BTV serotypes and genome. Agar gel immunodiffusion (AGID), competitive ELISA, and indirect ELISA can be used to identify the BTV antibodies. The concentration of BTV antibodies in ruminant serum is mostly assessed using the c-ELISA. Major group-specific antibodies against VP7 of BTV have been identified using the AGID assay as a precipitin line. An economical and sustainable approach for controlling vector-borne diseases like BT is vaccination. Inactivated adjuvanted pentavalent vaccination including BTV-1, BTV-2, BTV-10, BTV-16, and BTV-23 was developed by Reddy et al. (2010). This vaccine was found to be sterile, safe, and potent; it is presently used in India for control and prevention of BT.

10.19 Infectious Bovine Rhinotracheitis

Currently, infectious bovine rhinotracheitis (IBR), is a well-known respiratory disease of cattle, which is caused by Bovine herpesvirus 1 (BHV-1), belongs to the genus *Varicellovirus*, family *Herpesviridae* and subfamily *Alphaherpesvirinae* (Dannacher et al. 1980). The BHV-1 is also responsible for numerous other clinical manifestations like infectious pustular vulvovaginitis (IPV), conjunctivitis, abortion, balanoposthitis, mastitis, and encephalitis. Latency is one of the most striking feature of BHV-1 infection in cattle. The term "latency" refers to the masked persistence of virus in the host, which prevents it from being detected by standard virological techniques. Certain endogenous or external stimuli may unmask the virus from time to time. Thus, the virus may later get reactivated and occasionally reexcreted again. Many other viruses from family *Herpesviridae* exhibit the characteristic phenomenon of latency, but the BHV-1 infection of cattle is particularly interesting to investigate for two main reasons. First of all, BHV-1 shares this feature with Feline herpesvirus 1 in that it can be experimentally reactivated by the administration of glucocorticoids (dexamethasone). Clinical lesions often only noticed in the anterior respiratory tract, where they manifest as tracheitis and nasal exudation, but they can also affect the posterior respiratory system, where they manifest as bronchitis and pneumonia. The epithelium is injured as a result of viral multiplication lead to the destruction of epithelial cells. Transient intranuclear inclusion bodies formed during viral proliferation. Local clinical symptoms are preceded and accompanied by an intense hyperthermia. Numerous other symptoms, including conjunctivitis, abortion, metritis following a caesarean section, encephalitis in young calves, and rare cases of enteritis, are frequently associated with infectious bovine rhinotracheitis infection. Both the foetus and newborn animals are extremely susceptible to BHV-1 infection. If a fetus becomes infected, a generalized acute illness develops, which results in death and abortion of fetus (Stubbings and Cameron 1981).

The IBR/IPV is one of the endemic diseases in cattle in India brought on by crossbreeding programme. Mehrotra et al. (1976) was the first to describe the disease after isolating the IBR virus from the cases of keratoconjunctivitis in crossbred calves at an organized cattle herd in Uttar Pradesh. Since then, most of the Indian states have reported of this disease. It was reported that more prevalent of the disease in exotic and crossbred cattle than native breeds. The disease has been reported from the states of Uttar Pradesh, Odisha (Misra and Misra 1987), Kerala (Sulochana et al. 1982), Gujarat (Singh et al. 1983), Tamil Nadu (Manickam and Mohan 1987), Karnataka (Mohan Kumar et al. 1994), West Bengal (Ganguly et al. 2008), and Andhra Pradesh (Satyanarayana and Suri Babu 1987).

Madin et al. (1956) originally isolated the etiological agent for IBR, which was later identified and classified as a herpesvirus named BHV-1. The major mode of spreading the virus from an infected animal to an uninfected one is by contact with mucosal droplets. During an acute respiratory infection, the infectious virus is shed by the nose for 10–14 days. Abortion is a consequence of a respiratory BHV-1 infection. Following viremia, BHV-1 infects the fetus fatally by crossing the maternal-fetal barrier. The route of BHV-1 from placenta to foetus is unknown but since viral lesions are frequently found in the fetal liver, hematogenous transmission most likely occurs through the umbilical vein. The most common symptom of typical BHV-1 infection is conjunctivitis, which can be unilateral or bilateral, and is accompanied by excessive lacrimation. Animals showed photophobia, epiphora, and the hair beneath the eye become heavily soiled. Pus may be visible in the lacrimal discharge due to frequent secondary bacterial infections. Most of the time, the cornea remains unaffected, but if secondary bacterial infections happen, keratitis, corneal ulceration, and permanent corneal scarring are common (Turin and Russo 2003).

Innate and adaptive immune responses forms the host defense against BHV-1 infection. Strong immunological responses caused by BHV-1 during acute infection can prevent the systemic infection. Antiviral effects of IFNs, alternative complement pathway, and the local infiltration of lymphoid cells including, macrophages, neutrophils, and NK cells were participate in the innate immune responses. The IFN-α and IFN-β are detectable in secretions as soon as 5 h after BHV-1 infection, reach their peak levels 72–96 h after infection, and can persist for up to 8 days after infection. The IFN-α and IFN-β enhance leukocyte migration, activate macrophages, and increased NK cell activity shortly after infection. Cytolytic activities against virus-infected cells are stimulated by the activation of macrophages and increased NK cell activity.

By preventing the peptide transport, BHV-1 downregulates the MHC class I antigen expression pathway. Normally, viral proteins that have undergone proteasomal processing produce peptides that bind to the transporter-associated-with-peptide-transport 1 (TAP1) and TAP2, the subunits of TAP heterodimer. Following viral peptide binding, TAP1–TAP2 heterodimer undergoes conformational changes. Subsequently, peptides are transported into the endoplasmic reticulum and loaded onto MHC class I molecules to form MHC–peptide complexes, which are transported and presented on the antigen-presenting cell surface. The UL49.5 encoded envelope protein interacts with TAP in BHV-1-infected cells, which interferes the function of peptide transport results in TAP degradation (Lipinska et al. 2006). Consequently, by interfering with the MHC class I antigen pathway, BHV-1 transiently escapes host cellular immune surveillance and elimination during the initial phase of viral infection (Koppers-Lalic et al. 2005).

Neutralizing antibodies bind to virus particles and prevent productive infection as a result of humoral immune responses. The most potent inducers of virus-neutralizing antibodies are the envelope glycoproteins gB, gC, gD, and gH. Antibody-mediated cell cytotoxicity, also known as non-neutralizing antibody-mediated cell cytotoxicity, is the process of destroying cells that are expressing viral proteins on their membranes or enveloped viruses. Neutralizing and non-neutralizing antibodies produced against envelope proteins can inhibit virus infection by several different mechanisms, including (1) membrane attack complex lysis of virus envelope and virus-infected cells mediated by antibody and complement, (2) antibody-mediated cell cytotoxicity in which IgG interacts with Fc receptor-positive cells (macrophages), and (3) binding of C3b to IgM mediates binding to C3b receptor-positive cells (lymphocytes and macrophages). Virus-infected cells are lysed in all these cases. Systemic humoral immunity depends on IgG, whereas local/mucosal immunity depends on secreted neutralizing IgA antibodies.

Viral-infected cells that exhibit viral antigens on their cell surfaces are killed by cell-mediated immune (CMI) responses. Because cell-to-cell transfer in the upper respiratory epithelium happens before hematogenous spread, the CD8+ cytotoxic T lymphocyte (CTL) response is a crucial line of defense against BHV-1. Eight days after infection, cytotoxic T lymphocyte responses are found in the bloodstream. The gC and gD have been identified as targets for CTL responses in cattle, and gB DNA vaccines elicit a CTL response in cattle. Because only a limited number of BHV-1 proteins have been assessed for CTL activity, additional structural and non-structural viral proteins may also contribute to the CMI responses. In addition to destruction of infected cells, T lymphocytes release several lymphokines that modulate specific and non-specific immune responses. Cells expressing gB, gC or gD on their membranes have been identified as targets for CD4+ T cells. The CD4+ T cells are important for the development of antibody responses and for developing effective CD8+ T-cell memory. Therefore, antibodies, CD4+ and CD8+ T cells are required for long-term protection.

The reactivation of BHV-1 from latency can be prevented by interferons. Presence of the immune system in trigeminal ganglia after the establishment of latency may play an important role in maintaining the latency. Recent research has shown that CD8+ T lymphocytes release IFN-γ, which inhibits the reactivation from latency in sensory neurons. Recurrent herpetic lesions are controlled by IFN-α and IFN-γ (Jones 2003).

The BHV-1 causes widespread immunosuppression in infected cattle results in susceptibility to secondary viral and bacterial infections. There is impairment of function of macrophages, polymorphonuclear leukocytes (PMN), and lymphocytes (Tikoo et al. 1995); interleukin-2 (IL-2) receptor expression is downregulated; peripheral blood mononuclear cells (PBMCs) undergo less mitogenic activation; and reduced number of circulating T cells (Winkler et al. 1999). Due to the infection of monocytes and macrophages, there is decreased phagocytosis, antibody-dependent cell-mediated cytotoxicity (ADCC), and T-cells activation. The BHV-1 glycoprotein G (gG), a broad-spectrum chemokine-binding protein inhibits chemokine binding and activity, which mediates partly the effect of immunosuppression. The virus also affects CD4+ T cells, causing a loss of their CD4 expression and eventually these cells undergo apoptosis (Babiuk et al. 1996; Winkler et al. 1999). On the surface of infected cells, the BHV-1 is known to suppress the expression of MHC class I molecules (Hariharan et al. 1993). It most likely interferes with the protective role of CD8+ cytotoxic T lymphocytes (CTLs) in the lysis of BHV-1-infected cells (Denis et al. 1993). Other effector mechanisms likely to play a role are CD4+-mediated CTL activity, which is a strategy to provide the cellular protection during BHV-1 infection. It has been demonstrated that cytolytic effector cells, especially CD4+-activated CD8+ T lymphocytes, are capable of lysing the BHV-1-infected macrophages when PBMCs of cattle are stimulated by immunizing with attenuated live BHV-1 (Hariharan et al. 1993).

The BHV-1 can currently be detected in diagnostic virology laboratories using the following techniques: virus isolation, examination of tissues by fluorescent antibody technique (FAT) and immunoperoxidase test, and enzyme-linked immunosorbent assay (ELISA) for antigen detection. The development of new, extremely sensitive diagnostic techniques was aided by the frequently used virus isolation in cell culture. One of the molecular approaches used to detect the BHV-1 infection in the samples of semen and aborted foetus, calves, cows by polymerase chain reaction (PCR) (Takiuchi et al. 2005). Comparing this procedure to other diagnostic techniques including virus isolation, immunofluorescence, and nucleic acid hybridization has confirmed that PCR is more sensitive and specific (Kataria et al. 1997). Real-time PCR using primers of glycoprotein C gene provides satisfactory results for detection of BHV-1 in the extended semen with high specificity and sensitivity and significant reduction in time for detecting amplified products; further, it is a valuable alternative to the time and labour consuming virus isolation technique (OIE 2010).

10.20 Bovine Herpesvirus 4 Infection

Bovine herpesvirus 4 (BHV-4) belongs to the genus *Rhadinovirus* and family *Herpesviridae*. According to Thiry et al. (1989) and Donofrio et al. (2007), BHV-4 has been isolated from both healthy and clinically affected cattle. Most BHV-4 infections are subclinical. Infection with BHV-4 can cause reproductive diseases such as vulvovaginitis, endometritis, postpartum metritis, and abortion. In addition, it causes respiratory illnesses, conjunctivitis, and mastitis. The BHV-4 was initially isolated by Park and Kendrick (1973) from a case of bovine endometritis.

According to Donofrio et al. (2007), BHV-4 acts as a primary pathogen rather than merely a co-pathogen since it has a specific trophism for endometrial stromal and epithelial cells. But the pathophysiology of BHV-4 is still unknown (Donofrio et al. 2007). A simian virus 40 (SV40) immortalized endometrial stromal cell line (SV40BESC) was established for BHV-4 due to specific trophism. This cell line was stable, responsive to exogenous TNF-α, expressed TLRs 1 to 10. The TNF-α treated SV40BESC cell line showed increased BHV-4 replication and cytopathic effects.

BHV-4 seropositivity was associated with fetal infection and abortion (Czaplicki and Thiry 1998). The BHV-4 can infect both domestic and wild ruminants but most common in sheep, goats, African buffalo, and American bison (Opdenbosch et al. 1986). Additionally, BHV-4 has been isolated from lions, cats, chickens, owl monkeys (*Aotus trivirgatus*), and lions (Egyed et al. 1997; Kruger et al. 2000). Infection with BHV-4 has been experimentally reproduced in laboratory animals, particularly rabbits and guinea pigs (Egyed et al. 1997). African buffalo can be protected from malignant catarrhal fever by infection with BHV-4.

Polymerase chain reaction (PCR) can detect the BHV-4 viral DNA, but because of the inherent feature of herpesviruses like carrier/latency status, which lead to the presence of the virus that does not necessarily involve the causation of acute disease (Egyed et al. 1996; Boerner et al. 1999). Hence, the detection of BHV-4 may only reflect the presence of acute or latent infection. In endemic areas, both acute and latent BHV-4 infections are frequently present. For the detection of antibodies, serological diagnostic tests including ELISA and indirect immunofluorescence assays are useful. Serum neutralization test is less useful because cattle develop low titres of transient anti-BHV-4 neutralizing antibodies (Dubuisson et al. 1987). BHV-4 can be isolated from nasal and vaginal secretions using continuous or primary cell lines of bovine origin.

Vaccinations are not used very frequently. BHV-4 infection can be controlled in a farm by following hygienic measures. Seropositive animals are considered as latently infected, which must be removed. Post-parturient infected cows with metritis must be isolated from other animals because they can excrete high quantities of viruses in uterine discharges. Direct contact between seropositive and seronegative animals must be avoided because BHV-4 is mostly transmitted through the respiratory route (Thiry et al. 1989).

10.21 Epizootic/Enzootic Abortions

The Gram-negative intracellular bacterium *Chlamydia abortus* or *Chlamydophila abortus* is the cause of ovine chlamydiosis, also known as enzootic abortion of ewes (EAE) or ovine enzootic abortion (OEA). In many sheep-rearing regions of the world, particularly where flocks are closely congregated during the parturient period, chlamydial abortion during the late pregnancy is common results in significant economic losses (Longbottom and Coulter 2003; Aitken and Longbottom 2007). Abortion typically occurs in the last 2–3 weeks of pregnancy with the birth of stillborn lambs and grossly, placentitis was noticed. Fetal liver and lung lesions are milder, hypoxic brain damage, and severe placental injury may be seen (Buxton et al. 2002; Longbottom et al. 2013). The impairment of maternal-fetal gaseous and nutritional exchange, disturbance of hormonal regulation of pregnancy, and cytokine activation are likely to contribute to abortion (Entrican 2002). Chlamydial abortion also occurs to a similar extent in goats, but less frequently cattle, pigs, horses, and wild ruminants may be affected. Abortions in the late stages of pregnancy in sheep result in expulsion of necrotic fetal membranes, which is a characteristic diagnostic lesion.

The first line of defenses against chlamydia are the skin, mucosal lining, and body fluids. Innate immune cells, such as epithelial cells, monocyte/macrophages, and DCs, make up these defense barriers. Chlamydia are primarily epitheliotropic, where the bacteria can trigger an inflammatory response by producing the pro-inflammatory cytokines. These cytokines causes innate immune cells including neutrophils, NK cells, macrophages, and DCs to be recruited to the affected areas (Roan and Starnbach 2008). Innate immune cells may also be crucial in the spread of chlamydial infections because the location of chlamydial infection is frequently not the site of pathological lesion. One of the first cells to reach the site of a chlamydial infection are neutrophils (Register et al. 1986). These cells are normally short-lived and quickly eliminated by spontaneous apoptosis, and it is believed that they respond to chlamydial infection by releasing inflammatory mediators (Frazer et al. 2011). In vitro studies demonstrated that neutrophils can internalize chlamydia and are largely chlamydiacidal, however, some live bacteria were able to persist within these cells (Register et al. 1986). Recent research study has demonstrated that chlamydial infection can prolong the life of neutrophils by delaying the apoptosis, allowing the bacteria to multiply inside the cells (Frazer et al. 2011). The macrophages can engulf the neutrophils results in long-term survival, and neutrophils may also help to spread the bacterium from the infection site (Rupp et al. 2009). Additionally, it was discovered that neutrophils promoted the chlamydial replication in epithelial cells (Rodriguez et al. 2005). In vivo studies suggested that increased neutrophil recruitment was associated with the development of chlamydial pathogenesis and an increase in bacterial burden (Rodriguez et al. 2005; Frazer et al. 2011). It has been demonstrated that NK cells are recruited to the site of chlamydial infection, where they are believed to serve as an early source of IFN-γ (Tseng and Rank 1998). Further, NK cells have been identified in the induction of lysis of chlamydia-infected epithelial cells. According to research, chlamydia have been shown to suppresses the expression of MHC I on epithelial cells, which enables the bacterium to avoid being exposed to cells of the adaptive immune system. However, this suppression makes them targets for NK cells as MHC I is required for NK inhibitory receptors (Hook et al. 2004). Antigen-presenting cells called dendritic cells are crucial for the activation and polarization of T-cell response. Studies have shown that DCs are recruited to the site of chlamydial infection (Brunham and Rey-Ladino 2005), and bacteria can survive and persist inside the DCs. This implies that DCs may also be involved in the maintenance of persistent infections and dissemination (Rey-Ladino et al. 2007). The pathogen recognition receptors (PRRs), are the sentinels of the innate immune system. The PRRs are present on the surface or within the innate immune cells, and recognize specific molecular patterns, such as damage-associated molecular patterns (DAMPs) and pathogen-associated molecular patterns (PAMPs) (Seong and Matzinger 2004). Different PRR complements are expressed by cells, and when activated, they cause signaling pathways to be triggered inside the cells. These signaling pathways can result in the secretion of cytokines and chemokines, which activates the adaptive immune response and induces the cell death. Toll-like receptors (TLRs), nucleotide binding and oligomerization domain (NOD)-like receptors (NLRs), RIG-I-like receptors (RLRs), and C-type lectin receptors (CLRs) are the four major categories of PRRs. The TLRs and NLRs respond to the pathogenic bacteria independently and collaboratively (Oviedo-Boyso et al. 2014). Innate immune recognition triggers the production of cytokines and chemokines, which have a variety of important role in the host immunological defense against pathogens. Studies have identified that numerous innate immunity cytokines and chemokines, such as CXCL8, TNF-, IL-6, and IL-1β, have been found to be upregulated by a variety of innate immune cells in response to live chlamydial infection. The Th17 cells have recently been recognized as potential key immunological mediators in relation to chlamydial infection. The Th1-type CD4+ T cells are specific for antigen seem to be essential for mediating protective immunity to both primary and secondary chlamydial infection. Number of inflammatory cytokines including IFN-γ, IL-12, and IL-17 are produced in response to chlamydial infection. In vitro studies have shown that IFN-γ played a role in limiting intracellular chlamydial growth, which is crucial for the host defense but may also cause a persistent infection that is crucial for disease pathogenesis (Mascellino et al. 2011). The mechanism of action of IFN-γ is through tryptophan depletion. An essential cytokine that aids in the stimulation of Th1-type responses is IL-12. In general, it is believed that antibodies and B cells play a relatively little role in the protective immunity to primary infection. It is well documented that the host produces antibodies in response to primary chlamydial infection.

The clinical history of the flock and characteristic lesions in aborted placentae suggest a enzootic abortion. Diagnosis can be attempted by microscopic examination of smears made from affected chorionic villi or adjacent chorion. Smears are stained using modified Ziehl-Neelsen, Giemsa, brucella differential, or modified Macchiavello staining methods. Large numbers of small (300 nm) coccoid elementary bodies are visible singly or in clusters under a high-power microscope stained red against the blue background of cellular debris in positive cases. The elementary bodies appear light green under dark-ground illumination. Fluorescent antibody test (FAT) using a specific antiserum or monoclonal antibody may be used for identification of *C. abortus* in smears. However, However, polymerase chain reaction (PCR)-based tests are superior than FAT smears regarding sensitivity and specificity. The preferred technique for isolating the bacterium is cell culture. The causative agent of ovine chlamydiosis is zoonotic and thus isolation and identification procedures must be carried out with appropriate biosafety and containment procedures. The best transport medium is sucrose/phosphate/glutamate, also known as SPG medium, which contains sucrose (74.6 g/L), KH_2PO_4 (0.52 g/L), K_2HPO_4 (1.25 g/L), and L-glutamic acid (0.92 g/L). It is also supplemented with bovine serum albumin - fraction V (1 g/L), antibiotics (gentamycin and streptomycin are suitable, but not penicillin), and fungal inhibitor. A variety of cell types can be used to isolate *Chlamydia abortus* of ovine origin. The most commonly used cell types are McCoy, buffalo green monkey (BGM), or baby hamster kidney (BHK) cells. Because of great sensitivity and specificity of PCR, amplification of chlamydial DNA by PCR is the preferred method for confirming the presence of *Chlamydiae* in biological samples. The 16S-23S rRNA region or *pmp* genes are the targets of conventional PCR technique for the identification of *C. abortus* DNA (Everett and Andersen 1999; Laroucau et al. 2001). Real-time PCR has become the preferred method in diagnostic laboratories due to its high specificity, rapidity, high throughput and ease of standardisation (Sachse et al. 2009). For the precise detection and identification of microorganisms from clinical samples, real-time PCR and DNA microarray have been validated (Borel et al. 2008; Pantchev et al. 2010). PCR assays in combination with RFLP analysis or HRM (high resolution melting) analysis have been developed to differentiate the naturally infected from vaccinated animals (DIVA) (Laroucau et al. 2010; Wheelhouse et al. 2010). Several commercial ELISAs kits are available to diagnose the Chlamydia infection in ewes (Sachse et al. 2009). Care must be taken to select an appropriate ELISA for each diagnostic sample considering the different specificities and sensitivities.

Complement fixation test (CFT) has traditionally been the most widely used procedure for detecting EAE. However, *C. abortus* and *C. pecorum*, which is endemic in small ruminants, as well as with some Gram-negative bacteria (such as *Acinetobacter*), can exhibit antigenic cross-reactivity, which can result in false-positive CFT results. This is because chlamydial antigen contains LPS, which is an immunodominant component and common to all *Chlamydiaceae* species. Additionally, it has been demonstrated that CFT is less sensitive than alternative tests. As a result, CFT is no longer recommended as the preferred technique for the serological diagnosis of EAE, while it may still be used for herd diagnosis when no alternative tools are available and the limitations of CFT are taken into consideration.

Cattlemen frequently refer to epizootic bovine abortion (EBA) as "foothill abortion." The disease, was initially identified in the early 1950s and characterized by near-term abortions or the birth of weak calves by dams, who had been grazing in foothill regions of California during their first or second trimesters of pregnancy. The diagnosis was made based on the specific fetal pathology, higher serum immunoglobulin levels, and the geographical location of the dam in foothill terrain during the first half of pregnancy (Kennedy et al. 1983; Blanchard et al. 2014). The soft-shell tick *Ornithodoros coriaceus*, also called the pajaroella tick by Native Americans and early immigrants, was identified in the 1970s as the EBA vector. The etiologic agent of EBA was not identified until 2005. Using the cryopreserved thymus homogenate from a selected necropsied EBA-positive fetuses, researchers were able to develop a reproducible laboratory method to transmit the disease in 2000, which proves that the etiologic agent was an antibiotic-susceptible prokaryote (bacterium) (Stott et al. 2002). With this information and access to advanced molecular biological technologies, researchers were able to identify a unique bacterium belonging to the *Myxococcales* order, as the etiologic agent of EBA (King et al. 2005). This bacterium has tentatively been coined as *Pajaroellobacter abortibovis*. Immunohistochemistry (IHC; Anderson et al. 2006), PCR (King et al. 2005), and indirect fluorescent antibody test (IFAT) to detect the bacteria-specific antibody have been developed for the Identification of the etiologic agent (Blanchard et al. 2014).

10.22 Toxoplasmosis

Studies using knockout mice lacking B cells, CD4+, CD8+ T cells, and cytokines have shown the significance of the adaptive immune response in resistance to toxoplasmosis. Extremely high concentration of IFN-γ and IL-18 in mice causes lethal toxoplasmosis, whereas moderate concentrations of these cytokines result in non-lethal infection. Although tumor necrosis factor (TNF-α) plays a significant role in toxoplasmosis resistance, excessive amounts of this cytokine may also contribute to pathogenesis. Increased vascular permeability is caused by elevated levels of IL-18, IFN-γ, IL-12, and TNF-α, which can cause the multiple organ failure and death of the animal (Andrade et al. 2013; Wujcicka et al. 2014).

The ability of CD4+ T cells and CD8+ T lymphocytes to produce IFN-γ, a pro-inflammatory cytokine that is known to be a key mediator of resistance to

T. gondii, which are essential for the development of protective immunity and long-term survival during persistent infection. The IFN-γ production is necessary for the long-term survival, which was proved in mice by depleting this cytokine during the persistent phase of *T. gondii* infection. Extracellular tachyzoites can be destroyed in the presence of specific antibodies and complement pathway. Antibodies against *T. gondii* may also prevent the parasite from entering into the host cells (Andrade et al. 2013; Wujcicka et al. 2014).

Toxoplasma gondii is an obligatory intracellular protozoan parasite of public and animal health importance (Cenci-Goga et al. 2013; Cosendey-Kezenleite et al. 2014; Schluter et al. 2014). The high seroprevalence of *T. gondii* in flocks is a risk factor for the transmission of toxoplasmosis to humans through consumption of undercooked meat (Boughattas et al. 2014; Schluter et al. 2014). When sheep have primary *T. gondii* infection during pregnancy, they may develop reproductive problems including embryonic resorption, fetal mortality, mummification, stillbirth, abortion, or birth of debilitated animals (Esteban-Redondo and Innes 1997; Edwards and Dubey 2013). Due to the high prevalence of infection in sheep, abortion is one of the main symptoms of *T. gondii* infection and causes economic losses in many nations. Cats are the definitive hosts of *T. gondii*, and their feces contain oocysts. Sheep is the important intermediate hosts among most of the warm-blooded animals in the toxoplasmosis transmission cycle (Esteban-Redondo and Innes 1997). When pregnant ewes are infected with toxoplasma, typically following the consumption of oocysts, congenital infection can also happen. *T. gondii* rapidly multiply in the submucosa of the intestine, and reach associated lymph nodes and other organs through the lymph and blood circulation (Dubey 2010). Abortion in sheep has been reported from 60 to 90 days of gestation, mainly in ewes with primary infection (Dubey 2010).

Dendritic cells (DCs), monocytes, and neutrophils are recruited to the site of infection after a *T. gondii* challenge, and these cell types have been implicated to resistance to this parasite (Del Rio et al. 2001; Mordue and Sibley 2003; Liu et al. 2006; Dunay et al. 2008, 2010; Tait et al. 2010). One of the most critical functions of innate immune response against T. gondii is to sense the parasite and produce the cytokine IL-12, which stimulates NK cells and T cells to produce the cytokine IFN-γ (Gazzinelli et al. 1993, 1994; Hunter et al. 1994). The IFN-γ is a major mediator of *T. gondii* resistance and promotes various intracellular processes to kill the parasite and prevent its replication. Mice deficient in either IL-12 or IFN-γ who are infected with *T. gondii* succumb to acute disease and showed an inability to control the intracellular parasite burden. This Th1 immune response, defined by the production of IL-12 and IFN-γ, is characteristic of infection with many intracellular pathogens (Suzuki et al. 1988; Gazzinelli et al. 1994; Hunter et al. 1994). The innate production of IL-12 during toxoplasmosis requires that the parasite first be sensed by the host. Toll-like receptors (TLRs) are the innate immune receptors, participate in this process.

The TLRs are essential for the recognition of parasites via the innate immune response and for induction of antigen-specific responses by adaptive immune responses characterized by stimulation of naïve CD4+ helper T cells toward Th1 or Th2 phenotype, which is mediated by B and T cells. Therefore, mice lacking MyD88, an adaptor molecule necessary for downstream signaling from the majority of TLRs, are extremely susceptible to toxoplasmosis (Scanga et al. 2002). Specific TLRs implicated in the immune response to *T. gondii* include TLR-2, -4, -9, and -11. According to Jenkins et al. (2010), the TLR-11 reacts to a profilin-like protein that is conserved among protozoan parasites, whereas the TLR-2 and -4 detect glycosyl phosphatidylinositols on the surface of parasites (Debierre-Grockiego et al. 2007). Furthermore, after oral *T. gondii* infection, protozoan antigens translocate from the gut, and TLR-2, TLR-4, and TLR-9 respond to these parasite insults, thus contributing to the development of the Th1 immune response (Benson et al. 2009). The TLR-2 contributes to the resistance to high doses of *T. gondii* challenge in mice, whereas, TLR-11 and TLR-12 are crucial for regulating the immunological reactions. During the first trimester of pregnancy, TLR-4 is most prominently expressed in humans. This classic TLR-4 ligand recognizes the LPS of Gram-negative bacteria, suggesting a potential protective role for the dam (Wujcicka et al. 2014). The TLR-11 plays a dominant role in recognition of *T. gondii* in mice. However, TLR-11 is a pseudogene in humans, hence the major question of how innate and adaptive immune responses occur in the absence of TLR-11 remains unanswered. Neutrophils are an important source of IFN-γ, which is necessary for the defense against *T. gondii*, according to the studies in TLR-11 knockout mice. During the early stages of infection, monocytes, neutrophils, and DCs are recruited locally and are crucial for *T. gondii* resistance. The cytokine IL-12 is produced during innate immune responses, and it stimulates NK cells and T cells to release IFN-γ. To activate the adaptive immunological responses, *T. gondii* antigens are processed by MHC class II antigen-presenting cells and their peptides are delivered to CD4+ T cells (Wujcicka et al. 2014).

Since neutrophils have pre-stored IL-12 and can release this cytokine in vitro and in vivo in response to *T. gondii* (Bliss et al. 1999a, b, 2001). Additionally, there are reports that neutrophil depletion causes IL-12 levels to drop and parasite replication to increase (Bliss et al. 2001). Monocytes are crucial for toxoplasmosis resistance, as evidenced by the higher susceptibility of mice lacking the chemokine receptor CCR2 (CCR2 KO), which is required for monocyte recruitment to the site of infection (Robben et al. 2005; Dunay et al. 2010). Monocytes produce the cytokine IL-1 in response to soluble toxoplasma antigens, and this cytokine can enhance anti-toxoplasmic effector mechanisms in macrophages and astrocytes in vitro (Hammouda et al. 1995; Halonen et al. 1998). Further, IL-1 and IL-12 can work together to stimulate the production of IFN-γ from innate and adaptive sources (Hunter et al. 1995; Shibuya et al. 1998). Another innate population involved in immunity to *T. gondii* is the NK cells, and in mice lacking T cells, provide a limited ability of resistance due to decreased production of IFN-γ (Denkers et al. 1993; Johnson et al. 1993; Sher et al. 1993; Hunter et al. 1994). The NK cell activity is peak during early infection, and their activity is elevated during chronic toxoplasmosis, they do not appear to be significant contributor to immunity during the chronic stage of infection (Hauser et al. 1982; Denkers et al. 1993; Johnson et al. 1993; Sher et al. 1993; Hunter et al. 1994; Kang and Suzuki 2001). The NK cells additionally produce the cytokine IL-10, in addition to IFN-γ (Perona-Wright et al. 2009). The NK cells can also stimulate the adaptive immune responses in body. They can therefore aid the CD8+ T-cells response in the absence of CD4+ T cells (Combe et al. 2005). Increasing the synthesis of IL-12 from DCs through interactions with the molecule natural killer group 2D (NKG2D) is one way of assistance provided to CD8+ T-cells (Guan et al. 2007). The increased susceptibility of human patients with primary or acquired defects in T-cell function and mice with deficiencies in B cells, CD4+ T cells, or CD8+ T cells survive the acute stage of infection but ultimately show increased susceptibility to *T. gondii*, showing the importance of adaptive immune responses for resistance to *T. gondii* during human infection (Denkers et al. 1997; Kang et al. 2000; Johnson and Sayles 2002).

The CD4+ T cells provide several critical regulatory functions in mediating resistance to toxoplasmosis. The ability of these cells to control chronic infection may be related to their production of cytokines like IFN-γ or their expression of CD40L (also known as CD154), which can activate effector mechanisms in macrophages and other innate cells expressing CD40 on their surface (Johnson and Sayles 2002; Lutjen et al. 2006). They contribute optimal B-cells and CD8+ T-cells responses during the early stages of infection (Gazzinelli et al. 1992; Reichmann et al. 2000; Subauste and Wessendarp 2006; Subauste et al. 2007). Studies on knockout mice lacking B, CD4+, and CD8+ T cells as well as cytokines have shown the significance of adaptive immune responses in toxoplasmosis resistance. Extremely high concentrations of IFN-γ and IL-18 in mice cause lethal toxoplasmosis, whereas moderate concentrations of these cytokines result in non-lethal infection. Although high levels of TNF-α may contribute to the pathophysiology of the disease, optimal levels of TNF-α plays a critical role in toxoplasmosis resistance. Multiple organ failure and mortality can arise from increased vascular permeability caused by elevated levels of IL-18, IFN-γ, IL-12, and TNF-α (Wujcicka et al. 2014). The CD4+ and CD8+ T lymphocytes are essential for the development of protective immunity and long-term survival during persistent infection by stimulating IFN-γ production, which mediates resistance to *T. gondii*.

Continuous production of IFN-γ is necessary during the persistent phase of *T. gondii* infection for long-term survival in mice. Extracellular tachyzoites can be destroyed in the presence of specific antibodies and complement pathway. Antibodies to *T. gondii* may also prevent the parasite from entering into the cells (Wujcicka et al. 2014). It has long been known that *T. gondii* infection stimulates antibody production and that these antibodies can kill the parasite. Indeed, human patients have produced parasite-specific IgM, IgA, IgE, and IgG2 antibodies, and the identification of these antibodies is a useful diagnostic technique for distinguish freshly infected individuals from those infected chronically (Remington et al. 2004; Correa et al. 2007). Given that *T. gondii* is an intracellular pathogen, it is not surprising that CD8+ T cells, which are specialized to recognize and destroy cells infected with viral, bacterial, and parasitic organisms, also have a critical role in mediating CD8+ resistance to this infection. The T cells can control infection through the production of inflammatory cytokines such as IFN-γ through CD40/

CD40L interactions and through the perforin-mediated cytolysis of infected host cells (Gazzinelli et al. 1992; Denkers et al. 1997; Reichmann et al. 2000).

Mice and other species can develop immunopathology in the ileum after oral *T. gondii* infection, and this ileitis has been suggested as a model to investigate the causes of immune-mediated gastrointestinal disease in humans (Liesenfeld et al. 1996; Egan et al. 2011). The infection-induced ileitis is characterized by the development of severe necrosis and inflammatory foci, and is dependent upon the host's sex and genetic back ground (Liesenfeld et al. 1996, 2001; Egan et al. 2011). Factors that promote T cell responses such as CD40/CD40L interactions and the cytokines IL-12 and IL-23 also contribute to ileitis development (Li et al. 2002; Vossenkamper et al. 2004; Munoz et al. 2009). Other cytokines namely IFN-γ, TNF-α, IL-18, IL-22, and macrophage migration inhibitory factor have been linked in mediating the pathology (Liesenfeld et al. 1999; Vossenkamper et al. 2004; Munoz et al. 2009; Cavalcanti et al. 2011). Another example of severe pathology is seen in mice model of CD4+ T cells that have chronic toxoplasmic encephalitis. Although, T cells can cause severe central nervous system disease, they are also necessary for long-term resistance to *T. gondii*.

T. gondii can be diagnosed by immunohistochemical (IHC), biological, molecular, histological, serological, or combination of these methods (Da Motta et al. 2008; Dubey 2010). Modified agglutination test (MAT) and indirect immunofluorescence assay (IFA) can be used to detect in sheep fetus samples for *T. gondii* antibodies (Dubey and Desmonts 1987). The placenta and fetus with a special focus on the brain are sent to the laboratory for the diagnosis of parasitosis in cases of suspected toxoplasmosis abortion (Weissmann 2003). The agent can be isolated from the inoculation of placental and fetal tissues in mice (Dubey 2010; Edwards and Dubey 2013; Lopes et al. 2013). For molecular diagnostics, fetal tissue samples such as the placenta, brain, heart, spleen, liver, lungs, and spinal cord can be used (de Moraes et al. 2011). The IHC enables a conclusive diagnosis of toxoplasmosis when combined with pathology and clinical history (Da Motta et al. 2008; Dagleish et al. 2010). A risk factor for the spread of toxoplasmosis to sheep is the presence of cats (Andrade et al. 2013; Cosendey-Kezenleite et al. 2014).

10.23 Bovine Viral Diarrhea

Bovine viral diarrhoea (BVD) is a serious clinical disease in cattle caused by the Bovine viral diarrhea virus (BVDV), a *Pestivirus* belonging to the *Flaviviridae* family (Becher and Thiel 2011). Based on antigenic and genetic variations, BVDV is divided into two genotypes (BVDV-1 and BVDV-2) (Vilcek et al. 2005). The placenta can be crossed by the BVDV, which can infect the fetus. According to Houe (1999), infection with BVDV is known to cause significant financial loss due to the reproductive and immunosuppressive effects of acute infection. While immune-competent, healthy cattle (or late-term, immuno-competent fetuses) may suffer from an acute BVDV infection resulting in seroconversion, the disease is primarily spread and maintained in cattle populations by persistently infected (PI) individuals.

Persistency of infection arises from fetal infection with non-cytopathic (ncp) BVDV during early gestation, following acute infection in the dam (Grooms 2004). The establishment of fetal persistent infection results in adverse fetal developmental consequences, life-long viremia, and virus-specific immunotolerance. Based on the effects on cultured cells rather than the infected host, the BVDV is divided into non-cytopathogenic (ncp) and cytopathogenic (cp) biotypes. In contrast to ncp biotypes, the Cp biotypes cause apoptosis in cultured cells (Gamlen et al. 2010). However, non-cytopathogenic BVDV appears to be the cause of acute infections, which can spread through a variety of bodily fluids including saliva, tears, milk, urine, and fetal secretions (Meyling et al. 1990). Faeces are a poor source of BVD virus. Under experimental conditions, it has been demonstrated that the Cp BVDV can cause an acute infection (Lambot et al. 1997). The most important source of ncp BVDV infection is PI cattle and BVDV gains entry through the lymphocyte host cell membranes (Brownlie 1990; Maurer et al. 2004).

Infected pregnant animals with cp BVDV did not exhibit any interferon response. However, pregnant animals infected with ncp BVDV, IFN was found at greater concentrations (0.8–5.4 IU/mL). The type I interferon (IFN)-stimulated genes (ISGs) showed transient robust upregulation on 3–15 days after viral inoculation in heifers experimentally infected with ncp BVDV type 2 on 75 days of gestation. Following acute ncp BVDV infection in pregnant cattle, several signal transduction pathways are activated in PBMCs. The PI foetuses showed moderate chronic up-regulation of ISGs on 115 days post maternal infection. It was hypothesized that chronic stimulation of innate immune responses following infection of the fetus and placental production of type I IFNs contributes to up-regulation of ISGs in PI fetuses. On days 82–192 of gestation, there was a significant upregulation of the mRNAs (RIG-I and MDA5) that encode cytosolic dsRNA sensors. Detection of viral dsRNA by cytosolic sensors results in significant up-regulation of ISGs in fetal blood on 89, 97 and 192 days of gestation. Further, cotyledons from PI fetuses were shown to have a considerable upregulation of IFN-α and IFN-β at 192 days of gestation. In conclusion, fetuses respond to ncp BVDV infection during early gestation by induction of type I IFN signalling pathways results in chronic up-regulation of ISGs. Cotyledonary tissue is responsible for the up-regulation of ISGs by increased production of IFNs. Innate immune response can partially prevent viral replication in PI foetuses; however, virus-specific adaptive immune responses are required to eliminate the virus (Smirnova et al. 2008, 2012; Kelling and Topliff 2013).

Acute ncp BVDV infection of pregnant cattle during late stage of gestation results in transiently-infected fetus with upregulation of type I IFN genes in the blood of dams. The following genes are upregulated ISG15, ISG28, ISG44, dsRNA-dependent protein kinase R (PKR), 2',5'-oligoadenylate synthetase 1 (OAS-1), myxovirus resistance factor 2 (MX2), and JAK/STAT pathways (Kelling and Topliff 2013). Both humoral (antibodies) and cell mediated (T-cell) immune responses play major role against BVDV infection in cattle. The ncp BVDV infection during early gestation, produces a PI fetus, results in prolonged downregulation of chemokine receptor 4 (CXCR4), T cell receptor (TCR) signaling and CD8+ T lymphocytes in maternal blood. The CXCR4 downregulation was noticed during early infection at the time of viremia and remains downregulated for approximately 3 months, long after the dam has cleared the virus and seroconverted. The CXCL12/CXCR4 signaling are responsible for multiple biological processes and these signaling are downregulated during BVDV infection for an extended period of time, which could harm fetal and postnatal development (Smirnova et al. 2008, 2009).

Naive animal infected with BVDV develops a transient viremia that lasts 10–14 days after the infection (Howard 1990). This can be associated with thrombocytopenia (Marshall et al. 1996; Blanchard et al. 2010), apoptosis in the thymus (Raya et al. 2012), immunosuppression (Wilhelmsen et al. 1990), pyrexia (Baker 1995), and diarrhea (Muller-Doblies et al. 2004), and short-term leukopenia (Brownlie et al. 1987). The resultant immunosuppression, in turn, may allow other infectious agents to become established, or allow the recurrence of existing infections (Potgieter 1995). Direct effects of BVDV on circulating T and B lymphocytes and lymphocyte apoptosis in gut-associated lymphoid organs are linked to immunosuppression (Bolin et al. 1985; Chase 2013; Pedrera et al. 2012). Experimental BVDV infection of cattle causes immunosuppression results in isolation of *Bacillus* spp. from cattle blood. The fact that bacterial abortions and BVDV infections frequently co-occur, suggesting that BVDV infection may be one of the immunosuppressive diseases that frequently affect the pregnant cows. Experimental nasal infection of healthy calves with ncp BVDV led to the virus being localized in decreasing order of concentration in enterocytes, Peyer's patches, thymus, spleen, lymph nodes, tonsils, and liver (Pedrera et al. 2011). According to Liebler-Tenorio et al. (2004), there was significant lymphocyte apoptosis when the virus started to be cleared around 6 days after infection, and T cell-mediated destruction of infected lymphocytes caused the virus to be cleared by 9–13 days after infection. The ability of the immune system to react to other infectious agents is reduced by lymphocyte apoptosis (Wilhelmsen et al. 1990) and suppression of macrophage phagocytic function (Marshall et al. 1996) via inactivation of caspase-9 (Pedrera et al. 2012) in the lymph nodes, bronchiole-associated, and gut-associated lymphoid tissues. Mucosal disease only develops in PI cattle and is inevitably fatal. Disease is associated with the appearance of cp BVDV biotype arising from mutation of ncp BVDV already circulating in the PI animal (Brownlie et al. 1984).

Apoptosis is induced by the NS3 protease expressed by the cp BVDV (Gamlen et al. 2010). Double stranded RNA is produced by the virus in infected cells triggering apoptosis by intrinsic and extrinsic pathways (Yamane et al. 2006; Pedrera et al. 2012). Intrinsic pathways are regulated by the release of cytochrome C from mitochondria inducing activation of the death regulator, apoptotic protease-activating factor. Increased levels of tumur necrosis factor alpha (TNF-α), a crucial cytokine involved in the execution of apoptosis through the external pathway of apoptosis (Yamane et al. 2005). These changes mostly affect the Peyer's patches, where they cause lymphoid atrophy and lymphoid depletion. Over the Peyer's patches, microvilli disappear from the lamina propria. Cell debris and mucous accumulate in dilated intestinal gland crypts giving the appearance of necrosis. Necrosis of keratinocytes in the stratum spinosum leads to disruption of intercellular junctions in the keratinised epithelium of the skin, muzzle, oral cavity, esophagus, rumen, reticulum, and omasum (Bielefeldt-Ohmann 1995). A non-PI cow that is carrying a PI fetus is known colloquially as a "Trojan cow". In these situations, the dam appears immune to BVDV and healthy and thus a benign risk whilst, in fact, harbouring a potent source of infectious virus within the unborn fetal calf. Trojan cows have significantly higher antibody titres during mid-late stage of pregnancy than that of seropositive cows carrying normal calves (Brownlie et al. 1998; Lindberg and Alenius 1999).

Virus isolation, Ag detection [including Ag-enzyme-linked immunosorbent assay (ELISA) and immunohistochemistry (IHC)], nucleic acid probe hybridisation and reverse transcriptase-polymerase chain reaction (RT-PCR) used for the diagnosis of BVDV infection. Virus isolation is the 'gold standard' for BVDV diagnosis. Nowadays, use of RT-PCR has become increasingly common and widely accepted for BVDV diagnosis. Quantitative RT-PCR has been used for BVDV detection with excellent sensitivity and specificity. Ag-ELISA offers a quick and easy way to detect the PI animals, making it perfect for high throughput applications like herd screening (Mignon et al. 1991; Shannon et al. 1991; Horner et al. 1995). There are several antibody detection methods are available including microsphere-based immunoassay, an agarose gel immunodiffusion test, and an easy, affordable, reliable, quick dot-blot enzyme immunoassay (Hemmatzadeh and Amini 2009). However, the serum neutralization test (SNT) and the Ab-ELISA are by far the most commonly used techniques for detecting specific antibodies to BVDV (Dubovi 2013). The SNT is a highly specific test, but it is expensive and time consuming due to a need for tissue culture (Cho et al. 1991; Horner and Orr 1993; Houe et al. 2006).

10.24 Equine Viral Arteritis

Virus infections are the most common in humans, particularly acute respiratory infections. Equine herpesvirus-1 (EHV-1), equine herpesvirus-4 (EHV-4), equine influenza virus (EIV), and equine arteritis virus (EAV) are the most significant viral pathogens that cause respiratory infections in horses (Mumford 1992; Ostlund 1993). The EHV-1 is a ubiquitous pathogen of all breeds of horses and other equids worldwide. BHV-1 can cause respiratory and neurological disease as well as abortion in pregnant mares. The disease causes major economic losses and welfare problems in horses. Both humoral and cell-mediated immune responses, are crucial for defense against and recovery from EHV-1 infection. A research study (Goehring et al. 2010) suggested that virus-neutralizing (VN) antibodies stimulated by vaccination did reduce the cell-associated viremia, but the mechanism is unknown. For example, although virus neutralising antibody specific for EHV-1 in serum can be associated with a reduction in the amount and duration of virus shedding, there are no significant effects on cell-associated viremia (Hannant et al. 1993). Because most of the viruses become intracellular shortly after attachment on the respiratory mucosal surface, and cytotoxic T lymphocytes (CTL) are primarily responsible for killing of cell-associated viruses, this may be the reason for failure of the VN antibodies to eliminate the cell-associated viremia (Kydd et al. 2003; Allen et al.

2004). According to the research conducted by Kydd et al. (2006), EHV-1 infection both naturally and experimentally stimulates the CTLs, and it has been demonstrated that the frequency of CTL precursors (CTLp) is a key mediator of immunity to BHV-1 (Kydd et al. 2003). The infected lymphocytes migrate from lymph nodes into the circulation, resulting in a cell-associated viraemia from 4 to 6 days post infection, and then EHV-1 is transported by infected PBMCs and spreads throughout the body. The cell-associated virus may spread to internal organs with this method, including the nervous system and uterus. Infected lymphocytes adhere to the endothelial cells in the small blood vessels supplying the placenta in the uterus. Infected endothelial cells initiates the formation of blood clots, which causes thrombosis and vascular damage (Edington et al. 1991; Smith et al. 1992). Vasculitis, an inflammation of blood vessels develops, which damages the placenta as a result of which the virus spreads to the fetus and causes abortion (Smith and Borchers 2001; Smith et al. 2010). It is hypothesized that uterine disease and/or fetal injury initiates a physiological cascade that causes the placenta to separate from the endometrium (Smith et al. 2004; Kydd et al. 2006).

When EHV-1-infected PBMCs enter the nervous system and infect the vascular endothelia of small arterioles and venules, results in neurological disease. The investigation has found that the recovery of the virus from the central nervous system frequently fails, suggesting that immune complexes may be important in the pathophysiology of this disease (Platt et al. 1980). According to Edington et al. (1986), EHV-1 infection of endothelial cells of the blood vessels in the nervous system can result in vasculitis, thrombosis, hypoxia, and secondary ischemic damage, which compromises the blood supply to neurons and ultimately cause diseases of the nervous system. Following a primary infection, EHV-1 establishes latent infection and persists in its host, just like other members of subfamily *Alphaherpesvirinae*. During latency, expression of the EHV-1 genome is repressed and only a viral RNA transcribed from the immediate early (IE) gene occurs, results in a latency-associated transcript (LAT). However, the precise role of LAT is unclear, and no infectious virus is produced (Roizman et al. 1992). The trigeminal ganglion, lymphoid tissues draining the respiratory tract, and peripheral blood leukocytes have been identified as the sites of EHV-1 latency (Edington et al. 1994; Slater et al. 1994; Chester et al. 1997; Smith et al. 1998). According to Smith et al. (1998), the majority of EHV-1 latency was found in CD5+/CD8+ T lymphocytes in peripheral blood leukocytes. By identifying the latent transforming growth factor-β in alveolar macrophages in 2000, showed that alveolar macrophages were also a site of latency (Chesters et al. 2000). Both the local immune response at the primary site of replication and a systemic immunological response, which includes antibodies, cytokines, and cellular components, are typically involved in herpesvirus infection, particularly EHV-1 infection.

To measure the serum antibodies with VN and complement fixing (CF) activity in vitro, serological assays were developed. These diagnostic methods demonstrated virus neutralization, which is also known as serum neutralizing (SN) and CF antibodies, are detectable from 2 weeks after experimental EHV-1 infection up to 1 year or less than 3 months, respectively, in the sera of infected horses. The VN antibodies are mainly type specific for a foal immunised with an inactivated EHV-1 vaccine; however, there was cross reactivity after immunisation with inactivated EHV-4 (Fitzpatrick and Studdert 1984). The VN antibodies are directed primarily against epitopes on glycoproteins gB and gC recognized by the immune systems of horses with EHV-1 infection or vaccination are the target of the VN antibodies. The CF antibodies, in contrast to VN antibodies, are typically undetectable for 3 months after infection. The epitopes recognised by CF antibodies are cross reactive with EHV-1 and EHV-4 proteins, resulting in an inaccurate diagnosis using CF antibodies alone (Crabb and Studdert 1993). In the past, various techniques were used to detect EHV-1 antibodies in serum samples, including the serum neutralization (SN) test, which is comparable to the VN test, CF test, and the EHV-1 gG-specific enzyme-linked immunosorbent assay (ELISA). Breathnach et al. (2001) analysed EHV-1 specific antibody responses by monitoring equine IgGa, IgGb, IgG (T), IgA, and IgM in nasal wash samples from weanling foals after primary and recurrent experimental infections with a virulent EHV-1 using ELISA. The IgA was the major antibody isotype detected upto a period of 13 weeks in nasal mucosa. The studies have reported that IgA is the main antibody isotype in the nasal mucosa for protecting the horses against various upper respiratory tract pathogens, including *Streptococcus equi* and EIV (Nelson et al. 1998; Hannant et al. 1999).

Numerous studies have reported the role of cytokine responses to EHV-1 infection by screening for the presence of nucleic acid or protein of cytokines namely, IFN-γ, IFN-α, IL-4, IL-10, and TNF-α (Paillot et al. 2005, 2007; Coombs et al. 2006; Soboll Hussey et al. 2011). The first 10 days after experimental infection of ponies with EHV-1 revealed the presence of interferons in nasal secretions and serum (Edington et al. 1989). The IFN-α/β, which is a component of type I IFNs, was detected in the upper respiratory tract. Both of these IFNs are crucial for defense against viral infection in other species, because they increase the synthesis of MHC class I molecules in infected cells, rendering them more vulnerable to killing by CD8+ CTLs (Jung et al. 2008). A single type II IFN termed as IFN-γ plays a significant role in the adaptive immune responses against intracellular pathogens.

The intracellular EHV-1 is effectively controlled by the cellular immune response, which in turn reduce or eliminate the cell-associated viremia (Soboll et al. 2010). The evaluation of cellular immune responses can be done by using a various methods, including cytokine mRNA expression, measurement of antigen-specific T-cells proliferation, CTL activity detection, and EHV-1 specific IFN-γ production. Proliferation of lymphocytes is commonly used as an indicator of immune status because proliferation usually precedes the development of effector functions. In previous studies, the immune responses to primary EHV-1 infection was investigated by incubating lymphocytes from infected horses with EHV-1 antigens (virus-specific lymphocyte response) or with phytohemagglutinin (PHA), a lectin that stimulates a non-specific lymphocyte responses (Dutta et al. 1980; Bumgardner et al. 1982; Hannant et al. 1991), and by subsequent determination of the uptake of methyl tritiated thymidine uptake([3H]-thymidine). Generally, these studies showed the proliferation of lymphocytes from reputedly primary infected horses towards EHV-1 antigens, suggesting previous, undetected exposure. Non-specific lymphocyte proliferation was found to increase after the PHA response, according to Dutta et al. (1980) and Bumgardner et al. (1982); although, several other investigations reported a decreased non-specific lymphocyte proliferation (Hannant et al. 1991; Charan et al. 1997; Van Der Meulen et al. 2006). To date, there are no studies reported on the response of CTL effectors following a primary EHV-1 infection. The EHV-1 becomes intracellular in lymph nodes within hours of contact with host cells, suggesting the importance of the cell-mediated immune responses to EHV-1 in vivo. BHV-1 infection causes an increase in CD8+ T lymphocytes in the blood and lungs (Lunn et al. 1991; Kydd et al. 1996).

The EHV-1 has evolved immune evasion strategies to overcome the host immunity, like other herpesviruses (Favoreel et al. 2006; Van De Walle et al. 2007). Numerous in vitro research studies reported the EHV-1-induced immunomodulation (Stokes and Wardley 1988; Hannant et al. 1991; Huemer et al. 1995; Charan et al. 1997; Rappocciolo et al. 2003). However, there are only few studies on the in vivo EHV-1 immune evasion mechanisms by considering the clinical outcomes and viraemia (Nugent et al. 2006; Goodman et al. 2007). The following are few examples of immune evasive strategies. Following EHV-1 infection of ponies, immunosuppression by reducing the proliferation of PBMCs in vitro in response to mitogens and viral antigens (Hannant et al. 1991, 1999), escaping from the antibody-dependent immune responses by inhibiting the viral antigen expression on cell surfaces (Van Der Meulen et al. 2003), inducing downregulation of MHC class I expression on infected cells (Rappocciolo et al. 2003), and inhibiting the transporter associated with antigen processing (TAP) protein and blocking viral peptide transport to MHC class I molecules in the endoplasmic reticulum. Studies on adaptive immune responses to EHV-1 are numerous (Mumford et al. 1987; Hannant et al. 1991; Crabb and Studdert 1996; Allen et al. 1999; Slater and Hannant 2000; Breathnach et al. 2001; Rosas et al. 2006; Soboll Hussey et al. 2011). The EHV-1 stimulates cellular and humoral immune responses. The VN antibodies function to reduce the amount and duration of nasopharyngeal virus shedding (Mumford et al. 1987; Hannant et al. 1993), but they do not significantly play a role in reducing the cell-associated viremia. The VN antibodies first appear approximately 2 weeks after EHV-1 infection (Hannant et al. 1993). But according to a study, commercial vaccination that contains an inactivated virus stimulates the production of VN antibodies, which was effective in reducing the viremia (Goehring et al. 2010). It has been reported that the number of circulating CTLp offers an immunological correlation of protection from infection and recovery (O'Neill et al. 1999; Kydd et al. 2003). Cellular immune responses, particularly MHC class I restricted CD8+ CTLs, are most crucial in protection against EHV-1 infection (O'Neill et al. 1999; Kydd et al. 2003, 2006).

Clinical signs may be absent or may include rhinitis, conjunctivitis, pyrexia, depression, anorexia, leukopenia, leg edema, stiffness of gait, rhinorrhea, and epiphora. Edema of the periorbital and supraorbital areas, midventral regions, scrotum, prepuce, and mammary gland, urticarial rash, and abortion also occur. Less commonly, intermandibular and shoulder edema, ataxia, mucosal papular eruptions, submaxillary lymphadenopathy, and severe respiratory distress may be seen (Timoney and McCollum 1993). The EAV can be associated with epidemic abortion. The EAV can occasionally fatal in adults (Lopez et al. 1996) but more frequently can be fatal in foals (Timoney 1984; Cole et al. 1986; Timoney and McCollum 1993; Golnik et al. 1981; Freeman et al. 1989; Vaala et al. 1992; Wilkins et al. 1995; Del Piero et al. 1997). Hypoxia, hypercapnia, respiratory acidosis sometimes complicated by metabolic acidosis, neutropenia/neutrophilia, lymphopenia/lymphocytosis, thrombocytopenia, and hyperfibrinogenemia are clinical pathological findings that have been reported in affected foals with EVA (Freeman et al. 1989; Vaala et al. 1992; Wilkins et al. 1995; Del Piero et al. 1997).

The etiologic agent and seroconversion along with the presence of pathological lesions, are used to make the diagnosis of EVA. A reliable method for identifying the EAV infection in horses is the detection of seroconversion with complement-dependent viral neutralization carried out using the Bucyrus strain in EAV-infected animals. The RK-13 cells, Vero cells, and equine lung cells are the three tissue culture cell lines generally used to isolate EAV. Other molecular methods, such as reverse transcription-polymerase chain reaction, have been utilized especially for the detection of genital transmission of the virus. Immunohistochemistry is commonly used to detect the presence of EAV in the affected tissues (Starick 1998; Ramina et al. 1999).

10.25 Conclusion

Reproductive problems like infertility, fetal death, and economic losses to the farmers are caused by microbes and other infectious organisms, which are major concerns. Following the infection in the uterus, innate immunity, local immune cells, and pattern-recognition receptors contribute significantly to the host defensive mechanisms. The non-specific defense against microorganisms include physical barriers like the skin and mucosa is known as innate immunity. The host cell response involves the secretion of prostaglandins and cytokines, which provides certain type of immunity to the uterus. The uterine endometrium has very important function is the release of steroidal hormone and development of immunity, which have greater influence during the parturition. Parturition is a time when both mother and fetus are at significant risk. After parturition, the uterine immunity has very important role in the host defence mechanism because most of the uterine infections like pyometra and retention of foetal membranes are commonly seen in animals after the parturition. The main goal for the postpartum reproductive health in dairy cattle is the uterus to undergo complete involution, free from infection and to have cyclic activities in regular interval in cows and enter into the breeding period regularly. Very important reproductive diseases like metritis, endometritis, dystocia, and retention of fetal membranes may decrease the involution process of uterus and alter the fertility potential of cattle and buffalo. A critical factor in preventing uterine infections is uterine immunity. Innate immunity is mediated by hematopoietic cells such as monocytes, macrophages, neutrophils, and natural killer cells. By identifying the bacteria known as pathogen-related molecular patterns, the cells of the innate immune system were able to recognize the presence of pathogens.

Animal diseases that are mostly prevalent in India require a serious attention and needs improved research facilities especially in the field of epidemiology and huge funding. Valid, state-wise, comprehensive research data especially in the field of epidemiology are necessary for planning and control of diseases that are endemic in India, otherwise implementation of control measures will be difficult and eradication will be impossible. Animal diseases not only pose a threat to the Indian economy but are also crucial for human health because of zoonotic nature. During the recent years, majority of the infectious emerging diseases affecting the human are originated from animals. Thus, it is logical to say safeguarding the animal health is most important for maintenance of human health. Epidemiological forecasting, prompt and accurate diagnosis, safer and higher-quality vaccines, sanitation practices, adequate infrastructure facilities for cold storage, and transport facilities to reach the vaccines for the remote areas where end users are living are necessary for the successful control of diseases. Modern diagnostic tests have made it easier to diagnose and distinguish between various diseases. Door delivery of veterinary services and better extension services for greater awareness to farmers will significantly enhance the possibility of eradication of diseases thus helping in control programmes. An understanding of the immunopathology of abortions caused by many etiological agents will guide and optimise the diagnostic approaches. It will be possible to develop control strategies by using mouse model systems for investigating the mechanisms of cell-associated viremia, abortion, latency, immune evasion, persistence, and immunity to reinfection.

References

Abdelhameed AR, Ahmed WM, Ekhnawy KI, Khadrawi HH (2009) Strategy trials for prevention of retained foetal membranes in a Friesian herd in Egypt. J Glob Vet 3:63–68

Adler B, de la Pena Moctezuma A (2010) Leptospira and leptospirosis. Vet Microbiol 140:287–296

Aitken ID, Longbottom D (2007) Chlamydial abortion. In: Aitken ID (ed) Diseases of sheep, 4th edn. Blackwell Scientific Ltd., Oxford, pp 105–112

Akira S, Uematsu S, Takeuchi O (2006) Pathogen recognition and innate immunity. J Cell 124: 783–801

Allen GP, Kydd JH, Slater JD and Smith KC. 1999. Advances in understanding of the pathogenesis, epidemiology, and immunological control of equid herpes virus abortion. In: Wernery U, Wade JF, Mumford JA, Kaaden OR, Equine infectious diseases VIII. Proceedings of the 8th International Conference, R & W Publications, New Market, ON. pp. 129-146.

Allen GP, Kydd JH, Slater JD, Smith KC (2004) Equid herpesvirus-1 (EHV-1) and -4 (EHV-4) infections. In: Coetzer JAW, Tustin RC (eds) Infectious diseases of livestock, 2nd edn. Oxford Press, Cape Town, pp 829–859

Almeria S, Araujo RN, Darwich L, Dubey JP, Gasbarre LC (2011) Cytokine gene expression at the materno-foetal interface after experimental *Neospora caninum* infection of heifers at 110 days of gestation. Parasite Immunol 33(9):517–523

Almeria S, Serrano B, Yàniz JL, Darwich L, López-Gatius F (2012) Cytokine gene expression profiles in peripheral blood mononuclear cells from *Neospora caninum* naturally infected dams throughout gestation. Vet Parasitol 183(3–4):237–243

Anderson TD, Meador VP, Cheville NF (1986) Pathogenesis of placentitis in the goat inoculated with *Brucella abortus*. I. Gross and histological lesions. Vet Pathol 23:219–226

Anderson ML, Kennedy PC, Blanchard MT, Barbano L, Chiu P, Walker RL, Manzer M, Hall MR, King DP, Stott JL (2006) Histochemical and immunohistochemical evidence of a bacterium associated with lesions of epizootic bovine abortion. J Vet Diagn Investig 18(1):76–80

Andrade MMC, Carneiro M, Medeiros AD, Neto VA, Vitor RWA (2013) Sero prevalence and risk factors associated with ovine toxoplasmosis in Northeast Brazil. Parasite 20:1–5

Andre-Fontaine G (2006) Canine leptospirosis--do we have a problem? Vet Microbiol 117:19–24

Archambaud C, Nahori MA, Pizarro-Cerda J, Cossart P, Dussurget O (2006) Control of Listeria superoxide dismutase by phosphorylation. J Biol Chem 281:31812–31822

Aydintug MK, Leid RW, Widders PR (1990) Antibody enhances killing of *Tritrichomonas foetus* by the alternative bovine complement pathway. Infect Immun 58:944–948

Aydintug MK, Widders PR, Leid RW (1993) Bovine polymorphonuclear leukocyte killing of *Tritrichomonas foetus*. Infect Immun 61:2995–3002

Azawi OI (2008) Postpartum uterine infection in cattle. J Anim Reprod Sci 105:187–208

Babiuk LA, van Drunen L, Hurk S, Tikoo SK (1996) Immunology of bovine herpesvirus 1 infection. Vet Microbiol 53:31–42

Baker JC (1995) The clinical manifestations of bovine viral diarrhoea infection. Vet Clin N Am Food Anim Pract 11:425–446

Barbuddhe SB, Malik SVS, Chakurkar EB, Kalorey DR (2008) Listeria: an emerging zoonotic and food borne pathogen. Lead paper presented at: National Symposium on Zoonoses and Biotechnological Applications, 2008 Feb 4–5, Nagpur Veterinary College, Maharashtra. Souvenir, pp 31–41

Barbuddhe SB, Malik SVS, Kumar A, Kalorey DR, Chakraborty T (2012) Epidemiology and risk management of listeriosis in India. Int J Food Microbiol 154:113–118

Beauregard KE, Lee KD, Collier RJ, Swanson JA (1997) pH dependent perforation of macrophage phagosomes by listeriolysin O from Listeria monocytogenes. J Exp Med 186:1159–1163

Becher P, Thiel HJ (2011) Pestivirus (flaviviridae). In: Tidona CA, Darai G (eds) Springer index of viruses, 2nd edn. Springer, Heidelberg, pp 483–488

Bell MJ, Roberts DJ (2007) The impact of uterine infection on a dairy cow's performance. J Theriogenol 68:1074–1079

Benson A, Pifer R, Behrendt CL, Hooper LV, Yarovinsky F (2009) Gut commensal bacteria direct a protective immune response against Toxoplasma gondii. Cell Host Microbe 6(2):187–196

Bernard WV (1993) Leptospirosis. Vet Clin N Am Equine Pract 9:435–444

Bharti AR, Nally JE, Ricaldi JN, Matthias MA, Diaz MM, Lovett MA, Levett PN, Gilman RH, Willig MR, Gotuzzo E, Vinetz JM (2003) Leptospirosis: a zoonotic disease of global importance. Lancet Infect Dis 3(12):757–771

Bhudevi B, Weinstock D (2001) Fluorogenic RT-PCR assay (TaqMan) for detection and classification of bovine viral diarrhea virus. Vet Microbiol 83:1–10

Bielefeldt-Ohmann H (1995) The pathologies of bovine viral diarrhoea virus infection. Vet Clin N Am Food Anim Pract 1:447–476

Bilinski MJ, Thorne JG, Oh MJ, Leonard S, Murrant C, Tayade C, Croy BA (2008) Uterine NK cells in murine pregnancy. Reprod BioMed Online 16:218–226

Billard E, Dornand J, Gross A (2007) Interaction of *Brucella suis* and *Brucella abortus* rough strains with human dendritic cells. Infect Immun 75:5916–5923

Blanchard PC, Ridpath JF, Walker JB, Hietala SK (2010) An outbreak of late term abortions, premature births and congenital deformities associated with a bovine viral diarrhea virus 1 subtype b that induces thrombocytopenia. J Vet Diagn Investig 22:128–131

Blanchard MT, Anderson ML, Hoar BR, Pires AFA, Blanchard PC, Yeargan BV, Teglas MB, Belshaw M, Stott JL (2014) Assessment of a fluorescent antibody test for the detection of antibodies against epizootic bovine abortion. J Vet Diagn Investig 26:622–630

Bliss SK, Marshall AJ, Zhang Y, Denkers EY (1999a) Human polymorphonuclear leukocytes produce IL-12, TNF-alpha and the chemokines macrophage-inflammatory protein-1 alpha and -1 beta in response to *Toxoplasma gondii* antigens. J Immunol 162(12):7369–7375

Bliss SK, Zhang Y, Denkers EY (1999b) Murine neutrophil stimulation by *Toxoplasma gondii* antigen drives high level production of IFN-gamma-independent IL-12. J Immunol 163(4): 2081–2088

Bliss SK, Gavrilescu LC, Alcaraz A, Denkers EY (2001) Neutrophil depletion during *Toxoplasma gondii* infection leads to impaired immunity and lethal systemic pathology. Infect Immun 69(8): 4898–4905

Boerner B, Weigelt W, Buhk HJ, Castrucci G, Ludwig H (1999) A sensitive and specific PCR/Southern blot assay for detection of bovine herpesvirus 4 in calves infected experimentally. J Virol Methods 83(1/2):169–180

Bolin SR, McClurkin AW, Coria MF (1985) Effects of bovine viral diarrhoea virus on the percentages and absolute numbers of circulating B and T lymphocytes in cattle. Am J Vet Res 46:884–886

BonDurant RH, Corbeil RR, Corbeil LB (1993) Immunization of virgin cows with surface antigen TF1-17 of *Tritrichomonas foetus*. Infect Immun 61:1385–1394

Bondurant RH (1997) Pathogenesis, diagnosis and management of trichomoniasis in cattle. Vet Clin N Am Food Anim Pract 13:345–361

Bondurant RH (1999) Inflammation in the bovine female reproductive tract. J Anim Sci 77:101–110

Borel N, Kempf E, Hotzel H, Schubert E, Torgerson P, Slickers P, Ehricht R, Tasara T, Pospischil A, Sachse K (2008) Direct identification of chlamydiae from clinical samples using a DNA microarray assay – a validation study. Mol Cell Probes 22:55–64

Boschiroli ML, Foulongne V, O'Callaghan D (2001) Brucellosis: a worldwide zoonosis. Curr Opin Microbiol 4:58–64

Boughattas S, Ayari K, Sa T, Aoun K, Bouratbine A (2014) Survey of the parasite *Toxoplasma gondii* in human consumed ovine meat in Tunis City. PLoS One 9(1):e85044

Breathnach CC, Yeargan MR, Sheoran AS, Allen GP (2001) The mucosal humoral immune response of the horse to infective challenge and vaccination with equine herpesvirus-1 antigens. Equine Vet J 33:651–657

Bricker BJ (2002) PCR as a diagnostic tool for brucellosis. Vet Microbiol 90:435–446

Brownlie J (1990) Pathogenesis of mucosal disease and molecular aspects of bovine virus diarrhoea virus. Vet Microbiol 23:371–382

Brownlie J, Clarke MC, Howard CJ (1984) Experimental production of fatal mucosal disease in cattle. Vet Rec 114:535–536

Brownlie J, Clarke MC, Howard CJ, Pocock DH (1987) Pathogenesis and epidemiology of bovine virus diarrhoea infection of cattle. Annal Rech Vet 18:157–166

Brownlie J, Hooper LB, Thompson I, Collins ME (1998) Maternal recognition of foetal infection with bovine virus diarrhoea virus (BVDV) – the bovine pestivirus. Clin Diagn Virol 10:141–150

Brugere-Picoux J (2008) Ovine listeriosis. Small Rumin Res 76:12–20

Brunham RC, Rey-Ladino J (2005) Immunology of *Chlamydia* infection: implications for a *Chlamydia trachomatis* vaccine. Nat Rev Immunol 5:149–161

Bruun J, Ersbull AR, Alban L (2002) Risk factors for metritis in Danish dairy cows. J Prevent Vet Med 54:179–190

Buckley F, Dillon P, Mee JF (2010) Major management factors associated with the variation in the reproductive performance in Irish dairy herds. Final Report Project 5070. http://www.agresearch.teagasc.ie/moorepar

Bumgardner MK, Dutta SK, Campbell DL, Myrup AC (1982) Lymphocytes from ponies experimentally infected with equine Herpes virus 1: Subpopulation dynamics and their response to mitogens. Am J Vet Res 43:1308–1310

Butler JE (1983) Bovine immunoglobulins an augmented review. J Vet Immunol Immunopathol 43:43–52

Butt BM, Besser TE, Senger PL, Windders PR (1993) Specific antibody to Haemophilus somnus in the bovine uterus following intramuscular immunization. J Infect Immun 61:2558–2562

Buxton D, Anderson IE, Longbottom D, Livingstone M, Wattegadera S, Entrican G (2002) Ovine chlamydial abortion: characterization of the inflammatory immune response in placental tissues. J Comp Pathol 127:133–141

Campero CM, Ladds PW, Hoffmann D, Duffield B, Watson D, Fordyce G (1990) Immunopathology of experimental *Brucella abortus* strain 19 infection of the genitalia of bulls. Vet Immunol Immunopathol 24:235–246

Campero CM, Rodriguez Dubra C, Bolondi A, Cacciato C, Cobo E, Perez S, Odeon A, Cipolla A, Bondurant RH (2003) Two-step (culture and PCR) diagnostic approach for differentiation of non-*T. foetus* trichomonads from genitalia of virgin bulls in Argentina. Vet Parasitol 112:167–175

Campos MA, Rosinha GM, Almeida IC, Salgueiro XS, Jarvis BW, Splitter GA, Qureshi N, Bruna-Romero O, Gazzinelli RT, Oliveira SC (2004) Role of toll like receptor 4 in induction of cell-mediated immunity and resistance to *Brucella abortus* infection in mice. Infect Immun 72:176–186

Canton GJ, Katzer F, Benavides-Silván J, Maley SW, Palarea-Albaladejo J, Pang Y, Smith S, Bartley PM, Rocchi M, Innes EA, Chianini F (2013) Phenotypic characterisation of the cellular immune infiltrate in placentas of cattle following experimental inoculation with *Neospora caninum* in late gestation. Vet Res 44(1):60

Canton GJ, Konrad JL, Moore DP, Caspe SG, Palarea-Albaladejo J, Campero CM, Chianini F (2014) Characterization of immune cell infiltration in the placentome of water buffaloes (*Bubalus bubalis*) infected with *Neospora caninum* during pregnancy. J Comp Pathol 150(4):463–468

Capita R, Alonso-Calleja C, Moreno B, Garcia-Fernandez MC (2001) Occurrence of *Listeria* species in retail poultry meat and comparison of a cultural immunoassay for their detection. Int J Food Microbiol 65:75–82

Carpentier B, Cerf O (2011) Review: Persistence of *Listeria monocytogenes* in food industry equipment and premises. Int J Food Microbiol 145:1–8

Carvalho Neta AV, Stynen AP, Paixão TA, Miranda KL, Silva FL, Roux CM, Tsolis RM, Everts RE, Lewin HA, Adams LG, Carvalho AF, Lage AP, Santos RL (2008) Modulation of the bovine trophoblastic innate immune response by *Brucella abortus*. Infect Immun 76(5):1897–1907

Cavalcanti MG, Mesquita JS, Madi K, Feijo DF, Assuncao-Miranda I, Souza HS and Bozza MT. 2011. MIF participates in *Toxoplasma gondii*-induced pathology following oral infection.

Cenci-Goga BT, Ciampelli A, Sechi P, Veronesi F, Moretta I, Cambiotti V, Thompson PN (2013) Seroprevalence and risk factors for *Toxoplasma gondii* in sheep in Grosseto district, Tuscany, Italy. BMC Vet Res 9(25):1–8

Charan S, Palmer K, Chester P, Mire-Sluis AR, Meager A, Edington N (1997) Transforming growth factor-β induced by live or ultraviolet-inactivated equid herpes virus type-1 mediates immuno suppression in the horse. Immunology 90:586–591

Chase CCL (2013) The impact of BVDV infection on adaptive immunity. Biologicals 41:52–60

Chauhan RS, Rana JMS (2010) Recent advances in immuno biotechnology. IBT, Patwadangar

Chauhan HC, Biswas SK, Chand K, Rehman W, Das B, Dadawala AI, Chandel BS, Kher HN, Mondal B (2014) Isolation of bluetongue virus serotype 1 from aborted goat fetuses. Rev Sci Tech 33(3):803–812

Chester PM, Allsop R, Purewal A, Edington N (1997) Detection of latency-associated transcripts of equid herpesvirus 1 in equine leukocytes but not in trigeminal ganglia. J Virol 71:3437–3443

Chesters PM, Hughes A, Edington N (2000) Equid Herpesvirus 1: platelets and alveolar macrophages are potential sources of activated TGF-B1 in the horse. Vet Immunol Immunopathol 75:71–79

Cheville NF, Stevens MG, Jensen AE, Tatum FM, Halling SM (1993) Immune responses and protection against infection and abortion in cattle experimentally vaccinated with mutant strains of *Brucella abortus*. Am J Vet Res 54:1591–1597

Cho HJ, Masri SA, Deregt D, Yeo SG, Thomas EJ (1991) Sensitivity and specificity of an enzyme-linked immunosorbent assay for the detection of bovine viral diarrhea virus antibody in cattle. Can J Vet Res 55:56–59

Choy HA, Kelley MM, Chen TL, Moller AK, Matsunaga J, Haake DA (2007) Physiological osmotic induction of *Leptospira interrogans* adhesion: LigA and LigB bind extracellular matrix proteins and fibrinogen. Infect Immun 75(5):2441–2450

Cobo ER, Favetto PH, Lane VM, Friend A, Van Hooser K, Mitchell J, BonDurant RH (2007) Sensitivity and specificity of culture and PCR of smegma samples of bulls experimentally infected with *Tritrichomonas foetus*. Theriogen 68:853–860

Coetzee P, Stokstad M, Myrmel M, Mutowembwa P, Loken T, Venter EH, Van Vuuren M (2013) Transplacental infection in goats experimentally infected with a European strain of bluetongue virus serotype 8. Vet J 197(2):335–341

Cole JR, Hall RF, Gosser HS, Hendricks JB, Pursell AR, Senne DA, Pearson JE, Gipson CA (1986) Transmissibility and abortogenic effect of equine viral arteritis in mares. J Am Vet Med Assoc 189:769–771

Collado MC, Rautava S, Aakko J, Isolauri E, Salminen S (2016) Human gut colonisation may be initiated in utero by distinct microbial communities in the placenta and amniotic fluid. J Sci Rep 6:23129

Combe CL, Curiel TJ, Moretto MM, Khan IA (2005) NK cells help to induce CD8(+)-T-cell immunity against *Toxoplasma gondii* in the absence of CD4(+) T cells. Infect Immun 73(8): 4913–4921

Connor EE, Cates EA, Williams JL, Bannerman DD (2006) Cloning and radiation hybrid mapping of bovine toll like receptor 4 (TLR-4) signaling molecules. J Vet Immunol Immunopathol 112: 302–308

Coombs DK, Patton T, Kohler AK, Soboll G, Breathnach C, Townsend HG, Lunn DP (2006) Cytokine responses to EHV-1 infection in immune and non-immune ponies. Vet Immunol Immunopathol 111:109–116

Copin R, De Baetselier P, Carlier Y, Letesson JJ, Muraille E (2007) MyD88-dependent activation of B220-CD11b+LY-6C+ dendritic cells during *Brucella melitensis* infection. J Immunol 178: 5182–5191

Corbeil LB (1994) Vaccination strategies against *Tritrichomonas foetus*. Parasitol Today 10:103–106

Corbeil LB, Blau K, Inzana TJ, Nielsen KH, Jacobson RH, Corbeil RR, Winter AJ (1988) Killing of *Brucella abortus* by bovine serum. Infect Immun 56:3251–3261

Corbeil LB, Hodgson JL, Jones DW, Corbeil RR, Widders PR, Stephens LR (1989) Adherence of *Tritrichomonas foetus* to bovine vaginal epithelial cells. Infect Immun 57:2158–2165

Corbeil LB, Hodgson JL, Widders PR (1991) Immunoglobulin binding by *Tritrichomonas foetus*. J Clin Microbiol 29:2710–2714

Correa D, Canedo-Solares I, Ortiz-Alegria LB, Caballero-Ortega H, Rico-Torres CP (2007) Congenital and acquired toxoplasmosis: diversity and role of antibodies in different compartments of the host. Parasite Immunol 29(12):651–660

Cosendey-Kezenleite RIJ, Rodrigues de Oliveira FC, Frazao-Teixeira, Dubey JP, Nunes de Souza G, Ferreira AMR, Lilenbaum W (2014) Occurrence and risk factors associated to *Toxoplasma gondii* infection in sheep from Rio de Janeiro, Brazil. Tropical Animal Health and Production 46(8):1463–1466

Cossart P (2011) Illuminating the landscape of hostpathogen interactions with the bacterium *Listeria monocytogenes*. Proc Natl Acad Sci U S A 108:19484–19491

Crabb BS, Studdert MJ (1993) Epitopes of glycoprotein g of equine herpesviruses 4 and 1 located near the C termini elicit type specific antibody responses in the natural host. J Virol 67:6332–6338

Crabb BS, Studdert MJ (1996) Equine rhinopneumonitis (equine herpesvirus 4) and equine abortion (equine herpesvirus 1). In: Studdert MJ (ed) Virus infections of equines. Elsevier Sciences, Philadelphia, PA, pp 11–37

Crawford RP, Huber JD, Adams BS (1990) Epidemiology and surveillance. In: Nielsen K, Duncan JR (eds) Animal brucellosis. CRC Press, Boca Raton, FL, pp 131–151

Cronin JG, Turner ML, Goetze L, Bryant CE, Sheldon IM (2012) Toll like receptor 4 and MYD88-dependent signaling mechanisms of the innate immune system are essential for the response to lipopolysaccharide by epithelial and stromal cells of the bovine endometrium. J Biol Reprod 86: 51

Czaplicki G, Thiry E (1998) An association exists between bovine herpesvirus-4 seropositivity and abortion in cows. Prevent Vet Med 33(1/4):235–240

Czuczman MA, Fattouh R, van Rijn JM, Canadien V, Osborne S, Muise AM, Kuchroo VK, Higgins DE, Brumell JH (2014) *Listeria monocytogenes* exploits efferocytosis to promote cell-to-cell spread. Nature 509(7499):230–234

Da Motta AC, Vieira MI, Bondan C, Edelweiss MI, Dametto MA, Gomes A (2008) Ovine abortion associated with toxoplasmosis: serological, anatomo-pathological and immunohistochemistry characterization. Brazil J Vet Parasitol 17(Suppl 1):204–208

Dagleish MP, Benavides J, Chianini F (2010) Immunohistochemical diagnosis of infectious diseases of sheep. Small Rumin Res 92(1–3):19–35

Dannacher G, Fedida M, Perrin M, Moussa A, Coudert M (1980) Infectious bovine rhinotracheitis. Its place in respiratory pathology. Rev Med Vet 131:359–368

De Azevedo NL, De Souza W (1992) A cytochemical study of the interaction between *Tritrichomonas foetus* and mouse macrophages. Parasitol Res 78:545–552

De Azevedo NL, De Souza W (1996) An ultrastructural and cytochemical study of *Tritrichomonas foetus*-eosinophil interaction. J Submicrosc Cytol Pathol 28:243–249

Debierre-Grockiego F, Campos MA, Azzouz N, Schmidt J, Bieker U, Resende MG, Mansur DS, Weingart R, Schmidt RR, Golenbock DT, Gazzinelli RT, Schwarz RT (2007) Activation of TLR2 and TLR4 by glycosylphosphatidylinositols derived from *Toxoplasma gondii*. J Immunol 179(2):1129–1137

Del Piero F, Wilkins PA, Lopez JW, Glaser AL, Dubovi EJ, Schlafer DH, Lein DH (1997) Equine viral arteritis in newborn foals: clinical, pathological, serological, microbiological and immunohistochemical observations. Equine Vet J 29:178–185

Del Rio L, Bennouna S, Salinas J, Denkers EY (2001) CXCR2 deficiency confers impaired neutrophil recruitment and increased susceptibility during *Toxoplasma gondii* infection. J Immunol 167(11):6503–6509

Denis M, Slaoui M, Keil G (1993) Identification of different target glycoproteins for bovine herpesvirus-1 specific cytotoxic T lymphocytes depending on the method of *in vitro* stimulation. Immunology 78:7–13

Denkers EY, Gazzinelli RT, Martin D, Sher A (1993) Emergence of NK1.1+ cells as effectors of IFN-gamma dependent immunity to *Toxoplasma gondii* in MHC class I-deficient mice. J Exp Med 178(5):1465–1472

Denkers EY, Yap G, Scharton-Kersten T, Charest H, Butcher BA, Caspar P, Heiny S, Sher A (1997) Perforin-mediated cytolysis plays a limited role in host resistance to *Toxoplasma gondii*. J Immunol 159(4):1903–1908

Dhaliwal GS, Murray RD, Dobson H, Montgomery J, Ellis WA, Baker J (1996) Presence of antigen and antibodies in serum and genital discharges of cows from dairy herds naturally infected with Leptospira interrogans serovar hardjo. J Res Vet Sci 60:163–167

Diament D, Brunialti MK, Romero EC, Kallas EG, Salomao R (2002) Peripheral blood mononuclear cell activation induced by *Leptospira interrogans* glycolipoprotein. Infect Immun 70: 1677–1683

Disson O, Lecuit M (2013) *In vitro* and *in vivo* models to study human listeriosis: mind the gap. Microbes Infect 15:971–980

Donofrio G, Herath S, Sartori C, Cavirani S, Flammini CF, Sheldon IM (2007) Bovine herpesvirus 4 is tropic for bovine endometrial cells and modulates endocrine function. Reproduction 134: 183–187

Dramsi S, Biswas I, Maguin E, Braun L, Mastroeni P, Cossart P (1995) Entry of *Listeria monocytogenes* into hepatocytes requires expression of InIB, a surface protein of the internalin multigene family. Mol Microbiol 16:251–261

Dubey JP (2010) Toxoplasmosis of animals and humans, 2nd edn. CRC Press, Boca Raton, FL

Dubey JP, Desmonts G (1987) Serological responses of equids fed *Toxoplasma gondii* oocysts. Equine Vet J 19(4):337–339

Dubovi EJ (2013) Laboratory diagnosis of bovine viral diarrhea virus. Biologicals 41:8–13

Dubuisson J, Thiry E, Bublot M, Pastoret PP (1987) Role of complement in the neutralization of bovid herpesvirus 4. Ann Med Vet 131(1):69–73

Duenas AI, Orduna A, Crespo MS, Garcia-Rodriguez C (2004) Interaction of endotoxins with Toll-like receptor 4 correlates with their endotoxic potential and may explain the proinflammatory effect of *Brucella* spp. LPS. Int Immunol 16:1467–1475

Dunay IR, Damatta RA, Fux B, Presti R, Greco S, Colonna M, Sibley LD (2008) Gr1(+) inflammatory monocytes are required for mucosal resistance to the pathogen *Toxoplasma gondii*. Immunity 29(2):306–317

Dunay IR, Fuchs A, Sibley LD (2010) Inflammatory monocytes but not neutrophils are necessary to control infection with *Toxoplasma gondii* in mice. Infect Immun 78(4):1564–1570

Dussurget O, Pizarro-Cerda J, Cossart P (2004) Molecular determinants of *Listeria monocytogenes* virulence. Annu Rev Microbiol 58:587–610

Dutta SK, Myrup A, Bumgardner MK (1980) Lymphocyte responses to virus and mitogen in ponies during experimental infection with equine herpesvirus 1. Am J Vet Res 41:2066–2068

Eaglesome MD, Garcia MM (1992) Microbial agents associated with bovine genital tract infections and semen. Part 1. *Brucella, Leptospira, Campylobacter fetus* and *Tritrichomonas foetus*. Vet Bull 62:743–775

Edington N, Bridges CG, Patel JR (1986) Endothelial cell infection and thrombosis in paralysis caused by equid Herpesvirus-1: equine stroke. Arch Virol 90:111–124

Edington N, Bridges CG, Griffiths L (1989) Equine interferons following exposure to equid herpesvirus-1 or -4. J Interf Res 9:389–392

Edington N, Smyth B, Griffiths L (1991) The role of endothelial cell infection in the endometrium, placenta and foetus of equid herpesvirus 1 (EHV-1) abortions. J Comp Pathol 104:379–387

Edington N, Welch HM, Griffiths L (1994) The prevalence of latent equid herpesviruses in the tissues of 40 abattoir horses. Equine Vet J 26:140–142

Edwards JF, Dubey JP (2013) *Toxoplasma gondii* abortion storm in sheep on a Texas farm and isolation of mouse virulent atypical genotype *T. gondii* from an aborted lamb from a chronically infected ewe. Vet Parasitol 192(1–3):129–136

Egan CE, Cohen SB, Denkers EY (2011) Insights into inflammatory bowel disease using *Toxoplasma gondii* as an infectious trigger. Immunol Cell Biol 90(7):668–675

Egyed L, Ballagi-Pordany A, Bartha A, Belak S (1996) Studies of *in vivo* distribution of bovine herpesvirus type 4 in the natural host. J Clin Microbiol 34(5):1091–1095

Egyed L, Kluge JP, Batha A (1997) Histological studies of bovine herpesvirus type 4 infection in non-ruminant species. Vet Microbiol 51:283–289

Ellis WA, McParland PJ, Bryson DG, Thiermann AB, Montgomery J (1986) Isolation of leptospires from the genital tract and kidneys of aborted sows. Vet Rec 118:294–295

Ellis JA, Luedke AJ, Davis WC, Wechsler SJ, Mecham JO, Pratt DL, Elliott JD (1990) T lymphocyte subset alterations following bluetongue virus infection in sheep and cattle. Vet Immunol Immunopathol 24(1):49–67

Enright FM, Walker JV, Jeffers G, Deyoe BL (1984) Cellular and humoral responses of *Brucella abortus*-infected bovine fetuses. Am J Vet Res 45:424–430

Entrican G (2002) Immune regulation during pregnancy and host-pathogen interactions in infectious abortion. J Comp Pathol 126:79–94

Estavoyer JM, Racadot E, Couetdic G, Leroy J, Grosperrin L (1991) Tumor necrosis factor in patients with leptospirosis. Rev Infect Dis 13:1245–1246

Esteban-Redondo I, Innes EA (1997) *Toxoplasma gondii* infection in sheep and cattle. Comp Immunol Microbiol Infect Dis 20(2):191–196

Estes DM, Brown WC (2002) Type 1 and type 2 responses in regulation of Ig isotypes expression in cattle. J Vet Immunol Immunopathol 90:1–10

Everett KD, Andersen AA (1999) Identification of nine species of the Chlamydiaceae using PCR RFLP. Int J Syst Bacteriol 49:803–813

Favoreel HW, Van Minnebruggen G, Van De Walle GR, Ficinska J, Nauwynck HJ (2006) Herpesvirus interference with virus-specific antibodies: bridging antibodies, internalizing antibodies, and hiding from antibodies. Vet Microbiol 113:257–263

Felleisen RJ, Schimid-Lambelet N, Gottstein B (1997) Comparative evaluation of methods for the diagnosis of bovine *Tritrichomonas foetus* infection. J Protozool Res 7:90–101

Felleisen RSJ, Lambelet N, Bachmann P, Nicolet J, Muller N, Gottstein B (1998) Detection of *Tritrichomonas foetus* by PCR and DNA enzyme immunoassay based on rRNA gene unit sequences. J Clin Microbiol 36:513–519

Fitzgerald PR (1986) Bovine trichomoniasis in parasites: epidemiology and control. Vet Clin N Am Food Anim Pract 2:277–282

Fitzpatrick DR, Studdert MJ (1984) Immunologic relationships between equine herpesvirus type 1 (equine abortion virus) and type 4 (equine rhinopneumonitis virus). Am J Vet Res 45:1947–1952

Fortunato SJ, Menon R, Lombardi SJ (2001) Support for an infection induced apoptotic pathway in human fetal membranes. Am J Obstet Gynaecol 184:1392–1398

Foster NM, Luedke AJ, Parsonson IM, Walton TE (1991) Temporal relationships of viremia, interferon activity, and antibody responses of sheep infected with several bluetongue virus strains. Am J Vet Res 52(2):192–196

Fox JG, Rogers AB, Whary MT, Ge Z, Taylor NS, Xu S, Horwitz BH, Erdman SE (2004) Gastroenteritis in NF-κB-deficient mice is produced with wild-type *Campylobacter jejuni* but not with *C. jejuni* lacking cytolethal distending toxin despite persistent colonization with both strains. Infect Immun 72:1116–1125

Franasiak JM, Scott RT (2017) Endometrial microbiome. J Curr Opin Obstet Gynecol 29:146–152

Frazer LC, O'Connell CM, Andrews CW Jr, Zurenski MA, Darville T (2011) Enhanced neutrophil longevity and recruitment contribute to the severity of oviduct pathology during *Chlamydia muridarum* infection. Infect Immun 79:4029–4041

Freeman KP, Cline JM, Simmons R, Wilkins PA, Cudd TA, Perry BJ (1989) Recognition of bronchopulmonary dysplasia in a newborn foal. Equine Vet J 21:292–296

French LR, Northey DL (1983) Inhibitory effect of the bovine conceptus on lymphocyte stimulation. J Anim Sci 57:456–465

Funkhouser LJ, Bordenstein SR (2013) Mom knows best: the universality of maternal microbial transmission. PLoS Biol 11:1001631

Gamlen T, Richards KH, Mankouri J, Hudson L, McCauley J, Harris M, Macdonald A (2010) Expression of the NS3 protease of cytopathogenic bovine viral diarrhea virus results in the induction of apoptosis but does not block activation of the beta interferon promoter. J Gen Virol 91:133–144

Ganguly S, Mukhopadhya SK, Paul I (2008) Studies on seroprevalence of infectious bovine rhinotracheitis in cattle population of West Bengal. Indian journal of Comparative Microbiology. Immunol Infect Dis 29(1–2):12 16

Gault RA, Kvasnicka WG, Hanks D, Hanks M, Hall MR (1995) Specific antibodies in serum and vaginal mucus of heifers inoculated with a vaccine containing *Tritrichomonas foetus*. Am J Vet Res 56:454–459

Gautam G, Nakao T, Yusuf M, Koike K (2009) Prevalence of endometritis during postpartum period and its impact on subsequent reproductive performance in two Japanese dairy herds. J Anim Reprod Sci 116:175–187

Gautam G, Nakao T, Koike K, Long ST, Yusuf M, Kanasinghe RMSBK, Hayashi A (2010) Spontaneous recovery or persistence of postpartum endometritis and risk factors for its persistence in Holstein cows. J Theriogenol 73:163–179

Gazzinelli R, Xu Y, Hieny S, Cheever A, Sher A (1992) Simultaneous depletion of CD4+ and CD8+ T lymphocytes is required to reactivate chronic infection with *Toxoplasma gondii*. J Immunol 149(1):175–180

Gazzinelli RT, Hieny S, Wynn TA, Wolf S, Sher A (1993) Interleukin 12 is required for the T lymphocyte-independent induction of interferon gamma by an intracellular parasite and induces resistance in T-cell-deficient hosts. Proc Natl Acad Sci U S A 90(13):6115–6119

Gazzinelli RT, Wysocka M, Hayashi S, Denkers EY, Hieny S, Caspar P, Trinchieri G, Sher A (1994) Parasite-induced IL-12 stimulates early IFN-gamma synthesis and resistance during acute infection with *Toxoplasma gondii*. J Immunol 153(6):2533–2543

Gedde MM, Higgins DE, Tilney LG, Portnoy DA (2000) Role of listeriolysin O in cell-to-cell spread of *Listeria monocytogenes*. Infect Immun 68:999–1003

George LW (2002) Listeriosis. In: Smith BP (ed) Large animal internal medicine. Mosby, St Louis, MO, pp 946–949

Ghosh S, May MJ, Kopp EB (1998) NF kappa B and Rel proteins evolutionarily conserved mediators of immune responses. J Annu Rev Immunol 16:225–260

Gilbert RO, Shin ST, Guard CL, Erb HN, Frajblat M (2005) Prevalence of endometritis and its effect on reproductive performance in dairy cows. J Theriogenol 64:1879–1888

Goehring LS, Wagner B, Bigbie R, Hussey SB, Morley PS, Lunn DP (2010) Control of EHV-1 viremia and nasal shedding by commercial vaccines. Vaccine 28:5203–5211

Gogolin Ewens KJ, Lee CS, Mercer WR, Brandon MR (1989) Site directed differences in the immune response to the fetus. J Br Soc Immunol 66:312–317

Goldenberg RL, Hauth JC, Andrews WW (2000) Intrauterine infection and preterm delivery. N Engl J Med 342:1500–1507

Golding B, Scott DE, Scharf O, Huang LY, Zaitseva M, Laphan C, Eller N, Golding H (2001) Immunity and protection against *Brucella abortus*. Microbes Infect 3:43–48

Golnik W, Michalska Z, Michalak T (1981) Natural equine viral arteritis in foals. Schweiz Arch Tierheilkd 123:523–533

Goodman LB, Loregian A, Perkins GA, Nugent J, Buckles EL, Mercorelli B, Kydd JH, Palu G, Smith KC, Osterrieder N, Davis-Poynter N (2007) A point mutation in a herpesvirus polymerase determines neuropathogenicity. PLoS Pathog 3:e160

Gopalakrishnan A, Dimri U, Saminathan M, Yatoo MI, Bhuvana Priya G, Gopinath D, Sujatha V, Ajith Y, Suthar A, Lawrence C, Dhama K (2016) Virulence factors, intracellular survivability and mechanism of evasion from host immune response by Brucella: an overview. J Anim Plant Sci 26(6):1542–1555

Grant EJ, Lilly ST, Herath S, Sheldon IM (2007) Escherichia coli lipopolysaccharide modulates bovine luteal cell function. J Vet Rec 161:695–696

Grogono-Thomas R, Blaser MJ, Ahmadi M, Newell DG (2003) Role of S-layer protein antigenic diversity in the immune responses of sheep experimentally challenged with Campylobacter fetus subsp. fetus. Infect Immun 71(1):147–154

Grooms DL (2004) Reproductive consequences of infection with bovine viral diarrhea virus. Vet Clin N Am Food Anim Pract 20:5–19

Grooms DL (2006) Reproductive losses caused by bovine viral diarrhea virus and leptospirosis. Theriogenology 66:624–628

Guan H, Moretto M, Bzik DJ, Gigley J, Khan IA (2007) NK cells enhance dendritic cell response against parasite antigens via NKG2D pathway. J Immunol 179(1):590–596

Halonen SK, Chiu F, Weiss LM (1998) Effect of cytokines on growth of *Toxoplasma gondii* in murine astrocytes. Infect Immun 66(10):4989–4993

Hammouda NA, Rashwan EA, Hussien ED, Abo El-Naga I, Fathy FM (1995) Measurement of respiratory burst of TNF and IL-1 cytokine activated murine peritoneal macrophages challenged with *Toxoplasma gondii*. J Egypt Soc Parasitol 25(3):683–691

Hamon MA, Cossart P (2011) KC efflux is required for histone H3 dephosphorylation by *Listeria monocytogenes* listeriolysin O and other pore-forming toxins. Infect Immun 79:2839–2846

Hamon MA, Batsche E, Regnault B, Tham TN, Seveau S, Muchardt C, Cossart P (2007) Histone modifications induced by a family of bacterial toxins. Proc Natl Acad Sci U S A 104:13467–13472

Han YW, Redline RW, Li M, Yin L, Hill GB, McCormick TS (2004) *Fusobacterium nucleatum* induces premature and term stillbirths in pregnant mice implication of oral bacteria in preterm birth. J Microbiol Immunol Infect 72:2272–2279

Han YW, Shen T, Chung P, Buhimschi IA, Buhimschi CS (2009) Uncultivated bacteria as etiologic agents of intra-amniotic inflammation leading to preterm birth. J Clin Microbiol 47:38–47

Han YW, Fardini Y, Chen C, Iacampo KG, Peraino VA, Shamonki JM (2010) Term stillbirth caused by oral Fusobacterium nucleatum. J Clin Obstet Gynecol 115:442–445

Hannant D, O'Neill T, Jessett DM, Mumford JA (1991) Evidence for non-specific immunosuppression during the development of immune responses to equid herpesvirus-1. Equine Vet J 23:41–45

Hannant D, Jessett D, O'Neill T, Dolby CA, Cook RF, Mumford JA (1993) Responses of ponies to equid herpesvirus-1 ISCOM vaccination and challenge with virus to the homologous strain. Res Vet Sci 54:299–305

Hannant D, O'Neill T, Ostlund EN, Kydd JH, Hopkin PJ, Mumford JA (1999) Equid herpesvirus-induced immunosuppression is associated with lymphoid cells and not soluble circulating factors. Viral Immunol 12:313–321

Hansen PJ (1997) Interactions between the immune system and the bovine conceptus. J Theriogenol 47:121–130

Hansen LK, Becher N, Bastholm S, Glavind J, Ramsing M, Kim CJ (2014) The cervical mucus plug inhibits, but does not block, the passage of ascending bacteria from the vagina during pregnancy. Am J Obstet Gynecol 93:8–102

Hariharan MJ, Nataraj C, Srikumaran S (1993) Down regulation of murine MHC class I expression by bovine herpesvirus 1. Viral Immunol 6:273–284

Hartigan P (1997) Human brucellosis: epidemiology and clinical manifestations. Ir Vet J 50:179–180

Hauser WE Jr, Sharma SD, Remington JS (1982) Natural killer cells induced by acute and chronic toxoplasma infection. Cell Immunol 69(2):330–346

Hayashi F, Smith KD, Ozinsky A, Hawn TR, Yi EC, Goodlett DR, Eng JK, Akira S, Underhill DM, Aderem A (2001) The innate immune response to bacterial flagellin is mediated by Toll-like receptor 5. Nature 410:1099–1103

He Y (2012) Analyses of *Brucella* pathogenesis, host immunity, and vaccine targets using systems biology and bioinformatics. Front Cell Infect Microbiol 2:2

Hemmatzadeh F, Amini F (2009) Dot-blot enzyme immunoassay for the detection of bovine viral diarrhea virus antibodies. Veterinarski Arhiv 79:343–350

Herath S, Dobson H, Bryant CE, Sheldon IM (2006) Use of the cow as a large animal model of uterine infection and immunity. J Reprod Immunol 69:13–22

Hickey DK, Patel MV, Fahey JV, Wira CR (2011) Innate and adaptive immunity at mucosal surfaces of the female reproductive tract: stratification and integration of immune protection against the transmission of sexually transmitted infections. J Reprod Immunol 88:94–184

Hirata T, Osuga Y, Hirota Y, Koga K, Yoshino O, Harada M, Morimoto C, Yano T, Nishii O, Tsutsumi O, Taketani Y (2005) Evidence for the presence of toll like receptor 4 system in the human endometrium. J Clin Endocrinol Metab 90:548–556

Hodgson JL, Jones DW, Widders PR, Corbeil LB (1990) Characterization of *Tritrichomonas foetus* antigens by use of monoclonal antibodies. Infect Immun 58:3078–3083

Hook CE, Telyatnikova N, Goodall JC, Braud VM, Carmichael AJ, Wills MR, Gaston JS (2004) Effects of *Chlamydia trachomatis* infection on the expression of natural killer (NK) cell ligands and susceptibility to NK cell lysis. Clin Exp Immunol 138:54–60

Horner GW, Orr DM (1993) An enzyme-linked immunosorbent assay for detection of antibodies against bovine pestivirus. N Z Vet J 41:123–125

Horner GW, Tham KM, Orr D, Ralston J, Rowe S, Houghton T (1995) Comparison of an antigen capture enzyme-linked assay with reverse transcription– polymerase chain reaction and cell culture immunoperoxidase tests for the diagnosis of ruminant pestivirus infections. Vet Microbiol 43:75–84

Houe H (1999) Epidemiological features and economical importance of bovine virus diarrhoea virus (BVDV) infections. Vet Microbiol 64:89–107

Houe H, Lindberg A, Moennig V (2006) Test strategies in bovine viral diarrhea virus control and eradication campaigns in Europe. J Vet Diagn Investig 18:427–436

Howard CJ (1990) Immunological responses to bovine virus diarrhoea virus infections. Rev Sci Tech 9:95–103

Hu L, Bray MD, Osorio M, Kopecko DJ (2006) *Campylobacter jejuni* induces maturation and cytokine production in human dendritic cells. Infect Immun 74:2697–2705

Huemer HP, Nowotny N, Crabb BS, Meyer H, Hübert PH (1995) gp13 (EHV-gC): a complement receptor induced by equine herpesviruses. Virus Res 37:113–126

Humann J, Bjordahl R, Andreasen K, Lenz LL (2007) Expression of the p60 autolysin enhances NK cell activation and is required for *Listeria monocytogenes* expansion in IFN gamma responsive mice. J Immunol 178:2407–2414

Hunter CA, Subauste CS, Van Cleave VH, Remington JS (1994) Production of gamma interferon by natural killer cells from *Toxoplasma gondii*-infected SCID mice: regulation by interleukin-10, interleukin-12 and tumor necrosis factor alpha. Infect Immun 62(7):2818–2824

Hunter CA, Chizzonite R, Remington JS (1995) IL-1 beta is required for IL-12 to induce production of IFN-gamma by NK cells. A role for IL-1 beta in the T cell-independent mechanism of resistance against intracellular pathogens. J Immunol 155(9):4347–4354

Ikeda JS, BonDurant RH, Campero CM, Corbeil LB (1993) Conservation of a protective surface antigen of *Tritrichomonas foetus*. J Clin Microbiol 31:3289–3295

Jabbour HN, Sales KJ, Catalano RD, Norman JE (2009) Inflammatory pathways in female reproductive health and disease. J Reprod Fertil 138:903–919

Jagadeesan B, Koo OK, Kim KP, Burkholder KM, Mishra KK, Aroonnual A, Bhunia AK (2010) LAP, an alcohol acetaldehyde dehydrogenase enzyme in *Listeria*, promotes bacterial adhesion to enterocyte-like Caco-2 cells only in pathogenic species. Microbiology 156:2782–2795

Janakiraman V (2008) Listeriosis in pregnancy: diagnosis, treatment, and prevention. Rev Obstet Gynecol 1:179–185

Jenkins MC, Tuo W, Feng X, Cao L, Murphy C, Fetterer R (2010) *Neospora caninum*: cloning and expression of a gene coding for cytokine-inducing profilin. Exp Parasitol 125(4):357–362

Jiang X, Baldwin CL (1993) Effects of cytokines on intracellular growth of *Brucella abortus*. Infect Immun 61:124–134

Johansson J, Mandin P, Renzoni A, Chiaruttini C, Springer M, Cossart P (2002) An RNA thermosensor controls expression of virulence genes in *Listeria monocytogenes*. Cell 110: 551–561

Johnson LL, Sayles PC (2002) Deficient humoral responses underlie susceptibility to *Toxoplasma gondii* in CD4-deficient mice. Infect Immun 70(1):185–191

Johnson LL, Van der Vegt FP, Havell EA (1993) Gamma interferon-dependent temporary resistance to acute *Toxoplasma gondii* infection independent of CD4+ or CD8+ lymphocytes. Infect Immun 61(12):5174–5180

Jones C (2003) Herpes simplex virus type 1 and bovine herpesvirus 1 latency. Clin Microbiol Rev 16(1):79–95

Jones SM, Winter AJ (1992) Survival of virulent and attenuated strains of *Brucella abortus* in normal and gamma interferon-activated murine peritoneal macrophages. Infect Immun 60: 3011–3014

Jones MA, Totemeyer S, Maskell DJ, Bryant CE, Barrow PA (2003) Induction of proinflammatory responses in the human monocytic cell line THP-1 by *Campylobacter jejuni*. Infect Immun 71: 2626–2633

Jung A, Kato H, Kumagai Y, Kumar H, Kawai T, Takeuchi O, Akira S (2008) Lymphocytoid choriomeningitis virus activates plasmacytoid dendritic cells and induces a cytotoxic T-cell response via MyD88. J Virol 82:196–206

Kahn CM (2005) Listeriosis. The Merck veterinary manual, 9th edn. Merck and Co., Whitehouse Station, NJ, pp 2240–2241

Kang H, Suzuki Y (2001) Requirement of non-T cells that produce gamma interferon for prevention of reactivation of *Toxoplasma gondii* infection in the brain. Infect Immun 69(5):2920–2927

Kang H, Remington JS, Suzuki Y (2000) Decreased resistance of B cell-deficient mice to infection with *Toxoplasma gondii* despite unimpaired expression of IFN-gamma, TNF-alpha, and inducible nitric oxide synthase. J Immunol 164(5):2629–2634

Kataria RS, Tiwari AK, Gupta PK, Mehrotra ML, Rai A, Bandyopadhyay SK (1997) Detection of bovine herpesvirus 1 (BHV-1) genomic sequences in bovine semen inoculated with BHV-1 by polymerase chain reaction. Acta Virol 41(6):311–315

Kaufmann HE (1988) Listeriosis: new findings – current concerns. Microb Pathog 5:225–231

Keelan JA, Payne MS (2015) Vaginal microbiota during pregnancy: pathways of risk of preterm delivery in the absence of intrauterine Infection. J Proc Natl Acad Sci U S A 112:6414

Kelling CL, Topliff CL (2013) Bovine maternal, fetal and neonatal responses to bovine viral diarrhea virus infections. Biologicals 41(1):20–25

Kennedy P, Casaro A, Kimsey P, BonDurant R, Bushnell R, Mitchell G (1983) Epizootic bovine abortion: histogenesis of the fetal lesions. Am J Vet Res 44:1040–1048

Kim IH, Kang H (2003) Risk factors for post partum endometritis and effect of endometritis on reproductive performance in dairy cows in Korea. J Reprod Dev 49:485–491

Kim IH, Na KJ, Yang MP (2005) Immune response during the peripartum period in dairy cows with post-partum endometritis. J Reprod Dev 51:757–764

King D, Chen C, Blanchard M, Aldridge BM, Anderson ML, Walker R, Maas J, Hanks D, Hall M, Stott JL (2005) Molecular identification of a novel deltaproteobacterium as the etiologic agent of epizootic bovine abortion (foothill abortion). J Clin Microbiol 43:604–609

Kittel DR, Campero C, Van Hoosear KA, Rhyan JC, Bondurant RH (1998) Comparison of diagnostic methods for detection of active infection with *Tritrichomonas foetus* in beef heifers. J Am Vet Med Assoc 213:519–522

Klimpel GR, Matthias MA, Vinetz JM (2003) *Leptospira interrogans* activation of human peripheral blood mononuclear cells: preferential expansion of TCR gamma delta+ T cells vs TCR alpha beta+ T cells. J Immunol 171:1447–1455

Ko J, Splitter GA (2003) Molecular host–pathogen interaction in brucellosis: current understanding and future approaches to vaccine development for mice and humans. Clin Microbiol Rev 6:65–78

Konyves L, Szenci O, Jurkovich V, Tegzes L, Tirian A, Solymosi N, Gyulay G, Brydl E (2009) Risk assessment of postpartum uterine disease and consequences of puerperal metritis for subsequent metabolic status, reproduction and milk yield in dairy cows. J Acta Vet Hungarika 57:155–169

Koppers-Lalic D, Reits EA, Ressing ME, Lipinska AD, Abele R, Koch J, Marcondes Rezende M, Admiraal P, van Leeuwen D, Bienkowska-Szewczyk K, Mettenleiter TC, Rijsewijk FA, Tampe R, Neefjes J, Wiertz EJ (2005) Varicello viruses avoid T cell recognition by UL49.5-mediated inactivation of the transporter associated with antigen processing. Proc Natl Acad Sci U S A 102:5144–5149

Kruger JM, Venta PJ, Swenson CL, Syring R, Gibbons-Burgener SN, Richter M, Maes RK (2000) Prevalence of bovine herpesvirus-4 infection in cats in Central Michigan. J Vet Intern Med 14(6):593–597

Kurita T (2010) Developmental origin of vaginal epithelium. J Different 80:99–105

Kwak-Kim JY, Gilman-Sachs A, Kim CE (2005) T helper 1 and 2 immune responses in relationship to pregnancy, non-pregnancy, recurrent spontaneous abortions and infertility of repeated implantation failure. Chem Immunol Allergy 88:64–79

Kydd JH, Hannant D, Mumford JA (1996) Residence and recruitment of leucocytes to the equine lung after EHV-1 infection. Vet Immunol Immunopathol 52:15–26

Kydd JH, Wattrang E, Hannant D (2003) Pre-infection frequencies of equine herpesvirus-1 specific, cytotoxic T lymphocytes correlate with protection against abortion following experimental infection of pregnant mares. Vet Immunol Immunopathol 96:207–217

Kydd JH, Townsend HGG, Hannant D (2006) The equine immune response to equine Herpesvirus-1: the virus and its vaccines. Vet Immunol Immunopathol 111:15–30

Lambot M, Douart A, Joris E, Letesson JJ, Pastoret PP (1997) Characterization of the immune response of cattle against non-cytopathic and cytopathic biotypes of bovine viral diarrhoea virus. J Gen Virol 78:1041–1047

Laroucau K, Souriau A, Rodolakis A (2001) Improved sensitivity of PCR for *Chlamydophila* using *pmp* genes. Vet Microbiol 82:155–164

Laroucau K, Vorimore F, Sachse K, Vretou E, Siarkou VI, Willems H, Magnino S, Rodolakis A, Bavoil PM (2010) Differential identification of *Chlamydophila abortus* live vaccine strain 1B and *C. abortus* field isolates by PCR-RFLP. Vaccine 28:5653–5656

de Las Heras A, Cain RJ, Bielecka MK, Vazquez-Boland JA (2011) Regulation of *Listeria* virulence: PrfA master and commander. Curr Opin Microbiol 14:118–127

Leal-Klevezas DS, Lopez-Merino A, Martinez-Soriano JP (1995) Molecular detection of *Brucella* spp.: rapid identification of *B. abortus* biovar 1 using PCR. Arch Med Res 26:263–267

Lecuit M (2007) Human listeriosis and animal models. Microbes Infect 9:1216–1225

Leung ST, Derecka K, Mann GE, Flint APF, Wathes DC (2000) Uterine lymphocyte distribution and interleukin expression during early pregnancy in cows. J Reprod Fertil 119:25–33

Levett PN (2001) Leptospirosis. Clin Microbiol Rev 14:296–326

Lewis GS, Wulster-Radcliffe MC (2006) Prostaglandin F2alpha upregulates uterine immune defenses in the presence of the immunosuppressive steroid progesterone. Am J Reprod Immunol 56:102–111

Li Q, Verma IM (2002) NF kappa B regulation in the immune system. J Nat Rev Immunol 2:725–734

Li W, Buzoni-Gatel D, Debbabi H, Hu MS, Mennechet FJD, Durell BG, Noelle RJ, Kasper LH (2002) CD40/CD154 ligation is required for the development of acute ileitis following oral infection with an intracellular pathogen in mice. Gastroenterology 122(3):762–773

Liebler-Tenorio EM, Ridpath JF, Neill JD (2004) Distribution of viral antigen and tissue lesions in persistent and acute infection with the homologous strain of noncytopathic bovine viral diarrhoea virus. J Vet Diagn Investig 16:388–396

Liesenfeld O, Kosek J, Remington JS, Suzuki Y (1996) Association of CD4+ T cell-dependent, interferon-gamma-mediated necrosis of the small intestine with genetic susceptibility of mice to peroral infection with *Toxoplasma gondii*. J Exp Med 184(2):597–607

Liesenfeld O, Kang H, Park D, Nguyen TA, Parkhe CV, Watanabe H, Abo T, Sher A, Remington JS, Suzuki Y (1999) TNF-alpha, nitric oxide and IFN-gamma are all critical for development of necrosis in the small intestine and early mortality in genetically susceptible mice infected perorally with *Toxoplasma gondii*. Parasite Immunol 21(7):365–376

Liesenfeld O, Nguyen TA, Pharke C, Suzuki Y (2001) Importance of gender and sex hormones in regulation of susceptibility of the small intestine to peroral infection with *Toxoplasma gondii* tissue cysts. J Parasitol 87(6):1491–1493

Limmahakhun S, Chayakulkeeree M (2013) *Listeria monocytogenes* brain abscess: two cases and review of the literature. SE Asian J Trop Med Public Health 44:468–478

Lin YP, Greenwood A, Yan W, Nicholson LK, Sharma Y, McDonough SP, Chang YF (2009) A novel fibronectin type III module binding motif identified on C-terminus of *Leptospira* immunoglobulin-like protein, *LigB*. Biochem Biophys Res Commun 389(1):57–62

Lindberg ALE, Alenius S (1999) Principles for eradication of bovine viral diarrhoea virus (BVDV) infections in cattle populations. Vet Microbiol 64:197–222

Lipinska AD, Koppers-Lalic D, Rychlowski M, Admiraal P, Rijsewijk FA, Bienkowska-Szewczyk-K, Wiertz EJ (2006) Bovine herpesvirus 1 UL49.5 protein inhibits the transporter associated with antigen processing despite complex formation with glycoprotein M. J Virol 80:5822–5832

Liu CH, Fan YT, Dias A, Esper L, Corn RA, Bafica A, Machado FS, Aliberti J (2006) Cutting edge: dendritic cells are essential for *in vivo* IL-12 production and development of resistance against *Toxoplasma gondii* infection in mice. J Immunol 177(1):31–35

Longbottom D, Coulter LJ (2003) Animal chlamydioses and zoonotic implications. J Comp Pathol 128:217–244

Longbottom D, Livingstone M, Maley S, Van Der Zon A, Rocchi M, Wilson K, Wheelhouse N, Dagleish M, Aitchison K, Wattegedera S, Nath M, Entrican G, Buxton D (2013) Intranasal infection with *Chlamydia abortus* induces dose-dependent latency and abortion in sheep. PLoS One 8:e57950

Lopes WDZ, Rodriguez JD, Souza FA, dos Santos TR, dos Santos RS, Rosanese WM, Lopes WR, Sakamoto CA, da Costa AJ (2013) Sexual transmission of *Toxoplasma gondii* in sheep. Vet Parasitol 195(1-2):47–56

Lopez A, Hitos F, Perez A, Navarro-Fierro RR (1984) Lung lesions in bovine foetuses aborted by *Brucella abortus*. Can J Compar Med 48:275–277

Lopez JW, Del Piero F, Glaser A, Finazzi M (1996) Immunoperoxidase histochemistry as a diagnostic tool for detection of equine arteritis virus antigen in formalin fixed tissues. Equine Vet J 28:77–79

Lopez-Gatius F (2003) Is fertility declining in dairy cattle A retrospective study in Northeastern Spain. J Theriogenol 60:89–99

Low JC, Donachie W (1997) A review of *Listeria monocytogenes* and listeriosis. Vet J 153:9–29

Low BG, Hansen PJ, Drost M (1990) Expression of major histocompatibility complex antigens on the bovine placenta. J Reprod Fertil 90:235–243

Lun ZR, Gajadhar AA (1999) A simple and rapid method for staining *Tritrichomonas foetus* and *Trichomonas vaginalis*. J Vet Diagn Investig 11:471–474

Lunn DP, Holmes MA, Duffus WP (1991) Three monoclonal antibodies identifying antigens on all equine T lymphocytes, and two mutually exclusive T-lymphocyte subsets. Immunology 74:251–257

Lutjen S, Soltek S, Virna S, Deckert M, Schluter D (2006) Organ and disease-stage-specific regulation of *Toxoplasma gondii*-specific CD8-T-cell responses by CD4 T cells. Infect Immun 74(10):5790–5801

Macedo GC, Magnani DM, Carvalho NB, Bruna-Romero O, Gazzinelli RT, Oliveira SC (2008) Central role of MyD88-dependent dendritic cell maturation and proinflammatory cytokine production to control *Brucella abortus* infection. J Immunol 180:1080–1087

Maclachlan NJ, Osburn BI (2017) Teratogenic bluetongue and related orbivirus infections in pregnant ruminant livestock: timing and pathogen genetics are critical. Curr Opin Virol 27:31–35

Madin SH, York CJ, Mckercher DG (1956) Isolation of the infectious bovine rhinotracheitis virus. Science 124(721):722

Madoz LV, Ploentzke J, Albarracin D, Mejia M, Drillich M, Heuwieser W, De La Sota RL (2008) Prevalence of clinical and subclinical endometritis in dairy cows and the impact on reproductive performance. J Anim Reprod Sci 122:7–52

Manickam R, Mohan M (1987) Seroepidemiological studies on Infectious bovine rhinotracheitis (IBR) viral abortions in cows. Indian J Anim Sci 57:959–962

Mansfield LS, Bell JA, Wilson DL, Murphy AJ, Elsheikha HM, Rathinam VA, Fierro BR, Linz JE, Young VB (2007) C57BL/6and congenic interleukin-10-deficient mice can serve as models of *Campylobacter jejuni* colonization and enteritis. Infect Immun 75:1099–1115

Marangoni A, Aldini R, Sambri V, Giacani L, Di Leo K, Cevenini R (2004) Production of tumor necrosis factor alpha by *Treponema pallidum*, *Borrelia burgdorferis*. *L.* and *Leptospira interrogans* in isolated rat Kupffer cells. FEMS Immunol Med Microbiol 40(3):187–191

Marinho M, Langoni H, Oliveira SL, Lima VMF, Peiro JR, Perri SHV, Carreira R (2005) Role of cytokines, NO and H_2O_2 on the immunopathology of Leptospirosis in genetically selected mice. J Venom Anim Tox Incl Trop 11(2):198–212

Marinho M, Silva C, Lima VMF, Peiro JR, Perri SHV (2006) Cytokine and antibody production during murine leptospirosis. J Venom Anim Toxins Incl Trop Dis 12:595–603

Marinho M, Monteiro CMR, Peiro JR, Machado GF, Oliveira Junior IS (2008) TNF-a and IL-6 immunohistochemistry in rat renal tissue experimentally infected with *Leptospira interrogans* serovar Canicola. J Venom Anim Tox incl Trop Dis 14:533–540

Marinho M, Oliveira-Junior IS, Monteiro CM, Perri SH, Salomao R (2009) Pulmonary disease in hamsters infected with *Leptospira interrogans*: histopathologic findings and cytokine mRNA expressions. Am J Trop Med Hyg 80:832–836

Marshall DJ, Moxley RA, Kelling CL (1996) Distribution of virus and viral antigen in specific pathogen-free calves following inoculation with noncytopathic bovine viral diarrhea virus. Vet Pathol 33:311–318

Martius J, Eschenbach DA (1990) The role of bacterial vaginosis as a cause of amniotic fluid infection, chorioamnionitis and prematurity a review. J Arch Gynecol Obstet 247:1–13

Mascellino MT, Boccia P, Oliva A (2011) Immunopathogenesis in *Chlamydia trachomatis* infected women. ISRN Obstet Gynecol 2011:436936

Mateus T, Silva J, Maia RL, Teixeira P (2013) Listeriosis during pregnancy: a public health concern. ISRN Obstet Gynecol 2013:851712

Maurer K, Krey T, Moennig V, Thiel HJ, Rumenapf T (2004) CD46 is a cellular receptor for bovine viral diarrhoea virus. J Virol 78:1792–1799

Mayo C, Mullens B, Gibbs EP, MacLachlan NJ (2016) Overwintering of Bluetongue virus in temperate zones. Vet Ital 52(3-4):243–246

McGowan MR, Kirkland PD, Rodwell BJ, Kerr DR, Carroll CL (1993) A field investigation of the effects of bovine viral diarrhea virus infection around the time of insemination on the reproductive performance of cattle. J Theriogenol 39:443–449

Meador VP, Tabatabai LB, Hagemoser WA, Deyoe BL (1986) Identification of *Brucella abortus* in formalin-fixed, paraffin-embedded tissues of cows, goats, and mice with an avidin biotin-peroxidase complex immunoenzymatic staining technique. Am J Vet Res 47:2147–2150

Meador VP, Hagemoser WA, Deyoe BL (1988) Histopathologic findings in *Brucella abortus*-infected, pregnant goats. Am J Vet Res 49:274–280

Meador VP, Deyoe BL, Cheville NF (1989) Pathogenesis of *Brucella abortus* infection of the mammary gland and supramammary lymph node of the goat. Vet Pathol 26:357–368

Mehrotra ML, Rajya BS, Kumar S (1976) Infectious bovine rhinotracheitis (IBR) keratoconjunctivitis in calves. Indian J Vet Pathol 1:70–73

Mestecky J, Moldoveanu Z, Russell MW (2005) Immunological uniqueness of the genital tract: challenge for vaccine development. Am J Reprod Immunol 5:208–214

Meyling A, Houe H, Jensen AM (1990) Epidemiology of bovine virus diarrhoea virus. Rev Sci Tech 9:75–93

Mignon B, Dubuisson J, Baranowski E, Koromyslov I, Ernst E, Boulanger D, Waxweiler S, Pastoret PP (1991) A monoclonal ELISA for bovine viral diarrhoea pestivirus antigen detection in persistently infected cattle. J Virol Methods 35:177–188

Mineo TW, Oliveira CJ, Gutierrez FR, Silva JS (2010) Recognition by Toll-like receptor 2 induces antigen-presenting cell activation and Th1 programming during infection by *Neospora caninum*. Immunol Cell Biol 88(8):825–833

Misra PK, Misra A (1987) Infectious bovine rhinotracheitis virus infection and infertility in cows, heifers and bulls. Ind J Anim Sci 57:267–271

Mitchell RG (1996) *Listeria, Erysipelothrix*. In: Collee JG, Fraser AG, Marmion BP, Simmons A (eds) Mackie and McCartney practical medical microbiology, 14th edn. Churchill Livingstone, Edinburgh, pp 309–315

Mohan Kumar KM, Rajasekhar M, Krishnappa G (1994) Isolation of infectious bovine rhinotracheitis virus in Karnataka. Ind Vet J 71(2):109–113

Mor G, Cardenas I (2010) The immune system in pregnancy a unique complexity. Am J Reprod Immunol 63:425–433

de Moraes EPBX, Da Costa MM, Dantas AFM, Da Silvaa JCR, Mota RA (2011) *Toxoplasma gondii* diagnosis in ovine aborted fetuses and stillborns in the State of Pernambuco, Brazil. Vet Parasitol 183(1–2):152–155

Mordue DG, Sibley LD (2003) A novel population of Gr-1+- activated macrophages induced during acute toxoplasmosis. J Leukoc Biol 74(6):1015–1025

Moss N, Lean LJ, Reid SWJ, Hodgson DR (2002) Risk factors for repeat breeder syndrome in New South Wales dairy cattle. J Prevent Vet Med 54:91–103

Mukhufhi N, Irons PC, Michel A, Peta F (2003) Evaluation of a PCR test for the diagnosis of *Tritrichomonas foetus* infection in bulls: effects of sample collection method, storage and transport medium on the test. Theriogen 60:1269–1278

Muller-Doblies D, Arquint A, Schaller P, Heegaard PM, Hilbe M, Albini S, Abril C, Tobler K, Ehrensperger F, Peterhans E, Ackermann M, Metzler A (2004) Innate immune responses of calves during transient infection with a noncytopathic strain of bovine viral diarrhea virus. Clin Diagn Lab Immunol 11(2):302–312

Mumford JA (1992) Progress in the control of equine influenza. In: Plowright W, Rossdale PD, Wade JF (eds) Equine infectious diseases, VI. Proceedings of the 6th International Conference. R & W Publications, Newmarket, ON, pp 207–217

Mumford JA, Rossdale PD, Jessett DM, Gann SJ, Ousey J, Cook RF (1987) Serological and virological investigations of an equid herpesvirus 1 (EHV-1) abortion storm on a stud farm in 1985. J Reprod Fertil Suppl 35:509–518

Munoz M, Heimesaat MM, Danker K, Struck D, Lohmann U, Plickert R, Bereswill S, Fischer A, Dunay IR, Wolk K, Loddenkemper C, Krell HW, Libert C, Lund LR, Frey O, Holscher C, Iwakura Y, Ghilardi N, Ouyang W, Kamradt T, Sabat R, Liesenfeld O (2009) Interleukin (IL)-23 mediates *Toxoplasma gondii*-induced immunopathology in the gut via matrixmetalloproteinase-2 and IL-22 but independent of IL-17. J Exp Med 206(13):3047–3059

Nagaeva O, Jonsson L, Mincheva-Nilsson L (2002) Dominant IL-10 and TGF-β mRNA expression in γδT cells of human early pregnancy decidua suggests immunoregulatory potential. Am J Reprod Immunol 48:9–17

Nelson KM, Schram BR, Mcgregor MW, Sheoran AS, Olsen CW, Lunn DP (1998) Local and systemic isotype-specific antibody responses to equine influenza virus infection versus conventional vaccination. Vaccine 16:1306–1313

Nielsen K (2002) Diagnosis of brucellosis by serology. Vet Microbiol 90:447–459

Nielsen KH, Ewalt DR (2004) Bovine brucellosis. Office International des Epizooties. Manual of Standards for Diagnostic Tests and Vaccines. Office International des Epizooties, Paris, pp 328–345

Nugent J, Birch-Machin I, Smith KC, Mumford JA, Swann Z, Newton JR, Bowden RJ, Allen GP, Davis-Poynter N (2006) Analysis of equid herpesvirus 1 strain variation reveals a point mutation of the DNA polymerase strongly associated with neuropathogenic versus nonneuropathogenic disease outbreaks. J Virol 80:4047–4060

O'Neill T, Kydd JH, Allen GP, Wattrang E, Mumford JA, Hannant D (1999) Determination of equid herpesvirus 1-specific, CD8+, cytotoxic T lymphocyte precursor frequencies in ponies. Vet Immunol Immunopathol 70:43–54

OIE (2010) Infectious bovine rhinotracheitis/infectious pustular vulvovaginitis. Chapter 2.4.13. In: Manual of standards diagnostic tests and vaccines 2010. Office International des Epizooties, Paris

OIE (2014) *Listeria monocytogenes*. Chapter 2.9.7. Manual of diagnostic tests and vaccines for terrestrial animals. Office International des Epizooties, Paris, pp 1–18

Okada Y, Okutani A, Suzuki H, Asakura H, Monden S, Nakama A, Maruyama T, Igimi S (2011) Antimicrobial susceptibilities of *Listeria monocytogenes* isolated in Japan. J Vet Med Sci 73: 1681–1684

Oliveira LJ, Hansen PJ (2008) Deviations in populations of peripheral blood mononuclear cells and endometrial macrophages in the cow during pregnancy. Reproduction 136(4):481–490

Oliveira SC, Harms JS, Rech EL, Rodarte RS, Bocca AL, Goes AM, Splitter GA (1998) The role of T-cell subsets and cytokines in the regulation of intracellular bacterial infection. Braz J Med Biol Res 31:77–84

Oliveira SC, Soeurt N, Splitter G (2002) Molecular and cellular interactions between Brucella abortus antigens and host immune responses. J Vet Microbiol 90:417–424

Oliver SP, Jayarao BM, Almeida RA (2005) Food borne pathogens in milk and the dairy farm environment: food safety and public health implications. Foodborne Pathog Dis 2:115–129

Opdenbosch E, Wellemans G, Oudewater J (1986) Unexpected isolation of a bovine herpesvirus 4 from the lung of a sheep. Vlaams Diergeneeskundig Tijdschrift 55(6):432–433

Osterman B, Moriyon I (2006) International Committee on Systematics of Prokaryotes Subcommittee on the taxonomy of *Brucella*. Int J Syst Evol Microbiol 56:1173–1175

Ostlund EN (1993) The equine herpesviruses. Vet Clin N Am Equine Pract 9:283–294

Oviedo-Boyso J, Bravo-Patino A, Baizabal-Aguirre VM (2014) Collaborative action of Toll like and NOD-like receptors as modulators of the inflammatory response to pathogenic bacteria. Mediat Inflamm 2014:432785

Paillot R, Daly JM, Juillard V, Minke JM, Hannant D, Kydd JH (2005) Equine interferon gamma synthesis in lymphocytes after *in vivo* infection and *in vitro* stimulation with EHV-1. Vaccine 23:4541–4551

Paillot R, Daly JM, Luce R, Montesso F, Davis-Poynter N, Hannant D, Kydd JH (2007) Frequency and phenotype of EHV-1 specific, IFN-gamma synthesizing lymphocytes in ponies: the effects of age, pregnancy and infection. Dev Comp Immunol 31:202–214

Pantchev A, Sting R, Bauerfeind R, Tyczka J, Sachse K (2010) Detection of all *Chlamydophila* and *Chlamydia* spp. of veterinary interest using species-specific real-time PCR assays. Comp Immunol Microbiol Infect Dis 33:473–484

Park JB, Kendrick JW (1973) The isolation and partila characterization of a herpesvirus from a case of bovine metritis. Arch Gesamte Virusfrsch 41:211–215

Parker S, Campbell JR, Ribble C, Gajadhar AA (1999) Comparison of two sampling tools for diagnosis of *Tritrichomonas foetus* in bulls and clinical interpretation of culture results. J Am Vet Med Assoc 215:231–235

Parker S, Lun Z-R, Gajadhar A (2001) Application of a PCR assay to enhance the detection and identification of *Tritrichomonas foetus* in cultured preputial samples. J Vet Diagn Investig 13: 508–513

Parker S, Campbell J, Gajadhar A (2003) Comparison of the diagnostic sensitivity of a commercially available culture kit and a diagnostic culture test using Diamond's media for diagnosing *Tritrichomonas foetus* in bulls. J Vet Diagn Investig 15:460–465

Pedrera M, Gomez-Villamandos JC, Molina V, Risalde MA, Rodriguez-Sanchez B, Sanchez-Cordon PJ (2011) Quantification and determination of spread mechanisms of bovine viral diarrhoea virus in blood and tissues from colostrum-deprived calves during an experimental acute infection induced by a non-cytopathic genotype 1 strain. Transbound Emerg Dis 59:377–384

Pedrera M, Gomez-Villamandos JC, Risalde MA, Molina V, Sanchez-Cordon PJ (2012) Characterisation of apoptosis pathways (intrinsic and extrinsic) in lymphoid tissues of calves inoculated with non-cytopathic bovine viral diarrhoea virus genotype 1. J Comp Pathol 146:30–39

Perona-Wright G, Mohrs K, Szaba FM, Kummer LW, Madan R, Karp CL, Johnson LL, Smiley ST, Mohrs M (2009) Systemic but not local infections elicit immunosuppressive IL-10 production by natural killer cells. Cell Host Microbe 6(6):503–512

Platt H, Singh H, Whitwellm KE (1980) Pathological observations on an outbreak of paralysis in broodmares. Equine Vet J 12:118–126

Plontzke J, Madoz LV, De la Sota RL, Drillich M, Heuwieser W (2010) Subclinical endometritis and its impact on reproductive performance in grazing dairy cattle in Argentina. J Anim Reprod Sci 122:52–57

Poester FP, Samartino LE, Lage AP (2005) Diagnosis of the bovine undulant fever. Tech Exer Bk Vet Zootech 47:13–29

Poester FP, Gonçalves VSP, Paixao TA, Santos RL, Olsen SO, Schuring GG, Lage AP (2006) Efficacy of strain RB51 vaccine in heifers against experimental brucellosis. Vaccine 24:5327–5334

Poltorak A, He X, Smirnova I, Liu MY, Huffel CV, Du X, Birdwell D, Alejos E, Potter TJ, Guitian J, Fishwick J, Gordon PJ, Sheldon IM (1998) Risk factors for clinical endometritis in postpartum dairy cattle. J Theriogenol 74:127–134

Potgieter LN (1995) Immunology of bovine viral diarrhoea virus. Vet Clin N Am Food Anim Pract 11:501–520

Rae DO, Crews JE (2006) *Tritrichomonas foetus*. Vet Clin Food Anim 22:595–611

Raghupathy R (1997) TH-1 type immunity is incompatible with successful pregnancy. Immunol Today 10:478–482

Ramina A, Dalla Valle L, De Mas S, Tisato E, Zuin A, Renier M, Cuteri V, Valente C, Cancellotti FM (1999) Detection of equine arteritis virus in semen by reverse transcriptase polymerase chain reaction–ELISA. Comp Immunol Microbiol Infect Dis 22:187–197

Rappocciolo G, Birch J, Ellis SA (2003) Down-regulation of MHC class I expression by equine herpesvirus-1. J Gen Virol 84:293–300

Raya AI, Gomez-Villamandos JC, Sanchez-Cordon PJ, Bautista MJ (2012) Virus distribution and role of thymic macrophages during experimental infection with noncytopathic bovine viral diarrhea virus type 1. Vet Pathol 49:811–818

Reddy YK, Manohar BM, Pandey AB, Reddy YN, Prasad G, Chauhan RS (2010) Development and evaluation of inactivated pentavalent adjuvanted vaccine for bluetongue. Ind Vet J 87:434–436

Register KB, Morgan PA, Wyrick PB (1986) Interaction between *Chlamydia* spp. and human polymorphonuclear leukocytes *in vitro*. Infect Immun 52:664–670

Reichmann G, Walker W, Villegas EN, Craig L, Cai G, Alexander J, Hunter CA (2000) The CD40/CD40 ligand interaction is required for resistance to toxoplasmic encephalitis. Infect Immun 68(3):1312–1318

Reis O, Sousa S, Camejo A, Villiers V, Gouin E, Cossart P, Cabanes D (2010) LapB, a novel *Listeria monocytogenes* LPXTG surface adhesin, required for entry into eukaryotic cells and virulence. J Infect Dis 202:551–562

Remington JS, Thulliez P, Montoya JG (2004) Recent developments for diagnosis of toxoplasmosis. J Clin Microbiol 42(3):941–945

Rey-Ladino J, Jiang X, Gabel BR, Shen C, Brunham RC (2007) Survival of *Chlamydia muridarum* within dendritic cells. Infect Immun 75:3707–3714

Rhyan JC, Blanchard PC, Kvasnicka WG, Hall MR, Hanks D (1995) Tissue invasive *Tritrichomonas foetus* in four aborted bovine foetuses. J Vet Diagn Investig 7:409–412

Rhyan JC, Wilson KL, Wagner B, Anderson ML, Bondurant RH, Burgess DE, Mutwiri GK, Corbeil LB (1999) Demonstration of *Tritrichomonas foetus* in the external genitalia and of specific antibodies in preputial secretions of naturally infected bulls. Vet Pathol 36:406–411

Ribeiro LMM (1990) An efficient medium for the isolation of *Tritrichomonas foetus*. Onderstepoort J Vet Res 57:209–210

Ribet D, Hamon M, Gouin E, Nahori MA, Impens F, Neyret-Kahn H, Gevaert K, Vandekerckhove J, Dejean A, Cossart P (2010) *Listeria monocytogenes* impairs SUMOylation for efficient infection. Nature 464:1192–1195

Rinehart CL, Zimmerman AD, Buterbaugh RE, Jolie RA, Chase CC (2012) Efficacy of vaccination of cattle with the *Leptospira interrogans* serovar hardjo type hardjoprajitno component of a pentavalent Leptospira bacterin against experimental challenge with *Leptospira borgpetersenii* serovar hardjo type hardjo-bovis. Am J Vet Res 73(5):735–740

Roan NR, Starnbach MN (2008) Immune-mediated control of *Chlamydia* infection. Cell Microbiol 10:9–19

Robben PM, LaRegina M, Kuziel WA, Sibley LD (2005) Recruitment of Gr-1+ monocytes is essential for control of acute toxoplasmosis. J Exp Med 201(11):1761–1769

Rocourt J, Bille J (1997) Foodborne listeriosis. World Health Stat Q 50:67–73

Rodriguez N, Fend F, Jennen L, Schiemann M, Wantia N, Prazeres da Costa CU, Durr S, Heinzmann U, Wagner H, Miethke T (2005) Polymorphonuclear neutrophils improve replication of *Chlamydia pneumoniae in vivo* upon MyD88-dependent attraction. J Immunol 174:4836–4844

Roizman B, Desrosiers RS, Fleckenstein B, Lopez C, Minson AC, Studdert MJ (1992) The family herpesviridae: an update. Arch Virol 123:425–449

Rosas CT, Goodman LB, Von Einem J, Osterrieder N (2006) Equine herpesvirus type 1 modified live virus vaccines: *Quo vaditis*? Expert Rev Vacc 5:119–131

Rupp J, Pfleiderer L, Jugert C, Moeller S, Klinger M, Dalhoff K, Solbach W, Stenger S, Laskay T, van Zandbergen G (2009) *Chlamydia pneumoniae* hides inside apoptotic neutrophils to silently infect and propagate in macrophages. PLoS One 4:e6020

Sabet C, Toledo-Arana A, Personnic N, Lecuit M, Dubrac S, Poupel O, Poupel O, Gouin E, Nahori MA, Cossart P, Bierne H (2008) The *Listeria monocytogenes* virulence factor InlJ is specifically expressed *in vivo* and behaves as an adhesin. Infect Immun 76:1368–1378

Sachse K, Vretou E, Livingstone M, Borel N, Pospischil A, Longbottom D (2009) Recent developments in the laboratory diagnosis of chlamydial infections (Review). Vet Microbiol 135:2–21

Salmeron I, Rodrigue-Zapata M, Salmeron O, Manzano L, Vaquer S, Alvarez-Mon M (1992) Impaired activity of natural killer cells in patients with acute brucellosis. Clin Infect Dis 15:764–770

Samartino LE, Enright FM (1996) *Brucella abortus* differs in the multiplication within bovine chorioallantoic membrane explants from early and late gestation. Comp Immunol Microbiol Infect Dis 19:55–63

Saminathan M, Rana R, Ramakrishnan MA, Karthik K, Malik YS, Dhama K (2016) Prevalence, diagnosis, management and control of important diseases of ruminants with special reference to Indian scenario. J Exp Biol Agric Sci 4(3S):338–367

Saminathan M, Singh KP, Vineetha S, Maity M, Biswas SK, Reddy GBM, Milton AAP, Chauhan HC, Chandel BS, Ramakrishnan MA, Gupta VK (2018) Factors determining the clinical outcome of bluetongue virus infection in adult mice. Indian J Vet Pathol 42(4):239–248

Saminathan M, Singh KP, Rajasekar R, Malik YPS, Dhama K (2019) Role of type I interferons in the pathogenesis of bluetongue virus in mice and ruminants. J Exp Biol Agric Sci 7(6):513–520

Saminathan M, Singh KP, Khorajiya JH, Dinesh M, Vineetha S, Maity M, Rahman ATF, Misri J, Malik YS, Gupta VK, Singh RK, Dhama K (2020a) An updated review on Bluetongue virus: epidemiology, pathobiology, and advances in diagnosis and control with special reference to India. Vet Q 40(1):258–321

Saminathan M, Singh KP, Vineetha S, Maity M, Biswas SK, Manjunathareddy GB, Chauhan HC, Milton AAP, Ramakrishnan MA, Maan S, Maan NS, Hemadri D, Chandel BS, Gupta VK, Mertens PPC (2020b) Virological, immunological and pathological findings of transplacentally transmitted bluetongue virus serotype 1 in IFNAR1-blocked mice during early and mid gestation. Sci Rep 10(1):2164

Saminathan M, Singh KP, Maity M, Vineetha S, Manjunathareddy GB, Dhama K, Malik YS, Ramakrishnan MA, Misri J, Gupta VK (2021) Pathological and immunological characterization of bluetongue virus serotype 1 infection in type I interferons blocked immunocompetent adult mice. J Adv Res 31:137

Santos RL, Peixoto MTD, Serakides R, Costa GM, Martins NE (1998) Detection of *Brucella abortus* (sample B19) by the immunoenzymatic complex avidin-biotin-peroxidase in the testicle and in the epididymis of bovines inoculated experimentally. Anim Reprod Files 6:34–41

Satyanarayana K, Suri Babu T (1987) Comparative evaluation of enzyme linked immunosorbent assay (ELISA) and indirect haemagglutination (IHA) test in the detection of antibodies to Bovine herpes virus-1.(BHV-1) in cattle. Ind J Comp Microbiol Immunol Infect Dis 8:31 32

Sauret JM, Vilissova N (2002) Human brucellosis review. J Am Board Fam Pract 15:401–406

Scanga CA, Aliberti J, Jankovic D, Tilloy F, Bennouna S, Denkers EY, Medzhitov R, Sher A (2002) Cutting edge: MyD88 is required for resistance to *Toxoplasma gondii* infection and regulates parasite-induced IL-12 production by dendritic cells. J Immunol 168(12):5997–6001

Schaefer TM, Desouza K, Fahey JV, Beagley KW, Wira CR (2004) Toll-like receptor (TLR) expression and TLR-mediated cytokine, chemokine production by human uterine epithelial cells. J Immunol 112:428–436

Schlafer DH, Miller RB (2007) Female genital system. In: Maxie MG (ed) Jubb, Kennedy, and Palmer's pathology of domestic animals, vol 3. Elsevier, Saunders, Philadelphia, PA, pp 429–564

Schluter D, Daubener W, Schares G, Groß U, Pleyer Uand Luder C (2014) Animals are key to human toxoplasmosis. Int J Med Microbiol 304(7):917–929

Schnupf P, Portnoy DA (2007) Listeriolysin O: a phagosome specific lysin. Microbes Infect 9: 1176–1187

Schonmann MJ, Bondurant RH, Gardner LA, Van Hoosear K, Baltzer W, Kachulis C (1994) Comparison of sampling and culture methods for the diagnosis of *Tritrichomonas foetus* infection in bulls. Vet Rec 134:620–622

Schurig GG, Roop RM, Bagchi T, Boyle S, Buhrman D, Sriranganathan N (1991) Biological properties of RB51: a stable rough strain of *Brucella abortus*. Vet Microbiol 28:171–188

Semambo DK, Ayliffe TR, Boyd JS, Taylor DJ (1991) Early abortion in cattle induced by experimental intrauterine infection with pure cultures of Actinomyces pyogenes. J Vet Rec 129:12–16

Seong SY, Matzinger P (2004) Hydrophobicity: an ancient damage-associated molecular pattern that initiates innate immune responses. Nat Rev Immunol 4:469–478

Shannon AD, Richards SG, Kirkland PD, Moyle A (1991) An antigen-capture ELISA detects pestivirus antigens in blood and tissues of immunotolerant carrier cattle. J Virol Methods 34:1–12

Shaw AE, Ratinier M, Nunes SF, Nomikou K, Caporale M, Golder M, Allan K, Hamers C, Hudelet P, Zientara S, Breard E, Mertens P, Palmarini M (2013) Reassortment between two serologically unrelated bluetongue virus strains is flexible and can involve any genome segment. J Virol 87:543–557

Sheldon IM, Lewis GS, LeBlanc SJ, Gilbert RO (2006) Defining postpartum uterine disease in cattle. J Theriogenol 65:1516–1530

Sheldon IM, Cronin J, Goetze L, Donofrio G, Schuberth HJ (2009) Defining postpartum uterine disease and the mechanisms of infection and immunity in the female reproductive tract in cattle. J Biol Reprod 81:1025–1032

Sher A, Oswald IP, Hieny S, Gazzinelli RT (1993) *Toxoplasma gondii* induces a T-independent IFN-gamma response in natural killer cells that requires both adherent accessory cells and tumor necrosis factor-alpha. J Immunol 150(9):3982–3989

Shibuya K, Robinson D, Zonin F, Hartley SB, Macatonia SE, Somoza C, Hunter CA, Murphy KM, O'Garra A (1998) IL-1 alpha and TNF-alpha are required for IL-12-induced development of Th1 cells producing high levels of IFN-gamma in BALB/c but not C57BL/6 mice. J Immunol 160(4):1708–1716

Simpson H, Robson SC, Bulmer JN, Barber A, Lyall F (2002) Transforming growth factor β expression in human placenta and placental bed during early pregnancy. Placenta 23:44–58

Singh BK, Kant R, Tongaonkar SS (1983) Adaptation of Infectious bovine rhinotracheitis virus in Madin Darby bovine kidney cell line and testing of buffalo sera for neutralizing antibodies. Ind J Comp Microbiol Immunol Infect Dis 4:68

Skirrow SZ, BonDurant RH (1990) Immunoglobulin isotype of specific antibodies in reproductive tract secretions and sera in *Tritrichomonas foetus*-infected heifers. Am J Vet Res 51:645–653

Skirrow SZ, Bondurrant RH (1988) Bovine trichomoniasis. Vet Bull 58:591–603

Skopets B, Li J, Thatcher WW, Roberts RM, Hansen PJ (1992) Inhibition of lymphocyte proliferation by bovine trophoblast protein 1 (type 1 trophoblast interferon) and bovine interferon a1. J Vet Immunol Immunopathol 34:81–96

Slater J, Hannant D (2000) Equine immunity to viruses. Vet Clin N Am 16:49–68

Slater JC, Borchers K, Thackray AM, Field H (1994) The trigeminal ganglion is a site of equine herpesvirus-1 (EHV-1) latency and reactivation in the horse. J Gen Virol 75:2007–2016

van der Sluijs M, Timmermans M, Moulin V et al (2011) Transplacental transmission of Bluetongue virus serotype 8 in ewes in early and mid gestation. Vet Microbiol 149:113–125

van der Sluijs MT, de Smit AJ, Moormann RJ (2016) Vector independent transmission of the vector-borne bluetongue virus. Crit Rev Microbiol 42(1):57–64

Smirnova NP, Bielefeldt-Ohmann H, Van Campen H, Austin KJ, Han H, Montgomery DL, Shoemaker ML, van Olphen AL, Hansen TR (2008) Acute non-cytopathic bovine viral diarrhea virus infection induces pronounced type I interferon response in pregnant cows and fetuses. Virus Res 132(1–2):49–58

Smirnova NP, Ptitsyn AA, Austin KJ, Bielefeldt-Ohmann H, Van Campen H, Han H et al (2009) Persistent fetal infection with bovine viral diarrhea virus differentially affects maternal blood cell signal transduction pathways. Physiol Genomics 36:129–139

Smirnova NP, Webb BT, Bielefeldt-Ohmann H, Van Campen H, Antoniazzi AQ, Morarie SE, Hansen TR (2012) Development of fetal and placental innate immune responses during establishment of persistent infection with bovine viral diarrhea virus. Virus Res 167(2):329–336

Smith KC, Borchers K (2001) A study of the pathogenesis of equid herpesvirus-1 (EHV-1) abortion by DNA *in-situ* hybridization. J Comp Pathol 125:304–310

Smith KC, Whitwell KE, Binns MM, Dolby CA, Hannant D, Mumford JA (1992) Abortion of virologically negative foetuses following experimental challenge of pregnant pony mares with equid herpesvirus 1. Equine Vet J 24:256–259

Smith PM, Zhang Y, Jennings SR, O'Callaghan DJ (1998) Characterization of the Cytolytic T-lymphocyte response to a candidate vaccine strain of equine herpesvirus 1 in CBA mice. J Virol 72:5366–5372

Smith KC, Whitwell KE, Blunden AS, Bestbier ME, Scase TJ, Geraghty RJ, Nugent J, Davis-Poynter NJ, Cardwell JM (2004) Equine herpesvirus-1 abortion: atypical cases with lesions largely or wholly restricted to the placenta. Equine Vet J 36:79–82

Smith KL, Allen GP, Branscum AJ, Frank Cook R, Vickers ML, Timoney PJ, Balasuriya UB (2010) The increased prevalence of neuropathogenic strains of EHV-1 in equine abortions. Vet Microbiol 141:5–11

Soboll Hussey G, Hussey SB, Wagner B, Horohov DW, Van De Walle GR, Osterrieder N, Goehring LS, Rao S, Lunn DP (2011) Evaluation of immune responses following infection of ponies with an EHV-1 ORF1/2 deletion mutant. Vet Res 42:23

Soboll G, Schaefer TM, Wira CR (2006) Effect of toll-like receptor (TLR) agonists on TLR and microbicide expression in uterine and vaginal tissues of the mouse. Am J Reprod Immunol 55:434–446

Soboll G, Breathnach CC, Kydd JH, Hussey SB, Mealey RM, Lunn DP (2010) Vaccination of ponies with the IE gene of EHV-1 in a recombinant modified live vaccinia vector protects against clinical and virological disease. Vet Immunol Immunopathol 135:108–117

Soto P, Parma AE (1989) The immune response in cattle infected with *Tritrichomonas foetus*. Vet Parasitol 33:343–348

Starick E (1998) Rapid and sensitive detection of equine arteritis virus in semen and tissue samples by reverse transcription- polymerase chain reaction, dot blot hybridisation and nested polymerase chain reaction. Acta Virol 42:333–339

Stavru F, Bouillaud F, Sartori A, Ricquier D, Cossart P (2011) *Listeria monocytogenes* transiently alters mitochondrial dynamics during infection. Proc Natl Acad Sci U S A 108:3612–3617

Stevens MG, Pugh GW Jr, Tabatabai LB (1992) Effects of gamma interferon and indomethacin in preventing *Brucella abortus* infections in mice. Infect Immun 60:4407–4409

Stevenson B, Choy HA, Pinne M, Rotondi ML, Miller MC, Demoll E, Kraiczy P, Cooley AE, Creamer TP, Suchard MA, Brissette CA, Verma A, Haake DA (2007) *Leptospira interrogans* endostatin-like outer membrane proteins bind host fibronectin, laminin and regulators of complement. PLoS One 2(11):e1188

Stokes A, Wardley RC (1988) ADCC and complement-dependent lysis as immune mechanisms against EHV-1 infection in the horse. Res Vet Sci 44:295–302

Stott JL, Blanchard MT, Anderson M, Maas J, Walker RL, Kennedy PC, Norman BB, BonDurant RH, Oliver MN, Hanks D, Hall MR (2002) Experimental transmission of epizootic bovine abortion (foothill abortion). Vet Microbiol 88:161–173

Stubbings DP, Cameron IRD (1981) Bovine abortion associated with infectious bovine rhinotracheitis virus infection. Vet Rec 108:101–102

Subauste CS, Wessendarp M (2006) CD40 restrains *in vivo* growth of *Toxoplasma gondii* independently of gamma interferon. Infect Immun 74(3):1573–1579

Subauste CS, Andrade RM, Wessendarp M (2007) CD40-TRAF6 and autophagy-dependent antimicrobial activity in macrophages. Autophagy 3(3):245–248

Sulochana S, Pillai RM, Nair GK, Abdulla PKR (1982) Serological survey on the occurrence of infectious bovine rhinotracheitis in Kerala. Ind J Comp Microbiol Immunol Infec Dis 3:7–11

Suzuki Y, Orellana MA, Schreiber RD, Remington JS (1988) Interferon-gamma: the major mediator of resistance against *Toxoplasma gondii*. Science 240(4851):516–518

Tafuri A, Alferink J, Möller P, Hämmerling GJ, Arnold B (1995) T cell awareness of paternal alloantigens during pregnancy. Science 270:630–633

Tait ED, Jordan KA, Dupont CD, Harris TH, Gregg B, Wilson EH, Pepper M, Dzierszinski F, Roos DS, Hunter CA (2010) Virulence of *Toxoplasma gondii* is associated with distinct dendritic cell responses and reduced numbers of activated CD8+ T cells. J Immunol 185(3):1502–1512

Tajiki H, Salomao R (1996) Association of plasma levels of tumor necrosis factor alpha with severity of disease and mortality among patients with leptospirosis. Clin Infect Dis 23:1177–1178

Takiuchi E, Medici K, Alfieri A, Alfieri A (2005) Bovine herpesvirus type 1 abortions detected by a semi-nested PCR in Brazilian cattle herds. Res Vet Sci 79:85–88

Talbot JA, Nielsen K, Corbeil LB (1991) Cleavage of reproductive secretions by extracellular proteinases of *Tritrichomonas foetus*. Can J Microbiol 37:384–390

Thiry E, Bublot M, Dubuisson J, Pastoret PP (1989) Bovine herpesvirus 4 (BHV-4) infections of cattle. In: Wittmann G (ed) Herpesvirus diseases of cattle, horses, and pigs. Kluwer Academic Publishers, Norwell, MA, pp 96–115

Tikoo SK, Campos M, Babiuk LA (1995) Bovine herpesvirus 1 (BHV-1): biology, pathogenesis and control. Adv Virus Res 45:191–223

Timoney PJ (1984) Clinical, virological and epidemiological features of the 1984 outbreak of equine viral arteritis in the Thoroughbred population in Kentucky, USA. Proc Int Conf Thoroughbred Breed Organ: Equine Viral Arteritis 1984:24–33

Timoney PJ, McCollum WH (1993) Equine viral arteritis. Vet Clin N Am Equine Pract 9:295–309

Trichard CJ, Herr S, Bastianello SS, Roux D (1982) Unilateral orchitis in a bull caused by *Brucella abortus* biotype 1. J S Afr Vet Assoc 53:60–62

Tseng CT, Rank RG (1998) Role of NK cells in early host response to chlamydial genital infection. Infect Immun 66:5867–5875

Turin L, Russo S (2003) BHV-1 infection in cattle: an update. Vet Bull 73(8):15–21

Vaala WE, Hamir AN, Dubovi EJ, Timoney PJ, Ruiz B (1992) Fatal congenitally acquired infection with equine arteritis virus in a neonatal Thoroughbred. Equine Vet J 24:155–158

Van De Walle GR, May ML, Sukhumavasi W, Von Einem J, Osterrieder N (2007) Herpesvirus chemokine-binding glycoprotein G (gG) efficiently inhibits neutrophil chemotaxis *in vitro* and *in vivo*. J Immunol 179:4161–4169

Van Der Meulen KM, Nauwynck HJ, Pensaert MB (2003) Absence of viral antigens on the surface of equine herpesvirus-1-infected peripheral blood mononuclear cells: a strategy to avoid complement-mediated lysis. J Gen Virol 84:93–97

Van Der Meulen KM, Favoreel HW, Pensaert MB, Nauwynck HJ (2006) Immune escape of equine herpesvirus 1 and other herpesviruses of veterinary importance. Vet Immunol Immunopathol 111:31–40

Vander Wielen AL, King GJ (1984) Intraepithelial lymphocytes in the bovine uterus during the oestrus cycle early gestation. J Reprod Fertil 49:15–28

Vázquez-Boland JA, Kuhn M, Berche P, Chakraborty T, Domínguez-Bernal G, Goebel W, González-Zorn B, Wehland J, Kreft J (2001) Listeria pathogenesis and molecular virulence determinants. Clin Microbiol Rev 14(3):584–640

Vilcek S, Durkovic B, Kolesarova M, Paton DJ (2005) Genetic diversity of BVDV: consequences for classification and molecular epidemiology. Prevent Vet Med 72:31–35

Vinh T, Adler B, Faine S (1986) Glycolipoprotein cytotoxin from *Leptospira interrogans* serovar copenhageni. J Gen Microbiol 132:111–123

Vossenkamper A, Struck D, Alvarado-Esquivel C, Went T, Takeda K, Akira S, Pfeffer K, Alber G, Lochner M, Forster I, Liesenfeld O (2004) Both IL-12 and IL-18 contribute to small intestinal Th1-type immunopathology following oral infection with *Toxoplasma gondii*, but IL-12 is dominant over IL-18 in parasite control. Eur J Immunol 34(11):3197–3207

Voyich JM, Palecanda A, Burgess DE (2001) Antigen-specific T-cell responses in cattle immunized with antigens of Tritrichomonas foetus. J Parasitol 87(5):1040–1048

Watson RO, Galan JE (2005) Signal transduction in *Campylobacter jejuni*-induced cytokine production. Cell Microbiol 7:655–665

Watson ED, Diehl NK, Evans JF (1990) Antibody response in the bovine genital tract to intrauterine infusion of Actinomyces pyogenes. J Res Vet Sci 48:70–75

Watson RO, Novik V, Hofreuter D, Lara-Tejero M, Galan JE (2007) A MyD88-deficient mouse model reveals a role for Nramp1 in *Campylobacter jejuni* infection. Infect Immun 75:1994–2003

Weindl G, Naglik JR, Kaesler S, Biedermann T, Hube B, Korting HC (2007) Human epithelial cells establish direct antifungal defense through TLR4-mediated signaling. J Clin Investig 117:72–3664

Weiss DS, Takeda K, Akira S, Zychlinsky A, Moreno E (2005) MyD88, but not Toll like receptors 4 and 2, is required for efficient clearance of *Brucella abortus*. Infect Immun 73:5137–5143

Weissmann J (2003) Presumptive *Toxoplasma gondii* abortion in a sheep. Can Vet J 44(4):322–324

Werts C, Tapping RI, Mathison JC, Chuang TH, Kravchenko V, Saint Girons I, Haake DA, Godowski PJ, Hayashi F, Ozinsky A, Underhill DM, Kirschning CJ, Wagner H, Aderem A, Tobias PS, Ulevitch RJ (2001) Leptospiral lipopolysaccharide activates cells through a TLR2-dependent mechanism. Nat Immunol 2(4):346–352

Wheelhouse N, Aitchison K, Laroucau K, Thomson J, Longbottom D (2010) Evidence of *Chlamydophila abortus* vaccine strain 1B as a possible cause of ovine enzootic abortion. Vaccine 28(35):5657–5663

Wilhelmsen CL, Bolin SR, Ridpath JF, Cheville NF, Kluge JP (1990) Experimental primary postnatal bovine viral diarrhoea viral infections in six month-old calves. Vet Pathol 27:235–243

Wilkins PA, Del Piero F, Lopez J, Cline M (1995) Immunohistochemical diagnosis of equine arteritis infection in a foal. Equine Vet J 27:398

Winkler MTC, Doster A, Jones C (1999) Bovine herpesvirus 1 can infect CD4+ T lymphocytes and induce programmed cell death during acute infection of cattle. J Virol 73:8657–8668

Wira CR, Fahey JV, Sentman CL, Pioli PA, Shen L (2005) Innate and adaptive immunity in female genital tract cellular responses and interactions. J Inte Rev Immunol 206:306–335

Wira CR, Patel MV, Ghosh M, Mukura L, Fahey JV (2011) Innate immunity in the human female reproductive tract: endocrine regulation of endogenous antimicrobial protection against HIV and other sexually transmitted infections. Am J Reprod Immunol 65:196–211

Wooding FBP (1992) Current topic the synepitheliochorial placenta of ruminants: binucleate cell fusions and hormone production. Placenta J 13:101–113

Wujcicka W, Wilczynski J, Nowakowska D (2014) Do the placental barrier, parasite genotype and Toll-like receptor polymorphisms contribute to the course of primary infection with various *Toxoplasma gondii* genotypes in pregnant women? Eur J Clin Microbiol Infect Dis 33(5): 703–709

Wyckoff JH III (2002) Bovine T lymphocyte responses to *Brucella abortus*. Vet Microbiol 90:395–415

Xavier MN, Paixao TA, Poester FP, Lage AP, Santos RL (2009) Pathology, immunohistochemistry and bacteriology of tissues and milk of cows and foetuses experimentally infected with *Brucella abortus*. J Comp Pathol 140:149–157

Xue F, Zhao X, Yang Y, Zhao J, Yang Y, Cao Y, Hong C, Liu Y, Sun L, Huang M, Gu J (2013) Responses of murine and human macrophages to Leptospiral Infection. A study using comparative array analysis. PLoS Negl Trop Dis 7:2410–2477

Yamane D, Nagai M, Ogawa Y, Tohya Y, Akashi H (2005) Enhancement of apoptosis via an extrinsic factor, TNF alpha in cells infected with cytopathic bovine viral diarrhoea virus. Microbes Infect 7:1482–1491

Yamane D, Kato K, Tohya Y, Akashi H (2006) The double stranded RNA induced apoptosis pathway is involved in the cytopathogenicity of cytopathogenic bovine viral diarrhoea virus. J Gen Virol 87:2961–2970

Yang CW, Wu MS, Pan MJ, Hong JJ, Yu CC, Vandewalle A, Huang CC (2000) Leptospira outer membrane protein activates NF-kappaB and downstream genes expressed in medullary thick ascending limb cells. J Am Soc Nephrol 11(11):2017–2026

Yang H, Qiu L, Chen G, Ye Z, Lu C, Lin Q (2008) Proportional change of CD4+CD25+ regulatory T cells in decidua and peripheral blood in unexplained recurrent spontaneous abortion patients. Fertil Steril 89:656–661

Zanella G, Durand B, Sellal E, Breard E, Sailleau C, Zientara S, Batten CA, Mathevet P, Audeval C (2012) Bluetongue serotype 8: abortion and transplacental transmission in cattle in the Burgundy region, France, 2008–2009. Theriogenology 77:65–72

Zervomanolakis I, Ott HW, Hadziomerovic D, Mattle V, Seeber BE, Virgolini I (2007) Physiology of upward transport in the human female genital tract. Annal N Y Acad Sci 1101:1–20

Zuerner RL, Alt DP, Palmer MV, Thacker TC, Olsen SC (2011) A *Leptospira borgpetersenii* serovar Hardjo vaccine induces a Th1 response, activates NK cells, and reduces renal colonization. Clin Vaccine Immunol 18(4):684–691

Zwerdling A, Delpino MV, Pasquevich KA, Barrionuevo P, Cassataro J, García Samartino C, Giambartolomei GH (2009) *Brucella abortus* activates human neutrophils. Microbes Infect 11: 689–697

Immunopathology of Mastitis

Key Points

1. Mastitis is an inflammatory condition of the mammary gland.
2. Mastitis is most often associated with lactating mammals and caused by bacterial, viral, and fungal infections.
3. Mastitis incidence is higher in cows from third lactation and above, where in the optimum milk production occurs.
4. Beginning 3 weeks before parturition and continuing through early lactation, dairy cattle are particularly vulnerable to developing intramammary infections.
5. Mammary defense mechanisms are divided into nonspecific and specific defense mechanisms.
6. Keratin layer of the stratified squamous epithelium lining the teat duct provides barrier by exhibiting bacteriostatic properties.
7. The mammary gland microenvironment contains a number of soluble antibacterial peptides, proteins, and enzymes with known bactericidal and bacteriostatic properties.
8. California mastitis test (CMT) is frequently employed as a quick animal-side assay in conjunction with clinical symptoms for the diagnosis of mastitis.

11.1 Introduction

Mastitis is derived from the Greek words '*mastos*', which means breast, and '*itis*', which mean inflammation. It is an inflammatory condition of the mammary gland caused by bacterial, viral and fungal infections, most often associated with lactating mammals (Foxman et al. 2002; Inch and von Xylander 2000). Physical, chemical, and bacteriological alterations in milk are indicators of mastitis. It is a common disease of high milking cows like exotic breeds and crossbred. Buffaloes are not so predisposed. Mastitis incidence is higher in cows from third lactation and above, wherein optimum milk production occurs. Due to decreasing milk output and quality, treatment expenses, animal replacement costs, and challenges in marketing low-quality dairy products, it is the most expensive disease for dairy farmers and the business (Hujips et al. 2008; Hogeveen et al. 2011). The disease results from a complex interplay between infectious agents, managemental practices, and environmental factors. It is a reaction to an injury or infection that helps to eliminate the infectious agents, enhance healing, and eventually return to normal function (Wellenberg et al. 2002; Hillerton and Berry 2005). The most significant changes in the milk include discoloration and the presence of flakes.

11.2 Mastitis-Causing Pathogens

11.2.1 Bacteria

Innumerable genera and species of bacteria cause mastitis. Predominant organisms are *Staphylococcus aureus* (Figs. 11.1 and 11.2) followed by *Streptococcus agalactia* (Fig. 11.3). The other organisms include *E. coli* (Figs. 11.4 and 11.5), *Streptococcus uberis* (Fig. 11.6), *Streptococcus dysgalactiae*, *Streptococcus zooepidemicus*, *Streptococcus faecalis*, *Streptococcus pyogenes*, *Campylobacter jejuni*, *Haemophilus somnus*, *Streptococcus pneumoniae*, *Corynebacterium pyogenes*, *Corynebacterium bovis* (Fig. 11.6), *Corynebacterium ulcerans*, *Klebsiella* spp., *Enterobacter aerogenes*, *Mycobacterium bovis*, *Mycobacterium lacticola*,

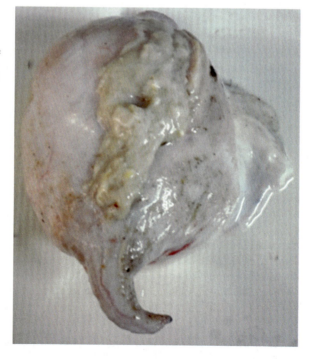

Fig. 11.1 Suppurative mastitis in an ewe caused by *Staphylococcus aureus*: the lactiferous sinus and ducts are filled with viscous thick grey colored pus and induration of udder

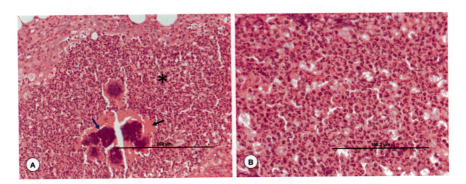

Fig. 11.2 Pyogranulomatous (botryomycotic) mastitis in mice caused by *Staphylococcus aureus*. (**a**) Marked infiltration of inflammatory cells especially intact and degenerate neutrophils (asterisk) with strongly eosinophilic, radiating material (Splendore-Hoeppli phenomenon; black arrow) containing large basophilic cocci in the center (blue arrow) in the mammary parenchyma. H&E ×200. (**b**) Higher magnification of Fig. (**a**). H&E ×400

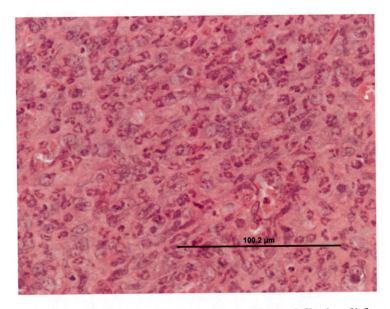

Fig. 11.3 Mixed mastitis in mice caused by *Streptococcus agalactiae*. Infiltration of inflammatory cells composed of mixed population of neutrophils, lymphocytes, and macrophages in the interstitium interspersed by fibrosis. H&E ×400

Mycobacterium bovigenitalium, *Mycoplasma*, *Acholeplasma laidlawii*, *Nocardia asteroids*, *N. farcinica*, *Leptospira interrogans* serovar *Pomona*, and *Leptospira interrogans hardjo* (Tables 11.1 and 11.2).

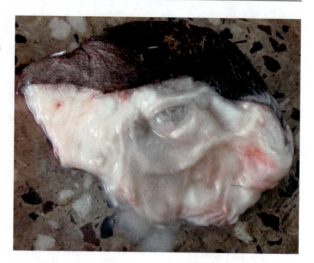

Fig. 11.4 Acute coliform mastitis in a buffalo: swelling of the gland, watery milk with small flakes that are barely visible nacked eyes

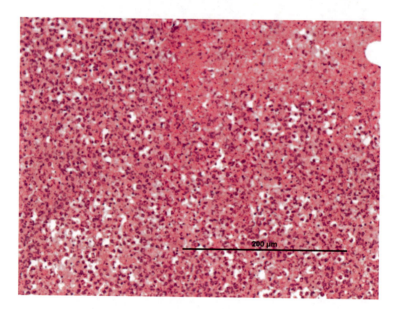

Fig. 11.5 Necrosuppurative mastitis in mice caused by *Escherichia coli*. Widespread areas of necrosis of the mammary parenchyma associated with marked infiltration of inflammatory cells especially intact and degenerate neutrophils and deposition of fibrin. H&E ×200

The fungal agents like *Trichophyton* species, *Aspergillus fumigatus*, *Aspergillus nidulans*, and *Pichia* species are responsible for causing mastitis. Mastitis causing yeast species are *Saccharomyces* spp., *Cryptococcus neoformans*, and *Candida* spp. Algae like *Prototheca irispora* and *Prototheca zopfii* are responsible for causing mastitis.

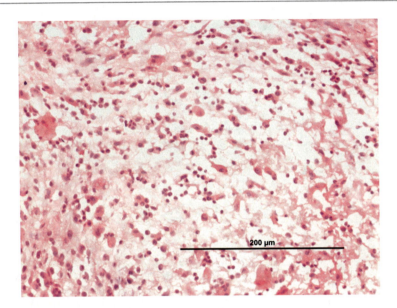

Fig. 11.6 Lymphoplasmacytic mastitis in mice. Infiltration of inflammatory cells composed of lymphocytes and plasma cells associated with fibrosis caused by *Streptococcus* spp., Coagulase-negative *Staphylococcus*, *Staphylococcus aureus*, *Corynebacterium bovis*, and *Streptococcus uberis*. H&E ×200

11.2.2 Viruses

Viruses causing mastitis are infectious bovine rhinotracheitis (IBR), bovine viral diarrhea (BVD), foot-and-mouth disease (FMD), cow pox, pseudo cowpox, and ulcerative mammillitis in cattle, which also predispose cows to bacterial mastitis.

More than 130 microorganisms can cause mastitis, although mastitis is usually caused by some groups of bacteria (Wellenberg et al. 2002; Hillerton and Berry 2005). Mastitis develops when pathogenic bacteria breach physical barriers, such as the teat, and enter into the mammary glands, which usually has sterile environment (Sordillo et al. 1997; Aitken et al. 2011a, b). Mastitis-causing microorganisms are typically classified as either contagious or environmental; although this distinction has recently been disputed (Zadoks 2014). The coliforms like *Klebsiella* or *Escherichia coli* (*E. coli*) and *Streptococci* have generally been classified as environmental pathogens and are the primary cause of clinical mastitis. On the other hand, contagious pathogens, such as *Staphylococcus aureus* (*S. aureus*) and *Streptococcus agalactiae*, are easily transmitted from the infected quarters to other quarters of the same cow or other cows (Bradley 2002; Atalla et al. 2010; Contreras and Rodriguez 2011).

The development of mastitis is partially related to the exposure of the mammary glands to bacterial pathogens. Mastitis is caused by a wide variety of Gram-positive

Table 11.1 Clinical manifestations of different types of mastitis and their etiological agents in cattle

Etiology	Type of mastitis	Clinical findings
Contagious pathogens		
Coagulase-positive *Staphylococcus aureus*	• Peracute, acute, and chronic (recurrent) clinical mastitis • Subclinical mastitis • Botryomycotic mastitis (Fig. 11.2)	• Chronic *S. aureus* mastitis is characterized by high SCC, gradual induration of udder, drop in milk yield, and atrophy with occasional appearance of clots in milk or wateriness • During early lactation, acute and peracute *S. aureus* mastitis are most common • Acute swelling of gland swelling accompanied by fever and heat; abnormal milk with thick clots, blood, and pus (Fig. 11.1); gangrene of the gland and teat; and occasionally, gas in the teat in peracute form
Streptococcus agalactiae	Subacute to acute mastitis	• Mastitis episodes recur frequently. Subacute to acute mastitis is most common • Swollen gland with warm temperature, transient fever, and watery milk with clots. If untreated, the udder will gradually indurate
Mycoplasma bovis	• Purulent interstitial mastitis • *Mycoplasma bovigenitalium* causes mild mastitis and spontaneously vanishes from the herd without affecting milk output	• Clinical mastitis that develops suddenly • Usually all four quarters are affected, milk production drops noticeably, and may stop lactation • Swelling of udder and severe abnormalities in the milk without clear symptoms of systemic infection. Eventually, the udder becomes atrophied and does not return to production • Secretion may be tinged pink with blood or show a gray or brown discoloration. Within a few days, secretion is frankly purulent or curdy, but there is absence of large, firm clots. This abnormal secretion persists for weeks or even months

(continued)

11.2 Mastitis-Causing Pathogens

Table 11.1 (continued)

Etiology	Type of mastitis	Clinical findings
Corynebacterium bovis	• Subclinical mastitis (89%) • Clinical mastitis (22%)	• Mild to moderate increase in SCC and little increase in the CMT score • Losses in milk production are typically undetectable
Environmental pathogens		
Escherichia coli, Klebsiella pneumonia, Enterobacter aerogenes	Coliform mastitis (Figs. 11.4 and 11.5)	**Acute mastitis**: Swelling of gland, watery milk that has small flakes (Fig. 11.2), mild systemic reaction, and recovery in few days
		Peracute mastitis: Agalactia and severe toxemia that develops suddenly, along with fever, tachycardia, impending shock, weakness, shivering, and even recumbency in the cows. The quarter may or may not be swollen and warm and the secretions are thin, serous, and contain extremely minute flakes that are hardly visible to the unaided eye. Hence, coliform mastitis may go unnoticed during the initial clinical examination. In a few days, animal may die
Environmental Streptococci (*Streptococcus uberis* and *S. dysgalactiae*)	Clinical mastitis (50%)	• Clinical findings are usually limited to abnormal secretion or abnormal gland, and usually no systemic signs • Recovery in two to three milkings with intramammary treatment • *S. uberis* mastitis has a higher milk SCC than *S. dysgalactiae* mastitis, indicating that *S. uberis* infections are more severe
Trueperella pyogenes (previously known as *Corynebacterium pyogenes, Actinomyces pyogenes*, and *Arcanobacterium pyogenes*)	• Clinical mastitis • Suppurative mastitis • Pyogenes mastitis • Summer mastitis	• The gland is sore, extremely hard, and severely swollen • Most often, only one quarter is affected • The secretion from infected quarter is initially watery with clots and thereafter purulent with a distinctive putrid odor

(continued)

Table 11.1 (continued)

Etiology	Type of mastitis	Clinical findings
		• Initially severe systemic symptoms, such as fever, lethargy, inappetence, tachycardia, depression, and mortality rate of up to 50% • If the cow survives from the initial infection, the affected quarter becomes severely indurated and abscessed. Later, the abscess ruptures through the floor of udder with drainage of purulent material at the base of the teat • There is an extremely higher SCC in the secretion of affected cows, which looks more like a purulent process than milk • A significant fly population is typically seen on affected cows • Function of the quarter is permanently lost, and recently calved cows may experience complete dryness • A common sequelae is severe thelitis with extreme thickening and obstruction of the teat
Teat skin opportunistic pathogens		
Coagulase-negative *Staphylococcus* spp.	Mild clinical and subclinical mastitis	Mild clinical disease (abnormal secretion only and occasionally abnormal gland)
Cattle mastitis related with less common infections		
Pseudomonas aeruginosa	Mild subacute or chronic mastitis (Fig. 11.7)	• Usually subacute, chronic, or mild, but can be clinically severe with a mortality rate of up to 17% of affected cows • Clinically, the condition manifests as a severe systemic reaction, acute enlargement of the gland, and the appearance of clotted, discolored milk; function of the gland is usually completely lost at the first attack

(continued)

11.2 Mastitis-Causing Pathogens

Table 11.1 (continued)

Etiology	Type of mastitis	Clinical findings
Mannheimia (formerly *Pasteurella*) *haemolytica* and *Pasteurella multocida*	Peracute gangrenous mastitis	• Severe mastitis accompanied by fever, severe toxemic shock, weak pulse, tachycardia, and recumbency • Affected quarter is extremely swollen, and the milk is watery, red-tinged color, and flakes are present • Internal bleeding may occur as a result of disseminated intravascular coagulopathy • All four quarters could be affected, leading to atrophy and fibrosis
Nocardia spp.	Nocardial mastitis	• Systemic reaction with high fever, depression, and anorexia • Fibrosis of the gland and development of clots in a viscous, greyish secretion that contains small white particles. Fibrosis may be diffuse but usually in the form of discrete masses of 2–5 cm in diameter • Severely affected glands become grossly enlarged and may rupture or develop sinus tracts to the exterior
Bacillus cereus and *B. subtilis*	Peracute to acute mastitis	• Clinically, one or more quarters affected and peracute to acute mastitis • Severe swelling, pain, and red-tinged secretion with serous consistency • Initially high fever and severe toxemia. Affected cows are weak and quickly become recumbent; death may occur in 24–36 h • If a cow survives, gangrene could develop, portions of affected glands would slough off, and recurrent chronic mastitis would continue
Campylobacter jejuni	Subclinical mastitis	Characterized by very high cell counts, transient episode of fever, swelling of the quarter, and fine granular clots in the milk

(continued)

Table 11.1 (continued)

Etiology	Type of mastitis	Clinical findings
Clostridium perfringens type A		• This is an uncommon form of mastitis • Characterized by high temperature, edematous swelling, and superficial hyperemia of the affected quarter, which are followed by gangrene, enlargement of the supramammary lymph nodes, thin, brown secretion that contains gas, and subcutaneous emphysema
Fusobacterium necrophorum	Mixed infections of *F. necrophorum* play a significant part in the summer mastitis brought on by *T. pyogenes*	• This is a rare type of mastitis but is likely to have a high incidence in the herd • A viscid, clotty, stringy secretion is present in the affected quarters, but there is little fibrosis
Histophilus somni (formerly known as *Haemophilus somnus*)	Mild chronic mastitis	Acute form with high fever, milk is stained with blood, and gangrenous form
Listeria monocytogenes	Subclinical mastitis	The majority of cases in cattle are subclinical, and abnormal milk is uncommon
Serratia marcescens	Mild chronic mastitis	Periodically, milk clots occur with swelling of the quarters

Table 11.2 Different types of mastitis and their etiological agents in cattle

Type of mastitis	Etiological agent
Severe necrotizing (gangrenous) mastitis	Virulent *Staphylococcus aureus* and *Streptococci* spp.
Suppurative mastitis	*Trueperella pyogenes*, *Mycoplasma bovis*, *Streptococcus dysgalactiae*
	Genera: *Bacteroides*, *Peptostreptococcus*, and *Fusobacterium*
Summer mastitis/Holstein udder plague	*Trueperella* (*Arcanobacterium*) *pyogenes* is a common pathogen along with *Bacteroides melaninogenicus*, *Fusobacterium necrophorum*, *Streptococcus dysgalactiae*, and *Peptostreptococcus indolicus*
Granulomatous mastitis	Algae (*Prototheca zopfii*), *Candida* species, atypical *Mycobacterium* species (other than *Mycobacterium bovis*), *Cryptococcus neoformans*, and *Nocardia asteroids*
Coliform mastitis	*Escherichia coli*, *Enterobacter aerogenes*, and *Klebsiella pneumoniae*; genera: *Citrobacter*, *Serratia*, and *Proteus*
Tuberculous mastitis	*Mycobacterium bovis*

Table 11.3 Innate or non-specific defenses of the mammary gland

Factors	Innate molecules
Physical factors	• Flushing action of milk
	• Sphincter and keratin of papillary orifice
Soluble factors	• Cytokines
	• Complement
	• Lysozyme
	• Lactoferrin
Cellular factors	• Natural killer cells
	• Neutrophils
	• Macrophages
	• Microbial recognition molecules

and Gram-negative bacteria. The expression of bacterial virulence factors determines the establishment and severity of mastitis. Various host-related factors, such as nutrition, genetics, oxidative stress, environmental stressors, and the physiological transition of the mammary gland from involution to lactation, determines the increased susceptibility to mastitis and the extent of severity of the disease (Sordillo and Streicher 2002; Sordillo and Aitken 2009; Sordillo et al. 2009; Contreras and Sordillo 2011). Dairy cattle are especially susceptible to intramammary infections beginning from 3 weeks prior to parturition through early lactation (Oliver and Sordillo 1988). The ability to control mastitis, especially during the periparturient period, is ultimately reliant upon an efficient immune system that rapidly clears the bacterial pathogens and restores the mammary gland function and milk production.

11.3 Immune Responses

The immune system of the mammary gland is constituted by the innate and adaptive (acquired) immune systems consist of various physical, cellular, and molecular factors. The primary line of defense is the innate immune system and already present in the mammary gland and promptly activated when exposed to microorganisms. Depending on the efficiency of the innate defense mechanisms, pathogens may be eliminated within minutes to hours following invasion. Frequently, there will not be any observable changes in mammary gland function or milk quality in cases of quick bacterial clearance. The efficiency of the innate arm of immune system not only determines occurrence of intramammary infections, but also influences the severity and duration of mastitis by modulating the adaptive immune responses. Innate defense mechanisms are made up of phagocytes (i.e., neutrophils and macrophages), pattern recognition receptors, a variety of soluble substances (i.e., cytokines, complement and lactoferrin), and non-specific physical barriers at the teat end (Table 11.3) (Aitken et al. 2011a, b).

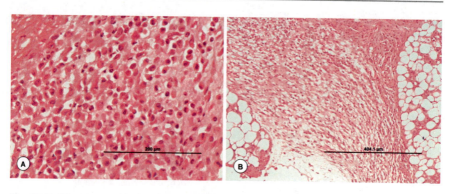

Fig. 11.7 Chronic mastitis in mice. (**a**) Marked infiltration of macrophages in the interstitium along with fibrosis. H&E ×200. (**b**) Marked fibrosis in the mammary parenchyma interspersed by inflammatory cells infiltrate. H&E ×100

When innate immune systems are unable to completely eliminate the pathogen, adaptive immune responses are activated. It is characterized by the development of antigen-specific memory cells and lymphocytes with the ability to recognize specific antigenic determinants of a pathogen. Immunological memory and clonal proliferation of antigen-specific effector cells in the mammary gland lead to a enhanced state of immune responsiveness upon re-exposure to the same antigen. Comparing to primary immune responses, adaptive immune responses frequently clears the invading microorganisms significantly quicker, much stronger, long lasting, and more efficiently. Due to the clonal expansion of B and T lymphocytes specific to the invading pathogens, adaptive immunity can take days to develop completely. Specific bacterial virulence factors are recognized and countered by antibodies, which are secreted by antigen-specific B lymphocytes. T lymphocytes produce cytokines that facilitate cell-mediated immunity by regulating the magnitude and duration of the immune responses. Both innate and adaptive immune defenses of the mammary gland must be highly interactive and coordinated in order to provide optimal protection from mastitis (Aitken et al. 2011a, b).

11.4 Host-Pathogen Interactions

The host-pathogen interactions within the mammary glands are variable and can result in acute or chronic symptoms that may presented as a range of mild from of subclinical to severe form of clinical mastitis. During intramammary infections, distinct mammary gland immune responses are elicited by Gram-positive and Gram-negative bacteria (Bannerman 2009). Different infectious agents produce differences in the magnitude and duration of host immune responses. For example, *Staphylococcus aureus* internalizes within the host cells to avoid the initial innate immune reactions, results in subclinical chronic mastitis. Further, coliform infections are associated with rapid bacterial growth, toxin release, eicosanoid biosynthesis, and cytokine production, which can cause severe acute clinical mastitis. Hence, the host immune responses to bacterial pathogens are determined by bacterial recognition and communication between different cell types within the mammary gland (Aitken et al. 2011a, b).

However, excessive immune responses may cause tissue damage. In order to prevent severe bystander tissue damage, the bacteria that cause mastitis must be quickly neutralized and eliminated. Therefore, delicate balances of pro-inflammatory and anti-inflammatory activities are critical to prevent inadvertent damage to the mammary gland and restore homeostasis to the immune systems. With better understanding the crucial host-pathogen interactions during infection, novel therapies aiming at enhancing the natural immunological defenses of mammary gland and preventing immune-related disease can be developed.

11.5 Mammary Immunology

The mammary defense mechanisms are divided into two types, namely, non-specific and specific defense mechanisms. The non-specific defense mechanisms include physical and chemical barriers of teat, endogenous soluble defenses or lactenins (i.e., cytokines, complement and lactoferrin), pattern recognition receptors, and phagocytes (i.e., neutrophils and macrophages).

11.6 Physical and Chemical Barriers of the Teat

The teat canal is the entry portal for bacterial pathogens. The patency of the sphincter muscles surrounding the teat end opening is directly associated to increased susceptibility to intramammary infections because they prevent bacterial penetration by maintaining a tight closure between periods of milk removal (Capuco et al. 1992). Keratin layer produced by the stratified squamous epithelium lining the teat duct provides barrier to invading pathogens between milking periods. During the non-lactating period, keratin plug completely occluded the teat canal, which physically traps bacteria and preventing subsequent migration into the gland cistern. In dairy cattle, keratin removal from the teat end was correlated to an increased bacterial colonization and invasion (Bramley and Dodd 1984; Capuco et al. 1992). Esterified and non-esterified fatty acids, which are lipid components of keratin, exhibits bacteriostatic properties. Intramammary infections still happens despite the ability of the teat to trap pathogens, and the mammary gland must rely on other antimicrobial defense mechanisms to inhibit the bacterial growth (Table 11.4) (Aitken et al. 2011a, b).

Table 11.4 Portals of entry into a mammary gland

Factors	Innate molecules
Physical factors	• Flushing action of milk
	• Sphincter and keratin of papillary orifice
Soluble factors	• Cytokines
	• Complement
	• Lactoferrin
	• Lysozyme
Cellular factors	• Natural killer cells
	• Neutrophils
	• Macrophages
	• Microbial recognition molecules

11.7 Endogenous Defenses

The mammary gland microenviroment contains a number of soluble antibacterial peptides, proteins, and enzymes with known bactericidal and bacteriostatic properties that can target the invading organisms. Lactoferrin, complement, lysozyme, cytokines, immunoglobulins (Ig), and other soluble molecules are some of the pre-existing antibacterial components. The composition of antibacterial components in mammary gland environment changes during different stages of lactation and have variable efficacy against different mastitis-causing pathogens (Aitken et al. 2011a, b).

11.8 Lactoferrin

Leukocytes and epithelial cells both produce lactoferrin, an iron-binding protein, which showed bacteriostatic properties. The presence of bicarbonate and lactoferrin sequester free ferric ions in milk and inhibits the growth of bacteria like staphylococci and coliforms, which require iron. It has been demonstrated that lactoferrin and immunoglobulins work synergistically to inhibit the growth of specific Gram-negative bacteria in ruminants (Chaneton et al. 2008). Lactoferrin may marginally neutralize the cytotoxic effects of endotoxin by binding the lipid A portion of lipopolysaccharide (LPS), thus potentially inhibit the course of Gram-negative intramammary infections (Pecorini et al. 2010).

Some bacteria are resistant to the antibacterial properties of lactoferrin. For example, after binding with citrate or cell surface receptors, *Streptococcus agalactiae* can use lactoferrin as an iron source, while *S. uberis* can use lactoferrin as a molecular bridge to adhere on mammary epithelial cell surfaces (Patel et al. 2009) resulting in internalization by cells and evading from the local immune defense mechanisms. Stage of lactation greatly influences the amount and effectiveness of antibacterial properties of lactoferrin. For example, the concentration of lactoferrin is low in the milk of healthy lactating mammary glands, but increases dramatically during involution and inflammation (Sordillo et al. 1987).

11.9 Complement

Complement is a component of the innate defense system and consists of collection of proteins synthesized mainly by hepatocytes and present in serum and milk. Colostrum, inflamed mammary glands, and during involution have the highest concentrations of complement (Riollet et al. 2000a, b). When the complement system is activated, various pro-inflammatory molecules are produced, of which the C5a molecule being particularly associated with mastitis (Rainard 2003). Direct bactericidal activities are due to the formation of membrane attack complex onto the surface of bacteria. *Escherichia coli* is a Gram-negative bacterium that causes mastitis, and particularly susceptible to complement-mediated lysis (Riollet et al. 2000a, b). Complement molecules opsonize the bacteria and activate the host immune cells for phagocytosis and intracellular killing. Complement is a potent chemoattractant for neutrophils and monocytes during the early stages of infection (Rainard 2003).

11.10 Cytokines

Cytokines play an important role in most of the aspects of inflammation and immunity (Sordillo et al. 1997; Riollet et al. 2000a, b; Alluwaimi 2004; Bannerman 2009; Watson et al. 2011). It is made up of a diverse group of proteins that are produced throughout the body by immune and non-immune cells. Individual cytokines can interact with other cytokines in a variety of ways, including additively, antagonistically, and synergistically on multiple cell targets. Due to the short half-lives of majority of the cytokines, their production and function typically happen in bursts of activity. Cytokines can influence the cellular functions through high affinity receptors for each cytokine located on the mammary gland epithelial cells. The concentration and composition of secreted cytokines within the mammary gland tissues changes dramatically during different physiological transitions of the mammary gland. For example, expression of IL-2 and IFN was lower during the periparturient period compared to fully involuted bovine mammary glands (Babiuk et al. 1991). In contrast, milk and mammary tissues were shown to express higher IL-4, IL-10, and TNF-α (Sordillo et al. 1995; Shafer-Weaver et al. 1999).

There is no evidence that cytokines have direct antibacterial effects, in contrast to other soluble defenses in the mammary gland. Instead, cytokines play a crucial role in host defense by orchestrating the antimicrobial activities of the mammary gland effector cell populations after exposure to invading pathogens. Therefore, preexisting concentrations of cytokines in the healthy mammary gland likely exert their biological effects by influencing the normal physiological functions and maintaining immunological homeostasis (Sordillo et al. 1997; Watson et al. 2011).

As a result, cytokines have a variety of effects on the defense mechanisms of mammary gland, including the induction of inflammation, escalation of innate and adaptive immune responses, and activation of leukocyte migration from blood into infected tissues after local cell populations recognize the bacteria. The pattern of cytokine expression by cells in the mammary gland will differ depending on the mastitis-causing pathogens that elicit their response (Bannerman 2009). However, in comparison to Gram-positive bacteria, which typically express weaker and slower cytokine responses during the early stage of infection, Gram-negative bacteria tend to initiate a greater magnitude of pro-inflammatory cytokine responses (i.e., IL-1, IL-6, IL-8, and TNF-α) (Aitken et al. 2011a, b).

11.11 Eicosanoids

Eicosanoids regulate various aspects of inflammation, including vascular permeability, leukocyte infiltration, localized edema, and fever (Harizi et al. 2008). Mastitic cows had higher eicosanoid concentrations in their milk and plasma (Zia et al. 1987; Maddox et al. 1991). Through the cyclooxygenase (COX), lipoxygenase (LOX), or P450 enzymatic pathways, fatty acids are oxygenated for the biosynthesis of eicosanoids. Certain eicosanoids can either exacerbate or suppress the inflammatory responses depending on the timing and intensity of expression. There are two main isoforms in the COX pathway. The COX1 synthesizes low amounts of prostaglandins (PG), such as prostacyclin (PGI2), which are necessary for the maintenance of normal physiological functions and vascular homeostasis. Conversely, COX2 is strongly induced in response to pro-inflammatory stimuli and is associated with the secretion of pro-inflammatory mediators such as PGE2, PGF2α, and thromboxane B2 (TXB2). Increased PGE2, PGF2α and TXB2 concentrations in milk were detected in both experimental and natural cases of mastitis (Atroshi et al. 1986, 1989; Peter et al. 1990; Boutet et al. 2003). However, increased COX2 expression during the resolution of inflammation is associated with the presence of metabolites, such as PGD2 and 15 d-PGJ2, which can inhibit leukocyte adhesion to endothelial cells and decrease cytokine expression by blocking nuclear factor kappa B (NF-kB) activation (Pattanaik and Prasad 1998). Non-steroidal anti-inflammatory drugs (NSAIDs) are commonly used to treat inflammatory-based disorders such as mastitis in dairy cows, which can inhibit the PG production by targeting the COX activity (Wagner and Apley 2004; Vangroenweghe et al. 2005; Banting et al. 2008; McDougall et al. 2009).

Arachidonic acid is metabolized through the 5LOX pathway, which produces the hydroxyl and hydroperoxy derivatives namely, 5-hydroxyeicosatetraenoic acid (HETE) and 5-hydroperoxyeicosatetraenoic acid (HPETE), respectively that are frequently increased during inflammation. The 15LOX1 isoform is characterized by an inducible enzyme expressed in endothelial cells, epithelial cells, reticulocytes, and macrophages with the ability to oxygenate polyunsaturated fatty acids (PUFA) during inflammation (Natarajan and Nadler 2004). Intercellular adhesion molecule 1 (ICAM1) expression and monocyte adherence in vessel walls were increased by

15LOX1 pathway metabolites (Spector et al. 1988; Reilly et al. 2004), thus enhancing the pro-inflammatory cytokines of endothelial cells. On the other hand, LOX pathways are also crucial for the production of lipoxins (LX), a special class of eicosanoids having dual anti-inflammatory and pro-resolving properties (Serhan et al. 2008). In contrast to acute mastitis, chronic mastitis results in an imbalance of LXA4:LTB4, which is thought to be caused by a sharp decline in LXA4 production within the infected mammary glands (Boutet et al. 2003).

11.12 Immunoglobulins

Immunoglobulins are produced by plasma cells and play a role in surveillance and early elimination of mastitis-causing pathogens from the mammary gland (Sordillo and Nickerson 1988). Some of the immunoglobulins found in colostrum and milk, in addition to plasma cells, which may be produced by mammary gland epithelial cells. Four classes of immunoglobulins are known to involve in the mammary gland defenses namely; IgG1, IgG2, IgA, and IgM. Immunoglobulin concentrations are often highest during colostrogenesis and intramammary infections. In healthy bovine mammary glands, IgG1 is a predominant isotype, while IgG2 significantly increases during mastitis. In fact, research findings suggested that low concentrations of IgG2 isotype correlated with an increased incidence of bovine mastitis (Sordillo and Streicher 2002). In Danish red cattle, IgG deficiency is characterized by increased susceptibility to pyogenic infection and gangrenous mastitis (Chauhan 1998). The IgA is found in highest concentrations in the milk of women, particularly during the immediate postpartum period. Increased susceptibility to mastitis in women is correlated with low concentrations of IgA in milk. The presence of immunoglobulin isotypes in the colostrum and milk can facilitate the antimicrobial defenses of the mammary gland. The IgG1, IgG2 and IgM act as opsonins to enhance the phagocytosis by neutrophils and macrophages. The IgM is effective at fixing the complement. The IgA play a role in bacterial agglutination, which can inhibit the spread of certain pathogens throughout the mammary gland and has ability to neutralize some bacterial toxins (Aitken et al. 2011a, b).

11.13 Pattern Recognition Receptors (PRRs)

Recognition of microbial pathogens by PRRs is an essential element of early host defense for initiation of innate immune responses and subsequent inflammation. Germline-encoded PRRs play a significant role in the activation of innate immune responses to invading pathogens. The pathogen-associated molecular patterns (PAMPs) are molecular structures that are largely shared among pathogens, which are recognized by the PRRs. The PAMPs include various viral and bacterial cell-wall and nuclear components including flagellin, bacterial DNA, viral double-stranded RNA, lipopolysaccharides, peptidoglycans, and lipopeptides (Singh et al. 2003). Upon PAMP recognition, PRRs initiate a series of signalling pathways that execute the first line of host defensive responses required for killing of infectious microbes (Medzhitov 2001; Takeda et al. 2003; Akira and Takeda 2004; Iwasaki and Medzhitov 2004; Takeuchi and Akira 2010; Kawai and Akira 2011; Prince et al. 2011). The expression of PRRs can occur intracellularly, on the cell surface, or by secretion (Jungi et al. 2011; Kumar et al. 2011). The PAMPs can distinguish a variety of bacterial components associated with bacteria that cause mastitis, such as lipopeptides from Gram-positive bacteria and LPS from Gram-negative bacteria. After binding to their ligand, the PRRs initiate intracellular signalling cascades that lead to the initiation of immune responses or can directly promote the antimicrobial action.

The Toll-like receptor (TLR) family was the first PRRs being identified. TLRs are best characterized PRRs and recognize a wide range of PAMPs. They are expressed either in association with intracellular vesicles or on the cell surface (Medzhitov 2001; Takeda and Akira 2004). To date, 10 functional TLRs have been identified in bovines, 10 in humans, and 12 in mice (Menzies and Ingham 2006). In bovines, these 10 TLRs and nucleotide-binding oligomerization domain (NOD) 1 and 2 were detected in tissues from alveolar, ductal, gland cistern and teat canal from infected and healthy quarters, with TLR8 having the least expression in comparison to other PRRs (Whelehan et al. 2011). Functional analysis of mammalian TLRs had revealed that they recognize specific patterns of microbial components that are conserved among pathogens (Takeda and Akira 2004).

The TLRs can work independently, antagonistically, or synergistically upon stimulation to modulate the immune responses (Trinchieri and Sher 2007). They consist of a leucine-rich repeat region that recognizes the PAMP and an intracellular Toll-interleukin 1 receptor (TIR) domain for downstream signalling. Toll-like receptors recruit TIR domain-containing adaptor molecules, such as MyD88, Toll/interleukin-1 receptor domain-containing adapter protein (TIRAP), Toll/interleukin-1 receptor domain-containing adapter inducing interferon-β (TRIF), and TIR domain-containing adaptor molecule-2 (TICAM-2), also known as TRIF-related adaptor molecule (TRAM), to activate downstream signalling pathways and pro-inflammatory mediator production, including apoptotic pathways.

Each TLR recognizes distinct PAMPs originating from parasites, fungus, bacteria, viruses, and mycobacteria. Lipoproteins are recognized by TLR1, TLR2, and TLR6; flagellin is recognized by TLR5; lipopolysaccharide is recognized by TLR4; and CpG DNA, a six-base DNA motif consisting of an unmethylated CpG dinucleotide motifs that are rarely found in higher vertebrates, is recognized by TLR9 (Medzhitov 2001; Takeda et al. 2003; Akira and Takeda 2004; Iwasaki and Medzhitov 2004; Takeda and Akira 2004; Takeuchi and Akira 2010; Kawai and Akira 2011). Both TLR2 and TLR4, which are typically activated in response to Gram-positive and Gram-negative infections, respectively, and are extremely important during bacterial mastitis infections.

It is known that all TLR signal transduction pathways activate NF-κB (Akira and Takeda 2004). Early-phase NF-κB response is associated with MyD88-dependent pathways, whereas late-phase NF-κB response is associated with MyD88-independent pathways. These NF-κB factors subsequently enter into the nucleus and bind to target promoters. Numerous pro-inflammatory regulated genes feature NF-κB attachment sites in their promoter region and transcription factor complex function as a major switch to orchestrate immune defense genes against bacterial infection due to the production of several pro-inflammatory cytokines. Thus, different PRRs are expressed on the surface of cells, in intracellular compartments, or secreted into the blood and tissue fluids, which are used by the innate immune system. Activation of the complement and coagulation cascades, opsonization, phagocytosis, and activation and induction of apoptosis are the main functions of PRRs (Medzhitov 2001).

11.14 Inflammation

Inflammation is a complex biological reaction of vascular tissues to adverse stimuli like bacterial pathogen or injury. The resident leukocytes and epithelial cells initiate the inflammatory reactions required to get rid of the invading bacteria soon after the bacterial entry through the teat canal (Paape et al. 2003; Rainard and Riollet 2006; Aitken et al. 2011a, b). Upon infection, resident cells that express PRRs become triggered by bacterial PAMPs and these cells release a variety of inflammatory mediators, including cytokines and eicosanoids, which initiates the inflammatory cascade. Initially, there is an increase in vasodilation, which enhances blood flow. The permeability of blood vessels increases causing the leakage of plasma components (i.e., serum albumin, complement and acute phase proteins) in to the localized areas of affected tissues, results in edema. Further, vascular endothelial cells are affected by cytokines and other mediator molecules, which enhance the leukocyte adherence and migration from the blood to the site of injury. Neutrophils are the predominant cell type to undergo extravasation and adhere to the local endothelium near the site of infection. Cytokines and eicosanoids further stimulate the adherent neutrophils to move between the endothelial cells and pass across the basement membrane into the damaged tissues. Chemotaxis related inflammatory molecules at the localized site of infection facilitate the movement of neutrophils. The somatic cell count (SCC) increases in milk. The SCC represents different cell types in milk, such as leukocytes and epithelial cells, of which neutrophils make up over 90% of the leukocyte population. The significant rise in milk SCC during infection is mostly caused by an influx of neutrophils to the mammary gland from the circulation. In contrast, healthy udder milk contains low numbers of neutrophil cell count (Paape et al. 2003; Pyorala 2003; Souza et al. 2012).

11.15 Mammary Vascular Endothelium

The mammary vascular endothelium has significant role in the pathogenesis of inflammatory-based diseases. Mammary gland capillary network forms a basket-like structure around alveoli, and these capillaries are lined with a single layer of endothelium. Capillary network allows the exchange of metabolites from the blood to the tissues. The mammary vascular system actively participates in the inflammatory response in addition to providing the nutrition to the mammary gland. Vascular endothelial cells are activated by a variety of stimuli, including those secreted by mammary gland cell populations, bacterial toxins, reactive oxygen and nitrogen species, and potent lipid mediators (Cao et al. 2000; Corl et al. 2010, 2008; Aitken et al. 2011a, b). The endothelium responds in a variety of ways, such as vasodilation, increased permeability, changes in vascular tone and blood flow to facilitate leukocyte adherence and emigration, production of pro-inflammatory cytokines and adhesion molecules, and production of reactive oxygen and nitrogen species crucial for intracellular signaling (Sordillo and Aitken 2009). Prolonged or excessive inflammation disrupts the endothelium homeostasis, results in loss of vascular barrier functions, which causes in the influx of serum components in to the lacteal secretions (Sordillo et al. 1987; Bannerman and Goldblum 2003). Therefore, the deterioration of vascular integrity may contribute to the development of severe or chronic mastitis. The outcome of intramammary infections may dependent upon on the functional integrity of mammary endothelial cells.

11.16 Localized Cellular Components of Inflammation

11.16.1 Epithelial Cells

Epithelial cells lining the teat canal, gland cistern and alveoli are the important epithelial cell to recognize the pathogens and participate in triggering of an inflammatory responses. In addition to physical and chemical barrier, the teat canal provides an early, active immune response to pathogens (Rinaldi et al. 2010; Whelehan et al. 2011). Following an experimental *E. coli* infection, the teat tissue underwent rapid and intense immune gene changes that were related to the pathways involved in the inflammatory responses, leukocyte recruitment, production of antimicrobial peptides, apoptosis, acute phase response, and bacterial recognition receptors (Rinaldi et al. 2010).

Alveolar epithelial cells participate in bacterial recognition and innate immune system activation. Following exposure to LPS, it was discovered that the bovine mammary epithelial cell line MAC-T expresses both TLR2 and TLR4 (Ibeagha-Awemu et al. 2008). Bovine mammary epithelial cells responded robustly to *E. coli*-induced activation of TLR4-dependent signaling pathways with the enhanced expression of pro-inflammatory cytokines such as TNF-α and IL-8 (Yang et al. 2008; Gunther et al. 2011). Further, TLR2 signalling was activated by *S. aureus* in mammary secretory epithelial cells (Yang et al. 2008). Bacterial pathogens can upregulate TLR on mammary epithelial cells, and they can also produce non-specific bactericidal substances including cytokines, chemokines, and β-defensins (Goldammer et al. 2004; Petzl et al. 2008). These results collectively suggested that mammary epithelial cells may differentially influence the overall inflammatory responses depending on how they recognize and respond to various bacterial PAMPs.

11.16.2 Somatic Cells

Mammary epithelial cells, lymphocytes, neutrophils, and macrophages primarily constitute the majority of somatic cells in milk from healthy glands. These cells do the surveillance of invading pathogens in the mammary gland. The composition of somatic cells in milk changes in response to bacterial infection. Neutrophil becomes the predominant cell type following release of chemoattractants (i.e., complement components, cytokines, and eicosanoids) by macrophages and epithelial cells. Pathogens are predominantly eliminated by neutrophils through phagocytosis and intracellular killing. Pathogens can be killed by neutrophils through the formation of neutrophil extracellular traps (NET), respiratory bursts, antibacterial peptides, and defensins. Neutrophils produce reactive oxygen species, including superoxide, hydrogen peroxide and hypochlorous acid, and release granule compounds into pathogen-containing vacuoles to kill the invading pathogens (Paape et al. 2003; Mehrzad et al. 2005; Rainard and Riollet 2006; Prince et al. 2011). Neutrophils become activated and initiate a respiratory burst after binding of complement components and immunoglobulin on neutrophil receptors.

Cathelicidins, hydrolases, proteases, and lysozyme are antibacterial peptides found in neutrophil granules. These phagocytic and oxidative burst functions of neutrophils are drastically reduced in the presence of milk due to the ingestion of fat and casein (Mehrzad et al. 2005). The formation of NET and other neutrophil functions are not appear to be affected in the presence of milk (Lippolis et al. 2006). The nuclear and granular materials are released by activated neutrophils in a web-like fashion, known as NET, which physically trap the bacteria. Bacterial entrapment by NET contains the pathogens and expose them in an environment with a high local concentration of antimicrobial compounds released by neutrophils to enhance the bacterial killing (Brinkmann et al. 2004). The NET may play a significant role in the bacterial killing by neutrophils during intramammary infections (Lippolis et al. 2006). Thus, the rapid influx of neutrophils to the site of infection is involved in rapid elimination of pathogens (Mehrzad et al. 2005). This significant role was demonstrated by Mehrzad et al. (2005) that somatic cell count (SCC) in moderate responder cows (moderate milk production loss) increases rapidly than colony forming units (CFU) of E. coli bacteria, whereas in severe responder cows the results were reversed.

Phagocytosis of microorganisms is carried out by macrophages. Upon bacterial recognition, macrophages stimulate the release of cytokines and other pro-inflammatory mediators, which activate the innate immune responses, including neutrophil emigration and bactericidal functions. It presents the bacterial antigens to the lymphocytes for initiation of specific immune responses. It also has a role in resolution of infection as well by phagocytizing the aged neutrophils (Sladek et al. 2005). Macrophages have several roles in mastitis and are critical to the bacterial recognition and elimination. Macrophages appear to play a significant role in *E. coli*-infected mammary epithelial cell invasion and colonization, which was proved in a murine model of mastitis (Gonen et al. 2007). Cellular communication between somatic and epithelial cells propagates the innate immune responses. Maintaining

Table 11.5 Reactions to the California Mastitis Test (CMT), corresponding somatic cell counts (SCC), and somatic cell scores (SCS) for cow milk

Test result	Observed reactions	Comparable milk SCC	Equivalent SCS
Negative	Mixture remains fluid without thickening or gel formation	0–200,000 cells/mL	0–4
Trace	• Slight slime formation • This reaction is most noticeable when the paddle is rocked from side to side	150,000–500,000 cells/mL	5
1+	• Distinct slime formation occurs immediately after mixing the solutions. This slime may dissipate over time • When the paddle is swirled, fluid does not form a peripheral mass and the surface of solution does not become convex or domed up.	400,000–1,500,000 cells/mL	6
2+	• Distinct slime formation occurs immediately after mixing the solutions • When the paddle is swirled, the fluid forms a peripheral mass and the bottom of the cup is exposed	800,000–5,000,000 cells/mL	7–8
3+	• Distinct slime formation occurs immediately after mixing the solutions • This slime may dissipate over time • When the paddle is swirled the surface of the solution becomes convex or domed up	>5,000,000 cells/mL	9

the health of each cell type is necessary to rapidly resolve the infection without causing irreversible mammary gland injury that will affect the subsequent milk production.

In order to diagnose mastitis, the California Mastitis Test (CMT) is frequently used as a rapid pen-side assay in conjunction with clinical symptoms. This basis for this test is the lysis of somatic cells by the CMT reagent (sodium lauryl sulphate) to precipitate the DNA and proteins of somatic cells. When this reagent is added to milk, the development of a change in viscosity of the reagent is directly correlated with the relative number of somatic cells in the milk. The milk sample can be semiquantitatively scored based on the viscosity change to enable the sample comparison and to facilitate the assessment of severity easier (Table 11.5).

11.17 Immunopathogenesis

Mammary gland immune responses are complex, interconnected, and essential for defense against mastitis-causing pathogens. Certain intramammary immune responses may cause a disease condition in certain circumstances. Failure of the

11.17 Immunopathogenesis

host defense mechanisms may result in immunopathogenesis. Failure of the local mammary gland defenses to detect and eliminate the pathogens may lead to widespread immune evasion resulting in chronic inflammation.

Uncontrolled activation and accumulation of inflammatory cells, like neutrophils and macrophages, can release excessive toxic levels of cytokines, lipid mediators, and reactive oxygen species that can severely damage the local host tissues along with possible systemic complications leading to death. Thus, a delicate balance between a robust immune response against mastitis causing pathogens and the anti-inflammatory mechanisms required to restore the mammary gland immune homeostasis influence the outcome of disease and the extent of immunopathology. An efficient immune response involves the accurate pathogen detection and complete elimination without excessive or prolonged inflammation (Aitken et al. 2011a, b).

Numerous bacterial species have the ability of epithelial invasion and colonization, which contributes to chronic mastitis. For example, *S. aureus* causing subclinical and chronic mastitis. They evade adaptive mammary gland defenses. The *S. aureus* infection in bovine teat canal tissue invades the epithelial cells, which causes the decreased expression of intracellular receptors, NOD1 and NOD2, but this infection did not cause significant change in cytokine gene expression like IL-1β and TNF-α across mammary tissues (Whelehan et al. 2011). Further, In primary bovine mammary epithelial cells, *S. aureus* infection fails to upregulate the inflammatory genes through TLR and MyD88-dependent activation (Gunther et al. 2011). In mammary epithelial cells, TLR2 and/or TLR4 signalling was activated by both *S. aureus* and *E. coli*, but neither *S. aureus* nor its active cell wall component lipoteichoic acid (LTA) could activate NF-κB. Conversely, a strong induction of pro-inflammatory gene expression of IL-8 and TNF-α by NF-κB mediated pathway was noticed during *E. coli* and LPS infection (Yang et al. 2008). Further, *S. aureus* exotoxin promotes immune evasion. Leukotoxins create pores in leukocytes, thus preventing bacteria from being phagocytosed and allowing them to persist within the mammary gland (Barrio et al. 2006). Reduced ability to recognize pathogens alone or in combination with a reduced immune response to bacterial invasion may contribute to the ability of some mastitis-causing pathogens to escape the innate immune responses and therefore result in subclinical and chronic mastitis.

In contrast to weak host immune responses, sometimes an excess inflammatory response also causes local tissue damage or systemic consequences in the mammary gland. Rapid bacterial growth is seen followed by an exaggerated inflammatory response in cases of severe coliform infections. Damage to the mammary tissue results from the release of bacterial toxins or bactericidal components by infiltrating inflammatory cells. Lipopolysaccharide from bacteria triggers cellular signaling and upregulation of pro-inflammatory molecules that, when produced in excess, may ultimately result in cellular damage or death (Sordillo and Peel 1992). A study reported that experimental *E. coli* infection increased the expression of apoptotic genes in mammary tissue (Long et al. 2001). Excess LPS release and NF-κB activation during coliform mastitis results in decreased milk production through mammary epithelial apoptosis. Further, during acute mastitis, there is a massive influx of leukocytes, which causes the production of reactive oxygen species such myeloperoxidase, free radicals, proteases, and lysozymes that cause indiscriminate damage to the surrounding mammary tissue (Zhao and Lacasse 2008). Mammary tissue injury and milk loss can be minimized by preventing an excessive leukocyte influx into the mammary gland.

The primary target of LPS produced by replicating or dying Gram-negative bacteria is the vascular endothelium. Endothelial cells can respond to LPS by either production of pro-inflammatory molecules or initiation of endothelial apoptosis. Excess LPS can cause enhanced production of IL-1, IL-6 and TNF-α. The TNF-α is attributed to cause severe clinical symptoms of coliform mastitis (Blum et al. 2000; Wenz et al. 2010) including vascular dysfunction resulting from enhanced leukocyte adhesion and transmigration, increased reactive oxygen and nitrogen species production, and ultimately apoptosis (Madge and Pober 2001). Oxidative stress is caused by an imbalance between the production of reactive oxygen species and the availability of antioxidants. Excess reactive oxygen species production results in direct cellular and tissue damage from unstable molecules interacting with cellular nucleic acids, lipids, and proteins or may indirectly trigger intracellular signaling and promote a pro-inflammatory or proapoptotic cellular phenotype (Castillo et al. 2005; Sordillo et al. 2007). Reactive oxygen species affect the endothelium in a number of ways, including via altering cellular signalling, increasing permeability, increasing the leukocyte adherence, and redox-regulation of transcription factors (Boueiz and Hassoun 2009). Vitamin E, selenium and micronutrients with antioxidant functions were found to decrease duration and severity of mastitis in the periparturient period (Erskine et al. 1989). The vascular endothelium is protected by antioxidant supplementation from either direct or indirect oxidant-induced damage.

Neutrophil migration is a multistep process and requires upregulation of adhesion molecules on both the immune cells and the endothelium. The severity of coliform mastitis is associated with delayed neutrophil emigration (Burvenich et al. 2003). Compared to selenium-deficient animals, selenium supplementation accelerated the speed of neutrophil emigration into the bovine mammary gland during *E. coli* infection (Erskine et al. 1989). Selenium deficiency causes oxidative stress, which increases the ICAM-1 expression and neutrophil adherence in bovine mammary and aortic endothelial cells (Sordillo et al. 2008). In bovine aortic endothelial cells that are deficient in selenium, the 15-HPETE increases the ICAM1 expression (Sordillo et al. 2008). Interestingly, 15LOX1 mRNA expression is significantly upregulated in early lactation cows compared to pre-partum cows (Aitken et al. 2009). Neutrophil-endothelial adhesion initiates the intracellular signaling through adhesion molecules, such as ICAM-1, and enhanced expression of ICAM-1 adhesion molecule is associated with pro-inflammatory conditions leads to severe pathology (Bonomini et al. 2008). Increased expression of adhesion molecules and tight neutrophil endothelial binding may indicate an inability to rapidly migrate to the infection site, thereby allowing bacterial growth and endotoxin release contributing to the severity of coliform mastitis.

Leukocyte transmigration across the endothelium is required for mounting an effective immune responses to infection. However, activation of immune cells in the process may have negative consequences on endothelial integrity. For example, pathogens can be killed by the formation of NET by active neutrophils (Medina 2009). It is possible that release of adhesion molecules and pro-inflammatory substances during the transmigration process may inadvertently cause endothelium damage. Endothelial damage during mastitis may be exacerbated by excessive neutrophil migration, NET formation, and endothelial activation. The speed of leukocyte influx into the mammary gland affects the outcome of mastitis. It is known that downregulation of neutrophil adhesion molecules increases mastitis susceptibility and periparturient immunosuppression (Burton et al. 1995). Other mechanisms may be involved in the rapid leukocyte migratory responses, such as activation of the uroplasminogen cascade that is involved with the breakdown of the basement membrane and extracellular matrix required for diapedesis and migration of leukocytes to the infection site (Aitken et al. 2011a, b).

In addition to inflammation, an increased influx of neutrophils can cause mammary gland tissue injury. Tissue injury causes the release of endogenous TLR ligands known as damage-associated molecular patterns (DAMPs). When there is tissue damage, they alert the host by acting in an autocrine manner. But occasionally, they themselves can exacerbate inflammation, resulting in further tissue damage (Prince et al. 2011). An apoptosis differentiation program promotes the resolution of neutrophil-mediated inflammation. Phagocytosis by neutrophils initiates the molecular cascade of events that accelerates the apoptosis of neutrophil leukocyte population. Therefore, rapid accumulation of neutrophils at the sites of infection can potentially cause severe tissue destruction, if they undergo necrosis, lysis and release of cytotoxic granules and reactive oxygen species onto the host tissues. Thus, the final stage of neutrophil-induced inflammation can be seen as apoptosis (Kobayashi et al. 2003).

The severity of mastitis is influenced by several factors, some of which are complement components. High concentrations of complement component C5a are produced during sepsis (Guo et al. 2004). In a recent experiment, C5a stimulated the TLR4 signalling in bovine neutrophils, which led to the production of IL-8 in the absence of other stimulatory factors (Stevens et al. 2011). The ability of complement components to initiate the TLR4 signaling may contribute to the severity of mastitis during chronic inflammation.

11.18 Conclusion

The immune responses of mammary gland are complex and highly interconnected. The primary functions of both innate and adaptive immune responses are the rapid elimination of pathogenic microbes and resolution of the gland tissue to its normal function with the minimal tissue damage. Failure of immune system to eliminate the insult results in damage to the glandular tissue leads to decreased milk quantity and quality. This failure of immune system can be attributed to immunosuppression, lack of tight regulation of immune system, and adaptation mechanisms of certain organisms. Animals are regularly exposed to toxic substances like pesticides, which include weedicides, insecticides, herbicides, rodenticides, fertilizers, etc. through water, air, and food. These toxins bioaccumulate in the body resulting in immunosuppression, thus increasing the incidences of infectious diseases in the present-day population. Furthermore, some pathogens that cause mastitis have intrinsic characteristics that allow to escape from the effective elimination by the immune system. As a result, attempts by local mammary gland defenses to achieve control frequently result in significant tissue damage and decreased milk production. Although the mainstay of mastitis treatment is antibiotic medication, the development of antibiotic resistance in the pathogens has reduced its efficiency and is also a major public health concern. Consequently, the development of alternative therapeutic strategies that target on the host immune responses is necessary. The strategy should specifically reduce the harmful host responses without compromising beneficial responses that facilitate the elimination of invasive pathogens. This will also minimize the risk of emergence of drug resistant bacteria associated with indiscriminate use of antibiotics.

References

Aitken SL, Karcher EL, Rezamand P, Gandy JC, Van de Haar MJ, Capuco AV, Sordillo LM (2009) Evaluation of antioxidant and proinflammatory gene expression in bovine mammary tissue during the periparturient period. J Dairy Sci 92(2):589–598

Aitken SL, Corl CM, Sordillo LM (2011a) Immunopathology of mastitis: insights into disease recognition and resolution. J Mammary Gland Biol Neoplasia 16:291–304

Aitken SL, Corl CM, Sordillo LM (2011b) Pro-inflammatory and proapoptotic responses of TNF-alpha stimulated bovine mammary endothelial cells. Vet Immunol Immunopathol 140(3–4):282–290

Akira S, Takeda K (2004) Toll-like receptor signalling. Nat Rev Immunol 4:499–511. https://doi.org/10.1038/nri1391

Alluwaimi AM (2004) The cytokines of bovine mammary gland: prospects for diagnosis and therapy. Res Vet Sci 77(3):211–222

Atalla H, Wilkie B, Gyles C, Leslie K, Mutharia L, Mallard B (2010) Antibody and cell-mediated immune responses to *Staphylococcus aureus* small colony variants and their parental strains associated with bovine mastitis. Dev Comp Immunol 34:1283–1290

Atroshi F, Parantainen J, Sankari S, Osterman T (1986) Prostaglandins and glutathione peroxidase in bovine mastitis. Res Vet Sci 40(3):361–366

Atroshi F, Rizzo A, Kangasniemi R, Sankari S, Tyopponen T, Osterman T, Parantainen J (1989) Role of plasma fatty acids, prostaglandins and antioxidant balance in bovine mastitis. J Veterinary Med Ser A 36(9):702–711

Babiuk LA, Sordillo LM, Campos M, Hughes HP, Rossi Campos A, Harland R (1991) Application of interferons in the control of infectious diseases of cattle. J Dairy Sci 74(12):4385–4398

Bannerman DD (2009) Pathogen-dependent induction of cytokines and other soluble inflammatory mediators during intramammary infection of dairy cows. J Anim Sci 87(13):10–25

Bannerman DD, Goldblum SE (2003) Mechanisms of bacterial lipopolysaccharide-induced endothelial apoptosis. Am J Phys Lung Cell Mol Phys 284(6):L899–L914

Banting A, Banting S, Heinonen K, Mustonen K (2008) Efficacy of oral and parenteral ketoprofen in lactating cows with endotoxin induced acute mastitis. Vet Rec 163(17):506–509

Barrio MB, Rainard P, Prevost G (2006) LukM/LukF'-PV is the most active Staphylococcus aureus leukotoxin on bovine neutrophils. Microbes Infect 8(8):2068–2074

Blum JW, Dosogne H, Hoeben D, Vangroenweghe F, Hammon HM, Bruckmaier RM, Burvenich C (2000) Tumor necrosis factor-alpha and nitrite/nitrate responses during acute mastitis induced by *Escherichia coli* infection and endotoxin in dairy cows. Domest Anim Endocrinol 19(4): 223–235

Bonomini F, Tengattini S, Fabiano A, Bianchi R, Rezzani R (2008) Atherosclerosis and oxidative stress. Histol Histopathol 23(3):381–390

Boueiz A, Hassoun PM (2009) Regulation of endothelial barrier function by reactive oxygen and nitrogen species. Microvasc Res 77(1):26–34

Boutet P, Bureau F, Degand G, Lekeux P (2003) Imbalance between lipoxin A4 and leukotriene B4 in chronic mastitis-affected cows. J Dairy Sci 86(11):3430–3439

Bradley A (2002) Bovine mastitis: an evolving disease. Vet J 164:116–128

Bramley AJ, Dodd FH (1984) Reviews of the progress of dairy science: mastitis control–progress and prospects. J Dairy Res 51(3):481–512

Brinkmann V, Reichard U, Goosmann C, Fauler B, Uhlemann Y, Weiss DS, Weinrauch Y, Zychlinsky A (2004) Neutrophil extracellular traps kill bacteria. Science 303(5663):1532–1535

Burton JL, Kehrli ME Jr, Kapil S, Horst RL (1995) Regulation of L-selectin and CD18 on bovine neutrophils by glucocorticoids: effects of cortisol and dexamethasone. J Leukoc Biol 57(2): 317–325

Burvenich C, Van Merris V, Mehrzad J, Diez-Fraile A, Duchateau L (2003) Severity of *E. coli* mastitis is mainly determined by cow factors. Vet Res 34(5):521–564

Cao YZ, Reddy CC, Sordillo LM (2000) Altered eicosanoid biosynthesis in selenium-deficient endothelial cells. Free Radic Biol Med 28(3):381–389

Capuco AV, Bright SA, Pankey JW, Wood DL, Miller RH, Bitman J (1992) Increased susceptibility to intramammary infection following removal of teat canal keratin. J Dairy Sci 75(8): 2126–2130

Castillo C, Hernandez J, Bravo A, Lopez-Alonso M, Pereira V, Benedito JL (2005) Oxidative status during late pregnancy and early lactation in dairy cows. Vet J 169(2):286–292

Chaneton L, Tirante L, Maito J, Chaves J, Bussmann LE (2008) Relationship between milk lactoferrin and etiological agent in the mastitic bovine mammary gland. J Dairy Sci 91(5): 1865–1873

Chauhan RS (1998) An introduction to immunopathology. G. B. Pant University of Agriculture & Technology, Pantnagar, p 52

Contreras GA, Rodriguez JM (2011) Mastitis: comparative etiology and epidemiology. J Mammary Gland Biol Neoplasia 16:339–356

Contreras GA, Sordillo LM (2011) Lipid mobilization and inflammatory responses during the transition period of dairy cows. Comp Immunol Microbiol Infect Dis 34(3):281–289

Corl CM, Gandy JC, Sordillo LM (2008) Platelet activating factor production and proinflammatory gene expression in endotoxin challenged bovine mammary endothelial cells. J Dairy Sci 91(8): 3067–3078

Corl CM, Contreras GA, Sordillo LM (2010) Lipoxygenase metabolites modulate vascular-derived platelet activating factor production following endotoxin challenge. Vet Immunol Immunopathol 136(1–2):98–107

Erskine RJ, Eberhart RJ, Grasso PJ, Scholz RW (1989) Induction of Escherichia coli mastitis in cows fed selenium-deficient or selenium-supplemented diets. Am J Vet Res 50(12):2093–2100

Foxman B, D'Arcy H, Gillespie B, Bobo JK, Schwartz K (2002) Lactation mastitis: occurrence and medical management among 946 breastfeeding women in the United States. Am J Epidemiol 155(2):103–114

Goldammer T, Zerbe H, Molenaar A, Schuberth HJ, Brunner RM, Kata SR, Seyfert HM (2004) Mastitis increases mammary mRNA abundance of beta-defensin 5, toll-like-receptor 2 (TLR2), and TLR4 but not TLR9 in cattle. Clin Diagn Lab Immunol 11(1):174–185

Gonen E, Vallon-Eberhard A, Elazar S, Harmelin A, Brenner O, Rosenshine I, Jung S, Shpigel NY (2007) Toll-like receptor 4 is needed to restrict the invasion of *Escherichia coli* P4 into mammary gland epithelial cells in a murine model of acute mastitis. Cell Microbiol 9(12): 2826–2838

Gunther J, Esch K, Poschadel N, Petzl W, Zerbe H, Mitterhuemer S, Blum H, Seyfert HM (2011) Comparative kinetics of *Escherichia coli-* and *Staphylococcus aureus*-specific activation of key immune pathways in mammary epithelial cells demonstrates that *S. aureus* elicits a delayed response dominated by interleukin-6 (IL-6) but not by IL-1A or tumor necrosis factor alpha. Infect Immun 79(2):695–707

Guo RF, Riedemann NC, Ward PA (2004) Role of C5a-C5aR interaction in sepsis. Shock 21(1): 1–7

Harizi H, Corcuff JB, Gualde N (2008) Arachidonic-acid-derived eicosanoids: roles in biology and immunopathology. Trends Mol Med 14(10):461–469

Hillerton JE, Berry EA (2005) Treating mastitis in the cow-a tradition or archaism. J Appl Microbiol 98:1250–1255

Hogeveen H, Hujips K, Lam TJ (2011) Economic aspects of mastitis: new developments. N Z Vet J 59:16–23

Hujips K, Lam TJ, Hogeveen H (2008) Costs of mastitis: facts and perception. J Dairy Res 75:113–120

Ibeagha-Awemu EM, Lee JW, Ibeagha AE, Bannerman DD, Paape MJ, Zhao X (2008) Bacterial lipopolysaccharide induces increased expression of toll-like receptor (TLR) 4 and downstream TLR signaling molecules in bovine mammary epithelial cells. Vet Res 39(2):11

Inch S, von Xylander S (2000) Mastitis: causes and management. World Health Organization (WHO) Department of child and adolescent health and development, Geneva

Iwasaki A, Medzhitov R (2004) Toll-like receptors and control of adaptive immune responses. Nat Rev Immunol 5:987–995. PMID: 11973138

Jungi TW, Farhat K, Burgener IA, Werling D (2011) Toll-like receptors in domestic animals. Cell Tissue Res 343(1):107–120

Kawai T, Akira S (2011) Toll-like receptors and their crosstalk with other innate receptors in infection and immunity. Immunity 34:637–650. https://doi.org/10.1016/j.immuni.2011.05.006

Kobayashi SD, Voyich, De Leo FR (2003) Regulation of the neutrophil-mediated inflammatory response to infection. Microbes Infect 5:1337–1344

Kumar H, Kawai T, Akira S (2011) Pathogen recognition by the innate immune system. Int Rev Immunol 30(1):16–34

Lippolis JD, Reinhardt TA, Goff JP, Horst RL (2006) Neutrophil extracellular trap formation by bovine neutrophils is not inhibited by milk. Vet Immunol Immunopathol 113(1–2):248–255

Long E, Capuco AV, Wood DL, Sonstegard T, Tomita G, Paape MJ, Zhao X (2001) *Escherichia coli* induces apoptosis and proliferation of mammary cells. Cell Death Differ 8(8):808–816

Maddox JF, Reddy CC, Eberhart RJ, Scholz RW (1991) Dietary selenium effects on milk eicosanoid concentration in dairy cows during coliform mastitis. Prostaglandins 42(4):369–378

Madge LA, Pober JS (2001) TNF signaling in vascular endothelial cells. Exp Mol Pathol 70(3): 317–325

McDougall S, Bryan MA, Tiddy RM (2009) Effect of treatment with the nonsteroidal anti-inflammatory meloxicam on milk production, somatic cell count, probability of re-treatment, and culling of dairy cows with mild clinical mastitis. J Dairy Sci 92(9):4421–4431

Medina E (2009) Neutrophil extracellular traps: a strategic tactic to defeat pathogens with potential consequences for the host. J Innate Immun 1(3):176–180

Medzhitov R (2001) Toll-like receptors and innate immunity. Nat Rev Immunol 1:135–145

Mehrzad J, Duchateau L, Burvenich C (2005) High milk neutrophil chemiluminescence limits the severity of bovine coliform mastitis. Vet Res 36(1):101–116

Menzies M, Ingham A (2006) Identification and expression of Toll-like receptors 1-10 in selected bovine and ovine tissues. Vet Immunol Immunopathol 109:23–30. PMID: 16095720

Natarajan R, Nadler JL (2004) Lipid inflammatory mediators in diabetic vascular disease. Arterioscler Thromb Vasc Biol 24(9):1542–1548

Oliver SP, Sordillo LM (1988) Udder health in the periparturient period. J Dairy Sci 71(9): 2584–2606

Paape MJ, Bannerman DD, Zhao X, Lee JL (2003) The bovine neutrophil: structure and function. Vet Res 34:597–627

Patel D, Almeida RA, Dunlap JR, Oliver SP (2009) Bovine lactoferrin serves as a molecular bridge for internalization of *Streptococcus uberis* into bovine mammary epithelial cells. Vet Microbiol 137(3–4):297–301

Pattanaik U, Prasad K (1998) Oxygen free radicals and endotoxic shock: effect of flaxseed. J Cardiovasc Pharmacol Ther 3(4):305–318

Pecorini C, Sassera D, Rebucci R, Saccone F, Bandi C, Baldi A (2010) Evaluation of the protective effect of bovine lactoferrin against lipopolysaccharides in a bovine mammary epithelial cell line. Vet Res Commun 34(3):267–276

Peter AT, Clark PW, Van Roekel DE, Luker CW, Gaines JD, Bosu WT (1990) Temporal changes in metabolites of prostanoids in milk of heifers after intramammary infusion of Escherichia coli organisms. Prostaglandins 39(4):451–457

Petzl W, Zerbe H, Gunther J, Yang W, Seyfert HM, Nurnberg G, Schuberth HJ (2008) *Escherichia coli*, but not *Staphylococcus aureus* triggers an early increased expression of factors contributing to the innate immune defense in the udder of the cow. Vet Res 39(2):18

Prince LR, Whyte MK, Sabroe I, Parker LC (2011) The role of TLRs in neutrophil activation. Curr Opin Pharmacol 11:397–403

Pyorala S (2003) Indicators of inflammation in the diagnosis of mastitis. Vet Res 34:565–578

Rainard P (2003) The complement in milk and defense of the bovine mammary gland against infections. Vet Res 34(5):647–670

Rainard P, Riollet C (2006) Innate immunity of the bovine mammary gland. Vet Res 37:369–400

Reilly KB, Srinivasan S, Hatley ME, Patricia MK, Lannigan J, Bolick DT, Vandenhoff G, Pei H, Natarajan R, Nadler JL, Hedrick CC (2004) 12/15-Lipoxygenase activity mediates inflammatory monocyte/endothelial interactions and atherosclerosis *in vivo*. J Biol Chem 279(10): 9440–9450

Rinaldi M, Li RW, Bannerman DD, Daniels KM, Evock-Clover C, Silva MV, Paape MJ, Van Ryssen B, Burvenich C, Capuco AV (2010) A sentinel function for teat tissues in dairy cows: dominant innate immune response elements define early response to E. coli mastitis. Funct Integr Genom 10(1):21–38

Riollet C, Rainard P, Poutrel B (2000a) Cells and cytokines in inflammatory secretions of bovine mammary gland. Adv Exp Med Biol 480:247–258

Riollet C, Rainard P, Poutrel B (2000b) Differential induction of complement fragment C5a and inflammatory cytokines during intramammary infections with *Escherichia coli* and *Staphylococcus aureus*. Clin Diagn Lab Immunol 7(2):161–167

Serhan CN, Chiang N, Van Dyke TE (2008) Resolving inflammation: dual anti-inflammatory and pro-resolution lipid mediators. Nat Rev Immunol 8(5):349–361

Shafer-Weaver KA, Corl CM, Sordillo LM (1999) Shifts in bovine CD4+ subpopulations increase T-helper-2 compared with Thelper-1 effector cells during the postpartum period. J Dairy Sci 82(8):1696–1706

Singh BP, Chauhan RS, Singhal LK (2003) Toll like receptors (TLRs) and their role in innate immunity. Curr Sci 85(8):1156–1164

Sladek Z, Rysanek D, Ryznarova H, Faldyna M (2005) Neutrophil apoptosis during experimentally induced *Staphylococcus aureus* mastitis. Vet Res 36(4):629–643

Sordillo LM, Aitken SL (2009) Impact of oxidative stress on the health and immune function of dairy cattle. Vet Immunol Immunopathol 128(1–3):104–109

Sordillo LM, Nickerson SC (1988) Quantification and immunoglobulin classification of plasma cells in nonlactating bovine mammary tissue. J Dairy Sci 71(1):84–91

Sordillo LM, Peel JE (1992) Effect of interferon-gamma on the production of tumor necrosis factor during acute *Escherichia coli* mastitis. J Dairy Sci 75(8):2119–2125

Sordillo LM, Streicher KL (2002) Mammary gland immunity and mastitis susceptibility. J Mammary Gland Biol Neoplasia 7(2):135–146

Sordillo LM, Nickerson SC, Akers RM, Oliver SP (1987) Secretion composition during bovine mammary involution and the relationship with mastitis. Int J Biochem 19(12):1165–1172

Sordillo LM, Pighetti GM, Davis MR (1995) Enhanced production of bovine tumor necrosis factor-alpha during the periparturient period. Vet Immunol Immunopathol 49(3):263–270

Sordillo LM, Shafer-Weaver K, De Rosa D (1997) Immunobiology of the mammary gland. J Dairy Sci 80(8):1851–1865

Sordillo LM, O'Boyle N, Gandy JC, Corl CM, Hamilton E (2007) Shifts in thioredoxin reductase activity and oxidant status in mononuclear cells obtained from transition dairy cattle. J Dairy Sci 90(3):1186–1192

Sordillo LM, Streicher KL, Mullarky IK, Gandy JC, Trigona W, Corl CM (2008) Selenium inhibits 15-hydroperoxyoctadecadienoic acid-induced intracellular adhesion molecule expression in aortic endothelial cells. Free Radic Biol Med 44(1):34–43

Sordillo LM, Contreras GA, Aitken SL (2009) Metabolic factors affecting the inflammatory response of periparturient dairy cows. Anim Health Res Rev 10(1):53–63

Souza FN, Blagitz MG, Penna CF, Della Libera AM, Heinemann MB, Cerqueira MM (2012) Somatic cell count in small ruminants: friend or foe? Small Rumin Res 107(2–3):65–75

Spector AA, Gordon JA, Moore SA (1988) Hydroxyeicosatetraenoic acids (HETEs). Prog Lipid Res 27(4):271–323

Stevens MG, Van Poucke M, Peelman LJ, Rainard P, De Spiegeleer B, Rogiers C, Van de Walle GR, Duchateau L, Burvenich C (2011) Anaphylatoxin C5a-induced Toll-like receptor 4 signaling in bovine neutrophils. J Dairy Sci 94(1):152–164

Takeda K, Akira S (2004) TLR signaling pathway. Semin Immunol 16:3–9. PMID: 14751757

Takeda K, Kaisho T, Akira S (2003) Toll-like receptors. Annu Rev Immunol 21:335–376

Takeuchi O, Akira S (2010) Pattern recognition receptors and inflammation. Cell 140:805–820. https://doi.org/10.1016/j.cell.2010.01.022

Trinchieri G, Sher A (2007) Cooperation of Toll-like receptor signals in innate immune defence. Nat Rev Immunol 7(3):179–190

Vangroenweghe F, Duchateau L, Boutet P, Lekeux P, Rainard P, Paape MJ, Burvenich C (2005) Effect of carprofen treatment following experimentally induced *Escherichia coli* mastitis in primiparous cows. J Dairy Sci 88(7):2361–2376

Wagner SA, Apley MD (2004) Effects of two anti-inflammatory drugs on physiologic variables and milk production in cows with endotoxin-induced mastitis. Am J Vet Res 65(1):64–68

Watson CJ, Oliver CH, Khaled WT (2011) Cytokine signalling in mammary gland development. J Reprod Immunol 88(2):124–129

Wellenberg GJ, Van Der Poela WHM, Oirschot JTV (2002) Viral infections and bovine mastitis: a review. Vet Microbiol 88:27–45

Wenz JR, Fox LK, Muller FJ, Rinaldi M, Zeng R, Bannerman DD (2010) Factors associated with concentrations of select cytokine and acute phase proteins in dairy cows with naturally occurring clinical mastitis. J Dairy Sci 93(6):2458–2470

Whelehan CJ, Meade KG, Eckersall PD, Young FJ, O'Farrelly C (2011) Experimental *Staphylococcus aureus* infection of the mammary gland induces region-specific changes in innate immune gene expression. Vet Immunol Immunopathol 140(3–4):181–189

References

Yang W, Zerbe H, Petzl W, Brunner RM, Gunther J, Draing C, von Aulock S, Schuberth HJ, Seyfert HM (2008) Bovine TLR2 and TLR4 properly transduce signals from *Staphylococcus aureus* and *E. coli*, but *S. aureus* fails to both activate NF-kappaB in mammary epithelial cells and to quickly induce TNF-alpha and interleukin-8 (CXCL8) expression in the udder. Mol Immunol 45(5):1385–1397

Zadoks R (2014) Understanding the sources, transmission routes and prognoses for mastitis pathogens. WCDS Adv Dairy Sci Technol 26:91–100

Zhao X, Lacasse P (2008) Mammary tissue damage during bovine mastitis: causes and control. J Anim Sci 86(13):57–65

Zia S, Giri SN, Cullor J, Emau P, Osburn BI, Bushnell RB (1987) Role of eicosanoids, histamine, and serotonin in the pathogenesis of *Klebsiella pneumoniae*-induced bovine mastitis. Am J Vet Res 48(11):1617–1625

Immunopathological Disorders of Kidneys

Key Points

1. Immunopathological conditions of kidneys mainly encompass immune-complex-mediated glomerulonephritis, membranoproliferative glomerulonephritis (MPGN), crescentic glomerulonephritis, IgA nephropathy, and postinfection glomerulonephritis.
2. Immunopathological condition of kidneys has wide range of causes such as immune complex formation, genetic, neoplasm, complement-mediated, autoimmune diseases, infectious causes, etc.
3. Glomerulonephritis is the inflammation of the glomerulus and other compartment of kidneys and mainly encompasses immune-mediated diseases.
4. Type I MPGN mainly occurs due to the localization of immune complex in the subendothelial space.
5. In Type II MPGN or dense deposit disease, deposition of the electron dense material is observed within the glomerular basement membrane of kidneys and choriocapillary—Bruch's membrane—retinal pigment epithelial interface.
6. Type III MPGN is characterized by disruption and lamination of the lamina densa of glomerular basement membrane due to the subendothelial and subepithelial deposition.
7. Histopathological lesions in immunopathological conditions of kidneys are inflammation of glomerulus, basement membrane thickening, and proliferation of glomerular cells.

12.1 Introduction

The kidneys are the oversized bean-shaped organs and act as a sewage treatment plant of our body that helps get rid of the waste products produced in the body. Basic structural and functional unit of kidneys is nephron. The excretion of fluid and solute is due to the complex interplay between tubular and vascular component within the nephron (Chmielewski 2003). Two main components of the nephron are glomerulus and tubule. Glomerulus produces the ultrafiltrate and act as filter of the blood. Ultrafiltrate finally converted to urine by the highly specialized tubules by performing two main functions, i.e., reabsorption and secretion (Preuss 1993). Other than producing urine, kidneys also perform other important functions like maintaining water and electrolyte balance of the body, maintenance of the blood pressure, produce hormones like erythropoietin and calcitriol, and maintenance of acid base balance of the body. There are various disorders that hinder the normal functioning of the kidneys. These disorders include various infections like bacterial, viral, and physical cause like obstruction, tumors, toxins like heavy metal toxicity, and immunopathological disorders (Table 12.1). Immunopathological disorders occur when there is a defect in either innate or acquired immune system or in both, which leads to autoimmune diseases, hypersensitivity reactions, and immunodeficiency disorders (Marshall et al. 2018).

12.2 Glomerulonephritis

Glomerulonephritis is the inflammation of the glomerulus and other compartments of kidneys and mainly encompasses immune-mediated diseases (Chadban and Atkins 2005). Basement membrane thickening and proliferation of glomerular cells are observed after the deposition of the immune complex in the glomeruli (Figs. 12.1 and 12.2). The proliferation is generally observed in any one or all of the cells, i.e., epithelial cells, endothelial cells, and mesangial cells of the glomerulus. Hence the lesions are generally considered as membranoproliferative glomerulonephritis (MPGN) (Tizard 2004). The MPGN-affected patients are presented with hematuria, nephritic range proteinuria, overt nephritic syndrome, hypertension, and some renal function impairment (Nakopoulou 2001). Renal function impairment progresses eventually to the end-stage renal disease (Licht and Mengel 2008). MPGN is classified into MPGN I, MPGN II, and MPGN III based on the electron microscopy. As this classification not able to give the pathophysiology of the disease, a newer classification based on the immunofluorescence staining is proposed. According to it, MPGN is classified into immune complex mediated, complement mediated, and chronic thrombotic microangiopathy mediated (Masani et al. 2014).

12.3 Type I Membranoproliferative Glomerulonephritis

Type I MPGN mainly occurs due to the localization of immune complex in the subendothelial space. The disorder is mainly associated with various disease conditions like viral, bacterial, etc., autoimmune diseases like lupus, and sometimes also due to malignant neoplasm like leukemia. Histopathologically, hyperlobulation is observed in the glomerular tuft due to increased cellularity and matrix of the mesangium along with infiltration of leukocytes and diffuse endocapillary

12.3 Type I Membranoproliferative Glomerulonephritis

Table 12.1 Common nephrotoxic agents of domestic animals

Category	Nephrotoxic agents
Heavy metals	• Mercury
	• Lead
	• Arsenic
	• Cadmium
	• Thallium
	• Bismuth
Antibacterial and antifungal agents	• Aminoglycosides (neomycin, kanamycin, gentamicin, streptomycin, tobramycin, amikacin)
	• Tetracyclines
	• Amphotericin B
	• Cephalosporins
	• Polymyxins
	• Sulfonamides (sulfapyridine, sulfathiazole, sulfadiazine)
Growth-promoting agents	• Monensin
Nonsteroidal anti-inflammatory drugs	• Aspirin
	• Phenylbutazone
	• Carprofen
	• Flunixin meglumine
	• Ibuprofen
	• Naproxen
Food and food contaminants	• Grapes or raisins
	• Melamine
	• Cyanuric acid
Bacterial and fungal toxins	• *Clostridium perfringens* type D, epsilon toxin (pulpy kidney)
	• Ochratoxin A
	• Citrinin
Plants	• Pigweed (*Amaranthus retroflexus*)
	• Oak and tannins (*Quercus* spp.)
	• *Isotropis* spp.
	• Yellow wood tree (*Terminalia oblongata*)
	• Lilies (*Zantedeschia* spp., *Lilium* spp., and *Hemerocallis* spp.)
	• *Lantana camara*
Oxalates	• Ethylene glycol (antifreeze)
	• Halogeton (*Halogeton glomeratus*)
	• Greasewood (*Sarcobatus vermiculatus*)
	• Rhubarb (*Rheum rhaponticum*)
	• Sorrel, dock (*Rumex* spp.)
Animal toxins	• Animal venoms
	• Cantharidin (blister beetle)
Vitamin D	• Vitamin D supplements
	• Calciferol-containing rodenticides
	• *Cestrum diurnum*
	• *Solanum* spp.

(continued)

Table 12.1 (continued)

Category	Nephrotoxic agents
	• *Trisetum* spp.
Vitamin K3	• Menadione
Anti-neoplastic compounds	• Cisplatin
	• Doxorubicin
	• Methotrexate
Volatile anesthetic	• Methoxyflurane
Herbicide and fertilizer	• Paraquat
	• Sodium fluoride
Endogenous	• Bile
	• Hemoglobin
	• Myoglobin
Others	• Chlorinated hydrocarbons
	• Contrast media

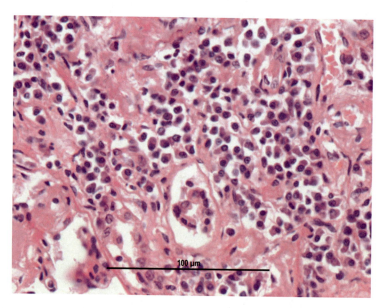

Fig. 12.1 Immune-mediated glomerulonephritis: Renal cortex showed severe infiltration of mononuclear cells, especially plasma cells. H&E ×400

proliferation. All this led to diffuse thickening and duplication of the glomerular basement membrane, which is also known as tam-tracking, splitting, or reduplication of the glomerular basement membrane (Alchi and Jayne 2009). Immune complex localized in the basement membrane activates the complement through classical pathway and sometimes mannose-binding lectin, which release chemotactic factors like C5a, opsonins like C3b, and membrane-attacking complex. Release of chemotactic factors such as C3a and C5a leads to the accumulation of the platelets and

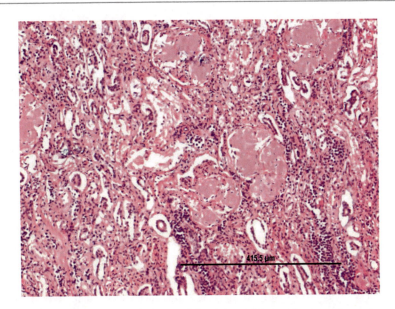

Fig. 12.2 Immune-mediated glomerulonephritis: Renal glomeruli and Bowman's capsule showing enlargement and with deposition of amorphous homogeneous to indistinctly fibrillar, eosinophilic, and acellular amyloid material. Cortex showing severe infiltration of mononuclear cells, especially plasma cells (secretory cells of amyloid). One of the causes is antigen-antibody reactions. H&E ×100

leukocytes. The latter again release the proteases and oxidants which cause in damage of the capillary wall leading to proteinuria and fall in glomerular filtration rate. Mesangial proliferation and matrix expansion are due to cytokines and growth factors released by both type of the glomerular cells, i.e., exogenous and endogenous (Schena and Alpers 2010).

12.4 Type II Membranoproliferative Glomerulonephritis

In type II MPGN, deposition of the electron dense material is observed within the glomerular basement membrane of kidneys and choriocapillary—Bruch's membrane—retinal pigment epithelial interface. So, type II MPGN is also known as dense deposit disease. Dense deposit is characterized by the dysregulation of the alternate complement pathway leading to the glomerular deposition of C3. Alternate dysregulation is mainly observed due to an autoantibody, i.e., C3 nephrotic factor, which stabilize the C3 convertase. Further, it is less likely observed due to mutation in the complement regulatory proteins like factor H and factor I (Servais et al. 2012). In 1989, Duvall-Young, MacDonald, and Mckechnie first described the retinal change in the type II MPGN. Renal biopsy is the only confirmatory diagnosis for the dense deposit disease (Cunningham and Kotagiri 2018). Clinically, the disease generally progresses to the end-stage renal disease (ESRD). Sometimes impaired visual acuity and field are also observed along with renal failure. Histologically, dense deposit is observed in the lamina densa of the glomerular basement membrane and is distributed in diffuse, discontinuous, and segmental pattern. It is also observed that characteristically C3 is deposited in ribbon-like pattern and as coarse granule or spherules in the glomerular capillary and mesangial region, respectively. When only outer surface of the deposit is stained, it appears along the capillary wall as double contour like linear railroad track and as a ring along the mesangial region (Appel et al. 2005).

12.5 Type III Membranoproliferative Glomerulonephritis

Type III membranoproliferative glomerulonephritis is characterized by disruption and lamination of the lamina densa of glomerular basement membrane due to the subendothelial and subepithelial deposition (Chae 2014). Spike formation due to deposition in the subepithelium is differentiating feature, which is present in MPGN III but absent in MPGN II (Nakopoulou 2001). As type III MPGN lesions are present only in later stage, so in early stage, it is sometimes mistaken for type I MPGN. Further, in type III MPGN, a nephritic factor of terminal pathway (NF_t) is identified in patients (Neary et al. 2002). At the time of biopsy, it is found that only patients with hypocomplementemia have subendothelial deposition, whereas subepithelial depositions are present in both patient with hypocomplementemia and normocomplementemia. Further, both subendothelial and subepithelial depositions are mainly associated with the presence of nephritic factor (West and McAdam 1998a, b). The NF_t activates C3 and terminal component slowly with the help of C3 convertase $C3B_n$, bB, P, and NF_t, which is stabilized with the help of properdin (West and McAdam 1998a, b).

12.6 Crescentic Glomerulonephritis

Crescentic glomerulonephritis is a rapidly progressive disease characterized by accumulation of the proliferated and dedifferentiated visceral and parietal cells in the bowmen capsule as principle histologic finding. It is clinically presented as hematuria, erythrocyte cast, proteinuria, and progressive loss of renal function (Moroni and Ponticelli 2014). It is classified into mainly three types, i.e., anti-glomerular basement membrane (GBM), immune complex-mediated, and pauci-immune (Parmer and Bahir 2019). Anti-glomerular basement membrane disease is characterized by linear deposit of IgG targeted against antigen present in the glomerular and alveolar basement membranes and increased serum anti-GBM antibody titers (Gupta et al. 2016). It is designated as Goodpasture syndrome when pulmonary hemorrhages are present along with glomerular lesions. The IgG autoantibodies are produced against the noncollagenous domain, i.e., NC1 domain of the α3 domain of type IV collagen. It is also known as Goodpasture antigen. The IgG1 is the prominent antibody present in the serum, but sometimes IgA autoantibody has also been reported. Codeposition of the other frequently occurring molecules are also there like mostly that of C3 followed by IgM. Histologically, there is glomerular basement membrane disruption, extravasation of the fibrin, and cellular crescent formation causing obliteration of the urinary space. Cellular crescent is formed mainly due to the aggregation of the histiocyte, lymphocyte, neutrophil, epithelial cell, and fibrin (Fischer and Lager 2006). There is a epitope spreading, after a primary response to α3 and sometimes serum and kidney tissue autoantibody against collagen chain α4 and α5 are also present.

Cell-mediated glomerular injury in the absence of humoral immune response is contributed by T cells (McAdoo and Pusey 2017). Immune complex-mediated crescentic glomerulonephritis is characterized by granular deposition of immune complex in mesangial and subendothelial regions. There is focal and segmental thickening of the glomerular basement membrane with injury to the epithelium, thickening of foot processes, and cellular or fibrocellular crescent formation (Alfaiw et al. 2018). The most common form of crescentic glomerulonephritis is pauci-immune glomerulonephritis caused by antineutrophilic cytoplasmic autoantibodies (ANCA)—associated vasculitis (AAV). The ANCA is produced against the proteinase 3 (PR3) and myeloperoxidase (MPO), which are the constituent of the granules of neutrophils and lysozyme of the monocyte (Tarzi et al. 2011). The AAV involves inflammation of all small arteries, arterioles, venules, and capillaries. The AAV in kidney includes microscopic polyangiitis, granulomatosis with polyangiitis, Churg–Strauss syndrome, and renal limited form. Binding of antigen PR3 and MPO with ANCA activates the neutrophils and promotes the binding of the neutrophils to the endothelial cells. The ROS and proteolytic enzyme releases from activated neutrophils cause vessel wall injury. Release of various cytokines exacerbates the injury (Kambham 2012). The ANCA-activated neutrophils also release neutrophil extracellular trap, which in conjugation with trapping and killing of the extracellular bacteria also contain targeted autoantigen PR3 and MPO and thus perpetuate the ANCA autoimmune response. There is also a protein called lysosome-associated membrane protein-2 (LAMP2), which colocalized with PR3 and MPO. The LAMP2 cross-reacts with the antibodies produced against FimH, i.e., the bacterial adhesion protein, and also becomes the cause of pauci-immune glomerulonephritis (Chen and Chen 2013). The PR3-ANCA-associated vasculitis had more necrotic lesions and more granulomatous lesions than MPO–ANCA-associated vasculitis, which is more sclerotic and less granulomatous in nature. The PR3 had HLA-DP genetic association and is more common in northern Europe, North America, and Australia. The MPO has HLA-DQ association and is more common in southern Europe, south USA, and Asia (Jennette and Nachman 2017).

12.7 IgA Nephropathy

The IgA nephropathy is an autoimmune disease and is one of the leading causes of chronic kidney disease and renal failure. The disease is characterized by the presence of circulating and depositing immune complex in glomeruli. Immune complex formed by the autoantibody IgG produced against hinge region O-glycan of IgA$_1$ and c$_3$. Immune complexes that are deposited contribute directly to the inflammation of the glomerulus and proliferation of the mesangium and thus are nephritogenic. Renal functions are further deteriorated by local and systemic renin and angiotensin system activation and complement activation (Rodrigues et al. 2017). Immunopathogenesis is explained by multi-hit hypothesis. First hit in the development of IgA nephropathy is the galactose-deficient IgA$_1$ production and production of IgG antibodies, which target the O-glycans is the second hit. Both are important in the production of immune complex. Thus, immune complex formed is deposited in the kidney and produces local inflammation, there which eventually progresses to the mesangial cell damage (Wu et al. 2018). The immune complex deposition is thought due to mesangial trapping and increased affinity of poor galactosylated IgA$_1$ antibody bind to extracellular matrix. Immune complex once bind to the activated mesangial cells results in proliferation of mesangial cells, deposition of extracellular matrix, formation of the glomerular crescent, and fibrosis of tubulointerstitial cells. All these occur due to increased release of cytokines like IL-6 and TGF-β and other pro-inflammatory and chemotactic factors. These factors further change the gene expression of podocytes and increased permeability of the glomerulus leading to the segmental sclerosis of glomerulus and damage of podocytes (Yeo et al. 2018). Environment and genetic factors contribute to the multi-hit system. Excess production of the glycosylated IgA is triggered by environmental factors like pathogenic and commensal bacteria in serum and glomerulus sample. Recently, the role of B-cell activation factor of the TNF family (BAFF) and A proliferation inducing ligand (APRIL) in the facilitation of the B-cell differentiation and proliferation in production of galactose-deficient IgA$_1$ has been identified (Penfold et al. 2018).

12.8 Postinfection Glomerulonephritis

Sometimes 2–20 days after the infection, when infection completely subsides, the symptoms of glomerulonephritis are observed, which mainly characterized by hematuria and proteinuria. As the symptoms of primary infection become subside, hence it is known as postinfection glomerulonephritis. The reason for the postinfection glomerulonephritis is the immune complex formation for the clearance of antigens (Table 12.2). Most of the immune complex gets phagocytized, but some of them get deposited in the glomerulus and cause postinfection glomerulonephritis. In poststreptococcal glomerulonephritis, two main antigens are responsible for the cause of glomerulonephritis, namely, nephritis-associated plasmin receptor (NAPlr) and cationic cysteine proteinase known as streptococcal pyrogenic exotoxin B (SPEB). Both of the antigens are able to activate the complement pathway and other chemotactic factors responsible for tissue damage (Iturbe and Musser 2008). Infection caused by *Borrelia burgdorferi* also induces lime disease associated with focal proliferated IgA nephropathy (Rolla et al. 2014). *Staphylococcus aureus*-associated glomerulonephritis occurs mainly during the active infection. Glomerulonephritis occurs because of the superantigen that activates massive T cells leading

Table 12.2 Causes of immune-mediated glomerulonephritis in domestic animals

Category	Etiology
Viral	• African swine fever virus
	• Aleutian mink disease virus
	• Bovine viral diarrhea virus
	• Canine adenovirus 1 (Infectious canine hepatitis)
	• Classical swine fever virus
	• Equine infectious anemia virus
	• Feline leukemia virus
Bacterial/fungal	• *Borrelia burgdorferi*
	• Canine pyometra
	• *Campylobacter fetus*
	• *Encephalitozoon cuniculi*
	• Septic valvular endocarditis
Protozoal	• African trypanosomiasis
	• *Babesia gibsoni*
	• *Leishmania infantum*
	• Coccidiosis
Helminths	• *Dirofilaria immitis*
Neoplasms	• Various neoplasms
Autoimmune	• Multiple autoimmune diseases suspected
Hereditary	• Abnormal complement system of Bernese Mountain dogs
	• Dense deposit disease of pigs
	• Hypocomplementemia of Brittany Spaniels
	• Hypocomplementemia in Finnish Landrace lambs

to cytokines release, overproduction of immunoglobulins by polyclonal B cells, and immune complex formed by the IgA. Deposition of *Staphylococcus* antigen results in vasculitis (Mahmood et al. 2018).

12.9 Conclusion

The immunopathological diseases of the kidneys, most of the time comprises of immune-complex-mediated glomerulonephritis. These complexes activate the complement system and release various cytokines and thus cause damage to the glomerular basement membrane. Autoimmune diseases like crescentic glomerulonephritis and IgA nephropathy are rapidly progressive diseases, which if not diagnosed in time become fatal within few days. Glomerulonephritis caused during infection or postinfection time due to immune complexes formation also become fatal, if not diagnosed properly. Damage to kidneys in all these immunopathological diseases is very severe and may result into the end-stage renal failure. Thus, proper diagnosis and treatment of such diseases in time is very important.

References

Alchi B, Jayne D (2009) Membranoproliferative glomerulonephritis. Pediatr Nephrol 25:1409–1418

Alfaiw A, Alghamdi G, Alsaad K, Aloudah N (2018) Immune complex-mediated rapidly progressive glomerulonephritis in a patient with family history of systemic lupus erythematosus. Saudi J Kidney Dis Transplant 29(5):1227–1231

Appel GB, Cook HT, Hageman G, Jennette JC, Kashgarian M, Kirschfink M, Lambris JD, Lanning L, Lutz HU, Meri S, Rose NR, Salant DJ, Sethi S, Smith RJH, Smoyer W, Tully HF, Tully SP, Walker P, Welsh M, Wurzner R, Zipfel PF (2005) Membranoproliferative glomerulonephritis type II (dense deposit disease): an update. J Am Soc Nephrol 16:1392–1404

Chadban SJ, Atkins RC (2005) Glomerulonephritis. Lancet 365:1797–1806

Chae DW (2014) New classification of membranoproliferative glomerulonephritis: a good start but a long way to go. Kidney Res Clin Pract 33:171–173

Chen YX, Chen N (2013) Pathogenesis of rapidly progressive glomerulonephritis: what do we learn? New Insight Glomerulonephritis 181:2017–2215

Chmielewski C (2003) Renal anatomy and overview of nephron function. Nephrol Nurs J 30(2):185–190

Cunningham A, Kotagiri A (2018) A long history of dense deposit disease. BMC Opthalmol 18(1):228

Fischer EG, Lager DJ (2006) Anti–glomerular basement membrane glomerulonephritis a morphologic study of 80 cases. Am J Clin Pathol 125:445–450

Gupta A, Agarwal V, Kaul A, Verma R, Pandey R (2016) Anti-glomerular basement membrane crescentic glomerulonephritis: a report from India and review of literature. Ind J Nephrol 26(5):335–339

Iturbe RB, Musser JM (2008) The current state of poststreptococcal glomerulonephritis. J Am Soc Nephrol 19:1855–1864

Jennette JC, Nachman PH (2017) ANCA glomerulonephritis and vasculitis. Clin J Am Soc Nephrol 12:1680–1691

Kambham N (2012) Crescentic glomerulonephritis: an update on pauci-immune and anti-GBM diseases. Adv Anat Pathol 19(2):11–124

Licht C, Mengel M (2008) Membranoproliferative glomerulonephritis. In: Geary DF, Schaefer F (eds) Comprehensive pediatric nephrology. Elsevier Publication, Amsterdam

Mahmood T, Puckrin R, Sugar L, Naimark D (2018) Staphylococcus-associated glomerulonephritis mimicking Henoch-Schönlein purpura and cryoglobulinemic vasculitis in a patient with an epidural abscess: a case report and brief review of the literature. Can J Kidney Health Dis 5:1–6

Marshall JS, Warrington R, Watson W, Kim HL (2018) An introduction to immunology and immunopathology. Allergy, Asthma Clin Immunol 14(2):49

Masani N, Jhaveri KD, Fishbane S (2014) Update on microproliferative GN. Clin J Am Soc Nephrol 9:600–608

McAdoo SP, Pusey CD (2017) Anti-glomerular basement membrane disease. Clin J Am Soc Nephrol 12:1162–1172

Moroni G, Ponticelli C (2014) Rapidly progressive crescentic glomerulonephritis: early treatment is a must. Autoimmun Rev 13(2014):723–729

Nakopoulou L (2001) Membranoproliferative glomerulonephritis. Naphrol Dial Transplantation 16(6):71–73

Neary J, Dorman A, Campbell E, Keogan M, Conlon P (2002) Familial membranoproliferative glomerulonephritis type III. Am J Kidney Dis 40(1):E1

Parmer MS, Bahir K (2019) Cresentic glomerulonephritis. StatPearls, Treasure Island, FL

Penfold PS, Prendecki M, McAdoo S, Tam FWK (2018) Primary IgA nephropathy: current challenges and future prospects. Int J Nephrol Renov Dis 11:137–148

Preuss HG (1993) Basic of renal anatomy and physiology. Clin Lab Med 13(1):1–11

Rodrigues JC, Haas M, Reich NH (2017) IgA nephropathy. Clin J Am Soc Nephrol 12:676–686

References

Rolla D, Conti N, Ansaldo F, Panaro L, Lusenti T (2014) Post-infectious glomerulonephritis presenting as acute renal failure in a patient with lyme disease. J Ren Inj Prev 3(1):17–20

Schena FP, Alpers CE (2010) Membranoproliferative glomerulonephritis, dense deposit disease, and cryoglobulinemic glomerulonephritis. In: Comprehensive clinical nephrology, 4th edn. Elsevier, Amsterdam

Servais A, Noel NH, Roumenina LT, Quintrec ML, Ngo S, Durey MAD, Macher MA, Zuber J, Karras A, Provot F, Moulin B, Grunfeld JP, Niaudet P, Lesavre P, Bacchi VF (2012) Acquired and genetic complement abnormalities play a critical role in dense deposit disease and other C3 Glomerulopathies. Kidney Int 86:454–464

Tarzi MR, Cook HT, Pusey CD (2011) Crescentic glomerulonephritis: new aspect of pathogenesis. Semin Nephrol 31(4):361–368

Tizard IR (2004) Veterinary immunology an introduction. Saunders, Philadelphia, PA

West CD, McAdam AJ (1998a) Glomerular para mesangial deposits: association with hypocomplementemia in membranoproliferative glomerulonephritis types I and III. Am J Kidney Dis 31(3):427–434

West CD, McAdam AJ (1998b) Membranoproliferative glomerulonephritis type III: association of glomerular deposits with circulating nephritic factor-stabilized convertase. Am J Kidney Dis 32(1):56–63

Wu MY, Chen CS, Yiang GT, Cheng PW, Chen YL, Chiu HC, Liu KH, Lee WC, Li CJ (2018) The emerging role of pathogenesis of IgA nephropath. J Clin Med 7:225

Yeo SC, Cheung CK, Barratt J (2018) New insights into the pathogenesis of IgA nephropathy. Pediatr Nephrol 33:763–777

Immunopathological Disorders of Joints 13

Key Points

1. Immunopathological conditions alter the natural cartilaginous structure, joint capsule, and synovial membrane in joints.
2. Immunopathological conditions of joints are rheumatoid arthritis, spondyloarthritis, osteoarthritis, psoriatic arthritis, and temporomandibular joint destruction.
3. Rheumatoid arthritis is one of the most common chronic inflammatory autoimmune diseases, which impairs the movement and causes discomfort in the joints.
4. Interleukin-7 is a potent immunoregulatory cytokine found in rheumatoid and juvenile idiopathic arthritis joints that correlates with the disease.
5. Domestic animals can get infectious arthritic conditions from a variety of bacterial, viral, protozoal, and fungal causes.
6. Immunopathological conditions in joints is potentially caused by various inflammatory mediators such as cytokines, interleukin-7, TNF-α, IL-8, nitric oxide etc. lead to the destruction of host tissue.
7. Arthritis is the main clinical manifestation of caprine arthritis encephalitis virus, which is a lentivirus infection.

13.1 Introduction

The immune system in the body has also evolved with the development of the microorganisms to shield us from their harmful effects. The immune system protects us not only from infectious organisms but also from poisonous and allergic substances (Chaplin 2010). There is a complex network of different organs, cells, proteins, humoral, and cellular factors functioning in cascade to maintain the normal homeostasis in the body. The immune system has three main pillars, including anatomical and physical barriers, innate immunity, and acquired immunity (Turvey and Broide 2010). In conjunction with each other, these three elements of the immune system provide protection against any harmful agents. Immunopathological disorder happens when one of these mechanisms has a flaw. This means that the defensive immune response can also cause tissue damage (Sell 1978). Accordingly, the study of diseases caused by the immune system is known as immunopathology, and the diseases are known as immunopathological disorders. Such conditions are mainly described by excessive immune responses, i.e., hypersensitivity; response to self-antigen, i.e., autoimmunity; and inadequate immune response, i.e., immunodeficiency. In joints, these immunopathological changes lead to the alteration in normal cartilaginous structure, joint capsule, and synovial membrane. However, the etiology of most of these conditions remains unknown, but it is suspected that both genetic and environmental influences play a pivotal role in the development of synovial inflammation as in disease like rheumatoid arthritis, spondyloarthritis, and osteoarthritis. Rheumatoid arthritis (RA) is an etiologically unknown, chronic inflammatory autoimmune disease. It is characterized by rheumatoid factor and peptide antibodies that are anticitrullinated. The inflammatory cycle ensemble between specific immune cells, cytokines, chemokines, proteases, matrix metalloproteinases (MMPs), and reactive oxidative stress plays crucial immunopathological roles in the joint environment's inflammatory cascade, resulting in clinical disability and RA (Chen et al. 2019). It is one of the most common chronic autoimmune diseases that cause pain, joint deterioration, and impairment (Silman and Pearson 2002; Aletaha and Smolen 2018). Various bacterial, viral, protozoal, and fungal agents are involved in the infectious arthritis of domestic animals (Table 13.1; Fig. 13.1).

Further, interleukin-7 is a potent immunoregulatory cytokine found in rheumatoid and juvenile idiopathic arthritis joints that correlates with disease parameters. In spondyloarthritis, the most prominent manifestation is chronic inflammation of musculoskeletal structures. More precisely, the spine, sacroiliac joints, and hips are affected by the axial disease, whereas peripheral disease involves peripheral arthritis, preferring asymmetric inflammation of lower limb joints and enthesitis, which is the development of inflammation at the places where ligaments and tendons are connected to the bone. Psoriatic arthritis (PsA) has several different clinical characteristics that distinguish it from rheumatoid arthritis. Some factors such as lentivirus, interleukin-7, arthritogenic alphavirus, tumor necrosis factor-alpha (TNF-α), interleukin-8 (IL-8), nitric oxide, etc. are also known to potentially cause immunopathological disorders in joints. Experimentally, an antigen-induced chronic monoarthritis of the temporomandibular joint (TMJ) was developed that results into synovium proliferation and cartilage destruction (Tominaga et al. 1999). Depending on the stage, the cytokines TNF-α and IL-8 were detected in synovial tissue and synovial fluid in TMJ disorders (Fu et al. 1995), RA, and osteoarthritis (Kaneko et al. 2000). Further, caprine arthritis encephalitis virus (CAEV), which is a lentivirus (Jackson et al. 1991), infects monocytes and macrophages and causes a complex of syndromes of disease in domestic goats including arthritis, pneumonia, mastitis, and encephalitis. Development of CAEV-induced arthritis is correlated with the dominance of immune responses that promote immunoglobulin development (Cheevers et al. 1991). Nitric oxide (NO) is an inflammatory mediator and acts as a biological signaling and effector molecule in inflammation and immunity. However, the

13.1 Introduction

Table 13.1 Common causes of infectious arthritis in domestic animals

Species	Etiology
Cattle	• *Chlamydophila pecorum* — chlamydial arthritis; *Escherichia coli* — coliform arthritis; *Histophilus somni* (previously known as *Haemophilus agni*, *Histophilus ovis*, or *Haemophilus somnus*); Mycoplasma arthritis—*Mycoplasma bovis* and *Mycoplasma mycoides* subsp. *Mycoides*; *Salmonella* spp.; *Streptococcus* spp.; *Trueperella pyogenes;* and *Borrelia burgdorferi*
Sheep	• *Chlamydophila pecorum* • *Erysipelothrix rhusiopathiae* — Fibrinopurulent polyarthritis • *Escherichia coli* • *Histophilus somni* • Contagious agalactia in sheep and goats — *Mycoplasma agalactiae* • *Staphylococcus aureus* • *Streptococcus dysgalactiae* • Visna/maedi virus
Goats	• Contagious caprine pleuropneumonia — *Mycoplasma capricolum* subsp. *capripneumoniae* • *Mycoplasma agalactiae*, *M. mycoides* subsp. *capri*, *M. capricolum* subsp. *capricolum*, and *M. putrefaciens* • Caprine arthritis-encephalitis virus
Horses	• *Actinobacillus equuli* • *Escherichia coli* • *Klebsiella* spp. • *Rhodococcus equi* • *Salmonella* spp. • *Streptococcus* spp. • *Borrelia burgdorferi*
Swine	• *Actinobacillus suis* • *Brucella suis* • *Erysipelothrix rhusiopathiae* — porcine erysipelas • *Escherichia coli* • *Haemophilus parasuis* — Glasser's disease/polyarthritis of pigs • *Mycoplasma hyosynoviae*, *M. hyopneumoniae*, and *M. hyorhinis* — polyarthritis in pigs • *Salmonella* spp. • *Staphylococcus aureus* • *Staphylococcus hyicus* subsp. *hyicus* — Staphylococcal arthritis • *Streptococcus dysgalactiae* subsp. *equisimilis* • *Streptococcus suis* — Streptococcal arthritis • *Trueperella pyogenes*
Dogs	• *Blastomyces dermatitidis* • *Borrelia burgdorferi* — Borreliosis/Lyme disease • *Ehrlichia ewingii* • *Escherichia coli* — rare • *Staphylococcus* spp. • *Streptococcus* spp. • *Mycoplasma spumans* and *Mycoplasma edwardii* — canine arthritis • Protozoal arthritis — *Leishmania donovani* or *Leishmania infantum* • Fungal arthritis — *Blastomyces*, *Histoplasma*, *Coccidioides*, *Cryptococcus*, and *Sporothrix* spp.

(continued)

Table 13.1 (continued)

Species	Etiology
Cats	• *Mycoplasma gateae* and *Mycoplasma felis* — feline polyarthritis • Feline calicivirus • Feline foamy (syncytium-forming) virus — chronic polyarthritis • Feline leukemia virus • *Chlamydophila felis* — rare

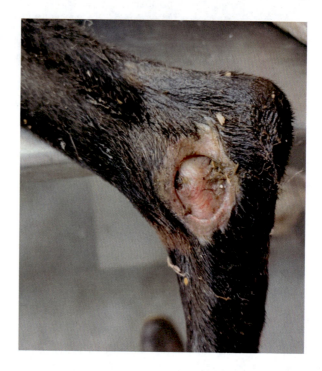

Fig. 13.1 Suppurative arthritis in hock joint of dog due to trauma

overproduction of NO results can be autotoxic and leads to tissue damage and has been implicated in tumor pathogenesis, infectious, autoimmune, and chronic degenerative diseases. Therefore, knowledge and understanding of new and updated immunopathological mechanisms are required for the development and discovery of new therapeutic and immune-modulatory agents to improve the quality of life and control of these types of diseases.

13.2 Normal Cartilage, Joint Capsule, and Synovium

Normal cartilage is a complex substance comprising of a dense matrix primarily composed of collagen and proteoglycan and saturated with water. It is not a homogeneous product. The interaction of physical and biochemical components of the cartilage is needed to enable the normal function of providing almost frictionless movement, wear resistance, joint congruence, and load transmission to subchondral bone. It is the duty of chondrocytes to synthesize and preserve this material (Johnston 1997).

The joint cavity is a joint capsule that invests the complete joint. The joint capsule can be classified into three layers: the synovial lining layer (also known as synovial intima or synovial membrane), the subsynovial layer (subintimal), and the fibrous joint capsule. For this region, nomenclature varies, and the term joint capsule referred to the fibrous joint capsule, and the term synovium is often used to the synovial lining and subsynovial layers (Walsh et al. 1997). The innermost layer is the synovial lining or synovial membrane. The fibrous layer is tough layer that contributes to the joint's structural stability or physical strength. The fibrous joint capsule contributes approximately 47% of maximum elastic strength during the normal range of motion of the feline carpus (Johns and Wright 1962). The subsynovial layer of the joint capsule is found between the synovial lining layer and the fibrous joint capsule. Fibroblasts are found in this layer, and, depending on the location, the stroma can be arranged into loose, areolar connective tissue or more fibrous tissue. The subsynovial layer is vascular, contains free ends of the nerve, and allows movement between the synovial membrane and the fibrous joint capsule (Mankin and Radin 1997).

The synovium is a layer that is connected to the bone's skeletal tissue, a cartilage network, which surrounds the joint cavities and the tendon sheaths and bursae of the joint. A healthy synovium comprises of a quite thin, one to two cell layers thick, an intimate layer of fibroblast-like synoviocytes and macrophages, and a sublining layer of loose connective tissue with blood vessels, lymph vessels, collagen fibers, nerve fibers, fibroblasts, and very less leukocytes. Inflamed synovial tissue shows three significant histological changes: intimate lining hyperplasia due to aggregation of macrophages and proliferation of fibroblast-like synoviocytes in an altered state of activation; neoangiogenesis with endothelial activation in synovial sublining; and substantial infiltration of inflammatory cells such as macrophages, lymphocytes, and dendritic cells (Sande and Baeten 2016). In this layer, two types of synoviocytes are found. Type A synoviocytes are macrophage-like cells that play role in removal of debris from joints and processing antigen. Type B synoviocytes are fibroblast-like cells that are responsible for hyaluronan production and also able to produce degradative enzymes. Both type A and B synoviocytes release cytokines and other mediators.

13.3 Synovium Function

The synovium actively prevents the large molecules such as proteins from reaching the joint cavity under normal conditions. Synovial fluid includes electrolytes and small molecules (such as lactate, glucose, and oxygen) in amounts identical to plasma, and synovial fluid is often referred to as plasma dialysate. There is natural fluid intake and egress across the synovial lining surface, allowing small molecules to be replenished within the synovial fluid reservoir. In regulating transsynovial exchange of small molecules, the interstitial space between synovial lining cells plays an important role. The release of inflammatory mediators including prostaglandins and cytokines, as with synovium or chondrocyte damage, results in increased synovial vasculature permeability. It leads to an increase in the synovial fluid's protein content, disrupting the usual oncotic balance, which helps to control the amount of synovial fluid. Increased synovial fluid development is frequently associated with injury or inflammation. The movement of small molecules across the synovial membrane rises as intrasynovial volume increases. This is likely due to the combination of thinning of the synovial membrane arising from the distended joint cavity and the increased synovial blood flow with synovitis. However, protein is removed from the joint by lymphatic drainage (Simkin and Benedict 1990). Protein clearance from the stifle of dogs with surgically transected cranial cruciate ligaments was approximately three times higher than that of the ordinary contralateral limb (Myers et al. 1996). This result has implications when calculating plasma or synovial fluid levels of cartilage breakdown products such as glycosaminoglycan or collagen fragments are considered a joint disease indicator. The increased rate of elimination of these molecules, together with variable release levels from cartilage, contributes to the inability to use these markers as measures of seriousness of disease (Liepold et al. 1989; Myers et al. 1995).

13.4 Rheumatoid Arthritis

Rheumatoid arthritis (RA) is an etiologically unknown, chronic inflammatory autoimmune disease. It is characterized by rheumatoid factor and peptide antibodies that are anticitrullinated. The inflammatory cycle ensemble between specific immune cells, cytokines, chemokines, proteases, matrix metalloproteinases (MMPs), and reactive oxidative stress plays crucial immunopathological roles in the joint environment's inflammatory cascade, resulting in clinical disability and RA (Chen et al. 2019). It is one of the most common chronic autoimmune diseases that cause joint deterioration, pain, and impairment (Silman and Pearson 2002; Aletaha and Smolen 2018). The initial symptoms are swelling and pain in the joints of hands and feet, particularly in metacarpophalangeal, metatarsophalangeal, and proximal interphalangeal joints. Large joints including the elbow, shoulder, ankle, and knee can also be involved (Aletaha and Smolen 2018). RA progresses to symmetric polyarthritis and damage the diarthrodial joints of the hands and knees, leading to disability, inability, and mortality in the absence of adequate treatment (Chen et al. 2019).

13.5 Immunopathological Mechanisms of Rheumatoid Arthritis

The important immunopathogenic pathways are the cascade responses of innate and adaptive immunity in the inflammatory process of RA (Holmdahl et al. 2014). Such growth is guided by an excess of inflammatory cytokines and autoantibodies and is supported by epigenetic changes in fibroblast-like synoviocytes, which promote more inflammation (Mateen et al. 2016; Harre and Schett 2017). In the intermediate stage, the synovial membrane and fluid are infiltrated by large numbers of various immune cells, including granulocytes, neutrophils, macrophages, B cells, and T cells. This intrusion results in massive release of cytokines, autoantibodies, chemokines, and reactive oxidative stress in the synovial membrane and space results in joint destruction by reactive oxygen species (ROS). The disease serological hallmark is high titers of rheumatoid factor, anticitrullinated peptide antigen, and antibodies (ACPAs) (Cohen et al. 1961; Scherer et al. 2018). It is also confirmed that RA's pathology is strongly associated with increased inflammatory activation of NLR family pyrin domain containing 3 (NLRP3) in vivo (Vande Walle et al. 2014).

13.6 Immune-Mediated Inflammation in Rheumatoid Arthritis

In RA, preliminary effector cells are neutrophils, which release high levels of oxidants and cytotoxic products like ROS and inflammatory agents such as proteases, TNF-α, phospholipases, myeloperoxidase, and defensins at the affected joint location. Th17 cells are involved in the induction of tissue inflammation through stimulation from recruited neutrophils in chronic RA inflammation. These activated Th17 cells produce neutrophil chemoattractants in the joint, such as TNF-α and IL-8 (Pelletier et al. 2010; Wright et al. 2011; Milanova et al. 2014; Navegantes et al. 2017).

Neutrophils in the joint then promote the activation of Th17 cells by secreting CCL20 and CCL2 and Th17-maintaining chemokines (Cua and Tato 2010). Neutrophils also play a role in natural killer (NK) cell activation. Neutrophil depletion can impair NK cells maturation, function, and homeostasis (Jaeger et al. 2012). Also activated macrophages play another pivotal role in the inflammatory process of RA, as these highly elastic cells can polarize into either the M1 or M2 phenotype; M1 cells secrete pro-inflammatory cytokines, while M2 cells secrete anti-inflammatory cytokines (Mantovani et al. 2002; Kennedy et al. 2011). In the course of promoting acute RA, M1 macrophages release pro-inflammatory cytokines such as TNF-α, IL-6, IL-12, IL-1β, IL-23, and low IL-10 and inflammatory enzymes. The M1 macrophages also trigger inflammatory chemokines like CXCL5, CXCL8, CXCL9, CXCL10, and CXCL13 to recruit additional leukocytes to the inflammatory site, resulting in more IL-1β, TNF-α, IL-6, matrix metalloproteinase (MMP), chemokine receptors, ROS, and inducible nitric oxide synthase in the joint, which leads to joint destruction (Navegantes et al. 2017). The primary feature of M2 macrophages is anti-inflammation. Therefore, through the development of IL-10, IL-12, expression of CD163, and CD206, M2 macrophages remodel and rebuild tissue, as well as release growth factors such as transforming growth factor-beta (TGF-β) and vascular endothelial growth factor (VEGF) during chronic inflammation (Wang et al. 2014; Roberts et al. 2015).

Calreticulin (CRT), a residential endoplasmic reticulum glycoprotein, plays a critical role in maintaining Ca2+ homeostasis intracellularly. Soluble CRT accumulates in the blood of RA patients (Michalak et al. 1999). Further, soluble oligomerized CRT may have a pathogenic effect in autoimmune diseases by inducing pro-inflammatory cytokines such as TNF-α and IL-6, by macrophages through the MAPK-NF-κB signaling pathway (Duo et al. 2014). Remarkably in RA, IL-17 (IL-17RA and IL-17RC) receptors are present in synovium and expressed on CD14+ monocytes and macrophages, while synoviocytes bind with IL-17 to induce more inflammation and synovium development of IL-6 and MMPs (Zrioual et al. 2008; Roberts et al. 2015). Furthermore, monocytes and macrophages from the inflamed arthritic joint's synovial fluid can promote the development of IL-17 in CD4+ T cells (Evans et al. 2009), indicating that subsequently recruited CD4 + T cells in the rheumatoid joint that develops into a Th17 lineage in combination with residential monocytes and macrophages. A reciprocal synchronous connection between Th17 cells, monocytes, and macrophages subsequently allows further inflammation (Alonso et al. 2011; Wang et al. 2018). Regulatory T cells (Tregs) are key players in controlling different immune responses. Tregs have the ability to guide macrophages with the functional and phenotypic characteristics of immune modulators to evolve into the M2 phenotype (Brennan et al. 2006). Tregs display novel surface receptors including CD83, neuropilin-1, and protein-coupled receptor 83, which have advanced our understanding of modulating mechanisms of Treg (Hansen et al. 2008). Therefore, there may be therapeutic potential in RA to address T-cell-macrophage interactions.

The IL-6R lead to IL-6 blockade therapy currently on RA is produced by a variety of cells such as endothelial cells, fibroblasts, keratinocytes, chondrocytes, some tumor cells, and immune cells including monocytes, macrophages, T cells, and B cells. The receptor IL-6 consists of two subunits. One is a receptor specific to IL-6 (IL-6R), and the other is a signal transducer (gp130). Both subunits are known as mIL-6R, sIL-6R, mgp130, and s130 in membrane-bound and soluble forms, respectively. Nevertheless, mIL-6R is only expressed on some leukocytes, while gp130 is present in many body cells. The IL-6 binds to mIL-6R and subsequently associates the complex with the signal transmission molecule gp130, which activates downstream signaling events in target cells through Janus kinase. Such interaction contributes to traditional pro-inflammatory signals. Alternatively, sIL-6R contributes to the anti-inflammatory pathway without transmembrane and cytoplasmic areas (Rose-John 2012; Mateen et al. 2016). High levels of IL-6 are found in most RA patient's blood and synovial fluid. The IL-6 facilities the ROS and proteolytic enzyme secretion from neutrophils, which increases the inflammation and eventually harm joints (Dayer and Choy 2010). The IL-6 causes inflammation and joint damage by secreting intermediate reactive oxygen and proteolytic enzymes from neutrophils. Additionally, through triggering either receptor activator of nuclear factor kappa-B ligand (RANKL)-dependent or RANKL-independent pathways, IL-6 promotes osteoclast differentiation (Yoshida and Tanaka 2014). The IL-6 enhances the synthesis of chemokines including monocyte chemotactic protein-1 and IL-8 from endothelial cells, mononuclear cells, and fibroblast-like synoviocytes; it also stimulates adhesion molecules like intercellular adhesion molecule 1 (ICAM-1) in endothelial cells and increases monocyte adhesion to endothelial cells in RA (Romano et al. 1997; Suzuki et al. 2010). The synergistic interaction of IL-6 with IL-1β and TNF-α stimulates the production of VEGF, an important cytokine in pannus organization and maintenance (Hashizume and Mihara 2011). Thus, knowledge and understanding of new and updated immunopathological mechanisms can result in the development and discovery of new therapeutic and immune-modulatory agents in order to improve the quality of life and control of diseases in RA.

13.7 Role of Interleukin-7 in Immunopathology of Rheumatoid Arthritis

Interleukin-7 is a potent immunoregulatory cytokine found in rheumatoid and juvenile idiopathic arthritis joints that correlates with disease parameters. Several types of synovial cells, such as macrophages, dendritic cells, and fibroblasts, which play an important role in inflammation and immunopathology, produce IL-7. The IL-7 induces cytokines produced by arthritogenic T cells (like interferon-γ and IL-17), T-cell differentiating factors (such as IL-12), chemokines capable of attracting inflammatory cells [macrophage inflammatory protein (MIP)-1a and macrophage-induced gene (MIG)], as well as molecules involved in cell adhesion, migration, and costimulation [lymphocyte function-associated antigen (LFA)-1, CD40 and CD80]. Furthermore, IL-7 can induce bone loss by stimulating osteoclastogenesis dependent on the nuclear factor kB ligand (RANKL) receptor activator. The IL-7 induces T-cell and macrophage-dependent activation/monocyte-dependent tumor necrosis factor (TNF-α). Importantly, results caused by IL-7 tend to be capable of operating independently of TNF-α. Together, this suggests that IL-7 is an essential cytokine that can induce inflammation and immunopathology under several rheumatic conditions. Thus, immunotherapy may be an important target (Hartgring et al. 2006).

13.8 Immune Target Therapy and Ongoing Immune-Modulated Therapy in Rheumatoid Arthritis

Disease-modifying antirheumatic drugs (DMARDs) target inflammatory processes by default and reduce subsequent damage in diseases like RA (Smolen et al. 2016). Over the past two decades, monoclonal antibodies have been commonly used in RA care clinical trials. TNF-α-blocking monoclonal antibodies in patients with RA have been clinically proven and used. The response time, however, is limited (Choy et al. 1995). Thereafter, several biological and immune targeting agents with therapeutic effects have developed in RA patients. In contrast, DMARD formulations combined with several immune-modulated agents and monoclonal antibodies have been preclinically and clinically tested to induce remission and control of the disease (Serio and Tovoli 2018). Inspiringly, several biological agents that target cytokines and cytokine networks have attained significant RA treatment successes. For more than a decade, rituximab, a monoclonal antibody against the CD20 expressed on the surface of B cells for B-cell depletion, has been used in RA. Some TNF-α targeting biological drugs, such as etanercept, infliximab, adalimumab, certolizumab, pegol, and golimumab, are approved for the treatment with RA. Nevertheless, a substantial minority of RA patients do not respond to these drugs, which required other biological agents to be created. Currently, tocilizumab, an anti-IL6R mAb; tofacitinib, a Janus kinase class inhibitor, inhibiting intracellular signaling; and abatacept, a soluble fusion protein consisting of the extracellular domain of cytotoxic T-lymphocyte-associated antigen 4 linked to the altered Fc portion of IgG1, interfering with T-cell activation, are used in clinical applications (Venuturupalli 2017).

13.9 Psoriatic Arthritis

Psoriatic arthritis (PsA) has several different clinical characteristics that distinguish it from RA. Nonetheless, recent research studies highlight new findings in PsA at genetic, cellular, and tissue levels that are the basis for a new understanding of this relatively common type of inflammatory arthritis. The cellular immunopathology reveals that perivascular distribution of cell infiltrate is predominant, while cells can migrate to the joint or epidermis lining layer. Furthermore, abundant B lymphocytes can form primitive germ centers; the role of these B cells is not clear because psoriasis and psoriatic arthritis (PsA) are not associated with increased circulating antibody levels (Veale et al. 1993; Laloux et al. 2001). There is a prominent T lymphocytic infiltrate in both tissues, which is found in the dermal papillae in the skin and the sublining stroma in the joint (Veale et al. 1993, 1994). Recent evidence indicates that the inflammatory enthesis exhibits a similar infiltration (Laloux et al. 2001). There is a concept of "three-cell interaction," i.e., effector CD8+ cells and regulatory CD4+ T cells both interacting with antigen-presenting cells (APCs), such as the Langerhans cell (Ridge et al. 1998). The T cells enter the joint by first attaching to activated endothelial cells through cell adhesion molecules (CAM) expressed on the surface.

There is a marked upregulation of ICAM-1 and vascular adhesion molecule-1 (VCAM-1) in the skin and the synovial membrane; however, E-selectin tends to be more upregulated in the skin than in the synovial PsA membrane (Veale et al. 1995). The CD4+ T cells are the most important lymphocytes in the tissue with a CD4+/CD8+ ratio of 2:1; this ratio, on the other hand, is reversed in the synovial fluid compartment and in entheses where CD8+ T cells are more common (Costello et al. 1999; Laloux et al. 2001). A dominant population of CD8+ T cells in synovial PsA fluid suggests that these cells may drive the joint's immune response (Costello et al. 2001). Cytokines, particularly TNF, TGF, and many others, are likely to be critically involved in driving the inflammatory process leading to cartilage and bone degradation. Affected skin and joint displayed increased vascularization, T cells, and expression of TNF-α in PsA. Nonetheless, functional interpretation of these results deserves caution, as T-cell-directed therapies such as alefacept tend to be very successful for psoriasis but not for PsA, indicating that specific molecular mechanisms are involved in the skin and joint (Sande and Baeten 2016). In general, the emergence of new biological antitumor necrosis factor, a therapy, has allowed further insight into psoriasis and PsA immunopathology.

13.10 Caprine Arthritis Encephalitis Virus-Induced Arthritis

Caprine arthritis encephalitis virus (CAEV) is a lentivirus (Jackson et al. 1991), which infects monocytes and macrophages, and causes a complex of syndromes of disease in domestic goats including arthritis, pneumonia, mastitis, and encephalitis (Table 13.1). Arthritis is the main clinical manifestation of CAEV infection (Cheevers and McGuire 1988). Development of CAEV-induced arthritis is correlated with the dominance of immune responses that promote immunoglobulin development (Cheevers et al. 1991). Vigorous humoral immune reactivity to CAEV antigens includes marked polyclonal IgG1 development in synovial fluid (SF) (Johnson et al. 1983), the involvement of plasma cells in inflamed synovium (Johnson et al. 1983), and the formation of secondary B-cell follicles in local lymph nodes (Cheevers and McGuire 1988). The recent phenotype studies have shown that SF of CAEV-infected arthritic carpal joints of goats showed few B lymphocytes infiltration and is enriched with IL-activated CD8+ T lymphocytes, which express little IL-2 receptor (IL-2R) for major histocompatibility class (MHC) (Wilkerson et al. 1995). The findings of the histological analysis of progressive arthritis indicate that CD5-B lymphocytes are the main component of CAEV-induced arthritis synovial tissue infiltrates and suggest unique immunopathogenesis mechanisms (Melinda et al. 1995). The B cells which expressed immunoglobulin existed in follicles and inflamed villi. In arthritic synovium, immunohistochemistry established CD45R+ CD5-B lymphocytes as the main component of most perivascular infiltrates. Clinical symptoms of arthritis involve periarticular swelling with abnormal deposition of SF comprising of inflammatory cells (Cheevers et al. 1991) and radiographic alterations like soft tissue mineralization and articular surface erosion (Wilkerson et al. 1995).

13.11 Temporomandibular Joint Destruction (TMJD)

Rheumatoid arthritis is a chronic inflammatory disorder of the joints, and around 30–50% of patients experience symptoms of temporomandibular joint (TMJ) arthritis with RA (Kopp 1994). Experimentally, an antigen-induced chronic monoarthritis of the TMJ was developed that results into synovium proliferation and cartilage destruction (Tominaga et al. 1999). The host reaction to infection or injury causes a cascade of events involving leukocyte recruitment and the release of multiple inflammatory mediators. Depending on the stage, the cytokines TNF-α and IL-8 were detected in synovial tissue and synovial fluid in TMJ disorders (Fu et al. 1995), RA, and osteoarthritis (Kaneko et al. 2000). TNF-α is a very potent pro-inflammatory cytokine that induces a potent immune and inflammatory responses and has various biological functions such as antibodies production from B cells, cytokines induction, prostaglandin E2 with macrophage activation, collagenase production in synovial cells, and osteoclastic bone resorption induction (Veale et al. 1994). The IL-8 activates leucocytes, and it is a member of ECR CXC chemokines (Laloux et al. 2001). In vitro, IL-8 also attracts the T lymphocytes. Both TNF-α and IL-8 are involved in angiogenesis, cartilage destruction, and acute stage of inflammation.

Further, an inflammatory mediator nitric oxide (NO) not only an important microbicidal agent in host defense but also acts as a biological signaling and effector molecule in inflammation and immunity. But the overproduction of NO can be autotoxic and leads to tissue destruction and has been implicated in tumor pathogenesis, infectious, autoimmune, and chronic degenerative diseases. One of this kind of chronic inflammatory syndrome includes TMJD, in which NOS and NO have been found in the synovial fluid (Suenaga et al. 2001) and in the synovial tissues leading to pain and tissue pathology (Homma et al. 2001).

13.12 Spondyloarthritis (SpA)

The most prominent manifestation of SpA disease is chronic inflammation of musculoskeletal structures. More precisely, the spine, sacroiliac joints, and hips are affected by the axial disease. Peripheral disease involves peripheral arthritis, preferring asymmetric inflammation of lower limb joints and enthesitis, which is the development of inflammation at the places where ligaments and tendons are connected to the bone. It has been shown in peripheral SpA that ankylosing spondylitis (AS), undifferentiated SpA, and PsA have identical synovial infiltration, characterized by increased levels of CD163 macrophages, neutrophils, and mast cells (Kruithof et al. 2005; De Rycke et al. 2005). The most prominent cellular population are of macrophages expressing CD163, which is a scavenger receptor for haem-haptoglobin complexes (Kristiansen et al. 2001). Increased vascularity and myogene signature are also shared among the different peripheral subtypes of SpA, suggesting that they reflect one pathophysiological entity (Yeremenko et al. 2013). In the spine, the inflammation of the vertebral body should be distinguished from that of the zygapophyseal joint. The inflammatory cells are mostly seen in annulus fibrosis in vertebral bodies and intervertebral spaces. In these structures, a prominent neovascularization also seen leads to formation of syndesmophytes (Cawley et al. 1972). The zygapophyseal joint is a synovial joint forming articulation between the vertebral bodies. These joints more frequently affected in SpA often results into bony ankylosis (de Vlam et al. 2000). The subchondral bone marrow and synovium are heavily infiltrated with inflammatory cells (Cawley et al. 1972), predominantly with T cells (both CD4 and CD8), but also with B lymphocytes (Appel et al. 2006a, b). However, the most typical site for SpA is the sacroiliac joint showing inflammatory infiltrate predominantly with T cells both CD4 and CD8 T cells and macrophages. The SpA affects not only the axial and peripheral joints but also extraarticular pathologies like skin psoriasis and inflammatory bowel disease (IBD)

(Rudwaleit and Baeten 2006). Comparison of synovial immunopathology with skin or gut shows some reveals many remarkable parallels but also significant difference. For example, in the gut-joint axis, an increase in CD163+ macrophages is seen not only in the joints of SpA patients but also in their intestines that mimicking the findings in Crohn's disease (Baeten et al. 2002; Demetter et al. 2005).

13.13 Ankylosing Spondylitis

Ankylosing spondylitis is the main subtype and a significant consequence of an interrelated rheumatic disease category now called spondyloarthritides. Clinical manifestation of this group involves inflammatory back pain, enthesitis, asymmetrical peripheral oligoarthritis (mostly of the lower limbs), and particular organ involvement like psoriasis, anterior uveitis, and chronic inflammatory bowel disease. In this, the subgroups are biologically related—the MHC class I molecule and HLA B27, which is the strongest known contributing factor, although others are still to be found (Braun and Siepe 2007). No doubt that the MHC, via HLA-B27 and possibly some other gene products, contributes significantly in the development of AS. Spondyloarthritides have a strong genetic effect, particularly in ankylosing spondylitis. Approximately one third of this impact is explained by HLA B27; the remainder, still largely unknown, is correlated with genes within and outside the MHC (Brown et al. 1997). The cartilaginous structures—collagen type II and proteoglycan—have been identified in ankylosing spondylitis as possible targets of an autoimmune response (Bollow et al. 2000). Mononuclear cells invade these cartilaginous structures of sacroiliac joints and intervertebral disks that cause destruction and ankylosis in patients suffering with this disease (Bardos et al. 2005). Not only in spondyloarthritides but also in other arthritides, T-cell responses to aggrecan have been seen (Guerassimov et al. 1998). In peripheral blood and synovial fluid samples of patients with ankylosing spondylitis, both CD4+ (Zou et al. 2003) and CD8+ (Zou et al. 2005) T-cell responses to aggrecan and collagen-derived peptides have been reported (Atagunduz et al. 2005). Both innate and adaptive immune responses could have a role in spondyloarthritides. The discovery that the tumor necrosis factor (TNF)-α was overexpressed in sacroiliac joints (Braun et al. 1995) offered a good justification for the use of TNF inhibitors, which are very active in spondyloarthritides. Osteoclasts are key element in inflammation-associated bone loss in rheumatic diseases (Walsh et al. 2005; Appel et al. 2006a, b). The anomalies found in AS humoral immunity vary from those seen in other rheumatic diseases such as systemic lupus erythematosus (SLE) and RA, which are thought to be immunologically mediated. The finding that subtyping of the HLA-B27 antigen with cytotoxic T cells and monoclonal antibodies revealed the presence of the HLA-B27 antigen may influence the function of polymorphonuclear cells.

13.14 Summary

Due to the impairment in the interrelated response of innate and acquired immunity, various immunopathological disorders arise. In joints, the process starts and continues through a series of definable steps that lead to an immunopathologic outcome. However, the etiology of most of these disorders remains unknown, but it is suspected that both genetic and environmental influences play a pivotal role in the development of synovial inflammation as in disease like rheumatoid arthritis, spondyloarthritis, psoriatic arthritis, osteoarthritis, and temporomandibular joint destruction. Some other factors such as lentivirus, interleukin-7, arthritogenic alphavirus, TNF-α, IL-8 and nitric oxide, etc. are also known to potentially cause immunopathological changes in joints and lead to the destruction of host tissue. Therefore, knowledge and understanding of new and updated immunopathological mechanisms are required for the development and discovery of new therapeutic and immune-modulatory agents to improve the quality of life and control of these types of diseases.

References

Aletaha D, Smolen JS (2018) Diagnosis and management of rheumatoid arthritis: a review. J Am Med Assoc 320:1360–1372

Alonso MN, Wong MT, Zhang AL, Winer D, Suhoski MM, Tolentino LL, Gaitan J, Davidson MG, Kung TH, Galel DM, Nadeau KC, Kim J, Utz PJ, Söderström K, Engleman EG (2011) T(H)1, T(H)2, and T(H)17 cells instruct monocytes to differentiate into specialized dendritic cell subsets. Blood 118:3311–3320

Appel H, Kuhne M, Spiekermann S et al (2006a) Immunohistologic analysis of zygapophyseal joints in patients with ankylosing spondylitis. Arthritis and Rheumatol 54:2845–2851

Appel H, Kuhne M, Spiekermann S et al (2006b) Immunohistochemical analysis of hip arthritis in ankylosing spondylitis: evaluation of the bone-cartilage interface and subchondral bone marrow. Arthritis Rheumatol 54:1805–1813

Atagunduz P, Appel H, Kuon W et al (2005) HLA-B27-restricted CD8+ T cell response to cartilage-derived self peptides in ankylosing spondylitis. Arthritis Rheumatol 52:892–901

Baeten D, Demetter P, Cuvelier CA et al (2002) Macrophages expressing the scavenger receptor CD163: a link between immune alterations of the gut and synovial inflammation in spondyloarthropathy. J Pathol 196:34350

Bardos T, Szabo Z, Czipri M et al (2005) A longitudinal study on an autoimmune murine model of ankylosing spondylitis. Ann Rheum Dis 64:981–987

Bollow M, Fischer T, Reisshauer H et al (2000) Quantitative analyses of sacroiliac biopsies in spondyloarthropathies: T cells and macrophages predominate in early and active sacroiliitis-cellularity correlates with the degree of enhancement detected by magnetic resonance imaging. Ann Rheum Dis 59:135–140

Braun J, Siepe J (2007) Ankylosing spondylitis. Seminar 369:1379–1389

Braun J, Bollow M, Neure L et al (1995) Use of immunohistologic and in situ hybridization techniques in the examination of sacroiliac joint biopsy specimens from patients with ankylosing spondylitis. Arthritis Rheumatol 38:499–505

Brennan FM, Foey AD, Feldmann M (2006) The importance of T cell interactions with macrophages in rheumatoid cytokine production. Curr Top Microbiol Immunol 305:177–194

Brown MA, Kennedy LG, MacGregor AJ et al (1997) Susceptibility to ankylosing spondylitis in twins: the role of genes, HLA, and the environment. Arthritis Rheumatol 40:1823–1828

Cawley MI, Chalmers TM, Kellgren JH et al (1972) Destructive lesions of vertebral bodies in ankylosing spondylitis. Ann Rheum Dis 31:345–358

Chaplin D (2010) Overview of immune response. J Allergy Clin Immunol 125(2):3–23

Cheevers WP, McGuire TC (1988) The lentiviruses: maedi/visna, caprine arthritis-encephalitis, and equine infectious anemia. Adv Virus Res 34:189–215

Cheevers WP, Knowles DP Jr, Norton LK (1991) Neutralization-resistant antigenic variants of caprine arthritis-encephalitis lentivirus associated with progressive arthritis. J Infect Dis 164:679–685

Chen SJ, Lin GJ, Chen JW, Wang KC, Tien CH, Hu CF, Chang CN, Hsu WF, Fan HC, Sytwu HK (2019) Immunopathogenic mechanisms and novel immune-modulated therapies in rheumatoid arthritis. Int J Mol Sci 20(6):1332

Choy EH, Panayi GS, Kingsley GH (1995) Therapeutic monoclonal antibodies. Br J Rheumatol 34:707–715

Cohen E, Nisonoff A, Hermes P, Norcross BM, Lockie LM (1961) Agglutination of sensitized alligator erythrocytes by rheumatoid factor(s). Nature 190:552–553

Costello P, Bresnihan B, O'Farrelly C, FitzGerald O (1999) Predominance of CD8+ T lymphocytes in psoriatic arthritis. J Rheumatol 26:1117–1124

Costello PJ, Winchester RJ, Curran SA, Peterson KS, Kane DJ, Bresnihan B et al (2001) Psoriatic arthritis joint fluids are characterized by CD8 and CD4 T cell clonal expansions appear antigen driven. J Immunol 166:2878–2886

Cua DJ, Tato CM (2010) Innate IL-17-producing cells: the sentinels of the immune system. Nat Rev. Immunol 10:479–489

Dayer JM, Choy E (2010) Therapeutic targets in rheumatoid arthritis: The interleukin-6 receptor. Rheumatology 49:15–24

De Rycke L, Baeten D, Foell D et al (2005) Differential expression and response to anti-TNF alpha treatment of infiltrating versus resident tissue macrophage subsets in autoimmune arthritis. J Pathol 206:1727

de Vlam K, Mielants H, Verstaete KL et al (2000) The zygapophyseal joint determines morphology of the enthesophyte. J Rheumatol 27:1732–1739

Demetter P, De Vos M, Van Huysse JA et al (2005) Colon mucosa of patients both with spondyloarthritis and Crohn's disease is enriched with macrophages expressing the scavenger receptor CD163. Ann Rheum Dis 64:3214

Duo CC, Gong FY, He XY, Li YM, Wang J, Zhang JP, Gao XM (2014) Soluble calreticulin induces tumor necrosis factor-α (TNF-α) and interleukin (IL)-6 production by macrophages through mitogen-activated protein kinase (MAPK) and NFκB signaling pathways. Int J Mol Sci 15(2):2916–2928

Evans HG, Gullick NJ, Kelly S, Pitzalis C, Lord GM, Kirkham BW, Taams LS (2009) In vivo activated monocytes from the site of inflammation in humans specifically promote Th17 responses. Proc Natl Acad Sci U S A 106(15):6232–6237

Fu K, Ma X, Zhang Z, Chen W (1995) Tumor necrosis factor in synovial fluid of patient with temporomandibular joint disorders. J Oral Maxillofac Surg 53:424–426

Guerassimov A, Zhang Y, Banerjee S et al (1998) Cellular immunity to the G1 domain of cartilage proteoglycan aggrecan is enhanced in patients with rheumatoid arthritis but only after removal of keratan sulfate. Arthritis Rheumatol 41:1019–1025

Hansen W, Westendorf AM, Buer J (2008) Regulatory T cells as targets for immunotherapy of autoimmunity and inflammation. Inflamm Allergy Drug Targets 7:217–223

Harre U, Schett G (2017) Cellular and molecular pathways of structural damage in rheumatoid arthritis. Semin Immunopathol 39:355–363

Hartgring SA, Bijlsma JW, Lafeber FP, van Roon JA (2006) Interleukin-7 induced immunopathology in arthritis. Ann Rheum Dis 65(3):69–74

Hashizume M, Mihara M (2011) The roles of interleukin-6 in the pathogenesis of rheumatoid arthritis. Arthritis 2011:765624

Holmdahl R, Malmstrom V, Burkhardt H (2014) Autoimmune priming, tissue attack and chronic inflammation—the three stages of rheumatoid arthritis. Eur J Immunol 44:1593–1599

Homma HT, Takahashi H, Seki M, Ohtani T, Kondoh M, Fukuda. (2001) Immunohisto-chemical localization of inducible nitric oxide synthase in synovial tissue of human temporomandibular joints with internal derangement. Arch Oral Biol 46:93–97

Jackson MK, Knowles DP, Stem TA, Harwood WG, Robinson MM, Cheevers WP (1991) Genetic structure of the pol-env region of the caprine arthritis-encephalitis lentivirus genome. Virology 180:389–394

Jaeger BN, Donadieu J, Cognet C, Bernat C, Ordonez-Rueda D, Barlogis V, Mahlaoui N, Fenis A, Narni-Mancinelli E, Beaupain B et al (2012) Neutrophil depletion impairs natural killer cell maturation, function, and homeostasis. J Exp Med 209:565–580

Johns RJ, Wright V (1962) Relative importance of various tissues in joint stiffness. J Appl Physiol 17:824

Johnson GC, Adams DS, McGuire TC (1983) Pronounced production of polyclonal immunoglobulin Gl in the synovial fluid of goats with caprine arthritis-encephalitis virus infection. Infect Immun 41:805–815

Johnston SA (1997) Osteoarthritis joint anatomy, physiology, and pathobiology. Vet Clin N Am Small Anim Pract 27(4):699–723

Kaneko S, Santoh T, Chiba J, Ju C, Inoue K, Kagawa J (2000) IL-6 and IL-8 levels in serum and synovial fluid of patients with osteoarthritis. Cytokines Cell Mol Ther 6:71–79

Kennedy A, Fearon U, Veale DJ, Godson C (2011) Macrophages in synovial inflammation. Front Immunol 2:51–52

Kopp S (1994) Temporomandibular joint and masticatory muscle disorders. In: Zarb GA, Carlsson GE (eds) Rheumatoid arthritis, 2nd edn. Munksgaard, Copenhagen, pp 346–366

Kristiansen M, Graversen JH, Jacobsen C et al (2001) Identification of the haemoglobin scavenger receptor. Nature 409:198–201

Kruithof E, Baeten D, De Rycke L et al (2005) Synovial histopathology of psoriatic arthritis, both oligo- and polyarticular, resembles spondyloarthropathy more than it does rheumatoid arthritis. Arthritis Res Ther 7:R56980

Laloux L, Voisin M, Allain J et al (2001) Immunohistological study of entheses in spondyloarthropathies: comparison in rheumatoid arthritis and osteoarthritis. Ann Rheum Dis 60:316–321

Liepold HR, Goldberg RL, Lust G (1989) Canine serum keratan sulfate and hyaluronate concentrations. Arthritis Rheumatol 32:312

Mankin HJ, Radin EL (1997) Structure and function of joints. In: Koopman WJ (ed) Arthritis and allied conditions, 13th edn. Williams & Wilkins, Baltimore, p 1969.49

Mantovani A, Sozzani S, Locati M, Allavena P, Sica A (2002) Macrophage polarization: tumor-associated macrophages as a paradigm for polarized M2 mononuclear phagocytes. Trends Immunol 23:549–555

Mateen S, Zafar A, Moin S, Khan AQ, Zubair S (2016) Understanding the role of cytokines in the pathogenesis of rheumatoid arthritis. Clin Chim Acta 455:161–171

Melinda J, Wilkerson MJ, Davis WC, Baszler TV, Cheevers WR (1995) Immunopathology of chronic lentivirus-induced arthritis. Am J Pathol 146(6):1433–1443

Michalak M, Corbett EF, Mesaeli N, Nakamura K, Opas M (1999) Calreticulin: one protein, one gene, many functions. Biochem J 344:281–292

Milanova V, Ivanovska N, Dimitrova P (2014) TLR2 elicits IL-17-mediated RANKL expression, IL-17, and OPG production in neutrophils from arthritic mice. Mediat Inflamm 2014:643406

Myers SL, Brandt KD, Eilam O (1995) Even low-grade synovitis significantly accelerates the clearance of protein from the canine knee. Arthritis Rheumatol 38:1085

Myers SL, O'Connor BL, Brandt KD (1996) Accelerated clearance of albumin from the osteoarthritic knee: implications for interpretation of concentrations of "cartilage markers" in synovial fluid. J Rheumatol 23:1744

Navegantes KC, de Souza GR, Pereira PAT, Czaikoski PG, Azevedo CHM, Monteiro MC (2017) Immune modulation of some autoimmune diseases: the critical role of macrophages and neutrophils in the innate and adaptive immunity. J Transl Med 15(1):36

Pelletier M, Maggi L, Micheletti A, Lazzeri E, Tamassia N, Costantini C, Cosmi L, Lunardi C, Annunziato F, Romagnani S, Cassatella MA (2010) Evidence for a cross-talk between human neutrophils and Th17 cells. Blood 115:335–343

Ridge JP, Di Rosa F, Matzinger P (1998) A conditioned dendritic cell can be a temporal bridge between a CD4+ T-helper and a T-killer cell. Nature 393:474–478

Roberts CA, Dickinson AK, Taams LS (2015) The interplay between monocytes/macrophages and CD4(+) T cell subsets in rheumatoid arthritis. Front Immunol 6:571

Romano M, Sironi M, Toniatti C, Polentarutti N, Fruscella P, Ghezzi P, Faggioni R, Luini W, van Hinsbergh V, Sozzani S, Bussolino F, Poli V, Ciliberto G, Mantovani A (1997) Role of IL-6 and its soluble receptor in induction of chemokines and leukocyte recruitment. Immunity 6:315–325

Rose-John S (2012) IL-6 trans-signaling via the soluble IL-6 receptor: importance for the pro-inflammatory activities of IL-6. Int J Biol Sci 8:1237–1247

Rudwaleit M, Baeten D (2006) Ankylosing spondylitis and bowel disease. Best Pract Res Clin Rheumatol 20:451–471

Sande MG, Baeten DL (2016) Immunopathology of synovitis: from histology to molecular pathways. Rheumatology 55:599–606

Scherer HU, Huizinga TWJ, Kronke G, Schett G, Toes REM (2018) The B cell response to citrullinated antigens in the development of rheumatoid arthritis. Nat Rev. Rheumatol 14: 157–169

Sell S (1978) Immunopathology. Am J Pathol 3:215–275

Serio I, Tovoli F (2018) Rheumatoid arthritis: new monoclonal antibodies. Drugs Today 54:219–230

Silman AJ, Pearson JE (2002) Epidemiology and genetics of rheumatoid arthritis. Arthritis Res Ther 4:S265–S272

Simkin PA, Benedict RS (1990) Iodide and albumin kinetics in normal canine wrists and knees. Arthritis Rheum 33:73

Smolen JS, Aletaha D, McInnes IB (2016) Rheumatoid arthritis. Lancet 388:2023–2038

Suenaga S, Abeyama K, Hamasaki A, Mimura T, Noikura T (2001) Temporomandibular disorders: relationship between joint pain and effusion and nitric oxide concentration in the joint fluid. Dentomaxillofac Radiol 30(4):214–218

Suzuki M, Hashizume M, Yoshida H, Mihara M (2010) Anti-inflammatory mechanism of tocilizumab, a humanized anti-IL-6R antibody: effect on the expression of chemokine and adhesion molecule. Rheumatol Int 30:309–315

Tominaga K, Alestergern P, Kurita H, Kopp S (1999) Clinical course of an antigen-induced arthritis model of the rabbit temporomandibular joint. J Oral Pathol Med 28:268–273

Turvey SE, Broide DH (2010) Innate immunity. J Allergy Clin Immunol 125(2):24–32

Vande Walle L, Van Opdenbosch N, Jacques P, Fossoul A, Verheugen E, Vogel P, Beyaert R, Elewaut D, Kanneganti TD, van Loo G, Lamkanfi M (2014) Negative regulation of the NLRP3 inflammasome by A20 protects against arthritis. Nature 512:69–73

Veale D, Yanni G, Rogers S, Barnes L, Bresnihan B, Fitzgerald O (1993) Reduced synovial membrane ELAM-1 expression, macrophage numbers and lining layer hyperplasia in psoriatic arthritis as compared with rheumatoid arthritis. Arthritis Rheum 36:893–900

Veale DJ, Barnes L, Rogers S, FitzGerald O (1994) Immunohistochemical markers for arthritis in psoriasis. Ann Rheum Dis 53:450–454

Veale D, Rogers S, Fitzgerald O (1995) Immunolocalization of adhesion molecules in psoriatic arthritis, psoriatic and normal skin. Br J Dermatol 132:32–38

Venuturupalli S (2017) Immune mechanisms and novel targets in rheumatoid arthritis. Immunol Allergy Clin N Am 37:301–313

Walsh DA, Sledge CB, Blake DR (1997) Biology of the normal joint. In: Kelly WN, Harris ED, Ruddy S (eds) Textbook of rheumatology, 5th edn. WB Saunders, Philadelphia, PA, p 1

Walsh NC, Crotti TN, Goldring SR, Gravallese EM (2005) Rheumatic diseases: the effects of inflammation on bone. Immunol Rev 208:228–251

Wang N, Liang H, Ze K (2014) Molecular mechanisms that influence the macrophage m1-m2 polarization balance. Front Immunol 5:614

Wang SP, Lehman CW, Lien CZ, Lin CC, Bazzazi H, Aghaei M, Memarian A, Asgarian-Omran H, Behnampour N, Yazdani Y (2018) Th1-Th17 ratio as a new insight in rheumatoid arthritis disease. Int J Mol Sci 17:68–77

Wilkerson MJ, Davis WC, Cheevers WP (1995) Peripheral blood and synovial fluid mononuclear cell phenotypes in lentivirus induced arthritis. J Rheumatol 22:8–15

Wright HL, Chikura B, Bucknall RC, Moots RJ, Edwards SW (2011) Changes in expression of membrane TNF, NF-{kappa}B activation and neutrophil apoptosis during active and resolved inflammation. Ann Rheum Dis 70:537–543

Yeremenko N, Noordenbos T, Cantaert T et al (2013) Disease-specific and inflammation-independent stromal alterations in spondylarthritis synovitis. Arthritis Rheum 65:174–185

Yoshida Y, Tanaka T (2014) Interleukin 6 and rheumatoid arthritis. Biomed Res Int 2014:698313

Zou J, Zhang Y, Thiel A et al (2003) Predominant cellular immune response to the cartilage autoantigenic G1 aggrecan in ankylosing spondylitis and rheumatoid arthritis. Rheumatology 42:846–855

Zou J, Appel H, Rudwaleit M, Thiel A, Sieper J (2005) Analysis of the CD8+ T cell response to the G1 domain of aggrecan in ankylosing spondylitis. Ann Rheum Dis 64:722–729

Zrioual S, Toh ML, Tournadre A, Zhou Y, Cazalis MA, Pachot A, Miossec V, Miossec P (2008) IL-17RA and IL-17RC receptors are essential for IL-17A-induced ELR+ CXC chemokine expression in synoviocytes and are overexpressed in rheumatoid blood. J Immunol 180:655–663

Immunopathology of Skin Ailments

14

Key Points

1. Skin is the largest organ in the body and possesses network of immune cells that serves as a primary immunological defense against the environment.
2. Epidermis is home to skin-resident immune cells like Langerhans cells and melanocytes, whereas dermis possesses dendritic cells, macrophages, mast cells, and various types of T cells.
3. Keratinocytes produce a significant number of antimicrobial peptides (AMPs).
4. Melanocytes have the ability to control local immunological responses by enhancing the phagocytosis of pathogens and the production of cytokines (IL-1, IL-6, TNF-alpha, and chemokines).
5. Immunopathological skin diseases in animals are allergic contact dermatitis, pemphigus foliaceus, vitiligo, canine atopic dermatitis, flea allergy dermatitis, Chediak-Higashi syndrome, and discoid lupus erythematosus.
6. Interaction of the allergen with the skin initiates the pathophysiology of contact allergic dermatitis.
7. Most typical autoimmune skin condition that affects dogs and cats is pemphigus foliaceus.
8. Atopy is an allergic reaction to environmental antigens (allergens) that are inhaled or absorbed via skin in genetically susceptible populations.
9. An acquired cutaneous condition called vitiligo causes uneven depigmentation of the skin and a progressive loss of melanocytes.

14.1 Introduction

The largest organ in the body is the skin. The main function is to serve as a barrier against physical and chemical assaults, pathogen entry, and excessive water loss in order to safeguard the internal organs (Table 14.1). The "skin immune system" is a complex network of immune cells that is the primary immunological defense in

Table 14.1 Host innate and adaptive defense mechanisms of the skin

Barriers	Innate and adaptive defenses
Skin	• Provides protective barrier against fluid loss, microbiological agents, chemicals, and physical injury • Regulates temperature and blood pressure • Produces vitamin D • Functions as a sensory organ • Stores nutrients • Absorptive surface • Participates in innate and adaptive immunity, inflammation, and repair
Barrier functions	• **Hair coat:** Physical and thermal protective barrier • **Tactile hairs and neurons:** Sensory function • **Claws, horns, and hooves:** Physical protective barrier • **Stratum corneum:** Barrier function • **Adnexal glandular secretions:** Barrier function • **Apocrine gland secretion:** Defense against excessive heat by sweating in horses and cattle • **Melanin:** Defense against ultraviolet radiation and camouflage • **Basement membrane zone:** Filter to macromolecules, barrier to invasion of neoplastic epidermal cells, and anchor epidermis to dermis • **Panniculus:** Barrier to temperature extremes
Resistance to mechanical forces	• **Hair follicles and dermal-epidermal interdigitations:** Anchor epidermis to dermis • **Stratum corneum:** Corneocyte, corneocyte envelope, and intercellular lipid adhesion • **Desmosomes and hemidesmosomes:** Intercellular and basement membrane adhesion • **Basement membrane:** Anchors epidermis to dermis • **Collagen and elastic tissues:** Resilience, strength, and support of adnexa and dermal structures • **Panniculus:** Shock absorption, facilitates movement, and anchors dermis to fascia

the body against the external environment (Bos and Kapsenberg 1986). An innate immune response and an adaptive immunological response are the two main components of the immune system. Immunological skin diseases can result from immune system dysfunction or abnormalities. Hypoimmunity can result in the infectious diseases and skin tumors, excessive and undesirable immune responses can lead to autoimmune diseases or hypersensitivity (Yuxiao et al. 2014).

In the body, immune system is located in major structural compartments: epidermis and dermis, and consists of several important immunocompetent cells. The epidermis is home to primary skin-resident immune cells like Langerhans cells (LCs) and melanocytes that produce melanin, while the dermis is the deeper layer and is home to other types of immune-specialized cells like different subpopulations of dendritic cells (DCs), macrophages, and various types of T cells. The efficacy of the skin immune system strongly depends on the close interplay and interaction between immune cells and the skin environment, such as adjacent keratinocytes and fibroblasts (Matejuk 2017).

The fundamental basis of protective immunity is the ability to distinguish between self and non-self antigens. This distinguishing ability is developed during the fetal growth. The main lymphoid organ thymus "educates" the fetal thymic lymphocytes those that enters the periphery (Laurel 1980). Naive immature thymic lymphocytes must come into contact with thymic epithelial cells in order to distinguish self from non-self. These cells significantly express the MHC antigens II and I in addition to variety of tissue antigens. The immature T cells are being "tested" for its ability to bind to self-MHC antigens. Those who are not bound at all are eliminated after being exposed to apoptotic induction. Similarly, those cells who bind too strongly are disposed off. The T cells are retained with the ability to recognize MHC of themselves, but not to bind strongly enough to produce a cytotoxic event (Beata and Katherine 2011).

Immune-mediated disease occurs in the normal system when the aforementioned process fails. Most of the challenging diseases in veterinary dermatology are immune-mediated diseases.

14.2 Cellular Components of the Skin

14.2.1 Keratinocytes

The majority of the cells in epidermis are keratinocytes. They serve as the first line of innate immune defense against pathogens of skin. They express pattern-recognition receptors (PRRs) called Toll-like receptors (TLRs), which recognize conserved molecules on pathogens and stimulate an inflammatory response.

Keratinocytes produce significant amounts of antimicrobial peptides (AMPs) and small cationic and amphipathic molecules together with neutrophils and epithelial cells (Harder et al. 1997; Matejuk et al. 2010). Keratinocytes produce AMPs called defensins and cathelicidins as a component of a highly conserved eukaryotic cell defense mechanism. To prevent the invasion of microorganisms, the injured epithelium expresses AMPs that kills bacteria, activate immune cells, and alter the cytokine profiles (Gilliet and Lande 2008). Keratinocytes produce cytokines such as IL-1, IL-6, IL-10, IL-17, IL-18, IL-22, and tumor necrosis factor-alpha (TNF-alpha). During an infection, IL-17 and IL-22 can stimulate keratinocytes to produce AMPs, which are constituent of an innate immune response. Under healthy physiological conditions, keratinocytes secrete IL-1 and activate biologically inactive form of IL-1. After inflammasomes have been activated in response to UV exposure, the IL-1 is released. The IL-1 appears to be involved in the induction of inflammatory lesions in psoriasis with neutrophils infiltration into the epidermis by increasing the expression of chemokine (C-C motif) ligand 20 (CCL20) by keratinocytes.

The expression of abnormal AMPs plays a role in the development of inflammatory skin diseases and increased susceptibility to microbial infections. Deficient function of some AMPs, including cathelicidin and β-defensins, may contribute to the development of atopic dermatitis lesions (Wollenberg et al. 2011). In atopic dermatitis, decreased AMP expression results in increased the risk of skin infections, whereas high AMP expression is seen in psoriatic lesions (De Jongh et al. 2005; Ong et al. 2002).

Keratinocytes can differentiate between the normal microbiota and potentially pathogenic agents and can identify the highly conserved pathogen-associated molecular pattern (PAMP) structures (Quaresma 2019a, b). PAMP-binding molecules are known as PPRs, which include TLRs (Lai and Gallo 2008). Binding of PAMPs results in activation of TLR pathways leads to a cascade of innate and adaptive immune responses. Epidermal keratinocytes are expressed by various TLRs and found on the surface of the keratinocytes (TLR1, TLR2, TLR4, TLR5, and TLR6) and endosomes (TLR3 and TLR9). Further, TLR3 activation by double-stranded RNA molecules involved in immunological responses to viruses can result in the expression of TLR7 (Lai and Gallo 2008).

14.2.2 Melanocytes

Melanocytes produce melanin, a pigment responsible for skin color and protects keratinocytes from harmful effects of UV radiation, which can cause DNA damage. Melanocytes are derived from the neural crest and can regulate the local immunological responses, including innate and adaptive immune responses, as well as increase the phagocytosis of pathogenic bacteria and the production of cytokines including IL-1, IL-6, TNF-alpha, and chemokines. During the pathophysiology of autoimmune diseases like vitiligo, melanocytes express MHC class II and perhaps other molecules recognized by cytotoxic T cells (Quaresma 2019a, b). Various studies have shown that activity of skin melanocytes can be impaired by infectious viruses like alphavirus, contagious ecthyma, sheeppox virus, goatpox virus, lumpy skin disease virus (Figs. 14.1 and 14.2), papillomavirus, foot-and-mouth disease virus, vesicular stomatitis virus, herpesvirus, varicella-zoster virus, parvovirus, and bacteria like *Mycobacterium leprae* and *Leptospira*. (Table 14.2) (Gasque and Jaffar-Bandjee 2015; Tsao et al. 2017).

14.2.3 Langerhans Cell

Langerhans cells (LCs) are one of the main cellular components involved in the innate and adaptive immune responses (Clausen and Kel 2010). The LCs are macrophage/dendritic cell (DC) family members that reside in the epidermis and create a dense network to interact with invading microorganisms. The LCs are specialized in "sensing" the environment, extending the dendritic processes to surveillance at the stratum corneum, the outermost layer of the skin through intercellular tight junctions (Kubo et al. 2009). They recognize the microenvironment, in which they encounter foreign antigens and, as a result, activate the appropriate level of immune responses. Under safe circumstances, LCs selectively encourage the activation and proliferation of skin-resident regulatory T cells (Seneschal et al. 2012; Van der Aar et al. 2013). In contrast, when LC is disrupted by "sensing"

14.2 Cellular Components of the Skin

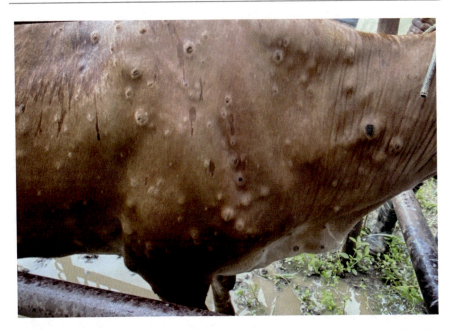

Fig. 14.1 Skin nodules in cattle caused by lumpy skin disease virus: Eruption of generalized firm, flat topped and circumscribed papules and nodules of variable sizes (0.5–5.0 cm size) in the skin all over the body

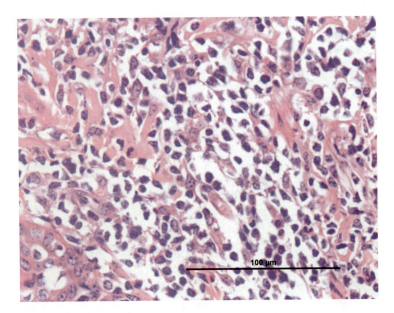

Fig. 14.2 Lumpy skin disease virus (LSDV) infected skin: Severe infiltration of mononuclear cells especially dendritic cells, lymphocytes and macrophages in dermis. H&E, ×400

Table 14.2 Most common viral infections of the skin in domestic animals

Diseases	Virus	Species affected
Contagious ecthyma	Parapoxvirus	Sheep, goats, cattle, and rarely dogs
Papular stomatitis		Cattle
Pseudocowpox (zoonotic)		Milking cows
Cowpox	Orthopoxvirus	Many species including cats and rarely dogs
Molluscum contagiosum	Molluscipoxvirus	Horses and rarely dogs
Sheeppox	Capripoxvirus	Sheep
Goatpox		Goat
Lumpy skin disease		Cattle
Swinepox	Suipoxvirus	Pigs
Ulcerative dermatosis of sheep	Unclassified poxvirus	Sheep
Granulomatous dermatitis	Equine herpesvirus 2	Horse
Pustular dermatitis of face	Equine herpesvirus 5	Horse
Bovine ulcerative mammillitis (bovine herpes mammillitis)	Bovine herpesvirus 2 (Dermatotropic)	Cattle
Pseudo-lumpy skin disease		Cattle
Bovine herpes mammary pustular dermatitis	Bovine herpesvirus 4 (Dermatotropic)	Cattle
Malignant catarrhal fever	Ovine herpesvirus 2	Cattle
Feline herpesvirus dermatitis	Feline herpesvirus 1	Cats
Papilloma (wart)	Papillomavirus	All species
Viral plaques		Horse, dog, and cat
Bowenoid in situ carcinoma (multicentric carcinoma in situ/Bowen's disease)		Cat and less in dog
In situ and invasive squamous cell carcinoma		Horse, dog, and cat
Fibropapilloma		Cattle
Sarcoid (fibropapilloma)		Horse and cat
Foot-and-mouth disease	Picornavirus	Ruminants and pigs
Swine vesicular disease		Pigs
Vesicular stomatitis	Rhabdovirus	Horses, cattle, and pigs
Vesicular exanthema	Calicivirus	Pigs
Feline calicivirus		Cats
Porcine parvovirus	Parvovirus	Piglets
Canine parvovirus 2		Puppies
Feline leukemia virus	Retrovirus	Cats
Feline immunodeficiency virus		Cats
Feline infectious peritonitis with rare concurrent dermatitis	Coronavirus (mutated)	Cats

danger in the form of microbial antigens, they quickly stimulate the innate antimicrobial defenses together with the epidermal keratinocytes, but crucially, they also activate the potent and specific adaptive response T-cell components (Seneschal et al. 2012; Polak et al. 2012; Klechevsky et al. 2008).

14.2.4 Macrophage

Macrophages are mononuclear phagocytes and are well known professional antigen-presenting cells because of their ability to present T-cells with antigen; however, macrophages do not have the ability to initiate primary immune responses (Steinman 1991; Hart 1997; Banchereau and Steinman 1998). The biological functions of activated macrophages are migration to sites of inflammation to encounter the pathogens and degrade them (Mosser and Handman 1992). Activated macrophages do not exhibit enhanced phagocytosis compared to resting cells, but they do have a markedly increased capacity to kill and destroy intracellular microorganisms through the production of toxic intermediates like nitric oxide (NO) and reactive oxygen intermediates (ROI). By binding PRRs like TLRs with microbial PAMPs, macrophages become activated. This process involves the production of pro-inflammatory cytokines in the classically activated macrophages, which triggers the production of inflammatory cytokines by T cells, which in turn acts on the macrophages to increase cytokine secretion, antigen presentation, and bactericidal activity (Trinchieri 1995; Raupach and Kaufmann 2001).

14.2.5 Mast Cells

One of the most numerous cell populations in the skin are mast cells, which express complement C5a (CD88) receptors (Kabashima et al. 2018). The position of mast cells in the dermis, their ability to release vasoactive and pro-inflammatory compounds, and the expression of IgE receptors on their surfaces suggest that mast cells play essential role in immune functions of the skin against infectious or harmful agents. Mast cells probably play a role in the mechanisms of fibroblast proliferation, blood flow regulation, and angiogenesis. These activities contribute to the remodeling of the extracellular matrix, cicatricial (scarring), and fibrotic processes associated with skin lesions (Quaresma 2019a, b).

14.3 Mechanism Regulating Immune-Mediated Skin Injury

The range of responses of the skin to injury is relatively limited regardless of the specific mechanism underlying the insult. An inflammatory and proliferative response is stimulated when the skin is exposed to irritants such xenobiotics, pathogenic agents, and ultraviolet (UV) radiation that might damage or disrupt defense barrier in an effort to restore this crucial defense function (Danilenko

2016). One of the primary functions of the skin is to serve as a physical and physiological protective barrier against the external injury and to prevent loss of water and solutes from the body. The epidermal keratinocytes and dendritic cells, including Langerhans cells, are crucial to the response to injurious stimuli in skin, particularly epidermis (Nickoloff 2006; Nestle et al. 2009).

Epidermal keratinocytes can recognize PAMPs of microbial origin and molecular risk-associated patterns, specifically damage-associated molecular patterns (DAMPs), such as xenobiotics and other irritants on their surface through TLRs, including TLR1, TLR2, TLR4, TLR5 and TLR6; whereas, TLR3 and TLR9 in their endosomes, and/or NLRs, thus trigger an inflammatory cascade and pro-inflammatory signaling pathways leading to secretion of antimicrobial peptides such as β-defensins, cathelicidins, and S100 family proteins; pro-inflammatory chemokines such as interleukin-8 (IL-8), CXCL1, CXCL9, CXCL10, CXCL11, CCL27, and CCL20; and pro-inflammatory cytokines such as IL-1β, tumor necrosis factor-α (TNF-α), IL-6, and IL-18. These chemokines and cytokines derived from keratinocytes further recruit and activate dendritic cells (DCs) and other leukocytes to produce additional cytokines and chemokines, such as interferon (IFN)-α from plasmacytoid DCs (pDCs) and dermal DCs produce IL-12 and IL-23, which further recruit and activate T lymphocytes of the Th1 lineage especially, the Th17/Th22 lineage to release pro-inflammatory cytokines such as IFN-γ, IL-17, and IL-22, thus converting the initial innate immune responses to an adaptive immune responses (Nestle et al. 2009).

The cytoplasmic PAMPs, DAMPs, and UV radiation are recognized by the nucleotide-binding domain, leucine-rich repeat-containing (NLR) proteins that are expressed by keratinocytes. NLRs initiate a pro-inflammatory signaling pathway through a large multiprotein complex called an inflammasome formed by an NLR, an adaptor protein called apoptosis-associated speck-like protein containing a caspase recruitment domain and procaspase 1 (Nestle et al. 2009). Caspase-1 is activated by inflammasome assembly, which in turn cleaves pro-IL-1β into active IL-1β.

14.4 Allergic Contact Dermatitis

Allergic contact dermatitis (ACD) is a type 4 or delayed-type hypersensitivity response (DTH) by the immune system of an individual to a small molecule (less than 500 daltons) or hapten (Luckett-Chastain et al. 2018). The interaction of the allergen with the skin initiates the pathophysiology of allergic contact dermatitis. Langerhans cells engulf the allergens when they enter into the stratum corneum (Simonsen et al. 2018). The antigens are then processed by Langerhans cells, and display them on their surface. Langerhans cells migrate to regional lymph nodes as part of the normal immunity of the body. The neighboring T lymphocytes are contact with the engulfed antigens by the Langerhans cells (Ameri et al. 2019). The processes of clonal expansion and cytokine-induced proliferation result in the development of antigen-specific T cells. Such lymphocytes can then enter the epidermis through the blood. This process is known as 'sensitization phase' of allergic contact dermatitis (Bil et al. 2018). After the antigen has been re-exposed again, the 'elicitation phase' occurs. The proliferation process is induced by cytokines when the antigen-containing Langerhans cells associate with the antigen-specific T lymphocytes. In turn, this proliferation process causes a localized inflammatory reaction.

It was observed that some dairy cattle have developed severe dermatitis that was suspected to have been caused by calcium cyanamide, which was added on the floor of the cattle shed to prevent environmental mastitis (Onda et al. 2008). Further, *Escherichia coli* can be drastically reduced by adding calcium cyanamide to a mixture of manure and sawdust (Minato et al. 2001).

14.5 Pemphigus Foliaceus

The most common autoimmune skin condition that affects dogs and cats is pemphigus foliaceus (PF). The epidermis below the stratum granulosum develops crusted spots and pustules as a result of the adverse immune response against desmosomes (Table 14.3). The keratinocytes lose their cellular anchors and develop into rounded acantholytic cells due to the action of specific antidesmoglein 1 antibodies. Among the desmosomal antigens reported, most commonly targeted antigen is desmoglein 1 (Rosenkrantz 2004).

Initially, the crusts and sometimes obvious pustules appear on the nose, periocular skin, and muzzle. The pustules frequently have a broad, irregular edges, and prominent peripheral erythema. The ears are commonly affected and the footpads can be affected by hyperkeratosis and caudal pad crusting in the dogs (Shaw 2013).

14.6 Vitiligo

Vitiligo is an acquired cutaneous disease, which is characterized by patchy depigmentation of the affected skin and progressive loss of melanocytes (Alikhan et al. 2011). It has been reported in brown and dark-skinned buffaloes (Cockrill 1981). Although the exact pathophysiology is yet unknown, it is thought that environmental, immunological, genetic, and neurological factors play a significant role in the etiology. Tyrosinase activity is reduced, as a result, decreased conversion of tyrosine to melanin results in abnormal hair pigmentation (Mude and SyaamaSundar 2009). Affected animals show depigmented lesions on their face, muzzle, limbs, and dorsal and ventral surfaces of the body (Singh et al. 2016). Serum biochemical study revealed that blood copper levels in the affected animals with vitiligo are lower than the normal. Since copper is a integral part of the enzyme tyrosinase, which converts tyrosine to melanin (Lerner and Fitzpatrick 1950). In livestock, copper deficiency is very common (Kachhawaha 2003). In the copper deficient areas, there is low blood levels of copper due to intake of copper-deficient forages and color coat of these animals is affected (Radostits et al. 2000).

Table 14.3 Clinical distribution of lesions in different types of immune-mediated dermatitis in domestic animals

Disorder	Species	Clinical distribution	Location of vesicles or bullae	Antigens	Relative prevalence
Pemphigus foliaceus (PF)[a]	Horse, goat, dog, cat	Skin	Subcorneal	**Dog:** Dsc 1 and Dsg 1	Common, but rare in goat
PF subtype (panepidermal pustular pemphigus)[a]	Dog	Skin, especially facial	Panepidermal	Not defined immunologically	Uncommon
Pemphigus vulgaris (PV)[a]	Horse, dog, cat	Mucosal or mucocutaneous types	Suprabasilar	**Dog:** Dsg 3 (mucosal) **Horse:** Dsg 3 and likely Dsg 1 (mucocutaneous)	Rare
Paraneoplastic pemphigus (PNP)[a]	Dog, cat	Oral, skin, mucocutaneous	Suprabasilar	Dsg 3, envoplakin, periplakin, desmoplakins	Rare, one putative case reported in cat
Acquired junctional epidermolysis Bullosa (AJEB)[b]	Dog	Oral, skin	Lower lamina lucida	Laminin-332	Rare
Bullous pemphigoid (BP)[b]	Horse, pig, dog, cat	Skin, mucosae, mucocutaneous, **Pigs:** Skin only	Upper lamina lucida	Collagen XVII	Rare, but seen in multiple species
Bullous subtype of systemic lupus erythematosus[b]	Dog	Oral, skin, mucocutaneous	Sublamina densa in anchoring fibrils	Collagen VII and nuclear antigens	Bullous subtype rare
Epidermolysis bullosa acquisita (EBA)[b]	Dog	Oral, mucocutaneous junctions, skin, areas of trauma	Sublamina densa in anchoring fibrils	Collagen VII	Rare, but one of the most common AISBDs in dogs
Linear IgA bullous dermatosis (LAD)[b]	Dog	Oral, skin of face and extremities	Upper lamina lucida	Processed extracellular form of collagen XVII	Rare
Mixed AISBD[b]	Dog	Skin and mucosae		Collagen VII Laminin-332	Rare

			Sublamina densa and/or lower lamina lucida		
Mucous membrane pemphigoid (MMP)[b]	Dog, cat	Mostly mucosae, mucocutaneous junctions	Lamina lucida	**Dog and cat:** Collagen XVII Laminin-332 **Dog:** BPAG 1	Rare, but one of the more common AISBDs in dogs

[a]Vesicles or bullae form within the epidermis or mucosal epithelium; *Dsc 1* desmocollin 1, *Dsg 1* desmoglein 1
[b]Vesicles or bullae form below the epidermis or mucosal epithelium; *AISBD* autoimmune subepidermal bullous dermatosis, *BPAG 1* bullous pemphigoid antigen 1

14.7 Canine Atopic Dermatitis (CAD)

Canine atopy is a hypersensitivity reaction against environmental antigens (allergens) that are inhaled or cutaneously absorbed by the genetically predisposed individuals. The main causes of CAD include molds, weeds, and pollen grains. Depending on the allergens involved, the initial characteristic sign of CAD is pruritus, which may manifest as scratching, rubbing, chewing, excessive grooming or licking, scooting, and head shaking. Pollen is one of the examples of a seasonal cause of pruritus, whereas dust mites and certain foods are the examples of a non-seasonal cause of pruritus (Zur et al. 2002). The IgE antibodies are mostly associated with the environmental (Halliwell 2006). Canine atopy has no specific pathognomonic signs that makes not possible to make a definitive diagnosis at the initial owner interview and clinical examination (Deboer and Hillier 2001). It has been proposed that canine atopic dermatitis serves as an animal model for human atopic dermatitis since its clinical, immunological, histological, and pathological features in humans are comparable to the canine counterpart (Mineshige et al. 2018).

14.8 Flea Allergy Dermatitis (FAD)

Flea allergy dermatitis is one of the common skin diseases in dogs and cats that are sensitized to flea bites. The dog flea (*Ctenocephalides canis*) and cat flea (*Ctenocephalides felis*), causes FAD in those dogs (Fig. 14.3) and cats allergic to flea saliva. Allergic patients will manifest in four typical patterns of cutaneous signs, including excoriation, self-induced alopecia, miliary dermatitis, and eosinophilic lesions in the head and neck (Hobi et al. 2011).

Flea allergy dermatitis is the hypersensitivity most often diagnosed in cats (Miller et al. 2013). Flea allergy dermatitis is typically observed in regions of the world, where fleas are prevalent and find the ideal environment in which they proliferate at low altitudes of geographical location with a temperatures of around 23 °C and a relative humidity of 78% (Reedy et al. 1999). Flea allergy dermatitis can occur in animals of any age group, while clinical signs can occur in animals of less than 6 months of age (Halliwell and Gorman 1989). Most common age of onset is 3 to 5 years (Scott et al. 2001). There is no predilection for sex or breed, although one study revealed a predisposition for certain breeds like Chow Chow, Labrit, Pyrenean Shepherd dogs, Setters, Fox-terriers, Beijing, and Spaniels (Carlotti and Costargent 1992).

The pupal stage of the *Hypoderma bovis* (warble fly) infection in cattle may rupture during its physical removal from the back of the animal, resulting in anaphylaxis. The rupture of pupal stage results in release of coelom fluid in the sensitized animal, which may cause acute reaction and occasionally death of animal. Biting of certain insects, such as black flies (*Simulium* spp.) and midges (*Culicoides* spp.), can cause allergic dermatitis, also known as Gulf coast itch, Queensland itch, or sweet itch. Further, helminth parasite infections like *Fasciola hepatica* can cause the production of IgE, which is responsible for allergy and anaphylactic reactions

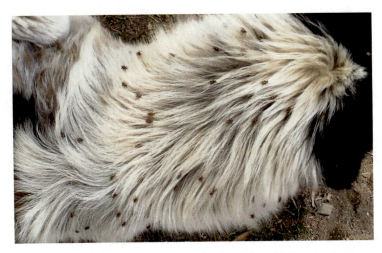

Fig. 14.3 Flea allergy dermatitis in dog: Severe infection of dog with *Ctenocephalides canis* (dog flea) in the neck and head region

(Chauhan and Joshi 2012). Sarcoptic mange is caused by a parasitic mite (*Sarcoptes scabiei*) that burrows just beneath the surface of the skin. Sarcoptes scabiei var canis infestation is a highly contagious disease of dogs that occurs worldwide. Female mites burrow into the stratum corneum to lay their eggs. Sarcoptic mange is readily transmissible between dogs by direct contact or indirect contact through combs, brushes etc. Intense pruritus is characteristic due to hypersensitivity to mite products. Primary lesions consist of papulo-crustous eruptions with thick, yellow crusts, excoriation, erythema, and alopecia. Secondary bacterial and yeast infections may develop. Typically, lesions develop on the ventral abdomen, chest, ears, elbows, and hocks. Infiltration of inflammatory cells, predominantly eosinophils and few neutrophils and mononuclear cells around the mite lesions (Fig. 14.4).

14.9 Chediak-Higashi Syndrome

Chediak-higashi syndrome (CHS) is a rare inherited disease has been reported in Hereford cattle and Japanese black heifers (Padgett et al. 1964). The disease is characterized by oculo-cutaneous albinism (decrease in melanin pigment of skin, hair, and eyes), photophobia, tendency to bleed, and increased susceptibility to infection. Bleeding diathesis is the main symptom due to defect in platelet aggregation (Shiraishi et al. 2002). In this syndrome, phagocytic cells including neutrophils, monocytes, and eosinophils have enlarged cytoplasmic granules. These large granular phagocytic cells become fragile and rupture result in tissue injury. Further, these cells exhibit defective motility, chemotaxis, and intracellular killing. The diagnosis can be made by the blood smear examination looking for large melanin granules in phagocytic cells or by examination of hair shafts for enlarged melanin granules.

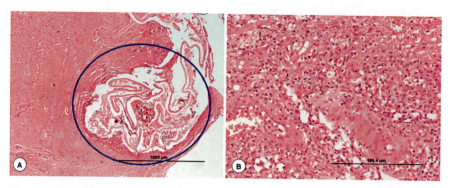

Fig. 14.4 Sarcoptic mange (canine scabies) in dogs. (**a**) Sarcoptic mange is caused by burrowing mite *Sarcoptes scabiei* var *canis* infestation and eggs in the upper dermis. H&E ×40. (**b**) Infiltration of inflammatory cells, predominantly eosinophils and few neutrophils and mononuclear cells in the upper dermis. H&E ×200

14.10 Discoid Lupus Erythematosus (DLE)

It is a common problem mainly affecting the nose in dogs. Unlike systemic lupus, DLE condition is solely cutaneous disease and affects the basal layer of the epidermis. It has many similarities with mucocutaneous pyoderma (MCP) both clinically and histopathologically, which makes a confusion and difficulty in diagnosis (Wiemelt et al. 2004). Breed predisposition had been identified in overrepresented collies; however, this condition typically affects older dogs. The etiology of the disease is probably UV exposure. The most typical early symptom is depigmentation around the nares, which is followed by the loss of the cobblestone pattern in the nasal leather and the appearance of ulceration and secondary scales. In advanced cases, the periocular skin, genital skin, and footpads may be affected, but this is rare.

The diagnosis can be made on the basis of typical histopathological findings and the typical clinical signs. In this case, an antibiotic pretreatment is required before a biopsy is carried out. However, some cases of cutaneous lupus erythematosus (CLE) respond only partially to antibiotics. Basal cell death and interface dermatitis should be seen on biopsy (Shaw 2013).

14.11 Conclusion

Immune-mediated diseases are large group of disorders with the common feature that they are caused by immune system dysfunctions. They can be broadly divided into autoimmune, hypersensitivity, and immunodeficiency diseases. The skin is a complex organ that acts as an arena for a wide variety of inflammatory processes, including immunity against infection, tumor immunity, autoimmunity, and allergies, in addition to acting as a strong barrier against external attacks. A number of cells works together to build a functional immune responses that are triggered by resident populations and develop by recruitment of additional cell populations into the skin. In addition to providing a passive physical barrier against infection, the skin also contains elements of innate and adaptive immune systems, which are activated when the tissue undergoes attack by invading pathogens. Any immune system disruption / defects can lead to immunological skin diseases in animals such as allergic contact dermatitis, pemphigus foliaceus, vitiligo, canine atopic dermatitis, flea allergy dermatitis, Chediak-Higashi syndrome, and discoid lupus erythematosus.

References

Alikhan A, Felsten LM, Daly M, Petronic-Rosic V (2011) Vitiligo: a comprehensive overview part I. introduction, epidemiology, quality of life, diagnosis, differential diagnosis, associations, histopathology, etiology, and work-up. J Am Acad Dermatol 65(3):473–491

Ameri AH, Moradi Tuchayi S, Zaalberg A, Park JH, Ngo KH, Li T, Lopez E, Colonna M, Lee RT, Mino-Kenudson M, Demehri S (2019) IL-33/regulatory T cell axis triggers the development of a tumor-promoting immune environment in chronic inflammation. Proc Natl Acad Sci U S A 116(7):2646–2651

Banchereau J, Steinman RM (1998) Dendritic cells and the control of immunity. Nature 392:245–252

Beata U, Katherine B (2011) Major histocompatibility complex (MHC) markers in conservation biology. Int J Mol Sci 12(8):5168–5186

Bil W, Van der Bent SAS, Spiekstra SW, Nazmi K, Rustemeyer T, Gibbs S (2018) Comparison of the skin sensitization potential of 3 red and 2 black tattoo inks using interleukin-18 as a biomarker in a reconstructed human skin model. Contact Dermatitis 79(6):336–345

Bos JD, Kapsenberg ML (1986) The skin immune-system—its cellular constituents and their interactions. Immunol Today 7(7–8):235–240

Carlotti DN, Costargent F (1992) Statistical analysis of positive skin tests in 449 dogs with allergic dermatitis. Eur J Companion Anim Pract 4:42–59

Chauhan RS, Joshi A (2012) Immunology for beginners. Kapish Prakashan, Gurgaon, Haryana

Clausen BE, Kel JM (2010) Langerhans cells: critical regulators of skin immunity. Immunol Cell Biol 88(4):351–360

Cockrill WR (1981) The water buffalo: a review. Br Vet J 137(1):8–16

Danilenko DM (2016) An overview of the pathogenesis of immune-mediated skin injury. Toxicol Pathol 44(4):536–544

De Jongh GJ, Zeeuwen PL, Kucharekova M (2005) High expression levels of keratinocyte antimicrobial proteins in psoriasis compared with atopic dermatitis. J Investig Dermatol 125: 1163–1173

Deboer DJ, Hillier A (2001) The ACVD task force on canine atopic dermatitis (XV), fundamental concepts in clinical diagnosis. Vet Immunol Immunopathol 81:6–271

Gasque P, Jaffar-Bandjee MC (2015) The immunology and inflammatory responses of human melanocytes in infectious diseases. J Infect 71(4):413–421

Gilliet M, Lande R (2008) Antimicrobial peptides and self-DNA in autoimmune skin inflammation. Curr Opin Immunol 20:401–407

Halliwell R (2006) Revised nomenclature for veterinary allergy. Vet Immunol Immunopathol 114: 8–207

Halliwell REW, Gorman NT (1989) Veterinary clinical immunology. W.B. Saunders, Philadelphia, PA

Harder J, Bartels J, Christophers E, Schröder JM (1997) A peptide antibiotic from human skin. Nature 387:861

Hart DN (1997) Dendritic cells: unique leukocyte populations which control the primary immune response. Blood 90:3245–3287

Hobi S, Linek M, Marignac G, Olivry T, Beco L, Nett C, Fontaine J, Roosje P, Bergvall K, Belova S (2011) Clinical characteristics and causes of pruritus in cats. A multicenter study on feline hypersensitivity associated dermatoses. J Vet Dermatol 22:406–413

Kabashima K, Nakashima C, Nonomura Y, Otsuka A, Cardamone C, Parente R, De Feo G, Triggiani M (2018) Biomarkers for evaluation of mast cell and basophil activation. Immunol Rev 282:114–120

Kachhawaha S (2003) Copper deficiency in Buffalo calves. Intas Polivet 4(2):238–239

Klechevsky E, Morita R, Liu M, Cao Y, Coquery S, Thompson-Snipes L (2008) 2008. Functional specializations of human epidermal Langerhans cells and CD14+ dermal dendritic cells. Immunity 29(3):497–510

Kubo A, Nagao K, Yokouchi M, Sasaki H, Amagai M (2009) External antigen uptake by Langerhans cells with reorganization of epidermal tight junction barriers. J Exp Med 206(13):2937–2946

Lai Y, Gallo RL (2008) Toll-like receptors in skin infections and inflammatory diseases. Infect Disord Drug Targets 8:144–155

Laurel JG (1980) Common canine autoimmune disorders, 3rd edn. National Academic Press, Washington DC, pp 216–219

Lerner AB, Fitzpatrick TB (1950) Biochemistry of melanin. Physiol Rev 30(1):91–126

Luckett-Chastain LR, Gipson JR, Gillaspy AF, Gallucci RM (2018) Transcriptional profiling of irritant contact dermatitis (ICD) in a mouse model identifies specific patterns of gene expression and immune-regulation. Toxicology 410:1–9

Matejuk A (2017) Skin immunity. Arch Immunol Ther Exp 66(1):45–54

Matejuk A, Leng Q, Begum MD (2010) Peptide-based antifungal therapies against emerging infections. Drugs Future 35:197

Miller WH, Griffin CE, Campbell KL (2013) Hypersensitivity disorders, Muller and Kirks small animal dermatology. Elsevier, St. Louis

Minato K, Tamura T, Maeta Y (2001) The effect of sterilisation on *Escherichia coli* in cattle manure by adding nitrolime. Bull Hokkaido Anim Res Cent 24:21–22

Mineshige T, Kamiie J, Sugahara G, Shirota K (2018) A study on periostin involvement in the pathophysiology of canine atopic skin. J Vet Med Sci 80:11–103

Mosser DM, Handman E (1992) Treatment of murine macrophages with interferon-gamma inhibits their ability to bind leishmania promastigotes. J Leukoc Biol 52:369–376

Mude S, SyaamaSundar N (2009) Vitiligo in buffaloes. Vet World 2(7):282

Nestle FO, Di Meglio P, Qin JZ, Nickoloff BJ (2009) Skin immune sentinels in health and disease. Nat Rev Immunol 9:679–691

Nickoloff BJ (2006) Keratinocytes regain momentum as instigators of cutaneous inflammation. Trends Mol Med 12:102–106

Onda K, Yagisawa T, Matsui T, Tanaka H, Yako J, Une Y, Wada Y (2008) Contact dermatitis in dairy cattle caused by calcium cyanamide. Vet Rec 163(14):418–422

Ong PY, Ohtake T, Brandt C (2002) Endogenous antimicrobial peptides and skin infections in atopic dermatitis. N Engl J Med 347:1151–1160

Padgett GA, Leader RW, Gorham JR, Omarry CC (1964) The familial occurrence of the Chediak-Higashi syndrome in mink and cattle. Genetics 49(3):505

Polak ME, Newell L, Taraban VY, Pickard C, Healy E, Friedmann PS (2012) CD70-CD27 interaction augments CD8+ T-cell activation by human epidermal Langerhans cells. J Investig Dermatol 132(6):1636–1644

Quaresma JAS (2019a) Organization of the skin immune system and compartmentalized immune responses in infectious diseases. Clin Microbiol Rev 32:e00034–e00018

Quaresma JAS (2019b) Skin immune system and infectious diseases. Clin Microbiol Rev 32(4):e00034–e00018

Radostits OM, Gay CC, Blood DC, Hinchcliff KW (2000) Textbook of the diseases of cattle, sheep, pigs, goats and horses, 9th edn. Elsevier, Amsterdam, pp 1487–1499

Raupach B, Kaufmann SH (2001) Immune responses to intracellular bacteria. Curr Opin Immunol 13:417–428

Reedy LH, Miller WH, Willemse T (1999) Arthropod hypersensitivity disorders. Allergic skin disease of dogs and cats. WB Saunders, Philadelphia, PA

Rosenkrantz WS (2004) Pemphigus: current therapy. Vet Dermatol 15:90–98

Scott DW, Miller WH, Griffin CE (2001) Muller and kirks small animal dermatology. WB Saunders, Philadelphia, PA

Seneschal J, Clark RA, Gehad A, Baecher-Allan CM, Kupper TS (2012) Human epidermal Langerhans cells maintain immune homeostasis in skin by activating skin resident regulatory T cells. Immunity 36(5):873–884

Shaw S (2013) Immune-mediated skin disease in the dog and cat. Companion Anim 18(7):322–326

Shiraishi M, Ogawah H, Ikeda M, Kawashima S, Ito K (2002) Platelet dysfunction in Chediak-Higashi syndrome-affected cattle. J Vet Med Sci 64(9):751–760

Simonsen AB, Foss-Skiftesvik MH, Thyssen JP, Deleuran M, Mortz CG, Zachariae C, Skov L, Osterballe M, Funding A, Avnstorp C, Andersen BL, Vissing S, Danielsen A, Dufour N, Nielsen NH, Thormann H, Sommerlund M, Johansen JD (2018) Contact allergy in Danish children: current trends. Contact Dermatitis 79(5):295–302

Singh VP, Motiani RK, Singh A, Malik G, Aggarwal R, Pratap K, Mohan R (2016) Water buffalo (*Bubalus bubalis*) as a spontaneous animal model of vitiligo. Pigment Cell Melanoma Res 29(4):465–469

Steinman RM (1991) The dendritic cell system and its role in immunogenicity. Annu Rev. Immunol 9:271–296

Trinchieri G (1995) Interleukin-12: a proinflammatory cytokine with immunoregulatory functions that bridge innate resistance and antigen-specific. Annu Rev Immunol 13:251–276

Tsao H, Fukunaga-Kalabis M, Herlyn M (2017) Recent advances in melanoma and melanocyte biology. J Invest Dermatol 137(3):557–560

Van der Aar AM, Picavet DI, Muller FJ, de Boer L, van Capel TM, Zaat SA (2013) Langerhans cells favor skin flora tolerance through limited presentation of bacterial antigens and induction of regulatory T cells. J Investig Dermatol 133(5):1240–1249

Wiemelt SP, Goldschmidt MH, Greek JS (2004) A retrospective study comparing the histopathological features and response to treatment in two canine nasal dermatoses, DLE and MCP. Veterinary Dermatol 15(6):341–348

Wollenberg A, Rawer HC, Schauber J (2011) Innate immunity in atopic dermatitis. Clin Rev. Allergy Immunol 41:272–281

Yuxiao H, Hong-Duo C, Xing-Hua G (2014) Immunological skin diseases: boundaries and relationships. Global Dermatol 1(1):3–5

Zur G, Ihrke PJ, White SD, Kass PH (2002) Canine atopic dermatitis: a retrospective study of 266 cases examined at the University of California, Davis, 1992-1998. Part I. clinical features and allergy testing results. J Vet Dermatol 13:89–102

Immunological Interventions for the Management of Coronavirus Disease 2019 (COVID-19)

Key Points

1. COVID-19 is caused by the emerging coronavirus known as severe acute respiratory syndrome coronavirus-2 (SARS-CoV-2) which belongs to the family *Coronaviridae* under the order *Nidovirales* and genus *Betacoronavirus*.
2. Aged patients, especially those with the history of health disorders like diabetes, hypertension, cardiovascular diseases, cerebrovascular diseases, chronic respiratory diseases, chronic obstructive pulmonary diseases, hepatic diseases, cancer, chronic kidney disease, etc. are having more risk for COVID-19 infection.
3. Incubation period of COVID-19 ranges from 1 to 14 days (average 5–6 days) in most of the patients.
4. SARS-CoV-2 infects airway epithelial cells of nasal cavity, and upper respiratory tract results in cytokine storm leading to inflammatory cascade.
5. Most common initial clinical signs of COVID-19 are fever, cough, nasal congestion, fatigue, symptoms of upper respiratory tract infection, progress to severe disease with dyspnea, asthenia, thrombocytopenia, and pneumonia.
6. Cytokine storm was associated with rampant inflammation resulting in the release of proinflammatory cytokines and chemokines, namely, IL-6, IL-2, IL-8, IL-10, TNF-α, IFN-γ, IL-1β, CXCL10/IP-10, G-CSF, MCP-1, and MIP-1A in severe cases.
7. Increased level of IL-6 has been frequently observed during the SARS-CoV-2 patients.
8. Tocilizumab is an antagonist of IL-6 recombinant monoclonal antibody, which is used for the treatment of SARS-CoV-2-induced cytokine release syndrome.
9. Convalescent plasma therapy (convalescent plasma from COVID-19 recovered patients) is effective and specific for COVID-19.
10. Histopathological lesions in lungs of COVID-19 patients are diffuse alveolar damage, acute fibrinous organizing pneumonia, hyaline membranes, multinucleated giant cells, perivascular and interstitial mononuclear cells infiltrate, and severe endothelial injury.

11. Convalescent plasma therapy; antagonists of IL-6, IL-1, JAK, ACE2, and GM-CSF-R; stem cell therapy; corticosteroids; remdesivir; chloroquine; and ivermectin are commonly used for treatment of COVID-19 patients.
12. FDA approved remdesivir for use in adults and pediatric patients for the treatment of COVID-19 to prevent the severity of disease progression.

15.1 Introduction

The coronavirus disease 2019 (COVID-19) pandemic has recently created huge global health concerns and because of significant morbidity, socio-economic impact, and mortality in immune-compromised and elderly patients, WHO announced COVID-19 as a global public health emergency. The COVID-19 is caused by the emerging coronavirus known as severe acute respiratory syndrome coronavirus-2 (SARS-CoV-2). The virus was originated from Wuhan, China, in December 2019 and caused severe outbreaks in many countries within a short period of time by crossing national borders across the globe. The ongoing pandemic of COVID-19 is one of the largest global threats to humanity after the Spanish flu pandemic. The SARS-CoV-2 rapidly spread to more than 215 countries with above 600.45 million confirmed cases and nearly 6.5 million deaths as on August 2022. The SARS-CoV-2/COVID-19 has toppled the world economy owing to enormous adverse effects, along with psychological, physiological, and socio-economic pressures, as well as stress and fear of losing lives (Ayittey et al. 2020; Li et al. 2020).

Various possible efforts were made to mitigate the COVID-19 pandemic by early diagnosis and prompt clinical care of affected individuals, along with adequate prevention and control measures. Various diagnostic tests such as reverse-transcription polymerase chain reaction (RT-PCR), quantitative RT-PCR (RT-qPCR), computed tomography (CT) imaging, genome sequencing, enzyme-linked immunosorbent assay (ELISA), lateral flow immunoassay (LFIA), automated chemiluminescence immunoassay (CLIA), point-of-care (POC)/bed-side testing, isothermal LAMP-based method for COVID-19 (iLACO), multiplex assays, and interactive web-based dashboard have been developed (Dong et al. 2020; Huang et al. 2020; Vashist 2020; Yu et al. 2020; Zhang et al. 2020a; Zhu et al. 2020). Many treatment options, including antivirals, protease inhibitors, and immunotherapeutics (neutralizing/monoclonal antibodies and convalescent plasma), and other therapeutics (antimalarial and antiparasitic drugs). However, these treatment options are not giving promising results. Hence, only prevention strategies to avoid virus infection and further transmission and spread may be considered. This reflects an urgent need for combined cooperation and collaborative efforts of common people, health workers, and research wings in a coordinated manner on regional, national, and international platforms (Qian et al. 2020). Many advanced therapeutic approaches, including clustered regularly interspaced short palindromic repeats (CRISPR) and artificial intelligence (AI)-based precautionary methods, are being explored to mitigate COVID-19. A collective "One Health" approach at the global level with appropriate monitoring and surveillance systems may serve the purpose to a great extent.

15.2 Etiology

Coronaviruses (CoVs) belong to the subfamily *Orthocoronavirinae* of the family *Coronaviridae* under the order *Nidovirales* and genus *Betacoronavirus*. The CoVs are reported to cause respiratory, nervous, and enteric diseases (de Wilde et al. 2017). The CoVs are enveloped, positive-sense, poly-A tailed single-stranded positive-sense RNA viruses with a genome of 26–32 kb, and largest genomes among all known RNA viruses till date (Rabaan et al. 2020). The SARS-CoV-2 is an enveloped virus measuring approximately 50–200 nm in diameter (Xu et al. 2020). The SARS-CoV-2 genome is approximately 29.90 kb size with a nucleocapsid buried inside the phospholipid bilayers that consist of three types of proteins, namely, envelope (E) protein, membrane (M) protein, and spike glycoprotein (S) (Wu et al. 2020). The S protein of SARS-CoV-2 showed 10–20 times higher affinity to human angiotensin-converting enzyme 2 (ACE2) receptors as compared to SARS-CoV resulted in more chances of human-to-human transmission. However, SARS-CoV-2 causes low mortality rate (3.4%) when compared to SARS (9.6%) and MERS. Molecular characterization of SARS-CoV-2 revealed a new beta coronavirus that belongs to the subgenus *Sarbecovirus* (Zhu et al. 2020). Phylogenetic analysis has shown that SARS-CoV-2 shares 79.50% and 50% sequence similarity with SARS-CoV and MERS-CoV, respectively (Zhou et al. 2020). Moreover, SARS-CoV-2 shares 89%, 82%, and 96.3% nucleotide similarity with SARS-like CoV ZXC21, SARS-CoV, and bat CoV RaTG13, respectively, suggesting a zoonotic origin of the virus (Chan et al. 2020; Paraskevis et al. 2020).

The RNA-dependent RNA polymerase enzyme of coronaviruses is responsible for error-prone replication, which resulted in frequent mutations and recombinations leading to the emergence of novel viral strains. Two different prevalent types of SARS-CoV-2, L-type strain (70% prevalence) and S-type strain (30%) were existed. The L type was derived from S type and is much more aggressive and highly transmissible (Tang et al. 2020). The S type is ancestral, less aggressive, and transmissible. It has been observed that during the initial times of the COVID-19 pandemic, L type was more prevalent, especially in Wuhan, China, whose circulation wilted due to human interventions and selection pressure (Tang et al. 2020).

15.3 Transmission of COVID-19

The SARS-CoV-2 is a deadly and rapidly transmitting virus (airborne and contact transmission) capable of producing sustained outbreaks, as the virus reproduction number (R_0 value) is more than one, resulting in a high global threat and panic situation across the globe (Chatterjee et al. 2020; Thompson 2020; Zheng 2020).

Moreover, the transmission of SARS-CoV-2 through asymptomatic carriers is another big concern (Riou and Althaus 2020; Rothe et al. 2020).

15.4 Predisposing Factors

Aged patients, especially those with the history of health disorders like diabetes (16–22%), hypertension (23.7–30%), cardiovascular diseases [e.g. coronary artery disease (5.8%), heart failure, pulmonary hypertension, cardiomyopathy], cerebrovascular diseases (2.3–22%), chronic respiratory diseases, chronic obstructive pulmonary diseases, hepatic diseases, cancer, chronic kidney disease (CKD), pro-inflammatory and pro-coagulative states, smoking etc. are having more risk for COVID-19 infection. Peoples aged between 40 and 64 years are at greatest risk of infection, followed by patients with 75 years and older, and 65 to 74 years of aged people. It has been reported that patients of hypertension and diabetes are mostly provided with angiotensin-converting enzyme (ACE) inhibitors and angiotensin II receptor blockers as part of their therapy but as they upregulate the ACE-2 receptor by inhibiting ACE, so these receptors became available for the SARS-CoV-2 to bind with, in order to enter the host cells, and hence, aggravate the pathogenesis of SARS-CoV-2 in such patients.

Overweight obese patients need more respiratory efforts and assistance due to their high body mass index and hence are at more risk for acquiring COVID-19. Cardiovascular disease patients are associated with three-fold increased odds of severe infection and an 11-fold increase in overall mortality (Aggarwal et al. 2020). Patients with hypertension have a 2.27-fold increased risk of severe disease and 3.48-fold more risk of mortality than patients without hypertension (Pranata et al. 2020). Male sex (18.4%) is having more risk of infection, disease progression, severe disease, mechanical ventilation, and increased mortality than females (13.3%). It has been hypothesized that this may be due to the presence of androgens or decreased levels of SARS-CoV-2 antibodies compared with females.

People with type 1 or gestational diabetes and type II diabetes have increased risk of severe illness. (Desai et al. 2020). The SARS-CoV-2 affects the immune regulation by producing the cytokine storm, which leads to pulmonary and endothelial dysfunction and may produce hypercoagulation. These immune mechanisms make diabetic patients more prone to COVID-19. Patients with diabetes are having two-fold increased risk of developing severe disease and mortality due to elevated C-reactive protein, age, and insulin use (Kumar et al. 2020). People with type I diabetes have 3.5 times the odds of mortality due to COVID-19, while people with type II diabetes are having 2.03 times the odds (Singh and Singh 2020). Patients with chronic kidney disease are also at increased risk of severe illness. Prevalence of preexisting end-stage kidney disease was 2.3%, and chronic kidney disease was 5.2% in COVID-19 patients. The prevalence of chronic liver disease was approximately 3% in COVID-19 patients.

15.5 Clinical Manifestations

The incubation period of COVID-19 ranges from 1 to 14 days (average 5–6 days) in most of the patients, and in some patients, it ranges from 0 to 24 days. The clinical manifestations of COVID-19 usually start within a week. Based on the degree of illness, patients with COVID-19 can be divided into five categories as per the Centers for Disease Control and Prevention (CDC) guidance: (a) patients with a positive result but have no symptom of infection (asymptomatic patients), (b) patients exhibiting mild symptoms such as flu, cough, and fever but have normal respiratory rate (mild ill patients); (c) patients with lower respiratory tract symptoms and have oxygen saturation (SpO_2) of $\geq 94\%$ (moderate ill patients); (d) patients with SpO_2 of $<94\%$ and respiratory frequency of less than 30 (severely ill patients); and (e) patients with respiratory failure, septic shock, and organ failure (sick critically patients).

The initial symptoms of fever with chills, dry cough, and malaise were reported in 83–98% of patients. Sputum production was reported in about one-third of patients. Other symptoms are breathing difficulties, headache, muscle pain, abdominal pain, diarrhea, sore throat, and vomiting in a few cases. If pulmonary inflammation worsens, hypoxemia occurs, which may lead to cardiac arrest. Studies revealed that COVID-19 can cause arrhythmia, myocardial injury, acute coronary syndrome, coagulopathy, and venous thromboembolism. Elderly patients and those with underlying diseases may develop critical and severe complications such as arrhythmia, shock, acute cardiac injury, acute respiratory distress syndrome (ARDS), acute renal failure, and neurological disturbances including dizziness, headache, peripheral nerve disorders, muscle incoordination, loss of sensory traits like inability to smell and taste impairment etc. Overall, the case fatality rate was estimated to be 2–3% (Rodriguez-Morales et al. 2020), while it was as high as 8–15% in older adults.

The most common initial clinical signs of COVID-19 disease are fever, cough, nasal congestion, fatigue, symptoms of upper respiratory tract infection, progress to severe disease with dyspnea, asthenia, thrombocytopenia, and progressing to pneumonic signs in approximately 75% of patients (Rabaan et al. 2020). Pneumonia usually occurs after the second or third week of the appearance of symptoms. Prominent signs of COVID-19-induced pneumonia are decreased oxygen saturation, blood gas deviation, lung lesions like ground-glass appearance, patchy consolidation, exudates in alveoli, and interlobular involvement, which were visible through chest imaging techniques and X-rays. Recently, gastrointestinal-related symptoms were also reported. Further, asymptomatic infections, especially in young children were also frequently reported.

15.5.1 Pathology

Initially, SARS-CoV-2 infects airway epithelial cells of nasal cavity, and upper respiratory tract results in cytokine storm leading to inflammatory cascade. Infection of alveolar type II cells results in development of pulmonary infiltrates, deciliation, diffuse alveolar damage with cellular fibromyxoid exudates, fibrin-rich hyaline membranes, and a few multinucleated giant cells (Dhama et al. 2020a). Significant cytopathic effects include multinucleated syncytial cells, atypical enlarged pneumocytes, interstitial mononuclear inflammatory infiltrates, and the presence of lymphocytes in the affected lungs (Dhama et al. 2020a). Aberrant wound healing may lead to more severe scarring, fibrosis, and ARDS. Grossly, bilateral multilobular subsegmental consolidation of lungs in early stages followed by multiple mottling and ground-glass opacity (Dhama et al. 2020a). In COVID-19 patients, histopathological lesions are diffuse alveolar damage, acute fibrinous organizing pneumonia (AFOP), hyaline membranes, few multinucleated giant cells, perivascular T-cell infiltrations, and severe endothelial injury (Xu et al. 2020). Pulmonary vessels of COVID-19-affected patients showed widespread thrombosis with microangiopathy. The lungs of COVID-19 patients showed neovascularization (enhanced growth of new blood vessels) by the mechanism of intussusceptive angiogenesis (Ackerman et al. 2020).

Patients dying of COVID-19 showed histopathologic findings of macrovesicular steatosis, mild acute hepatitis (lobular necroinflammation), and mild portal inflammation (Lagana et al. 2020). Heart showed myocarditis, and kidneys showed acute tubular injury, which was due to creatinine elevation (Barton et al. 2020). Placenta of women showed higher rates of decidual arteriopathy and other maternal vascular malperfusion (Shanes et al. 2020).

15.5.2 Clinical Pathology

There are hematological, biochemical, and immunological alterations in COVID-19 patients (Dhama et al. 2020a). Clinical laboratory findings include decreased white blood cell count (lymphopenia and leukopenia) in 70% patients, thrombocytopenia and prolonged prothrombin time in 58% patients, elevated lactate dehydrogenase (LDH) in 40% of patients, increased levels of liver enzymes (ALT, AST, CPK, γ-GT, and α-HBDH), and D-dimers. Increased levels of C-reactive protein (CRP), ESR, ferritin, and procalcitonin were noticed. The cytokine storm was associated with the rampant inflammation resulting in the release of pro-inflammatory cytokines and chemokines, namely, interleukin-6 (IL-6), IL-8, and IL-10; tumor necrosis factor-α (TNF-α); and IFN-γ, IL-1β, CXCL10/IP-10, G-CSF, MCP-1, and MIP-1A, which were reported in patients with severe cases and ICU admissions, which severely damage the pulmonary tissues leading to death (Chen et al. 2020b; Huang et al. 2020; Quin et al. 2020). Bilateral patchy consolidated areas were seen on chest radiograph, and ground-glass opacities are seen on chest CT scan.

Increased expression levels of IL-6, IL-2, and DD in the serum can help in the diagnosis of the severity of adult COVID-19 patients (Gao et al. 2020a, b; Singhai 2020). Studies showed that elevated levels of D-dimer could be an important marker in initial phase of hospitalized patients to decide the prognosis of COVID-19 patients. The D-dimer has a reference value of 250 ng/mL or 0.4 μg/mL. The risk of severe disease was two-fold higher, and mortality was four-fold higher

(2.0 μg/mL) in patients with increased D-dimer levels. Patients with elevated D-dimer levels have an increased risk of thrombosis (Kermali et al. 2020). The pooled prevalence of olfactory dysfunction (hyposmia or anosmia) was 53% and gustatory dysfunction (dysgeusia or ageusia) was 44% in COVID-19 patients. The incidence of anosmia was 73% before the diagnosis of COVID-19, and 26.6% of patients showed anosmia as the initial symptom of COVID-19 (Kaye et al. 2020).

15.5.3 Diagnosis

Diagnosis of COVID-19 should be suspected in patients with any acute respiratory distress, if they have been in contact with confirmed or suspected COVID-19 cases or with the history of travel to suspected areas or residence in a location reported to have community transmission of COVID-19 in the last 14 days before onset of symptoms. Molecular techniques such as RT-PCR and RT-qPCR are used for the rapid diagnosis of COVID-19 (Zhang et al. 2020d). Various serological tests such as LFIA, ELISA, and CLIA for early and accurate detection of COVID-19 have been developed. The most commonly used biomarkers for serological tests are IgM and IgG antibodies (Vashist 2020). The COVID-19 IgM/IgG rapid test is among the most prominent rapid immunoassays, which detect IgG and IgM antibodies in only 10 min. Culture of SARS-CoV-2 and detection of SARS-CoV-2 RNA is diagnostic from nasopharyngeal specimen; however, it requires biosafety level 3 facility and takes 3 days for specific cytopathic effects.

Recently, COVID-19 antigen test kits have been developed to handle the emergency situation. These test kits detect the fragments of proteins of the virus from samples of nasal swabs. The antigen test works faster than RT-PCR; however, it is peculiar for the virus and not a sensitive test. Hence, a negative result by the antigen test should be confirmed with the RT-PCR test. Reverse transcription loop-mediated isothermal amplification (RT-LAMP) is similar to RT-PCR but uses constant temperatures and produces more viral DNA when compared to RT-PCR. The RT-LAMP is a simple, quick test, newer technology, and there is less evidence for its use.

Metabolic profile of COVID-19 patients showed increased liver transaminases, D-dimer, fibrinogen, decreased albumin, prolonged prothrombin time, altered enzymes of renal impairment, and electrolyte derangements (Kunutsor and Laukkanen 2020). The D-dimer levels are increased during severe COVID-19 disease, and it is a useful biomarker for predicting COVID-19 disease progression (Kermali et al. 2020). Diagnosis of COVID-19-induced lung lesions by CT scan showed ground-glass opacity (GGO) in lungs, consolidation, interlobular septal thickening, and crazy-paving pattern with a lower lobe involvement are the more common lesions.

15.6 Immunological Interventions for the Management of COVID-19

Being a new viral disease, no specialized therapy was available for treating COVID-19 patients, and still various clinical and subclinical trials are currently going on in search of gold-standard therapeutic protocol, which should have high therapeutic efficacy along with less adverse effects on the patients. Potent antiviral drugs, such as remdesivir, lopinavir, ribavirin (Jones et al. 2004), umifenovir (Arbidol) (Zhang et al. 2020c), ritonavir, interferons or their combination (Omrani et al. 2014), and several other drugs, have been explored for their possible usage to tackle the COVID-19 outbreak (Dhama et al. 2020c; Li and De Clercq 2020; Rabaan et al. 2020; Yavuz and Ünal 2020).

Immunological therapies become indeed important for controlling the SARS-CoV-2 infections. Increased mortality of patients created a panic situation among the public for searching the treatment of COVID-19. Vaccine needs several clearances before getting administered in the patients of SARS-CoV-2, so the alternative treatments were taken in consideration. Previous infection of SARS and MERS has given clue for the treatment of SARS-CoV-2 infection. Although COVID-19 therapy clinical trials are being conducted, the outcomes of significant randomized investigations are still pending.

15.7 Immunological Interventions

15.7.1 Convalescent Plasma Therapy

Convalescent plasma therapy (convalescent plasma from COVID-19 recovered patients) is effective and specific for COVID-19. Convalescent plasma from recovered patients has been used for the treatment of various previous disease outbreaks like avian influenza, SARS, and Ebola virus infections (Chen et al. 2020a). The convalescent plasma reduces the clinical symptoms, viral load, and mortality in critically ill COVID-19 patients (Rajendran et al. 2020). Intravenous immunoglobulin (IVIG) administration in COVID-19 patients with severe disease as an adjuvant therapy within 48 h of admission reduces the mechanical ventilation use, hospital or intensive care unit stay, and 28-day mortality (Chen et al. 2020a; Jawhara 2020). A single dose of convalescent plasma with a high concentration of neutralizing antibodies (nAbs) rapidly reduced the viral load and eventually increased the clinical outcomes of COVID-19 patients (Duan et al. 2020). Transfusion of convalescent plasma led to increase in anti-SARS-CoV-2 nAb titers, resolution of ground-glass opacities, and consolidation in COVID-19 patients (Ye et al. 2020).

The SARS-CoV-2 monoclonal antibodies have been used for the prophylaxis and treatment of COVID-19-affected patients (Marovich et al. 2020). This antibody has completed the phase 1 studies. Recombinant human monoclonal neutralizing antibodies such as JS016 and LY-COV555 are used for the treatment of COVID-19-affected patients. These antibodies bind to the SARS-CoV-2 surface spike protein receptor-binding domain, which blocks the binding of the virus to the ACE-2 host cell surface receptor. Novel multi-antibody cocktail therapies (e.g., REGN-COV2) are in clinical trials for the prophylaxis or treatment of COVID-19-affected patients.

15.7.2 Antagonists of Interleukin 6 Receptor (IL-6R) and IL-6

Increased levels of IL-6 have been frequently observed in the SARS-CoV-2 patients. The IL-6 being a key inflammatory cytokine plays a significant role in the inflammatory cytokine storm. Tocilizumab, a recombinant monoclonal human antibody, and antagonist of IL-6 has been used for the treatment of SARS-CoV-2-induced cytokine release syndrome. The drug was extensively used for autoimmune disorder like rheumatoid arthritis (Choi et al. 2018). Tocilizumab efficiently binds to membrane-bound and soluble IL-6R, which blocks IL-6 from binding to IL-6R and inhibiting signal transduction (Xu et al. 2020). Tocilizumab is a first-line medication for the treatment of cytokine release syndrome or cytokine storm (quick and enormous release of cytokines into the blood from immune cells), particularly in COVID-19 patients with co-morbidities. Tocilizumab works on the mechanism of inhibiting the JAK-STAT signaling cascade and the synthesis of downstream inflammatory chemicals by binding to the membrane and soluble versions of the IL-6 receptors (Riegler et al. 2019). Treatment of COVID-19 patients with monoclonal antibody tocilizumab caused a 45% reduction in mortality of mechanically ventilated patients (Somers et al. 2020). In addition to tocilizumab, other monoclonal antibody inhibitors of the IL-6 signaling axis are clazakizumab and olokizumab (two humanized monoclonal antibodies against IL-6), sarilumab (monoclonal antibody against IL-6R), and siltuximab have received FDA approval against IL-6 for the treatment of SARS-CoV-2 infection (Ni et al. 2021).

15.7.3 Blockade of the IL-1 Pathway

Treatment for hyperinflammation pathway is blockade of IL-1 pathway. The recombinant IL-1 receptor antagonist, Anakinra was initially developed to combat the cytokine storm and accompanying tissue damage in severe sepsis patients (Shakoory et al. 2016). Therefore, blocking the IL-1 pathway has received a lot of interest. Previously used anakinra (an IL-1 antagonist) and canakinumab (an IL-1 inhibitor) are currently being used to combat the SARS-CoV-2 infection to avoid the respiratory dysfunction (Ong et al. 2020).

15.7.4 Inhibition of Janus Kinases (JAK)

The novel idea employed in systemic autoimmune or inflammatory disorders is the inhibition of Janus kinases (JAK) by small compounds. The JAKs are involved in the signaling of type 1 and type 2 IFN receptors, IL-6 receptor, and other cytokine receptors. They regulate the phosphorylation of transcription factors from the STAT family, which in turn leads to the production of pro-inflammatory cytokines. As a result, JAK inhibitors effectively reduce the cytokine expression and may help in managing the cytokine storm (Cron and Chatham 2020). The JAK1 and JAK2 kinase activity is specifically inhibited by the small molecule drug like baricitinib, ruxolitinib, and fedratinib (Zhong et al. 2020). Rheumatoid arthritis can be treated with baricitinib, which is approved for use in combination with one or more TNF inhibitors (Taylor 2019). In addition to controlling receptor-mediated endocytosis, cyclin G-related kinases are also able to bind to baricitinib (Titanji et al. 2021). In extreme situations of COVID-19, where immune-mediated lung damage and ARDS may ensue, the immunosuppressive action of baricitinib may improve the hyperactive immunological condition (Zhong et al. 2020; Titanji et al. 2021).

15.7.5 Recombinant Soluble ACE2

A key molecule for cell invasion is ACE2 receptor and its pharmacological blockade help in controlling the disease and viral clearance (Abassi et al. 2020). When the human ACE2 receptor on the surface of epithelial cells attaches to the spike glycoprotein of SARS-CoV-2, infection begins. The host transmembrane protease serine 2 (TMPRSS2) facilitates viral entrance into the cells (Hoffmann et al. 2020). The SARS-CoV-2 'S' protein has a 10 to 20 times more affinity for binding to ACE2 than the SARS 'S' protein, implying that SARS-CoV-2 may disseminate more easily from person to person (Wrapp et al. 2020). The major target cells for SARS-CoV-2 infection are alveolar macrophages that express ACE2 receptor. These activated macrophages might be significant in the COVID-19 hemophagocytic lymphohistiocytosis (HLH)-like cytokine storm. On the other hand, ACE2 is a crucial membrane protein and an AngII inactivator. During SARS-CoV-2 infection, virus occupied and endocytosed ACE2 receptors on the surface of target cells, which resulted in decreased ACE2 and increased serum AngII (Kuba et al. 2005). Future therapeutic interventions should include the administration of recombinant human ACE2 to deactivate virions, before they bind to the host cells.

15.7.6 Inhibition of Granulocyte Macrophage Colony-Stimulating Factor Receptor (GM-CSF-R)

Treatment of COVID-19 patients with mavrilimumab (anti-granulocyte–macrophage colony-stimulating factor receptor-alpha monoclonal antibody) resulted in improved clinical outcomes than normal treatment protocol in non-mechanically ventilated patients with systemic hyperinflammation and severe disease (De Luca et al. 2020).

15.7.7 Stem Cell Therapy

Recently, stem cell therapy is being investigated for the treatment of COVID-19 patients. Research reports showed that mesenchymal stem cells could reduce the pathological changes in the lungs and reduce the cell-mediated immune-inflammatory responses.

15.7.8 Corticosteroids

Corticosteroids including glucocorticoids were used in various primary and secondary forms of HLH. They used effectively for the treatment of acute respiratory distress syndrome. Recently, corticosteroids were also recommended for use in patients with severe COVID-19 by WHO to reduce hospital mortality; however, the same recommendations guided not to use corticosteroid with non-severe infection. There is substantial controversy about whether treating COVID-19 patients with corticosteroids would be beneficial. Others agreed that corticosteroids are potent inhibitors of the hyperinflammatory state, which is the primary cause of mortality in severe COVID-19 patients, and disagreed that corticosteroids would promote host immune suppression and postpone viral clearance (Ni et al. 2021). There are no controlled studies, and scant information is available on the effectiveness and safety of corticosteroids in ARDS, which is anecdotal and inconclusive. High-dosage corticosteroids cannot be universally advised for the treatment of COVID-19 due to their association with widely varying effects on pathogen clearance. Instead, low-dose regimens must be tested in formal and controlled investigations (Russell et al. 2020). Corticosteroid therapy elevates the glucose levels in 80% of COVID-19 patients. In diabetic patients, such poor glycemic control leads to hyperglycemic condition and ketoacidosis, which adversely affect pulmonary function; hence, corticosteroids are not advised in diabetic patients suffering with COVID-19.

15.7.9 Remdesivir

Recently, FDA approved remdesivir for use in adults and pediatric patients (12 years of age and older, and weighing at least 40 kg) for the treatment of COVID-19 on October 22, 2020. Remdesivir is recommended in COVID-19 patients to prevent the severity of disease progression as it alters functions of viral exonuclease and due to disturbed proofreading, viral genomic RNA replication, and virus production falls. Remdesivir prevents viral replication and, hence, used in the therapy of COVID-19 patients.

15.7.10 Chloroquine Phosphate and Hydroxychloroquine

The drug has long been used as antimalarial drug. Drug was also used for various infections like chikungunya, influenza, Q fever, and even for HIV. Chloroquine phosphate is the first drug that was found to be useful for the treatment of COVID-19 in China (Gao et al. 2020a). The analog of chloroquine, namely, hydroxychloroquine, is considered as an immunomodulatory drug for the systemic lupus erythematosus. The varied range of mode of action of hydroxychloroquine includes immunological control, anti-infection, antitumor, metabolic control, and antithrombosis. In vitro studies showed that hydroxychloroquine is more potent than chloroquine for the inhibition of SARS-CoV-2 (Yao et al. 2020). These medications elevate the endosomal pH, which is necessary for SARS-CoV-2 endocytosis and cell fusion. Chloroquine phosphate also interferes the glycosylation of ACE2, which is vital for viral attachment to host cells. Using an in vitro SARS-CoV-2-infected Vero-E6 cell culture model, chloroquine was initially discovered as strong COVID-19 inhibitor in 2020. However, due to the alkalization of the endosomes, there is marked reduction in proteolysis, phagocytosis, chemotaxis, and receptor recycling and showed the interference in the processing of epitopes by antigen-presenting cells (Ziegler and Unanue 1982; Devaux et al. 2020).

Studies suggested that the combination of hydroxychloroquine and azithromycin expressed synergistic antiviral effects in vitro against SARS-CoV-2 in clinical trials. Treatment of patients with combination of hydroxychloroquine and azithromycin had favorable impact and showed a marked decline in the death of COVID-19 patients. However, while using azithromycin, chloroquine, and hydroxychloroquine for managing SARS-CoV-2 infection in patients, all safety consideration should be taken into account. Clinical trials in combination of azithromycin and hydroxychloroquine showed some serious side effects in the function of the heart in COVID-19 patients (Devaux et al. 2020).

The recommended dosage of chloroquine for the treatment of COVID-19 is 500 mg of chloroquine twice daily for patients, who weigh more than 50 kg, and those who weigh less than 50 kg should consume 500 mg twice daily on the first 2 days and once daily for the next 5 days that follow at a dose rate of 200 mg of hydroxychloroquine sulfate three times daily (Zhao 2020). However, patients may be at a danger of dying, if given a high dose of chloroquine of more than 600 mg (Devaux et al. 2020; Ektorp 2020).

15.7.11 Ivermectin

Ivermectin is a broad-spectrum antiparasitic drug having multiple therapeutic applications in animals such as dogs. Recently, ivermectin has been shown to inhibit SARS-CoV-2 replication in vitro. It has received approval from the US Food and Drug Administration for use in COVID-19 patients (Caly et al. 2020). In addition, synergistic and consequential effects of ivermectin and hydroxychloroquine were also hypothesized for the treatment and chemoprophylaxis of COVID-19 when administered simultaneously in patients (Patrì and Fabbrocini 2020). Timely administration of ivermectin (within 48 h after the appearance of symptoms) in low-risk patients could reduce the further transmission of COVID-19.

15.7.12 Umifenovir (Arbidol)

Umifenovir is sold under the brand name Arbidol, which is an antiviral medication for the treatment of influenza infection used in Russia and China. Umifenovir inhibits or reduces the fusion of virus with target cell membrane and to prevent the entry of virus within the cell.

15.7.13 Low Molecular Weight Heparin (LMWH)

Anticoagulant therapy is found to be useful to reduce the mortality by the cardiovascular complications of COVID-19. Sepsis and hypoxia were reported to be responsible for coagulopathy. Low molecular weight heparin (LMWH) can be useful for the hospitalized patients by anticoagulant, anti-inflammatory, and endothelial protective effects.

15.7.14 Nonsteroidal Anti-inflammatory Drugs (NSAIDs)

The nonsteroidal anti-inflammatory drugs (NSAIDs) were also recommended for the management of pain associated with COVID-19; however, no curative results were reported using NSAIDs. Xu et al. (2020) reported the effectiveness of indomethacin at a dose of 1 mg/kg against SARS-CoV-2 through inhibition of viral RNA synthesis.

15.7.15 Anticancer Drugs

Anticancer drug bemcentinib is an orally available and selective inhibitor of the AXL receptor tyrosine kinase (UFO), with potential antineoplastic activity. Bemcentinib is currently used for various solid and hematological tumors as monotherapy and in combination with immunotherapy, chemotherapy, and targeted therapeutics. Bemcentinib has also been reported to have antiviral activity against SARS-CoV-2 in preclinical trials.

15.7.16 Other Antiviral Compounds

Antivirals, including oseltamivir, zanamivir, ganciclovir, acyclovir, peramivir, and ribavirin, were used earlier for the treatment of viral infections and, recently, which are screened for the usage against SARS-CoV-2; however, they are not recommended against SARS-CoV-2 (Li et al. 2020). Ritonavir and lopinavir combination used earlier for the treatment of human immunodeficiency virus and these compounds showed promising results in SARS and MERS. The ritonavir and lopinavir combination had also been recommended for the treatment of COVID-19 patients in China during the early stages of the pandemic (Chu et al. 2004; Arabi et al. 2018; Huang et al. 2020; Li et al. 2020).

15.7.17 CRISPR-Based Tools

The novel use of CRISPR-based tools and techniques such as SHERLOCK has been reported (Zhang et al. 2020e). The CRISPR could pave the way for developing highly precise and simple diagnostic tests as well as therapeutics. AI technology and computational calculations are being explored for rapidly developing drugs (Asai et al. 2020). Further, the enormous data available related to COVID-19 treatment, which require advanced machine learning-based methods for the analysis of therapeutic effects to provide improved and personalized clinical care to patients (Alimadadi et al. 2020).

15.8 Vaccines Against COVID-19

Researchers have developed effective vaccines (Table 15.1) and therapeutics/drugs to combat the COVID-19 pandemic within a short timeframe (Dhama et al. 2020c; Pathak et al. 2020; Rabaan et al. 2020; Yavuz and Ünal 2020; Zhang et al. 2020b). The use of effective vaccines, targeting epidemic and pandemic viruses, is an excellent approach to save the lives of people under this pandemic threat. Apart from developing vaccines to counter the present SARS-CoV-2, we need to consider universal vaccine concepts and that viruses are continuously evolving in multiple species, as evidenced by the recent threats during this century in the form of avian/bird flu, swine flu, Ebola, Zika, and Nipah virus diseases (Dhama et al. 2020a). Moreover, vaccines and vaccination policies dealing with coronaviruses that affect animals, wildlife, and poultry need to be strengthened to limit the chances of spread of the viruses and subsequent disease outbreaks and zoonotic events (Ella and Mohan 2020; Khamsi 2020).

The receptor-binding domain (RBD) of the SARS-CoV-2 is a potential antigen and is assumed to be responsible for the development of abundant neutralizing antibodies against SARS-CoV-2. Moreover, the RBD is a crucial candidate for subunit vaccine development against COVID-19 (Yi et al. 2020). A DNA plasmid-based vaccine, namely, INO-4800, by INOVIO Pharmaceuticals is being

15.8 Vaccines Against COVID-19

Table 15.1 SARS-CoV-2 vaccine candidates available for use in some regions of the world

Vaccine name	Vaccine type	Manufacturing company	Country	Target	Storage	Doses required	Immunization per dose	% Efficacy in preventing infection	Observations
BNT162b2 mRNA	Nucleic acid (or) RNA-based vaccine	Pfizer and BioNTech	Germany	Full-length S "Spike" protein with proline substitutions wrapped in a lipid nanoparticle using polyethylene glycol as a stabilizing agent	−70 °C up to 6 months, 2–8 °C up to 5 days Reconstituted up to 6 h	Three doses. Second dose 21–42 days after the first dose. Third dose 6–12 months after the second dose	100 and 30 μg (third dose)	95%. It was well tolerated and could induce neutralizing antibodies. Better protection for VOCs. High safety	The third dose is being evaluated in patients 18–55 years and 65–85 years
mRNA-1273	Nucleic acid (or) RNA-based vaccine	MODERNA	America	Full-length S-2P "Spike" protein wrapped in a lipid nanoparticle	−20 °C up to 6 months, 2–8 °C up to 30 days	Second dose 28 days after the first one	30 μg	94.1%. The vaccine showed 94.1% efficacy in preventing SARS-CoV-2	No safety concerns were identified. Better protection for VOCs
CVnCoV	RNA-based vaccine	CureVac/Bayer/GSK/Novartis	Germany	Full-length S-2P "Spike" protein wrapped in a lipid nanoparticle	2–8 °C up to 3 months	Second dose 28 days after the first one	12 μg	The vaccine could effectively induce immune response	Mexico is one of the countries selected for phase III
ARCoV	Nucleic acid (or) RNA-based vaccine	–	China	Encoding the RBD of S protein	2–8 °C up to 3 months	Second dose 28 days after the first one	–	Not reported	Not reported

(continued)

Table 15.1 (continued)

Vaccine name	Vaccine type	Manufacturing company	Country	Target	Storage	Doses required	Immunization per dose	% Efficacy in preventing infection	Observations
ZyCov-D	Nucleic acid (or) DNA-based vaccine	Cadila Healthcare	India	S protein	2–8 °C up to 3 months	Second dose 28 days after the first one	–	Vaccine has 66.6% efficacy from clinical trials	Not reported
INO-4800	Nucleic acid (or) DNA-based vaccine	INOVIO	America	S1 and S2 subunits	**2–8 °C up to 3 months**	Second dose 28 days after the first one	–	Vaccine induced a protective immune response	The vaccine showed excellent safety and tolerability
AZD1222 (ChAdOx1 nCoV-19)	Virus vector vaccine	AstraZeneca/Oxford	Britain	Chimpanzee adenovirus vectored vaccine (ChAdOx1) expressing S "Spike" protein	2–8 °C	Second dose 28 days after the first one	0.5×10^{11} Vp	82.4%. ChAdOx1 nCoV-19 is efficacious against symptomatic COVID-19	ChAdOx1 nCoV-19 has an acceptable safety profile
Ad5-nCov	Virus vector vaccine	CanSino Biological	China	Recombinant replication defective human type 5 adenovirus (Ad5) expressing S protein	2–8 °C	Single dose	0.5×10^{11} Vp	65.28%. Ad5-nCoV was well tolerated and could elicit neutralizing antibody responses	High safety
Sputnik V (Gam-COVID-Vac)	Virus vector vaccine	Gamaleya Research Institute	Russia	Recombinant Ad26 and recombinant Ad5 encoding full length S "Spike" protein	First vial frozen at −18° C Second vial lyophilized at 2–8 °C	Second dose 21 days after the first one	0.5 mL	92%. Well tolerated 91.6% efficacy against COVID-19	High safety

15.8 Vaccines Against COVID-19

Sputnik light vaccine	Virus vector vaccine	Gamaleya Research Institute	Russia	Recombinant Ad26 vector carrying the gene for SARS-CoV-2 S glycoprotein	2–8 °C	Second dose 21 days after the first one	—	Strong humoral and cellular immune responses both in seronegative and seropositive participants	Sputnik light vaccine has a good safety profile
Ad26.COV2.21S (JNJ-78436735)	Virus vector vaccine	Janssen Pharmaceutical Companies of Johnson & Johnson (J & J)	America	Recombinant replication incompetent adenovirus serotype 26 (Ad26) vector encoding full-length S protein	2–8 °C	Single dose, but second dose may be required depending on the patient's need	0.5×10^{11} Vp	72% in the USA and 61% in Latin America	The vaccine protected against symptomatic COVID-19 and asymptomatic SARS-CoV-2 infection. High safety
CoronaVac	Attenuated or inactivated virus	Sinovac	China	Whole inactivated SARS-CoV-2 with aluminum hydroxide adjuvant	2–8 °C	Second dose 14 days after the first one	3 µg	83.7% in Turkey, 50.3% in Brazil. The vaccine exhibited over 60% efficacy on average at preventing COVID-19 illness with favorable safety and immunogenicity profiles. Protection against VOCs is weakened and further immunization is needed	Immunization with Coronavac in a 0–14 schedule in adults is safe, induces anti-S1-RBD IgG with neutralizing capacity, activates T cells, and promotes the secretion of IFN-γ upon stimulation with SARS-CoV-2 antigens

(continued)

Table 15.1 (continued)

Vaccine name	Vaccine type	Manufacturing company	Country	Target	Storage	Doses required	Immunization per dose	% Efficacy in preventing infection	Observations
Covaxin (BBV152 A, B, C)	Attenuated or inactivated virus	Bharat Biotech/ Indian Council of Medical Research	India	Whole inactivated SARS-CoV-2 with Algel-IMDG adjuvant	2–8 °C	Second dose 28 days after the first one	3 μg	81%. A protective effect of 77.8% against symptomatic COVID-19. Effectively protects against VOCs	Vaccination was well tolerated with no safety concerns raised
Inactivated SARA-CoV-2 vaccine (Vero Cell)	Attenuated or inactivated virus	–	China	Whole inactivated SARS-CoV-2 with aluminum hydroxide adjuvant	2–8 °C	Second dose 28 days after the first one	–	Adults with inactivated SARS-CoV-2 vaccine significantly reduced the risk of symptomatic COVID-19	Serious adverse events were rare. Protection against VOCs is weakened
QazCovid-in (QazVac)	Attenuated or inactivated virus	Kazakh Biosafety Research Institute	Kazakhstan	Whole inactivated SARS-CoV-2	2–8 °C	Second dose 21 days after the first one	–	Preliminary results of studies demonstrate efficacy of the vaccine at 96%	High safety and potency
VLA2001 or Valneva COVID-19 vaccine	Attenuated or inactivated virus	Dynavax Technologies	Cooperation between France and Britain	Whole inactivated SARS-CoV-2 with high S-protein density	2–8 °C	Second dose 21 days after the first one	–	Not reported	S-protein in combination with two adjuvants, alum and CpG 1018

15.8 Vaccines Against COVID-19

BBIBP-CorV	Protein subunit or inactivated virus	Sinopharm/ Beijing Institute of Biological Products	China	Whole inactivated SARS-CoV-2	2–8 °C	Second dose 21 days after the first one	4 μg	79.34%. More than 75% of the vaccinators had seroconversion after the first vaccination	BBIBP-CorV is tolerable and immunogenic in healthy people
NVX-CoV2373	Protein subunit or recombinant protein vaccine	NOVAVAX	America	S protein with matrix-M adjuvant	2–8 °C	Second dose 21 days after the first one	5 μg SARS-CoV-2 rS + 50 μg of matrix-M1 adjuvant	96%. Original coronavirus 86% variant B.1.1.7 and 49% variant B.1.351	Nanoparticles containing the protein subunit S
ZF2001 (Recombinant SARS-CoV-2 vaccine)	Protein subunit or recombinant protein vaccine	Anhui Zhifei Longcom Biopharmaceutical Co./Government of Uzbekistan	China	Recombinant origin using CHO cell line to express protein S	2–8 °C	2–3 doses, 28 days after the first one	25 μg/0.5 mL	Have good tolerance, immunogenicity, and be effective in neutralizing VOCs	RBD-Dimer with alum adjuvant
Recombinant SARS-CoV-2 vaccine (Sf9 cell)	Recombinant protein vaccine	–	China	RBD with alum adjuvant	2–8 °C	Second dose 21 days after the first one	–	Not reported	Not reported
Nanocovax	Recombinant protein vaccine	Nanogen Pharmaceutical Biotechnology	Vietnam	Recombinant S protein with alum adjuvant	2–8 °C	Second dose 21 days after the first one	–	Not reported	Not reported
MVC-COV1901	Recombinant protein vaccine	Medigen Vaccine Biologics	America	Recombinant S protein with CpG 1018 and alum adjuvants	2–8 °C	Second dose 21 days after the first one	–	The vaccine could elicit promising immunogenicity responses	MVC-COV1901 has a good safety profile

(continued)

Table 15.1 (continued)

Vaccine name	Vaccine type	Manufacturing company	Country	Target	Storage	Doses required	Immunization per dose	% Efficacy in preventing infection	Observations
EpiVacCorona	Recombinant protein vaccine	VECTOR Center of Virology	Russia	Peptide antigens of SARS-CoV-2 proteins with alum adjuvant	2–8 °C	Second dose 21 days after the first one	–	Not reported	Not reported
CIGB-66 (RBD/ aluminum hydroxide)	Recombinant protein vaccine	–	ICGEB	RBD with aluminum hydroxide adjuvant	2–8 °C	Second dose 21 days after the first one	–	High efficiency	High safety
Razi Cov Pars	Recombinant protein vaccine	Iranian Razi Vaccine and Serum Research Institute	Razi Vaccine and Serum Research Institute	Recombinant S protein	2–8 °C	Second dose 21 days after the first one	–	Not reported	Not reported
FINLAY-FR-2 anti-SARS-CoV-2 Vaccine	Recombinant protein vaccine	Finlay Institute	Instituto Finlay de Vacunas	RBD with adjuvant	2–8 °C	Second dose 21 days after the first one	–	Not reported	Not reported

Note: *VOC* variants of interest, *CHO* Chinese Hamster Ovary planned to be administered in healthy individuals followed by electroporation after all the safety and efficacy studies are completed (Kim et al. 2020). An mRNA-based vaccine (mRNA1273-COVID-19 vaccine), which is being planned to be administered as an injection of mRNA encapsulated in lipid nanoparticles, is under phase 1 clinical trial (ClinicalTrials.gov: NCT04283461) and is considered to be highly safe (Kim et al. 2020). A chimpanzee adenovirus vector (ChAdOx1)-based vaccine is also being developed and has progressed to phase 1/2 clinical trial in a short period (NCT04324606) (Kim et al. 2020). Moreover, the ChAdOx1 is a non-replicating virus and is safe for use in children, people with comorbidities, and elderly people (Kim et al. 2020). The adenovirus type 5 (Ad5) vector-based vaccine (Ad5-nCoV) is genetically engineered vaccine candidate that uses a replication-defective Ad5 as a vector and most advanced DNA vaccine candidate against COVID-19 (Cohen 2020; Ella and Mohan 2020; Khamsi 2020).

Bacillus Calmette–Guérin vaccine is used to treat tuberculosis in humans for a century and, recently, used as an alternative treatment regimen in reducing COVID-19 morbidity and mortality (Miller et al. 2020). Inactivated SARS-CoV-2 virus (Sinovac®) vaccine was developed by China, which contained a chemically inactivated virus. The vaccine was found to induce a strong immunity in laboratory animals and non-human primates. The results of the challenge study with SARS-CoV-2 virus in monkeys revealed that vaccinated monkeys did not develop an infection. No virus was recovered from the throat, lungs, and rectum (Gao et al. 2020b). The mRNA-1273 is a novel vaccine that uses mRNA technology; however, these vaccines were not previously approved for human use. The mRNA encodes a full-length prefusion spike protein of SARS-CoV-2 and encapsulated by lipid nanoparticle formulation (Jackson et al. 2020). The BNT162b1 is a nucleoside-modified, mRNA-based, lipid nanoparticle-formulated vaccine that encodes spike glycoprotein RBD. The SARS-CoV-2 neutralizing and RBD-binding immunoglobulin G antibodies were detected from all the vaccinated persons at 28 days after two doses (Ella and Mohan 2020; Mulligan et al. 2020; Khamsi 2020).

15.9 Plant-Based Vaccines to Combat COVID-19

Plant-based vaccines have elicited promising immune responses against hepatitis B virus, Ebola virus, dengue fever virus, cholera, HIV, etc. in animals and humans (Nikhat and Fazil 2020). After obtaining the genetic sequence of the causative virus, SARS-CoV-2, a Canadian-based pharmaceutical company, Medicago, has successfully formulated virus-like particles (VLPs) by insertion of a spike protein-encoding genetic fragment into *Agrobacterium*, which is a soil bacterium taken up by plants. The developed plants produce the VLPs consisting of S protein and plant lipid membrane. Medicago used a tobacco plant, *Nicotiana benthamiana*, for producing the SARS-CoV2 VLPs, which are identical to actual coronavirus in terms of shape and size without the presence of nucleic acid. VLPs have undergone phase 1 clinical trials and are under process in the phase 2 clinical stage. The N-terminal fragment of S1 protein was subjected to expression in tobacco and tomato plants using

Agrobacterium-assisted nuclear expression strategies. Oral immunization of mice with developed transgenic tomato showed markedly enhanced concentrations of anti-SARS-CoV-1 IgA antibodies. The sera of transgenic tobacco injected mice revealed the existence of SARS-CoV-1-specific IgG. In another report, stabilized transgenic lettuce and tobacco plants were produced by the *Agrobacterium*-based approach. The chimeric antigen was also expressed in the chloroplasts of tobacco plants (Li et al. 2020; Nikhat and Fazil 2020). Three doses of nucleocapsid protein expressed in *N. benthamiana* in mice produced efficient B-cell differentiation and maturation, leading to enhanced levels of IgG1 and IgG2a. Moreover, IL-10 and IFN-γ were found to upregulate in splenocytes (Li et al. 2020).

15.10 Control Strategies

Continuous efforts are warranted to increase the testing of the mass population in the countries affected and to identify the hotspot areas of infection by rapid diagnostics, which would aid in adopting appropriate prevention and control strategies to mitigate the wave of the current pandemic (Abbott et al. 2020; Cheng et al. 2020; Dhama et al. 2020b; Pathak et al. 2020). Prevention and control measures, such as prompt diagnosis, isolation, quarantine, and strict vigilance on wet markets, may prove highly beneficial in the containment of COVID-19. In addition, temporary closure or ban on markets dealing with live or slaughtered wild and game animals, along with complete control over illegal and legal wildlife trading is also warranted (Rodriguez-Morales et al. 2020). Strengthening of healthcare facilities, identification of hotspot areas for probable emergence of zoonotic diseases, and strict surveillance and monitoring of wild and domestic animals are of utmost importance to prevent possible occurrences of new viruses and subsequent diseases. Recent emergence of Y453F mutation in SARS-CoV-2 in minks has further raised concerns. Proper preventive measures need to be taken to improve the mental health of front-line health workers and medical staffs as well as to relieve them from symptoms of anxiety occurred due to their direct exposure to infected patients while testing and treatment. To effectively contain this pandemic, strict surveillance of travelers, robust awareness campaigning, rapid communication with updates on current scenarios, prompt and appropriate clinical care, and implementation of updated strategies suggested by global health agencies are crucial (Harypursat and Chen 2020; Hellewell et al. 2020). Following national and international guidelines and protocols for minimizing the occurrence and spread of COVID-19 is essential especially in events involving crowd or travel.

Measures, such as intense epidemiological surveillance, quick diagnosis, isolation of positive cases, quarantine of suspected in-contact persons, social distancing, following prescribed sanitation and hygienic practices for environmental sanitation, and awareness campaigns by official health regulatory bodies through print-media and audio-visual aids at various online and offline platforms, are recommended for timely tackling of this rapidly spreading SARS-CoV-2 (Wilder-Smith and Freedman 2020; Ting et al. 2020).

15.11 Role of Artificial Intelligence in Controlling COVID-19 Spread

Artificial intelligence (AI), machine learning (ML), natural language processing (NLP), and computer vision applications are currently playing an important role in the medical field, such as drug development, diagnosis, monitoring, prevention of complications, etc. (Obeid et al. 2020; Ting et al. 2020). Therefore, AI and ML were also exploited in controlling COVID-19. It helped in contact tracing. A number of applications have been used for this purpose using GPS, GSM, and Bluetooth technologies. It also helped people to alert about areas where the infected individual has traveled or lived in the last 2 weeks to take extra precautionary measures during the stay in a particular area (Alimadadi et al. 2020; Obeid et al. 2020; Vaishya et al. 2020;). It is also utilized for the diagnosis of patients. For instance, AI utilized for the detection of COVID-19 associated pneumonia by examining chest CT. Their algorithm showed about 90% accuracy, with 10% of false-positive results. Additionally, AI is also playing an important role in the development of a proper vaccine for COVID-19 (Alimadadi et al. 2020; Obeid et al. 2020; Vaishya et al. 2020;). The easing of lockdown is progressing throughout the world, AI is also helping to monitor the temperature of peoples and facial mask-wearing and has a record through facial recognition. This monitoring is important for the further spread of disease in the high populous areas, where it is difficult to monitor through human workforce. However, there are some concerns about the privacy of the public using such applications.

Artificial intelligence (AI) is a potentially powerful tool in the fight against the COVID-19 pandemic (Bullock et al. 2020; Petropoulos 2020). Main applications of AI in COVID-19 pandemic are early detection and diagnosis of the infection, monitoring the treatment, contact tracing of the individuals, projection of cases and mortality, development of drugs and vaccines, reducing the workload of healthcare workers, and prevention of the disease (Vaishya et al. 2020; Naudé 2020). Proper application of AI using both existing and novel machine learning approaches may be pivotal to eliminating the COVID-19 cases (Obeid et al. 2020; Ting et al. 2020).

15.12 One Health Approach to Counter Future Pandemics of SARS-CoV-2

The SARS-CoV-2 has been implicated to have originated in animals, showing spillover events and zoonosis, with bats and pangolins suspected to have played a role in its origin and subsequent human-to-human transmission (Dhama et al. 2020b). There is a need to enforce a complete ban on wildlife trade, restrict habitat destruction of wildlife fauna, and alter food habits. Animal and wildlife markets, where different species of domestic animals, poultry, and wildlife animals are sold, must be considered as a potent source of any new emerging viruses in the future, as SARS-CoV-2 may have emerged from such places, leading to a devastating pandemic (Bonilla-Aldana et al. 2020; Daszak et al. 2020). Further, recent studies of SARS-CoV-2 infection in tigers, cats, dogs, and other animal species, although mild, warrant the timely need to carry out surveillance studies in domestic animals and wildlife species to identify the zoonotic links and spillover events associated with this virus that led to its transmission to humans (Chen et al. 2020a, b; Contini et al. 2020; Daly 2020; Dhama et al. 2020b). Because of various activities of humans, the balance of nature has been disrupted, and multiple calamities and severe disease outbreaks have occurred and are well documented in history. Increasing human-animal interface events need to be taken care of by adopting the "One Health" concept (Bonilla-Aldana et al. 2020; Heymann et al. 2020).

15.13 Conclusion

Following the emergence of SARS-CoV-2, researchers sought effective therapeutic and prophylactic candidates to address the ongoing pandemic. Vaccines play a key role as a primary means of prevention, while drugs serve as therapeutic agents. Several vaccines have been introduced to the market, and numerous others, alongside drugs, are currently in the final stages of validation and approval by regulatory authorities. Regular hygiene, respiratory etiquette, physical distancing, and disinfection appear to be the primary steps in COVID-19 mitigation. A holistic approach with an increased focus on the "One Health" concept and a thorough investigation of probable causes of this and earlier pandemics and possible solutions are of utmost necessity to prevent the occurrence of such pandemics soon. Moreover, a global effort is required for dealing with the increased risk of future pandemics. The development of infrastructure by countries for managing future pandemics will be of utmost importance as reflected in the present COVID-19 crisis. The global expansion of human activities, including deforestation, wildlife trade, and intensification of agriculture, is the major driver of such diseases. These activities have led to an enormous increase in the frequency of animal-human conflicts and the subsequent emergence of novel diseases, suggesting that more frequent and devastating pandemics may be encountered in the future. Providing appropriate funding for supporting coronaviruses research programs along with undertaking collaborative and cooperative approaches at the national and international levels will help to tackle the current pandemic as well as create preparedness plans for future pandemics.

References

Abassi ZA, Skorecki K, Heyman SN, Kinaneh S, Armaly Z (2020) Covid-19 infection and mortality: a physiologist's perspective enlightening clinical features and plausible interventional strategies. Am J Physiol Lung Cell Mol Physiol 318(5):L1020–L1022. https://doi.org/10.1152/ajplung.00097.2020. Epub 2020 Mar 24. PMID: 32207983; PMCID: PMC7200872

Abbott TR, Dhamdhere G, Liu Y, Lin X, Goudy LE, Zeng L, Chemparathy A, Chmura S, Heaton N, Debs R and Pande T (2020) Development of CRISPR as a prophylactic strategy to combat novel coronavirus and influenza. bioRxiv

References

Ackerman CM, Myhrvold C, Thakku SG, Freije CA, Metsky HC, Yang DK, Ye SH, Boehm CK, Kosoko-Thoroddsen TS, Kehe J, Nguyen TG (2020) Massively multiplexed nucleic acid detection using Cas13. Nature 582:277. https://doi.org/10.1038/s41586-020-2279-8

Aggarwal G, Cheruiyot I, Aggarwal S et al (2020) Association of cardiovascular disease with coronavirus disease 2019 (COVID-19) severity: a meta-analysis. Curr Probl Cardiol 45:100617

Alimadadi A, Aryal S, Manandhar I, Munroe PB, Joe B, Cheng X (2020) Artificial intelligence and machine learning to fight COVID-19. Physiol Genomics 52(4):200–202. https://doi.org/10.1152/physiolgenomics.00029.2020

Arabi YM, Alothman A, Balkhy HH, Al-Dawood A, Al Johani S, Al Harbi S, Kojan S, Al Jeraisy M, Deeb AM, Assiri AM, Al-Hameed F, Al Saedi A, Mandourah Y, Almekhlafi GA, Sherbeeni NM, Elzein FE, Memon J, Taha Y, Almotairi A, Maghrabi KA, Qushmaq I, Al Bshabshe A, Kharaba A, Shalhoub S, Jose J, Fowler RA, Hayden FG, Hussein MA, And the MIRACLE trial group (2018) Treatment of Middle East Respiratory Syndrome with a combination of lopinavir-ritonavir and interferon-β1b (MIRACLE trial): study protocol for a randomized controlled trial. Trials 19(1):81. https://doi.org/10.1186/s13063-017-2427-0

Asai A, Konno M, Ozaki M, Otsuka C, Vecchione A, Arai T, Kitagawa T, Ofusa K, Yabumoto M, Hirotsu T, Taniguchi M, Eguchi H, Doki Y, Ishii H (2020) COVID-19 drug discovery using intensive approaches. Int J Mol Sci 21(8):2839. https://doi.org/10.3390/ijms21082839

Ayittey FK, Ayittey MK, Chiwero NB, Kamasah JS, Dzuvor C (2020) Economic impacts of Wuhan 2019-nCoV on China and the world. J Med Virol 92:473. https://doi.org/10.1002/jmv.25706

Barton LM, Duval EJ, Stroberg E, Ghosh S, Mukhopadhyay S (2020) Covid-19 autopsies, Oklahoma, USA. Am J Clin Pathol 153(6):725–733

Bonilla-Aldana DK, Dhama K, Rodriguez-Morales AJ (2020) Revisiting the one health approach in the context of COVID-19: a look into the ecology of this emerging disease. Adv Anim Vet Sci 8(3):234–237

Bullock J, Pham KH, Lam CSN and Luengo-Oroz M (2020) Mapping the landscape of artificial intelligence applications against COVID-19. arXiv preprint arXiv:2003.11336

Caly L, Druce JD, Catton MG, Jans DA, Wagstaff KM (2020) The FDA-approved drug ivermectin inhibits the replication of SARS-CoV-2 in vitro. Antivir Res 178:104787. https://doi.org/10.1016/j.antiviral.2020.104787

Chan JF, Yuan S, Kok KH, To KK, Chu H, Yang J, Xing F, Liu J, Yip CC, Poon RW, Tsoi HW, Lo SK, Chan KH, Poon VK, Chan WM, Ip JD, Cai JP, Cheng VC, Chen H, Hui CK, Yuen KY (2020) A familial cluster of pneumonia associated with the 2019 novel coronavirus indicating person-to-person transmission: a study of a family cluster. Lancet 395(10223):514–523. https://doi.org/10.1016/S0140-6736(20)30154-9

Chatterjee P, Nagi N, Agarwal A, Das B, Banerjee S, Sarkar S, Gupta N, Gangakhedkar RR (2020) The 2019 novel coronavirus disease (COVID-19) pandemic: a review of the current evidence. Indian J Med Res 151:147. https://doi.org/10.4103/ijmr.IJMR_519_20

Chen L, Xiong J, Bao L et al (2020a) Convalescent plasma as a potential therapy for COVID-19. Lancet Infect Dis 20(4):398–400

Chen N, Zhou M, Dong X, Qu J, Gong F, Han Y, Qiu Y, Wang J, Liu Y, Wei Y, Yu T (2020b) Epidemiological and clinical characteristics of 99 cases of 2019 novel coronavirus pneumonia in Wuhan, China: a descriptive study. Lancet 395(10223):507–513

Cheng MP, Papenburg J, Desjardins M, Kanjilal S, Quach C, Libman M, Dittrich S, Yansouni CP (2020) Diagnostic testing for severe acute respiratory syndrome–related coronavirus-2: a narrative review. Ann Intern Med 172:726. https://doi.org/10.7326/M20-1301

Choi IA, Lee SJ, Park W, Park SH, Shim SC, Baek HJ, Yoo DH, Kim HA, Lee SK, Lee YJ, Park YE, Cha HS, Lee EY, Lee EB, Song YW (2018) Effects of tocilizumab therapy on serum Interleukin-33 and Interleukin-6 levels in patients with rheumatoid arthritis. Arch Rheumatol 33(4):389–394. https://doi.org/10.5606/ArchRheumatol.2018.6753. PMID: 30874247; PMCID: PMC6409174

Chu CM, Cheng VC, Hung IF, Wong MM, Chan KH, Chan KS, Kao RY, Poon LL, Wong CL, Guan Y, Peiris JS, Yuen KY, HKU/UCH SARS Study Group (2004) Role of lopinavir/ritonavir in the treatment of SARS: initial virological and clinical findings. Thorax 59(3):252–256. https://doi.org/10.1136/thorax.2003.012658

Cohen J (2020) Vaccine designers take first shots at COVID-19. Science 368(6486):14–16. https://doi.org/10.1126/science.368.6486.14

Contini C, Di Nuzzo M, Barp N, Bonazza A, De Giorgio R, Tognon M, Rubino S (2020) The novel zoonotic COVID-19 pandemic: an expected global health concern. J Infect Dev Ctries 14(3):254–264. https://doi.org/10.3855/jidc.12671

Cron RQ, Chatham WW (2020) The rheumatologist's role in COVID-19. J Rheumatol 47(5):639–642. https://doi.org/10.3899/jrheum.200334. Epub 2020 Mar 24

Daly N (2020) Tiger tests positive for coronavirus at Bronx Zoo, first known case in the world. https://www.nationalgeographic.com/animals/2020/04/tiger-coronavirus-covid19-positive-test-bronx-zoo/

Daszak P, Olival KJ, Li H (2020) A strategy to prevent future pandemics similar to the 2019-nCoV outbreak. Biosaf Health 2020(2):6–8

De Luca G, Cavalli G, Campochiaro C et al (2020) GM-CSF blockade with mavrilimumab in severe COVID-19 pneumonia and systemic hyperinflammation: a single-Centre, prospective cohort study. Lancet Rheumatol 2(8):e465–e473

de Wilde AH, Snijder EJ, Kikkert M, van Hemert MJ (2017) Host factors in coronavirus replication. Curr Top Microbiol Immunol 419:1–42

Desai R, Singh S, Parekh T et al (2020) COVID-19 and diabetes mellitus: a need for prudence in elderly patients from a pooled analysis. Diabetes Metab Syndr 14(4):683–685

Devaux CA, Rolain JM, Colson P, Raoult D (2020) New insights on the antiviral effects of chloroquine against coronavirus: what to expect for COVID-19? Int J Antimicrob Agents 55:105938. https://doi.org/10.1016/j.ijantimicag.2020.105938

Dhama K, Sharun K, Tiwari R, Sircar S, Bhat S, Malik YS, Singh KP, Chaicumpa W, Bonilla-Aldana DK, Rodriguez-Morales AJ (2020a) Coronavirus disease 2019—COVID-19. Clin Microbiol Rev 33(4):e0028. https://doi.org/10.20944/preprints202003.0001.v1

Dhama K, Patel SK, Sharun K, Pathak M, Tiwari R, Yatoo MI, Malik YS, Sah R, Rabaan AA, Panwar PK, Singh KP, Michalak I, Chaicumpa W, Bonilla-Aldana DK, Rodriguez-Morales AJ (2020b) SARS-CoV-2: jumping the species barrier, lessons from SARS and MERS, its zoonotic spillover, transmission to humans, preventive and control measures and recent developments to counter this pandemic virus. Travel Med Infect Dis 37:101830. https://doi.org/10.20944/preprints202004.0011.v1

Dhama K, Sharun K, Tiwari R, Dadar M, Malik YS, Singh KP, Chaicumpa W (2020c) COVID-19, an emerging coronavirus infection: advances and prospects in designing and developing vaccines, immunotherapeutics, and therapeutics. Hum Vaccin Immunother 16(6):1–7. https://doi.org/10.1080/21645515.2020.1735227

Dong E, Du H, Gardner L (2020) An interactive web-based dashboard to track COVID-19 in real time. Lancet Infect Dis S1473-3099(20):30120–30121. https://doi.org/10.1016/S1473-3099(20)30120-1

Duan K, Liu B, Li C, Zhang H, Yu T, Qu J, Zhou M, Chen L, Meng S, Hu Y, Peng C (2020) Effectiveness of convalescent plasma therapy in severe COVID-19 patients. Proc Natl Acad Sci 117(17):9490–9496

Ektorp E (2020) Death threats after a trial on chloroquine for COVID-19. Lancet Infect Dis 20(6):661. https://doi.org/10.1016/S1473-3099(20)30383-2. Erratum in: Lancet Infect Dis 2020 Aug;20(8):e180. PMID: 32473139; PMCID: PMC7255234

Ella KM, Mohan VK (2020) Coronavirus vaccines: light at the end of the tunnel. Indian Pediatr 15:S097475591600163

Gao J, Tian Z, Yang X (2020a) Breakthrough: chloroquine phosphate has shown apparent efficacy in treatment of COVID-19 associated pneumonia in clinical studies. Biosci Trends 14(1):72–73

Gao Q, Bao L, Mao H et al (2020b) Development of an inactivated vaccine candidate for SARS-CoV-2. Science 369(6499):77–81

Harypursat V, Chen YK (2020) Six weeks into the 2019 Coronavirus disease (COVID-19) outbreak- it is time to consider strategies to impede the emergence of new zoonotic infections. Chin Med J 133:1118. https://doi.org/10.1097/CM9.0000000000000760

Hellewell J, Abbott S, Gimma A, Bosse NI, Jarvis CI, Russell TW, Munday JD, Kucharski AJ, Edmunds WJ, Centre for the Mathematical Modelling of Infectious Diseases COVID-19 Working Group, Funk S, Eggo RM (2020) Feasibility of controlling COVID-19 outbreaks by isolation of cases and contacts. Lancet Glob Health 8(4):e488–e488. https://doi.org/10.1016/S2214-109X(20)30074-7

Heymann DL, Shindo N, WHO Scientific and Technical Advisory Group for Infectious Hazards (2020) COVID-19: what is next for public health? Lancet 395(10224):542–545. https://doi.org/10.1016/S0140-6736(20)30374-3

Hoffmann M, Kleine-Weber H, Schroeder S, Krüger N, Herrler T, Erichsen S, Schiergens TS, Herrler G, Wu NH, Nitsche A, Müller MA, Drosten C, Pöhlmann S (2020) SARS-CoV-2 cell entry depends on ACE2 and TMPRSS2 and is blocked by a clinically proven protease inhibitor. Cell 181(2):271–280.e8. https://doi.org/10.1016/j.cell.2020.02.052. Epub 2020 Mar 5. PMID: 32142651; PMCID: PMC7102627

Huang C, Wang Y, Li X, Ren L, Zhao J, Hu Y, Zhang L, Fan G, Xu J, Gu X, Cheng Z, Yu T, Xia J, Wei Y, Wu W, Xie X, Yin W, Li H, Liu M, Xiao Y, Gao H, Guo L, Xie J, Wang G, Jiang R, Gao Z, Jin Q, Wang J, Cao B (2020) Clinical features of patients infected with 2019 novel coronavirus in Wuhan, China. Lancet 395(10223):497–506

Jackson LA, Anderson EJ, Rouphael NG et al (2020) An mRNA vaccine against SARS-CoV-2: preliminary report. N Engl J Med 383(20):1920–1931

Jawhara S (2020) Could intravenous immunoglobulin collected from recovered coronavirus patients protect against COVID-19 and strengthen the immune system of new patients? Int J Mol Sci 21(7):2272

Jones BM, Ma ESK, Peiris JSM, Wong PC, Ho JCM, Lam B, Lai KN, Tsang KWT (2004) Prolonged disturbances of in vitro cytokine production in patients with severe acute respiratory syndrome (SARS) treated with ribavirin and steroids. Clin Exp Immunol 135(3):467–473

Kaye R, Chang CWD, Kazahaya K et al (2020) COVID-19 anosmia reporting tool: initial findings. Otolaryngol Head Neck Surg 163(1):132–134

Kermali M, Khalsa RK, Pillai K et al (2020) The role of biomarkers in diagnosis of COVID-19: a systematic review. Life Sci 254:117788

Khamsi R (2020) If a coronavirus vaccine arrives, can the world make enough? Nature 580(7805):578–580

Kim YC, Dema B, Reyes-Sandoval A (2020) COVID-19 vaccines: breaking record times to first-in-human trials. NPJ Vaccines 5:34. https://doi.org/10.1038/s41541-020-0188-3

Kuba K, Imai Y, Rao S, Gao H, Guo F, Guan B, Huan Y, Yang P, Zhang Y, Deng W, Bao L, Zhang B, Liu G, Wang Z, Chappell M, Liu Y, Zheng D, Leibbrandt A, Wada T, Slutsky AS, Liu D, Qin C, Jiang C, Penninger JM (2005) A crucial role of angiotensin converting enzyme 2 (ACE2) in SARS coronavirus-induced lung injury. Nat Med 11(8):875–879. https://doi.org/10.1038/nm1267. Epub 2005 Jul 10. PMID: 16007097; PMCID: PMC7095783

Kumar A, Arora A, Sharma P et al (2020) Is diabetes mellitus associated with mortality and severity of COVID-19? A meta-analysis. Diabetes Metab Syndr 14(4):535–545

Kunutsor SK, Laukkanen JA (2020) Markers of liver injury and clinical outcomes in COVID-19 patients: a systematic review and meta-analysis. J Infect 82(1):159–198

Lagana SM, Kudose S, Iuga AC, Lee MJ, Fazlollahi L, Remotti HE, Del Portillo A, De Michele S, de Gonzalez AK, Saqi A, Khairallah P (2020) Hepatic pathology in patients dying of COVID-19: a series of 40 cases including clinical, histologic, and virologic data. Mod Pathol 33(11):2147–2155

Li G, De Clercq E (2020) Therapeutic options for the 2019 novel coronavirus (2019-nCoV). Nat Rev Drug Discov 19(3):149–150. https://doi.org/10.1038/d41573-020-00016-0

Li H, Liu SM, Yu XH, Tang SL, Tang CK (2020) Coronavirus disease 2019 (COVID-19): current status and future perspective. Int J Antimicrob Agents 55:105951

Marovich M, Mascola JR, Cohen MS (2020) Monoclonal antibodies for prevention and treatment of COVID-19. JAMA 324:131–132

Miller A, Reandelar MJ, Fasciglione K, Roumenova V, Li Y, Otazu GH (2020) Correlation between universal BCG vaccination policy and reduced morbidity and mortality for COVID-19: an epidemiological study. medRxiv

Mulligan MJ, Lyke KE, Kitchin N, et al (2020) The incidence and outcomes of COVID-19 in IBD patients: a rapid review and meta-analysis phase 1/2 study to describe the safety and immunogenicity of a COVID-19 RNA vaccine candidate (BNT162b1) in adults 18 to 55 years of age: interim report. medRxiv

Naudé W (2020) Artificial intelligence against COVID-19: an early review. IZA Paper No. 13110, pp 1–14

Ni Y, Alu A, Lei H, Wang Y, Wu M, Wei X (2021) Immunological perspectives on the pathogenesis, diagnosis, prevention and treatment of COVID-19. Mol Biomed 2(1):1. https://doi.org/10.1186/s43556-020-00015-y. Epub 2021 Jan 20. PMID: 34766001; PMCID: PMC7815329

Nikhat S, Fazil M (2020) Overview of Covid-19; its prevention and management in the light of Unani medicine. Sci Total Environ 728:138859

Obeid JS, Davis M, Turner M, Meystre SM, Heider PM, O'Bryan EC, Lenert LA (2020) An artificial intelligence approach to COVID-19 infection risk assessment in virtual visits: a case report. J Am Med Inform Assoc 27(8):1321–1325

Omrani AS, Saad MM, Baig K, Bahloul A, Abdul-Matin M, Alaidaroos AY, Almakhlafi GA, Albarrak MM, Memish ZA, Albarrak AM (2014) Ribavirin and interferon alfa-2a for severe Middle East respiratory syndrome coronavirus infection: a retrospective cohort study. Lancet Infect Dis 14(11):1090–1095. https://doi.org/10.1016/S1473-3099(14)70920-X

Ong EZ, Chan YFZ, Leong WY, Lee NMY, Kalimuddin S, Haja Mohideen SM, Chan KS, Tan AT, Bertoletti A, Ooi EE, Low JGH (2020) A dynamic immune response shapes COVID-19 progression. Cell Host Microbe 27(6):879–882.e2. https://doi.org/10.1016/j.chom.2020.03.021. Epub 2020 Apr 30. PMID: 32359396; PMCID: PMC7192089

Paraskevis D, Kostaki EG, Magiorkinis G, Panayiotakopoulos G, Sourvinos G, Tsiodras S (2020) Full-genome evolutionary analysis of the novel corona virus (2019-nCoV) rejects the hypothesis of emergence as a result of a recent recombination event. Infect Genet Evol 79:104212. https://doi.org/10.1016/j.meegid.2020.104212

Pathak M, Patel SK, Rana J, Tiwari R, Dhama K, Sah R, Rabaan AA, Bonilla-aldana K, Rodriguez-Morales AJ (2020) Global threat of SARS-CoV-2/COVID-19 and the need for more and better diagnostic tools. Arch Med Res 51:450. https://doi.org/10.1016/j.arcmed.2020.04.003

Patrì A, Fabbrocini G (2020) Hydroxychloroquine and ivermectin: a synergistic combination for COVID-19 chemoprophylaxis and/or treatment? J Am Acad Dermatol S0190-9622(20):30557–30550. https://doi.org/10.1016/j.jaad.2020.04.017

Petropoulos G (2020) Artificial intelligence in the fight against COVID-19. Bruegel (23 march)

Pranata R, Lim MA, Huang I et al (2020) Hypertension is associated with increased mortality and severity of disease in COVID-19 pneumonia: a systematic review, meta-analysis and meta-regression. J Renin-Angiotensin-Aldosterone Syst 21(2):1470320320926899

Qian X, Ren R, Wang Y, Guo Y, Fang J, Wu ZD, Liu PL, Han TR, Members of Steering Committee, Society of Global Health, Chinese Preventive Medicine Association (2020) Fighting against the common enemy of COVID-19: a practice of building a community with a shared future for mankind. Infect Dis Poverty 9(1):34. https://doi.org/10.1186/s40249-020-00650-1

Quin C, Zhou L, Hu Z, Zhang S, Yang S, Tao Y (2020) Dysregulation of immune response in patients with COVID-19 in Wuhan, China. Clin Infect Dis 248:1–7

Rabaan AA, Al-Ahmed SH, Sah R, Tiwari R, Yatoo MI, Patel SK, Pathak M, Malik YS, Dhama K, Singh KP, Bonilla-Aldana DK, Haque S, Rodriguez-Morales AJ (2020) SARS-CoV-2/COVID-19 and advances in developing potential therapeutics and vaccines to counter this emerging pandemic virus: a review. Ann Clin Microbiol Antimicrob 19(1):40

Rajendran K, Narayanasamy K, Rangarajan J et al (2020) Convalescent plasma transfusion for the treatment of COVID-19: systematic review. J Med Virol 92(9):1475–1483

Riegler LL, Jones GP, Lee DW (2019) Current approaches in the grading and management of cytokine release syndrome after chimeric antigen receptor T-cell therapy. Ther Clin Risk Manag 15:323–335. https://doi.org/10.2147/TCRM.S150524. PMID: 30880998; PMCID: PMC6400118

Riou J, Althaus CL (2020) Pattern of early human-to-human transmission of Wuhan 2019 novel coronavirus (2019-nCoV), December 2019 to January 2020. Euro Surveill 25(4):2000058. https://doi.org/10.2807/1560-7917.ES.2020.25.4.2000058. Erratum in: euro Surveill. 2020 Feb;25(7)

Rodriguez-Morales AJ, Bonilla-Aldana DK, Balbin-Ramon GJ, Rabaan AA, Sah R, Paniz-Mondolfi A, Pagliano P, Esposito S (2020) History is repeating itself, a probable zoonotic spillover as a cause of an epidemic: the case of 2019 novel coronavirus. Infez Med 28(1):3–5

Rothe C, Schunk M, Sothmann P, Bretzel G, Froeschl G, Wallrauch C, Zimmer T, Thiel V, Janke C, Guggemos W, Seilmaier M, Drosten C, Vollmar P, Zwirglmaier K, Zange S, Wolfel R, Hoelscher M (2020) Transmission of 2019-nCoV infection from an asymptomatic contact in Germany. N Engl J Med 382:970–971. https://doi.org/10.1056/NEJMc2001468

Russell CD, Millar JE, Baillie JK (2020) Clinical evidence does not support corticosteroid treatment for 2019-nCoV lung injury. Lancet 395(10223):473–475. https://doi.org/10.1016/S0140-6736(20)30317-2. Epub 2020 Feb 7. PMID: 32043983; PMCID: PMC7134694

Shakoory B, Carcillo JA, Chatham WW, Amdur RL, Zhao H, Dinarello CA, Cron RQ, Opal SM (2016) Interleukin-1 receptor blockade is associated with reduced mortality in sepsis patients with features of macrophage activation syndrome: reanalysis of a prior phase III trial. Crit Care Med 44(2):275–281. https://doi.org/10.1097/CCM.0000000000001402. PMID: 26584195; PMCID: PMC5378312

Shanes ED, Mithal LB, Otero S, Azad HA, Miller ES, Goldstein JA (2020) Placental pathology in COVID-19. Am J Clin Pathol 154(1):23–32

Singh AK, Singh R (2020) Does poor glucose control increase the severity and mortality in patients with diabetes and COVID-19? Diabetes Metab Syndr 14(5):725–727

Singhai T (2020) A review of the coronavirus disease-2019. Indian J Pediatr 87:281–286

Somers EC, Eschenauer GA, Troost JP et al (2020) Tocilizumab for treatment of mechanically ventilated patients with COVID-19. Clin Infect Dis 73(2):e445–e454

Tang X, Wu C, Li X, Song Y, Yao X, Wu X, Duan Y, Zhang H, Wang Y, Qian Z, Cui J, Lu J (2020) On the origin and continuing evolution of SARS-CoV-2. Natl Sci Rev 7(6):1012–1023

Taylor PC (2019) Clinical efficacy of launched JAK inhibitors in rheumatoid arthritis. Rheumatology (Oxford) 58(Suppl 1):i17–i26. https://doi.org/10.1093/rheumatology/key225. PMID: 30806707; PMCID: PMC6390878

Thompson R (2020) Pandemic potential of 2019-nCoV. Lancet Infect Dis 20(3):280. https://doi.org/10.1016/S1473-3099(20)30068-2

Ting DSW, Carin L, Dzau V, Wong TY (2020) Digital technology and COVID-19. Nat Med 26(4): 459–461

Titanji BK, Farley MM, Mehta A, Connor-Schuler R, Moanna A, Cribbs SK, O'Shea J, DeSilva K, Chan B, Edwards A, Gavegnano C, Schinazi RF, Marconi VC (2021) Use of Baricitinib in patients with moderate to severe coronavirus disease 2019. Clin Infect Dis 72(7):1247–1250

Vaishya R, Javaid M, Khan IH, Haleem A (2020) Artificial intelligence (AI) applications for COVID-19 pandemic. Diabetes Metab Syndr Clin Res Rev 14:337

Vashist SK (2020) In vitro diagnostic assays for COVID-19: recent advances and emerging trends. Diagnostics (Basel) 10(4):E202. https://doi.org/10.3390/diagnostics10040202

Wilder-Smith A, Freedman DO (2020) Isolation, quarantine, social distancing and community containment: pivotal role for old-style public health measures in the novel coronavirus (2019-nCoV) outbreak. J Travel Med 27(2):taaa020. https://doi.org/10.1093/jtm/taaa020

Wrapp D, Wang N, Corbett KS, Goldsmith JA, Hsieh CL, Abiona O, Graham BS, McLellan JS (2020) Cryo-EM structure of the 2019-nCoV spike in the prefusion conformation. Science 367(6483):1260–1263. https://doi.org/10.1126/science.abb2507. Epub 2020 Feb 19. PMID: 32075877; PMCID: PMC7164637

Wu F, Zhao S, Yu B, Chen YM, Wang W, Hu Y, Song ZG, Tao ZW, Tian JH, Pei YY, et al (2020) Complete genome characterisation of a novel coronavirus associated with severe human respiratory disease in Wuhan, China China. BioRxiv

Xu X, Han M, Li T, Sun W, Wang D, Fu B, Zhou Y, Zheng X, Yang Y, Li X, Zhang X, Pan A, Wei H (2020) Effective treatment of severe COVID-19 patients with tocilizumab. Proc Natl Acad Sci U S A 117(20):10970–10975. https://doi.org/10.1073/pnas.2005615117. Epub 2020 Apr 29. PMID: 32350134; PMCID: PMC7245089

Yao X, Ye F, Zhang M, Cui C, Huang B, Niu P, Liu X, Zhao L, Dong E, Song C, Zhan S, Lu R, Li H, Tan W, Liu D (2020) *In vitro* antiviral activity and projection of optimized dosing design of hydroxychloroquine for the treatment of severe acute respiratory syndrome coronavirus 2 (SARS-CoV-2). Clin Infect Dis 71:ciaa237. https://doi.org/10.1093/cid/ciaa237

Yavuz S, Ünal S (2020) Antiviral treatment of COVID-19. Turk J Med Sci 50:611. https://doi.org/10.3906/sag-2004-145

Ye M, Fu D, Ren Y, Wang F, Wang D, Zhang F, Xia X, Lv T (2020) Treatment with convalescent plasma for COVID-19 patients in Wuhan, China. J Med Virol 92:1890

Yi C, Sun X, Ye J, Ding L, Liu M, Yang Z, Lu X, Zhang Y, Ma L, Gu W, Qu A, Xu J, Shi Z, Ling Z, Sun B (2020) Key residues of the receptor binding motif in the spike protein of SARS-CoV-2 that interact with ACE2 and neutralizing antibodies. Cell Mol Immunol 17:621. https://doi.org/10.1038/s41423-020-0458-z

Yu L, S Wu, X Hao, X Li, X Liu, S Ye, H Han, X Dong, X Li, J Li, J Liu, N Liu, W Zhang, V Pelechano, W-H Chen, X Yin (2020). Rapid colorimetric detection of COVID-19 coronavirus using a reverse transcriptional loop-mediated isothermal amplification (RT-LAMP) diagnostic plat-form: Ilaco. medRxiv. doi: https://doi.org/10.1101/2020.02.20.20025874

Zhang N, Wang L, Deng X, Liang R, Su M, He C et al (2020a) Recent advances in the detection of respiratory virus infection in humans. J Med Virol 92(4):408–417

Zhang J, Zeng H, Gu J, Li H, Zheng L, Zou Q (2020b) Progress and prospects on vaccine development against SARS-CoV-2. Vaccines (Basel) 8(2):E153. https://doi.org/10.3390/vaccines8020153

Zhang J, Zhou L, Yang Y, Peng W, Wang W, Chen X (2020c) Therapeutic and triage strategies for 2019 novel coronavirus disease in fever clinics. Lancet Respir Med 8(3):e11–e12

Zhang W, Du R-H, Li B, Zheng X-S, Yang X-L, Hu B et al (2020d) Molecular and serological investigation of 2019-nCoV infected patients: implication of multiple shedding routes. Emerg Microbes Infect 9(1):386–389

Zhang F, Abudayyeh OO and Jonathan SG (2020e) A protocol for detection of COVID-19 using CRISPR diagnostics. (v.20200321)

Zhao M (2020) Cytokine storm and immunomodulatory therapy in COVID-19: role of chloroquine and anti-IL-6 monoclonal antibodies. Int J Antimicrob Agents 55(6):105982. https://doi.org/10.1016/j.ijantimicag.2020.105982. Epub 2020 Apr 16. PMID: 32305588; PMCID: PMC7161506

Zheng J (2020) SARS-CoV-2: an emerging coronavirus that causes a global threat. Int J Biol Sci 16(10):1678–1685. https://doi.org/10.7150/ijbs.45053

Zhong J, Tang J, Ye C, Dong L (2020) The immunology of COVID-19: is immune modulation an option for treatment? Lancet Rheumatol 2(7):e428–e436. https://doi.org/10.1016/S2665-9913(20)30120-X. Epub 2020 May 20. PMID: 32835246; PMCID: PMC7239618

Zhou D, Dai SM, Tong Q (2020) COVID-19: a recommendation to examine the effect of hydroxychloroquine in preventing infection and progression. J Antimicrob Chemother 75:dkaa114. https://doi.org/10.1093/jac/dkaa114

Zhu N, Zhang D, Wang W, Li X, Yang B, Song J, Zhao X, Huang B, Shi W, Lu R, Niu P, Zhan F, Ma X, Wang D, Xu W, Wu G, Gao GF, Tan W (2020) China novel coronavirus investigating and research team. A novel coronavirus from patients with pneumonia in China, 2019. N Engl J Med 382(8):727–733. https://doi.org/10.1056/NEJMoa2001017

Ziegler HK, Unanue ER (1982) Decrease in macrophage antigen catabolism caused by ammonia and chloroquine is associated with inhibition of antigen presentation to T cells. Proc Natl Acad Sci U S A 79(1):175–178. https://doi.org/10.1073/pnas.79.1.175. PMID: 6798568; PMCID: PMC345685

Immunopathology of Parasitic Diseases of Animals

16

Key Points

1. Cell-mediated immune responses regulate the intracellular protozoal infections, whereas antibody-mediated immune responses guard against external protozoa.
2. Immune responses against helminths are mainly due to the production of parasite antigen-specific IgE antibodies by B cells in response to IL-4 stimulation by Th2 cells, and interaction mast cells could lead to release of preformed granules and cytokines (IL-4, IL-5, IL-9, IL-10, and IL-13).
3. T and B lymphocytes are the representative cells of adaptive immunity against parasites.
4. Eosinophilia is a classical sign of helminth infection.
5. Immunological molecules like GM-CSF, IL-2, IFN-γ, and epithelial growth factor can enhance the multiplication and pathogenesis of *Leishmania amazonensis* and *Trypanosoma brucei*.
6. Coccidial protozoa are extremely host specific.
7. Some parasites like *Trypanosoma* may evade from the humoral and cellular adaptive immune effector mechanisms of their host to allow for reproduction.
8. Intestinal epithelial cells and goblet cells play a role in the helminth removal from the intestine.

16.1 Introduction

Mostly, parasites can cause damage to the host and produces disease directly (e.g., *Fasciola*) and/or indirectly due to host reaction. Predominantly, excessive number of parasites cause disease by exploiting the nutrition of the host. Limited number of parasites cause mild depletion of nutrition without causing harm to the host or triggering effective immune responses. Some parasites escape from the host immune system. Mostly, parasitic infections including helminths and protozoal infections cause production losses. Immunological molecules like granulocyte-macrophage colony-stimulating factor (GM-CSF) and interleukin-2 (IL-2) can enhance the multiplication and pathogenesis of *Leishmania amazonensis*, and interferon-gamma (IFN-γ) and epithelial growth factor can promote the multiplication and pathogenesis of *Trypanosoma brucei*. Helminthic infestations cause eosinophilia and it induces cytokines, which are responsible for the significant inflammatory responses. The pathology and protective immunity to most of the helminths and protozoal infections are believed to be caused by T lymphocytes, B lymphocytes, mast cells and macrophages. Infections with helminth parasites induce immune effector mechanisms resulting in IgE antibody production, tissue and peripheral blood eosinophilia, and infiltration of inflammatory mediator–rich tissue mast cells. Further, these responses can also induce pathologic reactions, in addition to mediating the protective immunity to the helminth parasites.

16.2 Innate Immunity Against Parasites

The innate immune responses against parasites are similar to that of bacterial and viral infections. However, parasitic species and host species play a major role in the disease induction. For example, *Trypanosoma brucei*, *T. congolense*, and *T. vivax* do not cause disease in the wild ungulates, but these cause severe disease and death in domestic cattle. Likewise, coccidia are extremely host specific; for example, *Eimeria necatrix* and *E. tenella* are most pathogenic in chickens and not in cattle. Pathogenicity is influenced by species of the parasites, host species, age and genetics of the host, breed, nutritional status, and concurrent diseases. African breed of cattle N'Dama is resistant to pathogenic trypanosome infections (trypanotolerance), which results in selection of resistant animals over many generations leading to control of infections and production losses. Increased IL-4 and immunoglobulin G (IgG) and less IL-6 production levels and increased response of γ/δ T cells to trypanosome antigens in the N'Dama cattle than non-native or susceptible cattle are responsible for trypanotolerant animals. Trypanotolerant animals produce high levels of IgG against *T. congolense* cysteine protease. Since this enzyme contributes to the pathology of infection, and these antibodies may partially account for their tolerance.

16.3 Parasites Recognition

The pathogen-associated molecular patterns (PAMPs) are recognized by pattern recognition receptors (PRRs) of various types, which have been reported among human parasitic diseases, but none has been described that is exclusive to parasites, i.e., those receptors are also engaged by other organisms (McGuinness et al. 2003; Male et al. 2007). Some extracellular receptors have been linked to the identification of parasites among the PRRs family. For example, *Plasmodium falciparum* proteins on the infected erythrocytes (Klabunde et al. 2002; Garred et al. 2003), mannose-binding lectin (MBL) (Turner 1996) binds mannose-rich lipophosphoglycan (LPG) from *Leishmania* (Green et al. 1994; Ambrosio and de Messias-Reason 2005), and C-reactive protein (CRP) binds to Leishmania LPG molecules and enhances parasite entry into macrophages by opsonization (Culley et al. 1996).

In addition, Toll-like receptors (TLRs) are a type of PRRs that play a role in innate immunity against infections (Akira et al. 2006). The TLR-2 on dendritic cells (DCs) and its interaction with *Schistosoma mansoni* lysophosphatidylserine induce a Th2 response. Binding of glycophosphatidylinositol (GPI) from *Trypanosoma cruzi* with TLR-2 stimulates Th1 responses (McGuinness et al. 2003). The TLR appears to activate the synthesis of tumor necrosis factor-alpha (TNF-α) by macrophages via GPI anchor proteins from *T. cruzi*, *P. falciparum*, and *Toxoplasma gondii* (Denkers et al. 2004). The TLR activation has also been suggested as a possible cause of some immunopathology linked with parasite infections, such as anemia and nephritis produced by autoantibodies in malaria (Daniel-Ribeiro and Zanini 2000).

16.4 Adaptive Immunity to Parasites

The T and B lymphocytes are the representative cells of adaptive immunity against diseases, including parasites. Depending on the stimulus, naïve CD4+ T cells can differentiate into either Th1 or Th2 cells, and they produce their characteristic cytokines. These cytokines activate different effector cells depending on the Th phenotype, which then generate more Th-response specific cytokines and chemokines (Brenier-Pinchart et al. 2001; Dixon et al. 2006; Teixeira et al. 2006). Protective responses against protozoa (mostly intracellular) are often carried out by Th1 and are mediated predominantly by IFN-γ; however, helminths, which are extracellular organisms, require Th2 responses, and the important cytokines include IL-4, IL-5, and IL-13 (Chen et al. 2002; Meresse and Cerf-Bensussan 2009).

16.5 Protozoa Induced Adaptive Immunity

Interferons production by $CD4^+$ T cells, as well as $CD8^+$ T cells, leads to the activation of effector mechanisms that successfully eradicate the parasites through macrophage stimulation to destroy the phagocytosed parasites (e.g., *T. cruzi*) (Teixeira et al. 2006). This feature is essential because many protozoa, such as *Toxoplasma* (Morisaki et al. 1995) and *Leishmania* (Suzuki et al. 2002; Handman and Bullen 2002), bypass humoral defense by invading within macrophages. Interferons enhance the expression of MHC-I and MHC-II molecules, which help $CD8^+$ cytotoxic T cells to recognize and eliminate the intracellular protozoa and cross presentation to $CD4^+$ T cells (Handman and Bullen 2002). The role of $CD8^+$ T lymphocytes in Chagas disease is also important to control the infection (Miyahira et al. 1999). *T. cruzi* infection has been suggested as a model for $CD8^+$ T cell-mediated vaccine development against intracellular infections (Miyahira 2008). Antibodies are produced in response to all protozoal infections, even though they do not appear to be the predominant control mechanism in parasite diseases with intracellular stages. On the other hand, antibody production appears to play a key role in African trypanosomiasis, owing to the fact that *T. brucei* is an extracellular parasite (Magez et al. 2008). Although IgM levels are high in African trypanosomes, IgG play a critical role in infection management than IgM. Different subclasses of IgG are produced at each stage of infection due to the presence of variable surface glycoprotein or variant surface glycoprotein (VSG) (Black et al. 1982; Sendashonga and Black 1982; Diffley 1985).

Other anti-protozoal immune mechanisms include direct lysis of protozoa through antibodies, which were observed in *T. cruzi* infection (Gazzinelu et al. 1991) and complement mediated destruction in *Plasmodium* gametocytes (Healer et al. 1997) or *T. cruzi* trypomastigotes (Almeida et al. 1991). Further, antibodies assist macrophages and other phagocytic cells with Fc receptors to phagocytose parasites, resulting in better parasite clearance, for example, phagocytosis of *P. falciparum*-infected erythrocytes through macrophages (Kumaratilake et al. 1997; Tebo et al. 2002).

16.6 Helminths Induced Adaptive Immunity

Helminths are large extracellular parasites, and the immune response against these pathogens is exerted through differentiation of Th2 cells and their cytokines (IL-4, IL-5, IL-9, IL-10, and IL-13) (Kopf et al. 1993). Immune responses against helminths include the production of parasite antigen-specific IgE antibodies by B cells in response to IL-4 stimulation, which is mostly generated by Th2 cells. Interaction of IgE and mast cells could lead to activation and release of preformed cytoplasmic granules (e.g., histamine). These released chemical mediators can expel the GI helminths through increased mucus production and peristaltic activity (Maizels and Holland 1998; Abass et al. 2007).

Eosinophilia is a classical sign of helminth parasitic disease (Leder and Weller 2000). But, still the exact role of eosinophils in these infections is not yet clarified. The IL-4 and IL-13 (Mochizuki et al. 1998; Fallon et al. 2000), as well as other chemokines including eotaxin (Rankin et al. 2000; Mir et al. 2006) and RANTES (Cooper et al. 2000), circulate in the bloodstream and attract eosinophils to parasitic infection sites. Other immunoglobulins, such as IgG or IgA, which behave as opsonin, can bind to Fc receptors on eosinophils and promote degranulation (Capron et al. 1981; Bracke et al. 2000; Woerly et al. 2004). Destruction of opsonized parasites was carried out by cytoplasmic granules like lysosomal hydrolases, eosinophil peroxidase or specific eosinophil proteases such as major basic protein (MBP), and eosinophil cationic protein (Glauert and Butterworth 1977; Butterworth et al. 1979; Specht et al. 2006). Eosinophilia is more chronic in helminth infections with tissue migration in their life cycle, such as *Ascaris lumbricoides* or *Trichinella spiralis*. Phenotypic modification of macrophage is another feature of Th2 responses against helminths. Classical macrophage phenotype was modified into "alternatively activated macrophages" (Rodríguez-Sosa et al. 2002), and these changes are induced by Th2 cells-mediated cytokines (IL-4 and IL-13). This modified phenotype differs from other classical macrophages by (1) increased expression of mannose receptors, (2) synthesis of arginase-1, (3) inhibition of nitric oxide synthase (iNOS), and (4) collagen deposition (Stein et al. 1992; Goerdt and Orfanos 1999; Stempin et al. 2009).

Intestinal epithelial cells and goblet cells are two other cells that play a role in helminth removal in the intestine. It has been demonstrated that epithelial cell turnover was enhanced during the immunological responses in order to aid intestinal helminths clearance (Cliffe et al. 2005). Goblet cell hyperplasia may contribute to worms expulsion through increased production of mucin (Nawa et al. 1994; McKenzie et al. 1998). Several studies identified the upregulation of intestinal epithelial cells (Pemberton et al. 2004) and goblet cells (Knight et al. 2004) specific genes. Increased expression of intelectin genes can enhance their secretion, and it favors to expel parasites by binding to parasite surface residues (Pemberton et al. 2004). The REsistin-like molecule (RELM), which is produced mostly by goblet cells, is thought to be involved in intestinal helminth evacuation (Artis et al. 2004).

The regulatory T-cell (Treg) population is another T-cell subset that has gained attention in chronic helminth infections. Treg cells restrict the Th2 responses and regulate the tissue damage produced by Th2-mediated immune responses (van Riet et al. 2007). In *S. mansoni* and protozoa, such as Leishmania, these Treg cells appear to be important in limiting the pathology generated by Th2 immune responses to parasites (Aseffa et al. 2002; Hesse et al. 2004). The IL-10 has been shown to modulate immunoregulation during parasitic infections like filariasis and schistosomiasis and protozoal infections like leishmaniasis and toxoplasmosis (King et al. 1996; Mahanty et al. 1997). Natural Treg and other cells, such as DCs or conventional T and B lymphocytes, produce IL-10. During parasite infections, T regulatory type 1 (Tr1) cells are the key source of IL-10 cytokine, although it is produced from other cells, such as DCs or conventional T and B lymphocytes (Doetze et al. 2000; Mills and McGuirk 2004). It has been postulated that Treg-mediated immunoregulatory response aids in protective role against exaggerated Th2 responses mediated allergic reactions (Maizels 2005; Wilson et al. 2005).

16.7 Evasion of Immune Responses by Parasites

Parasites can bypass humoral and cellular adaptive immune effector mechanisms. The fact that helminth parasites may survive for long periods of time inside mammalian host suggests that they have developed complex strategies to avoid the cytotoxic effects of immune systems. Complement system (soluble factor) existing in the host confronts a first line of defense against extracellular parasites. Inactivation of the alternative complement pathway at various enzyme levels is the most common strategy adopted by parasites to evade the complement-mediated death. Complement inactivation by *T. cruzi* is achieved by acquiring complement regulatory proteins fixed to their surface, such as glycoproteins like decay-accelerating factor (DAF) proteins in host cells, which speed up the dissociation of the C3/C4b convertase (Beucher and Norris 2008). Blocking of membrane attack complex (MAC) proteins

(C5–C9) or preventing pore formation by some alternative ways of parasites avoids complement-mediated lysis (Farkas et al. 2002).

Another well-studied soluble mediator, which avoids parasites to penetrate inside the host, is trypanosome lytic factor (TLF) or trypanolytic factor. It is present in the human serum, which protects primates against infection by *T. brucei* (Lugli et al. 2004). Intracellular adaptation is another important mechanism exerted by the parasites to escape from the serum component recognition. Parasites have evolved many methods to avoid being killed by the lysosomal hydrolytic environment. *T. gondii* and *Leishmania* parasites have the potential to shift cellular compartmentalization to prevent the union of parasitophorous vacuoles (PV) with endosomes or lysosomes (Mordue et al. 1999; Dermine et al. 2000).

Intracellular parasites can also impede phagocytic processes by affecting the reactive oxygen species-mediated elimination. Through suppression of enzymes involved in the process, the malarial pigment hemozoin has been shown to perform as a strong regulator of macrophage oxidative phagocytic function (Carney et al. 2006).

Many parasites, such as *T. cruzi* have been reported to impede DCs activation. *T. cruzi* penetration inside the DCs worsens their activation process and reduction in TNF-α and IL-12 upregulation. Antigenic shift allows *P. falciparum* and African trypanosomes parasites to avoid being recognized by circulating antibodies, allowing them to escape from humoral responses (Van Overtvelt et al. 1999).

16.8 Trichomoniasis

The most important Tritrichomonas species is *Tritrichomonas foetus*, which is the primary cause of bovine venereal tritrichomonas, an infection spread through sexually and can cause infertility and abortion. The *T. foetus* is a flagellate protozoan parasite and the normal host for *T. foetus* is cattle (*Bos taurus* and *B. indicus*). Major routes of transmission are spread from asymptomatic bulls to cows at the time of coitus or by artificial insemination using contaminated semen. Normally in bulls, infection persists for years without clinical signs. The protozoa are frequently found in the preputial cavity and occasionally found in the deeper portions of the urogenital system. The parasites invade and colonize the vagina, uterus, and oviduct after infecting the cows. Transient or permanent infertility may occur as a result of endometritis and uterine catarrh. If conception takes place, abortion typically occurs early in pregnancy (6–16 weeks).

Cows typically recover from their infection and develop immunity, at least throughout that particular breeding season. Studies on the immune responses to *T. foetus* infection in bulls are scarce. Young animals are more resistant to infection due to the microscopic structure of the lining of the penis and foreskin rather than effective immune responses. The immunological responses against *T. foetus* can be effectively developed in females. The parasite causes a mild inflammatory reaction associated with the abortion. An immunological system mediates the inflammation, which frequently eliminates the infection. This immune system most likely fails in carrier cows, which maintains the infection in the herd. Bovine females respond to the initial *T. foetus* infection by producing IgG and IgA immunoglobulins locally in the cervico-vaginal mucus produced by the uterus. Elimination of infection is probably mediated by the specific immunoglobulins, since the organism is an extracellular parasite. Monoclonal antibodies cause agglutination and complement-mediated lysis, which prevents the protozoa from adhering to vaginal epithelial cells and facilitates the phagocytosis of *T. foetus* by monocytes. The combination of specific anti-*T. foetus* antibodies and complement enhances the killing the parasites by polymorphonuclear leukocytes.

Bovine immune sera and monoclonal antibodies targeted against *T. foetus* surface epitopes are the main mechanisms of complement-dependent killing of the parasite in vitro. By colonizing in the female reproductive tract, which serves as a niche where only modest levels of complement are present, *T. foetus* is able to evade from the host immunological defenses. Bovine immunoglobulins can be cleaved by extracellular and membrane-bound cysteine proteinases from *T. foetus*. The *T. foetus* proteinases effectively cleaved the IgG1 and IgG2, which have been shown to kill *T. foetus* in vitro via complement-mediated and independent immune effector mechanisms result in the clearance of the parasite in vivo. However, IgA was either little or not at all proteolyzed in vitro. The binding and internalization of antibodies on the surface of parasites is the another potential defense strategy against the immune responses of host. The non-specific binding and exposition of IgG on the surface of *T. foetus* may be a key molecular mimicry strategy for the masking of parasite antigens. Additionally, it was proposed that *T. foetus* exhibits antigenic variation as a potentially significant method of immune evasion. The antigenic variation of the protective superficial antigen TF1.17 served as the basis for this hypothesis. Animals that recovered from a *T. foetus* infection exhibited some degree of temporary resistance to re-infection. Since *T. foetus* is mostly found in the lumen of reproductive organs and on the surface of the mucosal tissues of its host in adult cattle, it can be hypothesized that the mucosal immune system is crucial in recognizing and combating the *T. foetus* infection.

16.9 Neosporosis

Neospora caninum is an apicomplexan protozoan infection that causes significant economic losses in cattle through abortions. Worldwide, *N. caninum* is a significant contributor of abortion and reproductive failure in cattle. The most common route of *N. caninum* infection appears to be transplacental (vertical) transfer of the parasite from mother to fetus, which can lead to abortion or the birth of clinically normal but persistently infected offspring. An important factor in determining the transplacental transfer of parasites to the fetus and subsequent abortion in cattle is the immunological responses or immunomodulation seen during pregnancy. Experimental *N. caninum* tachyzoites infection in heifers by intravenous route at 110 days of gestation showed cytokine gene expressions at the materno-fetal interface. Real-time RT-PCR analysis of infected heifers revealed increased Th1, Th2, and Treg cytokine gene expressions in the maternal (caruncle) and fetal (cotyledon) placentas. The IFN-γ, IL-12p40, IL-6, and IL-10 were elevated in the caruncle; whereas, cotyledon showed upregulated expression of IFN-γ and downregulation of TGF-β. This cytokine production pattern was linked to live transplacentally infected fetuses, suggesting a protective effect for fetus survival; however, it could have a role in the transplacental transmission of parasites. The key to understanding the process of abortion and/or transplacental transmission to the fetus may lie in the immunological control of the parasite in the placenta or by the fetus. Furthermore, it is still unknown that why some infected animals abort and others not.

Cell-mediated immunity is crucial in preventing *N. caninum* proliferation and lowering parasitemia. The Th1 cytokines including IFN-γ and IL-12 are known to play the significant protective immunological responses against *N. caninum* in pregnant cattle. The IFN-γ is produced as a result of the Th1 immune responses at the materno-fetal interface, which is characterized by the infiltrations of CD4+ T cells, γδ-T cells, macrophages, and NK cells. Strong Th1 cytokine responses are incompatible with a successful pregnancy and the survival of the fetus, but they have important consequences for pregnancy in cattle by causing destruction of the placental tissues. Pro-inflammatory Th1 responses during pregnancy protects the dam by significantly inhibiting the multiplication of *N. caninum* tachyzoites. The development of protective immune responses against the abortion during a second Neospora exposure in chronically infected cows has been shown. When cattle are first time infected with *N. caninum*, the likelihood of abortion is 3–7 times higher than that of subsequent pregnancies. Neosporosis affected animals are less likely to abort during subsequent pregnancies. This shows that after infection, certain level of protective immunity develops.

When compared to seronegative animals, the *N. caninum*-infected-aborted cows showed upregulated mRNA gene expression of pro-inflammatory Th1 cytokines such as IFN-γ, TNF-α, IL-4, IL-12p40, and Treg cytokine IL-10 in PBMCs and antigen-specific cell proliferation. Chronically infected cattle showed significantly greater levels of IFN-γ are essential for controlling infection and providing protection. Activation of the host immunological responses, including inflammatory pathways during *N. caninum* infection in cattle causes placental damage and abortion. It is not well known that whether water buffaloes are susceptible to neosporosis; however, vertical transmission and fetal death have been reported in buffaloes.

Although, the intracellular nature of *N. caninum* induces cell-mediated immune (CMI) responses in the host, which is probably crucial to protect the host and this response could also be the cause of placental damage leading to abortion. Cattle experimentally challenged with *N. caninum* on 70 days of gestation showed development of strong CMI responses in dams and fetuses, infiltrations of more numbers of immune cells, and increased levels of expression of IFN-γ mRNA in the placenta lead to fetal death and abortion.

16.10 Toxoplasmosis

Toxoplasma gondii is an apicomplexan protozoan that infects humans and other warm-blooded animals and birds worldwide. This intracellular parasite has a facultative, indirect life cycle, reproduce sexually in enterocytes of definitive host and asexually in nucleated cells of intermediate host. Felids are the only definitive host for *T. gondii*, which contaminates the environment with oocysts excreted in feces. The *T. gondii* has three infectious stages: (1) tachyzoites (rapidly multiplying form); (2) bradyzoites (slow division form present in tissue cysts); and (3) sporozoites (mature or sporulated oocysts). The *T. gondii* is transmitted by the consumption of infectious oocysts from the contaminated environment, or consumption of tissue cysts from the infected meat, and by transplacental transfer of tachyzoites from mother to fetus. The *T. gondii* replicates in the entero-epithelial tissues of unexposed felids after ingestion of uncooked tissues containing cysts. Bradyzoites are released from the tissue cysts after digestion in the stomach and small intestine, which invades the intestinal epithelium and undergoes the asexual and sexual replication, results in the release of oocysts (~10 mcm in diameter) in the feces.

The oocysts are first evident in the feces, 3 days after infection and may be released for up to 20 days. Oocysts sporulate (become infectious) outside the cat within 1–5 days, depending on the aeration and temperature, and remain viable in the environment for several months. Cats generally develop immunity to *T. gondii* after the initial infection, and they shed oocysts only once in their life-time; however, immunocompromised animals can re-shed oocysts. Felids are also intermediate host for extraintestinal asexual multiplication of the parasite, especially in the nervous system. Neurologic and ocular lesions can develop in immunocompromised and aged cats.

Tachyzoites are transmitted systemically and cause interstitial pneumonia, myocarditis, hepatic necrosis, meningoencephalomyelitis, chorioretinitis, lymphadenopathy, and myositis. The clinical signs include fever, diarrhea, cough, dyspnea, icterus, seizures, and death. *T. gondii* is also an important cause of abortion and stillbirth in sheep, goats, cervids, and sometimes pigs. After infection of pregnant ewes, tachyzoites are transmitted via the bloodstream to placental cotyledons and causing necrosis. Tachyzoites may also be transmitted to the fetus, causing necrosis in multiple organs. Finally, immunocompromised adult animals are extremely susceptible to acute generalized toxoplasmosis, which is manifested as neurologic and respiratory disorders. The immunocompromised individuals may develop generalized toxoplasmosis with multi-organ failure. The *T. gondii* may be transmitted vertically and produce fetal lesions and abortions.

Studies using the knock-out mice lacking B cells, CD4+ and CD8+ T cells, and cytokines showed a failure in the development of adaptive immune responses against toxoplasmosis. Extremely high concentrations of IFN-γ and IL-18 in mice cause lethal toxoplasmosis, whereas moderate concentrations of these cytokines result in non-lethal infection. Although, tumor necrosis factor (TNF-α) plays a significant role in toxoplasmosis resistance, excessive amounts of this cytokine may also contribute to pathogenesis. Increased vascular permeability is caused by the elevated levels of IL-18, IFN-γ, IL-12, and TNF-α, which can cause the multiple organ failure and death of the animal.

The ability of CD4+ and CD8+ T lymphocytes to produce IFN-γ, a pro-inflammatory cytokine that is known to be a key mediator of resistance to *T. gondii*, which are essential for the development of protective immunity and long-term survival during persistent infection. The IFN-γ production is necessary for the long-term survival, which was proved in mice by depleting this cytokine during the persistent phase of *T. gondii* infection. Extracellular tachyzoites can be destroyed in the presence of specific antibodies and complement pathway. Antibodies against *T. gondii* may also prevent the parasite from entering into the host cells. Dendritic cells (DCs), monocytes, and neutrophils are recruited to the site of infection after a *T. gondii* challenge, and these cell types have been implicated to resistance to this parasite. One of the most critical functions of the innate immune responses against *T. gondii* is to sense the parasite and produce the cytokine IL-12, which stimulates the NK cells and T cells to produce the cytokine IFN-γ. The IFN-γ is a major mediator of *T. gondii* resistance and promotes various intracellular processes to kill the parasite and prevent its replication. Mice deficient in either IL-12 or IFN-γ who are infected with *T. gondii* succumb to acute disease and showed an inability to control the intracellular parasite burden. This Th1 immune responses, defined by the production of IL-12 and IFN-γ, is characteristic of infection with many intracellular pathogens. The innate production of IL-12 during toxoplasmosis requires that the parasite first be sensed by the host. Toll-like receptors (TLRs) are the innate immune receptors, participate in this process.

Since neutrophils have pre-stored IL-12 and can release this cytokine in vitro and in vivo in response to *T. gondii*. Additionally, there are reports that neutrophil depletion causes IL-12 levels to drop and parasite replication to increase. Monocytes are crucial for toxoplasmosis resistance, as evidenced by the higher susceptibility of mice lacking the chemokine receptor CCR2 (CCR2 knock-out), which is required for the monocyte recruitment to the site of infection. Monocytes produce the cytokine IL-1 in response to soluble toxoplasma antigens, and this cytokine can enhance the anti-toxoplasmic effector mechanisms in macrophages and astrocytes in vitro. Furthermore, IL-1 and IL-12 can work together to stimulate the production of IFN-γ from the innate and adaptive responses. Another innate population involved in immunity to *T. gondii* is the NK cells, and in mice lacking T cells, provide a limited ability of resistance due to decreased production of IFN-γ. The NK cell activity is peak during early infection, and their activity is elevated during chronic toxoplasmosis, they do not appear to be significant contributor to immunity during the chronic stage of infection. The NK cells additionally produce the cytokine IL-10, in addition to IFN-γ. The NK cells can also stimulate the adaptive immune responses in body. They can therefore aid the CD8+ T cells response in the absence of CD4+ T cells. Increasing the synthesis of IL-12 from DCs through interactions with the molecule natural killer group 2D (NKG2D) is one way of assistance provided to CD8+ T cells. The increased susceptibility of human patients with primary or acquired defects in T cell function and mice with deficiencies in B cells, CD4+ T cells, or CD8+ T cells survive the acute stage of infection but

16.11 Fasciolosis

ultimately show increased susceptibility to *T. gondii*, showing the importance of adaptive immune responses for resistance to *T. gondii* during human infection.

16.11 Fasciolosis

Fasciolosis is mostly caused by the liver fluke *Fasciola hepatica* and affects sheep and cattle. Hepatic fascioliasis can be found in places where the climate is favorable for the survival of aquatic snails, which act as intermediate hosts for the parasites. These places are often low marshy environments. Adult *F. hepatica* parasites live in the biliary system, which are leaf-shaped. Their eggs pass through the bile from the digestive tract to the feces. Then, in the intermediate host snail, miracidium develops (genus *Lymnaea*). Cercariae come out from the snail, encyst and settle on vegetation, where they grow into infectious metacercariae. The ruminant host consumes metacercariae, which then pass through the wall of the duodenum to reach the peritoneal cavity and then the liver. Before settling inside the bile ducts, they move within the liver. Hemorrhagic tracts in the necrotic liver parenchyma are produced when immature flukes migrate across the liver. These tracts are grossly visible and are initially dark red during acute infection, they eventually become paler than the adjacent parenchyma. These migrations can cause a number of unfavorable sequelae, such as acute peritonitis, hepatic abscesses, and death of the host due to acute, widespread hepatic necrosis produced by a significant infiltration of immature flukes. Bacillary hemoglobinuria or infectious necrotic hepatitis is caused by the growth of *Clostridium haemolyticum* or *Clostridium novyi* spores in necrotic tissues, respectively.

Microscopically, concentric fibrosis, markedly thickened larger intrahepatic bile ducts, which are typically dilated and frequently with papillary projections of the biliary epithelium into the lumen. The ducts frequently have mild to moderate inflammatory infiltrations of neutrophils and macrophages, while the portal tracts have an infiltrate of neutrophils, lymphocytes, and plasma cells. Eosinophils are rarely found. When adult Fasciola ova lodge in affected tissues, trigger an inflammatory response, results in the development of granulomatous lesions of the liver, pancreas, intestines, and mesentery. Fasciolosis causes liver fibrosis, cirrhosis, cancer, and significant economic losses. An infection with the liver fluke results in the dominant Th2/T regulatory type immune responses, and it is well known for the modulating of the host immune responses through a number of mechanisms, such as alternate activation of macrophages and the production of immunosuppressive cytokines, increased stimulation of regulatory T cells, and the modulation of differentiation and function of dendritic cells. However, the immune responses to *F. gigantica* infection is a mix of Th1/Th2 response, with a Th2-biased pattern predominating.

Fasciola hepatica infection in lambs can induce dominant Th2-biased immune responses along with suppression of Th1/Th17 responses, and can negatively impact Th1 responses to bystander infections, such as during co-infection with *Mycobacterium tuberculosis*. Buffaloes can exhibit a combination of Th1 and Th2 cytokine expression patterns in response to *F. gigantica* infection. The development of local immune responses in the liver of large ruminants infected with *F. gigantica* is indicated by the infiltrations of T and B lymphocytes, plasma cells, eosinophils, and mast cells in hepatic lesions. This reaction was most likely brought on by the increased antigen load that the developing flukes were releasing. In addition, the continuous immune responses might be explained by tissue damage and the subsequent production of autoantigens. In bovine and bubaline *F. gigantica* infection, the T lymphocytes may aid and assist in selecting the particular antibody responses, in producing cell-mediated responses, and recruit and activate macrophages and granulocytes. The T cell responses in the liver of large ruminants displayed various patterns. While the quantity of T cells in buffaloes gradually increased, it started to decline in cattle after 3 weeks. This shows that there was increasing host responsiveness to the antigenic products released by the flukes and to the stimulus induced by the necrotic tissues in the liver in buffaloes; whereas, in cattle, the T cell responses may be depressed to a certain extent after 3 weeks. Proliferative responses of lymphocytes from sheep infected with *F. hepatica* to concanavalin A were reduced after 4 weeks of infection. *Fasciola gigantica* may have either inhibited the proliferation of T lymphocytes or suppressed the local cellular responses to a certain degree in cattle to facilitate their migration through the hepatic parenchyma. As leucocyte infiltration was hampered in sheep with fasciolosis, there may be a decrease of the local inflammatory and immunological responses in the infected liver to permit their migration across the hepatic parenchyma. The rapid migration of *F. hepatica* in goats was thought of as a possible mechanism of immune evasion by the parasite.

Fasciola hepatica employs a variety of ways to alter the host immune responses, rendering it ineffective to kill the parasites. The stimulation of T regulatory cells (Foxp3) is a strategy shared by other helminths, which promotes the parasite survival and modulates the tissue damage. The majority of helminth parasite infections result in a potent type-2 immune responses with an early production of IL-4 over IFN-γ, which is thought to play a dominating role in the protective immunity of the host and associated with a reduction in both worm burden and disease severity. In previous studies, it has been reported that *F. hepatica* is able to downregulate the Th1 immune responses and upregulate the Th2 responses at early stages of infection in sheep, mice, and chronic stages in cattle. Regulatory cytokines and cells that modify and/or decrease inflammatory responses mediate this imbalance toward a Th2 immune profile. The induction of a regulatory environment by the expression of cytokines such as IL-10 and TGF-β has been shown as a common strategy used by the parasites and microorganisms to extend their survival. The expression of Foxp3 T cells are elevated as the outcome of this regulatory environment. Particularly, it has been demonstrated that Foxp3 T lymphocytes play a decisive role in *F. hepatica* infection, contributing to the parasite survival throughout the migratory stages. In addition, *F. hepatica* develops other mechanisms to evade the immune responses of host during the early stages in sheep where larvae can induce apoptosis of peritoneal leukocytes, allowing the migration of larvae through the peritoneum.

In both vaccinated and non-immunized sheep, upregulation of Foxp3 along with overexpression of IL-10 and TGF-β indicates that *F. hepatica* induces a modulation of the host responses during the initial stages of infection to facilitate the survival of parasites during these crucial phases of the disease. However, while cytokine qPCR analysis showed elevated levels of IL-10, IL-12, IL-13, IL-23, and TGF-β in comparison to uninfected animals at 18 days post-infection, this suggested that the immune response is muted and has not yet been skewed toward a Th2-type response that is linked to chronic disease. The most severe liver damage and cirrhosis were seen in goats with numerous hepatic calcareous granulomas. These goats also had a striking infiltrate of CD3+ T lymphocytes and lambda IgG+ plasma cells that replaced large areas of the hepatic parenchyma, where there was a clear hypertrophy of the smooth endoplasmic reticulum of hepatocytes. These results were primarily seen in the goats that received multiple infective doses. These studies provided the first evidence to suggest that the induction of an early type-1 immune responses in the natural host sheep may be responsible for the resistance to liver fluke infection.

16.12 *Spirocerca lupi*

Spirocerca lupi belongs to the phylum Nematoda, class Scerenenta, and superfamily Spiroidea. Adult *S. lupi* worms are spirally coiled, bright red color and size ranges from 30 to 80 mm. Adult worms are generally located within the nodules of the esophageal wall and causes spirocrecosis. They primarily infect the host of Canidae family like dogs, but occasionally found in cats and wild felids. They are found in the tropical and subtropical areas of the world and follows indirect lifecycle. The intermediate host is dung beetle and many vertebrates like rodents, birds, reptiles, and rabbits act as paratenic host. Dogs are infected by eating an intermediate host or paratenic host.

The *S. lupi* larvae penetrate the gastric mucosa and migrate along the wall of the celiac arteries to the aorta, then subintimally to the caudal thoracic area, where they usually live for several weeks of infection, approximately for 3 months. The final preferred location of adult parasites is the esophageal wall and form characteristic oesophageal sarcoma (Fig. 16.1a) containing pleomorphic fibroblasts. Larvated eggs are passed in feces approximately for 5–6 months after infection, which can be detected using zinc sulphate fecal flotation technique (Fig. 16.1b). Adult parasites can live for more than 2 years.

Most of the dogs infected with *S. lupi* do not show clinical signs; however, when signs are present, the most common are vomiting, weight loss, coughing, regurgitation, and dyspnea. When esophageal lesions are severe, especially neoplastic, dogs may have difficulty in swallowing and may vomit repeatedly after trying to eat. Affected dogs may salivate profusely and eventually become emaciated. The *S. lupi* infection can cause esophageal neoplasia, enlargement of salivary gland, and thickening of thoracic limb bones due to hypertrophic osteopathy in dogs. The most common and pathognomonic lesions for spirocercosis are spondylitis of the thoracic vertebrae, nodules of variable size around worms in the esophagus, and

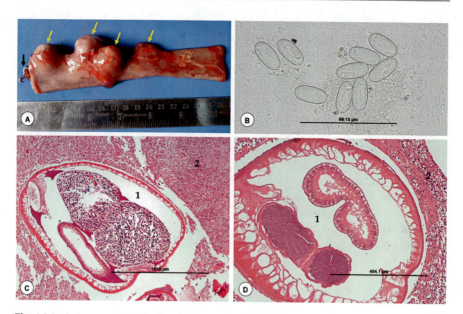

Fig. 16.1 *Spirocerca lupi* infection in the esophagus of dog. (**a**) Multiple variable sized nodules (yellow arrow) in the wall of esophagus with coiled round worms present in the lumen (black arrow). (**b**) Microscopic examination of feces revealed numerous capsule shaped, thick shelled *S. lupi* eggs (30–37 × 11–15 μm) with larvae. (**c**) Oesophageal submucosa and muscularis showed cross section of female *S. lupi* worm and uterus filled with numerous embryonated eggs (1), proliferation of fibroblasts, and infiltration of inflammatory cells (2). H&E, ×40. (**d**) Oesophageal submucosa showed cross section of *S. lupi* (1) along with marked infiltration of inflammatory cells, especially neutrophils and plasma cells and proliferation of fibroblasts (2). H&E ×100

aortic lesions, especially aneurysm of the thoracic aorta. Occasionally, aberrant migration of larvae results in neurologic signs and sudden mortality due to hemorrhages into the thorax after rupture of the aorta damaged by the developing worms. Migrating larvae produces hemorrhages, necrosis with eosinophilic inflammation, scaring, and formation of fibrotic nodules on aorta, which may cause stenosis or even rupture in severe cases.

The *S. lupi* has been associated with the formation of fibrosarcomas in canids, with the reports of malignant transformation of oesophageal nodules in approximately 25% of infected dogs. The fibrosarcoma, osteosarcoma, chondrosarcoma, or undifferentiated sarcomas are the most common malignant neoplasms diagnosed in *S. lupi* infection. The analysis of non-neoplastic nodules consists of adult worms, eggs, and migratory tracts when compared to neoplastic nodules. The esophageal neoplastic lesions are divided into three phases: inflammatory, preneoplastic, and neoplastic with potential metastasis. (1) Early inflammatory phase composed of lymphoblastic inflammation, inactive fibrocytes, and marked deposition of collagen; (2) preneoplastic phase consist of activated and atypical fibroblasts, reduced collagen and lymphoblastic inflammation with high mitosis index; (3) neoplastic phase is characterized by neutrophils and plasma cells infiltration, fibrin deposition, mitotic cells, multinucleated giant cells, and necrosis (Fig. 16.1c, d). This process of neoplastic transformation can be triggered by chronic inflammation due to direct mechanical damage induced by the worms or *S. lupi* excretory and secretory products (Sl-ESP), and constant repair of the tissues.

Chronic inflammation during spirocercosis is characterized by neutrophils infiltration around the parasites, generating oxygen, and nitric oxide reactive species involved in the oxidation of the DNA of host cell. This can lead to chromosomal aberrations and subsequent malignant transformation. Increased mutation rate precedes alterations in oncogenes and tumor suppressor genes, which in combination with prosurvival signals, the inhibition of apoptosis, and the stimulation of proliferation pathways induced by Sl-ESP such as galectin, 14-3-3 protein, HSP70, and HSP90, may promote the neoplastic nodule formation.

Clinical pathological findings in *S. lupi* infected dogs are mild anemia in approximately 50% of cases. Dogs with sarcomas showed microcytic hypochromic anemia due to chronic blood loss and melaena as result of ulceration of the esophageal mass. Dogs with early phase of disease showed normocytic normochromic anemia and advanced stage of disease showed leucocytosis, especially in oesophageal osteosarcomas. Monocytosis was common, whereas eosinophilia was uncommon. There was no correlation between the white blood cell counts and the existence of any associated inflammatory conditions such as spondylitis and it thus appears that the inflammatory response is as a result of the granuloma itself. Dogs with early phase of disease showed mildly elevated levels of creatine kinase. However, once neoplastic transformation has occurred, increased alkaline phosphatase, creatine kinase, amylase, and lactate dehydrogenase have been reported.

In tissues, the *S. lupi* worms are surrounded by highly vascularized loose connective tissue and proliferating fibroblasts, fibrin-rich fluid, infiltration of neutrophils and plasma cells, and necrosis. Doramectin is the current drug of choice, which effectively kills the adult worms and decreases the shedding of eggs.

16.13 *Cysticercus fasciolaris*

The adult tapeworm (Cestoda), *Taenia taeniaeformis* occurs in the small intestines of the definitive host, cat, and related carnivores all over the world. In intermediate host rat and mice, the prevalence of this parasite ranges from 4.3% to 67.7%. The infected definitive host excretes thousands of eggs daily (average 12,000 partially developed eggs, called as oncospheres) into the host feces from the proglottids of the adult parasite. The intermediate host, rodents and less frequently lagomorphs become infected through contaminated environment, feed, and water containing viable oncospheres. Common intermediate host species are laboratory, urban, and wild rodents such as rats (*Rattus norvegicus* and *R. rattus*) and mice (*Mus musculus*).

The metacestode or bladder worm or larval stage, *Cysticercus fasciolaris* also known as *Strobilocercus fasciolaris*, *Hydatigera fasciolaris,* and *Taenia crassicolis* develops in the liver of the infected rodents. Occasionally, the cysts also develop in the abdominal wall and kidneys, filled with purulent exudate without larvae. Under experimental conditions, 1-month old mice infected with low numbers of *T. taeniaeformis* eggs (200–500) developed 11–250 metacestodes in the liver. The *T. taeniaeformis* eggs lose their membrane in the stomach or intestine of intermediate host, soon after being ingested and release the larvae, which pass through the intestinal wall. Larvae then migrate via the hepatic portal system and reach the liver. Laboratory rodents that have been experimentally infected with *C. fasciolaris* have a prepatent period of 34–80 days (41.1 ± 5.9); at the end of this period, the ingested larvae become fully developed and infectious. The *T. taeniaeformis* life cycle is completed when the definitive host cats consume infected intermediate host rodents or any other intermediate host containing larval stage in their liver.

The parasite is of zoonotic significance and human beings can act as accidental intermediate host. Adult parasites and metacestodes have been detected in intestines and liver of people from Czech Republic, Argentina, Denmark, Sri Lanka, and Taiwan. Infection of the rat liver by *C. fasciolaris* may cause fibrosarcomas. The cat tape worm *T. taeniaeformis* produce cysts with fibrous tissue capsule around in the intermediate host rat liver with marked infiltration of inflammatory cells especially mononuclear cells and eosinophils (Fig. 16.2a–d).

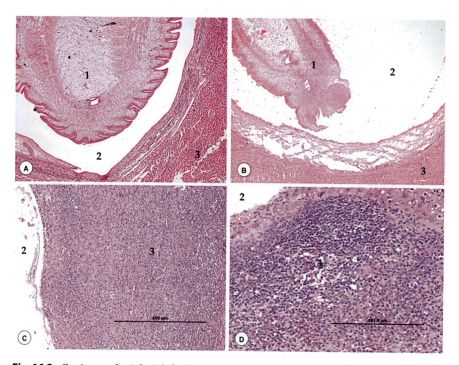

Fig. 16.2 *Cysticercus fasciolaris* infection in a rat liver. (**a**) The larval stage *Cysticercus fasciolaris* (1) in the cystic cavity (2) of liver (3). H&E ×40. (**b**) The mature larval stage *C. fasciolaris* showed oral suckers (1) in the cystic cavity (2) of liver (3). H&E ×40. (**c**) Liver showed *C. fasciolaris* cyst (2) and marked infiltration of inflammatory cells especially mononuclear cells and few eosinophils (3). H&E ×100. (**d**) Higher magnification of Fig. (**c**). H&E ×200

16.14 Diarrheal Parasites

Research findings have revealed that Cryptosporidium activates nuclear factor kappa B (NF-κB) in the infected biliary epithelial cells, which inhibits apoptosis, provides protection to parasite, and promotes propagation of the parasite in the infected cells. Researchers have reported that Cryptosporidium escapes the host immune system by residing in the parasitophorus vacuoles. Trichuris causes necrosis of the cells with inflammation and infiltration of cells. Strongyloides penetrates the intestinal mucosa and damages the mucosa. It causes ulcerative enteritis along with marked inflammatory response, which is responsible for diarrhea.

16.15 Conclusion

Parasitic infections affect both animals and humans across the world. Parasitic diseases remain one of the major causes of morbidity and mortality. The parasite derives nourishment and shelter from the host. An imbalance between host–parasite interaction results in pathogenicity, which depends upon the host immune system and parasite species. Host immune response forms a three-tier barrier against the parasitic infections: (1) first line of innate immune defense, including the non-specific anatomic barriers of the body, (2) second line of innate immune defenses are inflammation, phagocytosis and complement activation, (3) third line of adaptive immunity includes humoral and cell-mediated immune responses. Antigen presenting cells are macrophages and dendritic cells engulf the parasites, process and present its antigen on surface MHC class II. Formation of antigen-MHC complex activates CD4+T cells, which differentiate into either Th1 or Th2 subtypes. The Th1-mediated immune responses target the intracellular parasites, whereas Th2-mediated humoral immune response targets the extracellular parasites. Immune responses against parasites involve B cells (production of antibodies), T cells, macrophages, mast cells, and NK cells (production of pro-inflammatory cytokines including IL-6, IL-12, TNF-α, and nitric oxide). Elimination of parasites requires a well-coordinated operation of both humoral and CMI responses, type-I hypersensitivity, inflammation, eosinophilia, high IgE levels, and mast cell degranulation. The parasites may survive inside the host by evading the host immune system by several ways. Some of the immune evasion strategies are prevention of phagosome formation and maturation, inhibit phagolysosome fusion, inactivate macrophages and complement proteins, and inhibit oxidative burst (to avoid phagocytosis) inside the host body. This book chapter highlights the parasite–host interactions, immune responses, and disease pathology and effective strategies to control the parasitic infections.

References

Abass EM, Mansour D, el Harith A (2007) Demonstration of agglutinating anti-Leishmania antibodies in lymph node aspirate for confirmation of kala-azar serodiagnosis. J Med Microbiol 56:1256–1258

Akira S, Uematsu S, Takeuchi O (2006) Pathogen recognition and innate immunity. Cell 124(4):783–801

Almeida IC, Milani SR, Gorin PA, Travassos LR (1991) Complement-mediated lysis of Trypanosoma cruzi trypomastigotes by human anti-alpha-galactosyl antibodies. J Immunol 146(7):2394–2400

Ambrosio AR, de Messias-Reason IJT (2005) Leishmania (Viannia) braziliensis: interaction of mannose-binding lectin with surface glycoconjugates and complement activation. An antibody-independent defence mechanism. Parasite Immunol 27(9):333–340

Artis D, Wang ML, Keilbaugh SA, He W, Brenes M, Swain GP, Knight PA, Donaldson DD, Lazar MA, Miller HR, Schad GA (2004) RELMβ/FIZZ2 is a goblet cell-specific immune-effector molecule in the gastrointestinal tract. Proc Natl Acad Sci 101(37):13596–13600

Aseffa A, Gumy A, Launois P, MacDonald HR, Louis JA, Tacchini-Cottier F (2002) The early IL-4 response to Leishmania major and the resulting Th2 cell maturation steering progressive disease in BALB/c mice are subject to the control of regulatory CD4+ CD25+ T cells. J Immunol 169(6):3232–3241

Beucher M, Norris KA (2008) Sequence diversity of the Trypanosoma cruzi complement regulatory protein family. Infect Immun 76(2):750–758

Black SJ, Hewett RS, Sendashonga CN (1982) Trypanosoma brucei variable surface antigen is released by degenerating parasites but not by actively dividing parasites. Parasite Immunol 4(4):233–244

Bracke M, van de Graaf E, Lammers JWJ, Coffer PJ, Koenderman L (2000) *In vivo* priming of FcαR functioning on eosinophils of allergic asthmatics. J Leukoc Biol 68(5):655–661

Brenier-Pinchart MP, Pelloux H, Derouich-Guergour D, Ambroise-Thomas P (2001) Chemokines in host–protozoan-parasite interactions. Trends Parasitol 17(6):292–296

Butterworth AE, Wassom DL, Gleich GJ, Loegering DA, David JR (1979) Damage to schistosomula of Schistosoma mansoni induced directly by eosinophil major basic protein. J Immunol 122(1):221–229

Capron M, Capron A, Goetzl EJ, Austen KF (1981) Tetrapeptides of the eosinophil chemotactic factor of anaphylaxis (ECF-A) enhance eosinophil fc receptor. Nature 289(5793):71–73

Carney CK, Schrimpe AC, Halfpenny K, Harry RS, Miller CM, Broncel M, Sewell SL, Schaff JE, Deol R, Carter MD, Wright DW (2006) The basis of the immunomodulatory activity of malaria pigment (hemozoin). J Biol Inorg Chem 11(7):917–929

Chen Y, Chou K, Fuchs E, Havran WL, Boismenu R (2002) Protection of the intestinal mucosa by intraepithelial γδ T cells. Proc Natl Acad Sci 99(22):14338–14343

Cliffe LJ, Humphreys NE, Lane TE, Potten CS, Booth C, Grencis RK (2005) Accelerated intestinal epithelial cell turnover: a new mechanism of parasite expulsion. Science 308(5727):1463–1465

Cooper PJ, Beck LA, Espinel I, Deyampert NM, Hartnell A, Jose PJ, Paredes W, Guderian RH, Nutman TB (2000) Eotaxin and RANTES expression by the dermal endothelium is associated with eosinophil infiltration after ivermectin treatment of onchocerciasis. Clin Immunol 95(1):51–61

Culley FJ, Harris RA, Kaye PM, McAdam KP, Raynes JG (1996) C-reactive protein binds to a novel ligand on Leishmania donovani and increases uptake into human macrophages. J Immunol 156(12):4691–4696

Daniel-Ribeiro CT, Zanini G (2000) Autoimmunity and malaria: what are they doing together? Acta Trop 76(3):205–221

Denkers EY, Butcher BA, Del Rio L, Bennouna S (2004) Neutrophils, dendritic cells and toxoplasma. Int J Parasitol 34(3):411–421

References

Dermine JF, Scianimanico S, Privé C, Descoteaux A, Desjardins M (2000) Leishmania promastigotes require lipophosphoglycan to actively modulate the fusion properties of phagosomes at an early step of phagocytosis. Cell Microbiol 2(2):115–126

Diffley P (1985) Trypanosoma brucei: immunogenicity of the variant surface coat glycoprotein of virulent and avirulent subspecies. Exp Parasitol 59(1):98–107

Dixon H, Blanchard C, Deschoolmeester ML, Yuill NC, Christie JW, Rothenberg ME, Else KJ (2006) The role of Th2 cytokines, chemokines and parasite products in eosinophil recruitment to the gastrointestinal mucosa during helminth infection. Eur J Immunol 36(7):1753–1763

Doetze A, Satoguina J, Burchard G, Rau T, Löliger C, Fleischer B, Hoerauf A (2000) Antigen-specific cellular hyporesponsiveness in a chronic human helminth infection is mediated by Th3/Tr1-type cytokines IL-10 and transforming growth factor-β but not by a Th1 to Th2 shift. Int Immunol 12(5):623–630

Fallon PG, Richardson EJ, McKenzie GJ, McKenzie AN (2000) Schistosome infection of transgenic mice defines distinct and contrasting pathogenic roles for IL-4 and IL-13: IL-13 is a profibrotic agent. J Immunol 164(5):2585–2591

Farkas I, Baranyi L, Ishikawa Y, Okada N, Bohata C, Budai D, Fukuda A, Imai M, Okada H (2002) CD59 blocks not only the insertion of C9 into MAC but inhibits ion channel formation by homologous C5b-8 as well as C5b-9. J Physiol 539(2):537–545

Garred P, Nielsen MA, Kurtzhals JA, Malhotra R, Madsen HO, Goka BQ, Akanmori BD, Sim RB, Hviid L (2003) Mannose-binding lectin is a disease modifier in clinical malaria and may function as opsonin for plasmodium falciparum-infected erythrocytes. Infect Immun 71(9): 5245–5253

Gazzinelu R, Pereira MES, Romanha A, Gazzinelli G, Brener Z (1991) Direct lysis of Trypanosoma cruzi: a novel effector mechanism of protection mediated by human anti-gal antibodies. Parasite Immunol 13(4):345–356

Glauert AM, Butterworth AE (1977) Morphological evidence for the ability of eosinophils to damage antibody-coated schistosomula. Trans R Soc Trop Med Hyg 71(5):392–395

Goerdt S, Orfanos CE (1999) Other functions, other genes: alternative activation of antigen-presenting cells. Immunity 10(2):137–142

Green PJ, Feizi T, Stoll MS, Thiel S, Prescott A, McConville MJ (1994) Recognition of the major cell surface glycoconjugates of Leishmania parasites by the human serum mannan-binding protein. Mol Biochem Parasitol 66(2):319–328

Handman E, Bullen DV (2002) Interaction of Leishmania with the host macrophage. Trends Parasitol 18(8):332–334

Healer J, McGuinness D, Hopcroft P, Haley S, Carter R, Riley E (1997) Complement-mediated lysis of plasmodium falciparum gametes by malaria-immune human sera is associated with antibodies to the gamete surface antigen Pfs230. Infect Immun 65(8):3017–3023

Hesse M, Piccirillo CA, Belkaid Y, Prufer J, Mentink-Kane M, Leusink M, Cheever AW, Shevach EM, Wynn TA (2004) The pathogenesis of schistosomiasis is controlled by cooperating IL-10-producing innate effector and regulatory T cells. J Immunol 172(5):3157–3166

King CL, Medhat A, Malhotra I, Nafeh M, Helmy A, Khaudary J, Ibrahim S, El-Sherbiny M, Zaky S, Stupi RJ, Brustoski K (1996) Cytokine control of parasite-specific anergy in human urinary schistosomiasis. IL-10 modulates lymphocyte reactivity. J Immunol 156(12): 4715–4721

Klabunde J, Uhlemann AC, Tebo AE, Kimmel J, Schwarz RT, Kremsner PG, Kun JF (2002) Recognition of plasmodium falciparum proteins by mannan-binding lectin, a component of the human innate immune system. Parasitol Res 88(2):113–117

Knight PA, Pemberton AD, Robertson KA, Roy DJ, Wright SH, Miller HR (2004) Expression profiling reveals novel innate and inflammatory responses in the jejunal epithelial compartment during infection with Trichinella spiralis. Infect Immun 72(10):6076–6086

Kopf M, Gros GL, Bachmann M, Lamers MC, Bluethmann H, Köhler G (1993) Disruption of the murine IL-4 gene blocks Th2 cytokine responses. Nature 362(6417):245–248

Kumaratilake LM, Ferrante A, Jaeger T, Morris-Jones SD (1997) The role of complement, antibody, and tumor necrosis factor alpha in the killing of plasmodium falciparum by the monocytic cell line THP-1. Infect Immun 65(12):5342–5345

Leder K, Weller PF (2000) Eosinophilia and helminthic infections. Best Pract Res Clin Haematol 13(2):301–317

Lugli EB, Pouliot M, Portela MDPM, Loomis MR, Raper J (2004) Characterization of primate trypanosome lytic factors. Mol Biochem Parasitol 138(1):9–20

Magez S, Schwegmann A, Atkinson R, Claes F, Drennan M, De Baetselier P, Brombacher F (2008) The role of B-cells and IgM antibodies in parasitemia, anemia, and VSG switching in trypanosoma brucei–infected mice. PLoS Pathog 4(8):e1000122

Mahanty S, Ravichandran M, Raman U, Jayaraman K, Kumaraswami V, Nutman TB (1997) Regulation of parasite antigen-driven immune responses by interleukin-10 (IL-10) and IL-12 in lymphatic filariasis. Infect Immun 65(5):1742–1747

Maizels RM (2005) Infections and allergy—helminths, hygiene and host immune regulation. Curr Opin Immunol 17(6):656–661

Maizels RM, Holland MJ (1998) Parasite immunity: pathways for expelling intestinal helminths. Curr Biol 8(20):R711–R714

Male D, Brostoff J, Roth DB, Roitt I (2007) Immunology, 7th edn. MMVI Elsevier Limited, an Elsevier Imprint, Edinburgh

McGuinness DH, Dehal PK, Pleass RJ (2003) Pattern recognition molecules and innate immunity to parasites. Trends Parasitol 19(7):312–319

McKenzie GJ, Bancroft A, Grencis RK, McKenzie AN (1998) A distinct role for interleukin-13 in Th2-cell-mediated immune responses. Curr Biol 8(6):339–342

Meresse B, Cerf-Bensussan N (2009) Innate T cell responses in human gut. In: Seminars in immunology, 21(3). Academic Press, London, pp 121–129

Mills KH, McGuirk P (2004) Antigen-specific regulatory T cells—their induction and role in infection. In: Seminars in immunology, 16(2), Academic Press, London, pp. 107–117

Mir A, Benahmed D, Igual R, Borras R, O'Connor JE, Moreno MJ, Rull S (2006) Eosinophil-selective mediators in human strongyloidiasis. Parasite Immunol 28(8):397–400

Miyahira Y (2008) Trypanosoma cruzi infection from the view of CD8+ T cell immunity—an infection model for developing T cell vaccine. Parasitol Int 57(1):38–48

Miyahira Y, Kobayashi S, Takeuchi T et al (1999) Induction of CD8+ T cell-mediated protective immunity against Trypanosoma cruzi. Int Immunol 11:133–141

Mochizuki M, Bartels J, Mallet AI, Christophers E, Schröder JM (1998) IL-4 induces eotaxin: a possible mechanism of selective eosinophil recruitment in helminth infection and atopy. J Immunol 160(1):60–68

Mordue DG, Desai N, Dustin M, Sibley LD (1999) Invasion by toxoplasma gondii establishes a moving junction that selectively excludes host cell plasma membrane proteins on the basis of their membrane anchoring. J Exp Med 190(12):1783–1792

Morisaki JH, Heuser JE, Sibley LD (1995) Invasion of toxoplasma gondii occurs by active penetration of the host cell. J Cell Sci 108(6):2457–2464

Nawa Y, Ishikawa N, Tsuchiya K, Horii Y, Abe T, Khan AI, Shi B, Itoh H, Ide H, Uchiyama F (1994) Selective effector mechanisms for the expulsion of intestinal helminths. Parasite Immunol 16(7):333–338

Pemberton AD, Knight PA, Wright SH, Miller HR (2004) Proteomic analysis of mouse jejunal epithelium and its response to infection with the intestinal nematode, Trichinella spiralis. Proteomics 4(4):1101–1108

Rankin SM, Conroy DM, Williams TJ (2000) Eotaxin and eosinophil recruitment: implications for human disease. Mol Med Today 6(1):20–27

Rodríguez-Sosa M, Satoskar AR, Calderón R, Gomez-Garcia L, Saavedra R, Bojalil R, Terrazas LI (2002) Chronic helminth infection induces alternatively activated macrophages expressing high levels of CCR5 with low interleukin-12 production and Th2-biasing ability. Infect Immun 70(7):3656–3664

Sendashonga CN, Black SJ (1982) Humoral responses against Trypanosoma brucei variable surface antigen are induced by degenerating parasites. Parasite Immunol 4(4):245–257

Specht S, Saeftel M, Arndt M, Endl E, Dubben B, Lee NA, Lee JJ, Hoerauf A (2006) Lack of eosinophil peroxidase or major basic protein impairs defense against murine filarial infection. Infect Immun 74(9):5236–5243

Stein M, Keshav S, Harris N, Gordon S (1992) Interleukin 4 potently enhances murine macrophage mannose receptor activity: a marker of alternative immunologic macrophage activation. J Exp Med 176(1):287–292

Stempin CC, Dulgerian LR, Garrido VV, Cerban FM (2009) Arginase in parasitic infections: macrophage activation, immunosuppression, and intracellular signals. J Biomed Biotechnol 2010:683485

Suzuki E, Tanaka AK, Toledo MS, Takahashi HK, Straus AH (2002) Role of β-D-galactofuranose in Leishmania major macrophage invasion. Infect Immun 70(12):6592–6596

Tebo AE, Kremsner PG, Luty AJF (2002) Fc receptor-mediated phagocytosis of plasmodium falciparum-infected erythrocytes *in vitro*. Clin Exp Immunol 130:300–306

Teixeira MJ, Teixeira CR, Andrade BB, Barral-Netto M, Barral A (2006) Chemokines in host–parasite interactions in leishmaniasis. Trends Parasitol 22(1):32–40

Turner MW (1996) Mannose-binding lectin: the pluripotent molecule of the innate immune system. Immunol Today 17(11):532–540

Van Overtvelt L, Vanderheyde N, Verhasselt V, Ismaili J, De Vos L, Goldman M, Willems F, Vray B (1999) Trypanosoma cruzi infects human dendritic cells and prevents their maturation: inhibition of cytokines, HLA-DR, and costimulatory molecules. Infect Immun 67(8):4033–4040

van Riet E, Hartgers FC, Yazdanbakhsh M (2007) Chronic helminth infections induce immunomodulation: consequences and mechanisms. Immunobiology 212(6):475–490

Wilson MS, Taylor MD, Balic A, Finney CA, Lamb JR, Maizels RM (2005) Suppression of allergic airway inflammation by helminth-induced regulatory T cells. J Exp Med 202(9):1199–1212

Woerly G, Decot V, Loiseau S, Loyens M, Chihara J, Ono N, Capron M (2004) CD28 and secretory immunoglobulin A-dependent activation of eosinophils: inhibition of mediator release by the anti-allergic drug, suplatast tosilate. Clin Exp Allergy 34(9):1379–1387

Immunopathological Disorders of Cattle and Buffalo

Key Points

1. Bovine leukocyte adhesion deficiency, transient hypogammaglobulinemia, and Chediak-Higashi syndrome are examples of primary immunodeficiencies in cattle and buffalo.
2. Chediak-Higashi syndrome is a rare inherited disease reported in Hereford cattle and Japanese black heifer.
3. Chediak-Higashi syndrome is characterized by oculocutaneous albinism, photophobia, bleeding diathesis, and increased susceptibility for infection due to enlarged cytoplasmic granules of phagocytic cells which results in defective chemotaxis, motility, and intracellular killing.
4. Diagnosis of Chediak-Higashi syndrome can be done by blood smear and hair shafts examination for large melanin granules of phagocytic cells.
5. Bovine leukocyte adhesion deficiency is an autosomal recessive congenital disease, commonly seen in Holstein cattle characterized by recurrent bacterial infections, delayed wound healing, and persistent neutrophilia.
6. Indirectly or directly, some medications, neoplastic illnesses, nutritional deficiencies, metabolic disorders, environmental afflictions, and infectious agents can suppress the immune system and cause secondary immunodeficiency.
7. Acquired or secondary immunodeficiency is caused by some viruses such as bovine viral diarrhea virus, bovine immunodeficiency virus, and bovine herpes virus 1 in cattle and buffalo.
8. Bronchial asthma, allergic rhinitis, allergic dermatitis, milk allergy, insect bite allergy, allergic conjunctivitis, and acute systemic anaphylaxis are examples of type I hypersensitivity reactions in cattle and buffalo.
9. Tuberculin reaction is the important example of type IV hypersensitivity reaction.
10. Tuberculin reaction is the standard method to diagnose the bovine tuberculosis.

11. Johnin testing is the delayed-type hypersensitivity reaction produced in animals after intradermal injection of Johnin PPD for the detection of paratuberculosis.
12. Vitiligo is an autoimmune disorder and reported in cattle and buffalo.

17.1 Introduction

The immune system deals with the collection of cells and proteins of our body that functions to protect the skin, respiratory passages, intestinal tract, and other areas from foreign antigens such as bacteria, viruses, fungi, parasites, cancer cells, and toxins. In basic terms, immune system can be viewed as having two "lines of defense": innate immunity and adaptive immunity. Innate immunity is entitled as the first line of defense toward any intruding pathogen as it is the rapid immune response that is used by the host instantly or within hours of encountering an antigen. The innate immune response is an antigen-independent (nonspecific) defense mechanism and has no immunologic memory. Therefore, it is unable to recognize or "memorize" the reexposure of the same antigen that has once encountered in the body. The adaptive immunity is also known as acquired immunity, as it is acquired during the life-time of an individual. It is antigen-dependent and antigen-specific and, therefore, involves a lag time between exposure to the antigen and maximal response. The most important thing of adaptive immunity is its capacity to create immunological memory, which enables the host to produce more rapid and effective immune responses upon subsequent exposure to the antigen. Innate and adaptive immunity are not mutually exclusive mechanisms of host defense but rather are complementary, with defects in either system can result in defenselessness of host (Murphy et al. 2007; Bonilla and Oettgen 2010; Turvey and Broide 2010).

Certain diseases, i.e., immunopathological diseases, take place when there is defect in either system. Immunopathology is the study of diseases caused by immune reaction; therefore, the word immunopathology connotes that protective immune response may cause tissue damage and disease (Sell 1978). Immunopathological diseases are characterized into immunodeficiency, hypersensitivity, and autoimmunity. Immunodeficiency disorders have been described as diseases caused by one or more defects of the immune system, leading to increased susceptibility to infections (Raje and Dinakar 2015). Hypersensitivity reactions are immune response that are exaggerated or inappropriate against an antigen or allergen and classified into type I, i.e., anaphylaxis; type II, i.e., cytotoxic; type III, i.e., immune mediated; and type IV, i.e., T-cell-mediated (Justiz 2018). Type I, Type II, and Type III are also known as antibody-mediated hypersensitivity, whereas Type IV is also known as cell-mediated hypersensitivity. Autoimmune diseases occur when the immune system attack self-molecule as a result of breakdown of immunologic tolerance to autoreactive immune cells (Smith and Germolec 1999).

17.2 Immunodeficiency

Immunodeficiency is the condition of body in which the ability of immune system is compromised or entirely absent to fight against infectious diseases. In other words, it can be defined as the failure or absence of elements of the immune system including lymphocytes, phagocytes, and complement system (Pac and Bernatowska 2016). Immunodeficiency disorders are broadly classified into congenital, i.e., primary immunodeficiency, and acquired, i.e., secondary immunodeficiency.

17.3 Primary Immunodeficiency

Primary immunodeficiency (PID) also known as congenital immunodeficiency presents in animals since their birth. This type of immunodeficiency mainly occurs due to intrinsic defects in the immune cells including T cells, complement components, and phagocytes (Notarangelo 2010). The PIDs are now known to include a group of heterogeneous disorders with immune system abnormalities characterized by various combinations of recurrent infections, autoimmunity, lymphoproliferation, granulomatous process, atopy, and malignancy (Raje and Dinakar 2015). Primary immunodeficiencies in cattle and buffalo include diseases such as Chediak-Higashi syndrome, bovine leukocyte adhesion deficiency, and transient hypogammaglobulinemia.

17.4 Chediak-Higashi Syndrome

Chediak-Higashi syndrome is a rare inherited disease reported in Hereford cattle (Padgett et al. 1964) and Japanese black heifer (Umemura et al. 1983). The disease is characterized by oculocutaneous albinism (reduction in melanin pigment of skin, hair, and eyes), photophobia, tendency to bleed, and increased susceptibility for infection. Bleeding diathesis is the main symptom due to defect in aggregation of platelets (Shiraishi et al. 2002). In this syndrome, the cytoplasmic granules of phagocytic cells like neutrophils, monocytes, and eosinophils become enlarged. Such phagocytic cells with large granules become fragile, and their rupture results in the tissue damage. Further, they show defective chemotaxis, motility, and intracellular killing.

Diagnosis can be done by the blood smear examination for large melanin granules of phagocytic cells or by the examination of hair shafts for enlarged melanin granules.

17.5 Bovine Leukocyte Adhesion Deficiency

Bovine leukocyte adhesion deficiency (BLAD) is an autosomal recessive congenital disease characterized by recurrent bacterial infections, delayed wound healing, and retarded growth, along with persistent marked neutrophilia. This condition is commonly seen in Holstein cattle.

There is a single point mutation (adenine to guanine) at position 383 of the CD18 gene, which caused substitution of glycine in place of aspartic acid at amino acid 128 (D128G) in the adhesion molecule CD18. The neutrophil of affected cattle shows impaired expression of the β2 integrin (CD11a, b, c/CD18) of the leukocyte adhesion molecule. The clinical findings include severe ulcers on oral mucous membrane, periodontitis, loss of teeth, chronic pneumonia, and recurrent or chronic diarrhea. Due to the infectious complications, affected cattle may die at early age. Holstein bulls, including carrier sires that had a mutant BLAD gene in heterozygote, were controlled from dairy cattle for a decade. The BLAD gene in Holstein cattle can be controlled by avoiding the mating between BLAD carriers and was found to be successful (Shuster et al. 1992; Nagahata 2004).

17.6 Transient Hypogammaglobulinemia

Transient hypogammaglobulinemia is associated with the delayed onset of immunoglobulin synthesis, i.e., suggestive of primary specific IgG2 deficiency in the newborn without any apparent deficiency in T-cell function. No other abnormality of the immune system was found. Typically, cattle with IgG2 deficiency show decreased resistance to infections caused by pyogenic bacteria. Clinical manifestations of disease are seen at the age of 6 months to 3 years, and lung infections are most commonly observed. The pulmonary lesions observed in the heifer were those typically caused by chronic infection with inhaled bacterial pathogens, such as mycoplasma.

17.7 Acquired Immunodeficiency

Acquired immunodeficiencies are also known as secondary immunodeficiencies, and it is more common in domesticated animals and humans than primary immunodeficiency. It results from a variety of factors that can affect the host with an intrinsically normal immune system. These deficiencies of immunity are clinically manifested by an increased frequency or unusual complications of common infections and occasionally by the occurrence of opportunistic infections (Chinen and Shearer 2010). For example, certain drugs, neoplastic condition, deficiency of nutrition, metabolic diseases, environmental conditions, and infectious agents directly or indirectly can cause suppression of immune system. Commonly used drugs such as steroids or alkylating agents can induce very specific abnormalities in both granulocytes and lymphocytes. A variety of neoplasms, including lymphomas and multiple myeloma, can result in immunologic dysfunction. Protein malnutrition or single nutrient deficiencies such as zinc or iron deficiency can have significant immunologic manifestations. However, infectious agents are commonly responsible to induce immunodeficiency; the mechanisms by which viruses induce alterations in immunity are not yet completely understood (Rouse and Horohov 1986). Some viruses such as bovine viral diarrhea (BVD), bovine immunodeficiency virus (BIV), and bovine herpes virus 1 (BHV-1) are suggested to induce immunosuppression in cattle and buffalo. In general, there are four distinct mechanisms through which viruses can cause immunosuppression: (1) direct (cytotoxic) effect of virus replication on cells of the immune system; (2) effect of an immunosuppressive, soluble, and viral product; (3) induction of soluble immunosuppressive substances by host cells; and (4) imbalance of immunoregulatory cell subsets. The specific cells affected by these processes will determine the disease which will be manifested (Reimann and Letvin 1993).

17.8 Bovine Viral Diarrhea Virus

Bovine viral diarrhea virus (BVDV) is the *Pestivirus* genus of family *Flaviviridae*. The BVDV has two biotypes non-cytopathogenic (ncp) and cytopathogenic (cp) according to their effects on tissue cell culture rather than in the infected host. The Cp biotypes induce apoptosis in cultured cells (Gamlen et al. 2010), while ncp biotypes of BVDV induce acute infections and can be transmitted through body fluids, including nasal discharge, urine, milk, semen, saliva, tears, and fetal fluids (Meyling et al. 1990), whereas Cp of BVDV has also been shown to be capable of inducing acute infection under experimental conditions (Lambot et al. 1997). Animals persistently infected with BVDV are generally much more efficient transmitters of virus than transiently or acutely infected animals, because they are capable of shedding large quantities of virus throughout their lives and are considered primary reservoirs for BVDV (Khodakaram-Tafti and Farjanikish 2017). However, the cattle persistently infected with BVDV become immunotolerant and do not show lymphocytopenia (Falkenberg et al. 2018).

Cattle infected with BVDV show transient immunosuppression as a result of predilection of virus for the cells. In acute phase of the infection, there will be reduction of CD4 and CD8 T lymphocytes, B lymphocytes, and neutrophils in the circulation, and functional activities of these cells also get suppressed (Brewoo et al. 2007). The CD46 has been shown to be the receptor on macrophage and lymphocyte host cell membranes, where BVDV gains entry (Maurer et al. 2004). Infection of animal with BVDV results in a transient viremia in a duration of 10–14 days (Howard 1990), and the disease can be associated with short-term leukopenia, lymphopenia and/or thrombocytopenia, apoptosis in the thymus, immunosuppression, pyrexia, and diarrhea (Lanyon et al. 2014). The resultant immunosuppression, in turn, can allow the chances of infection of other infectious agents or allow the reoccurrence of existing infections (Potgieter 1995). Immunosuppression is associated with direct effects of BVDV on circulating T and B lymphocytes (Bolin

Table 17.1 Commonly used adjuvants in veterinary vaccines

Commercial vaccine	Viral/bacterial strain	Adjuvant
Raksha ovac	Foot-and-mouth disease (O, A, C, and Asia 1)	Mineral oil
Raksha biovac	Foot-and-mouth disease (O, A, and Asia 1) + hemorrhagic septicemia (HS)	Double emulsion oil adjuvant (mineral oil)
Raksha monovalent	Foot-and-mouth disease O strain	Aluminum hydroxide and saponin
Raksha bivalent	Foot-and-mouth disease (O and A)	Aluminum hydroxide and saponin
HS vaccine	Inactivated *Pasteurella multocida* organism	Aluminum hydroxide
Raksha HS+ black quarter (BQ) vaccine	Inactivated culture of *Pasteurella multocida* and *Clostridium chauvoei*	Aluminum hydroxide
Enterotoxemia (ET) vaccine	*Clostridium perfringens* type D and epsilon toxoid	Aluminum hydroxide
Botulinum vaccine	Toxoid of *Clostridium* type C and D	Aluminum hydroxide
Raksharab	Inactivated rabies virus	Aluminum hydroxide
Botuthrax	Inactivated alum precipitated toxoids of *Clostridium botulinum* types C and D	Aluminum hydroxide
Rotavec corona	Inactivated bovine rotavirus, coronavirus, and *E. coli* K99 antigens	Aluminum hydroxide and mineral oil
Equilis prequenza	Purified haemagglutinin/neuraminidase subunits from equine influenza viruses	Purified saponin
Pulpyvax	*Clostridium perfringens* type D toxoids	Aluminum hydroxide

et al. 1985; Chase 2013) and apoptosis of lymphocytes in gut-associated lymphoid tissue (Pedrera et al. 2012). The disease is characterized by poor fertility, diarrhea, stillbirth, abortions, mummified fetus, anorexia, and fever. Vaccination plays important role in prevention of infectious diseases of ruminants (Table 17.1).

17.9 Bovine Immunodeficiency Virus Infection

Bovine immunodeficiency virus (BIV) is a *Lentivirus* of the family *Retroviridae* and causes persistent viral infection in cattle and buffalo. Infection with BIV has never been linked to a specific disease or clinically identifiable syndrome, but it has been associated with lymphadenopathy, lymphocytosis, central nervous system lesions, progressive weakness, decreased milk yield, decreased lymphocytic blastogenic response, and bovine paraplegic syndrome, though there are many experimental evidences, which are available to believe that BIV can cause immune dysfunction, therefore making animals susceptible to secondary infections (Bhatia et al. 2013).

The bovine immunodeficiency (BID) virus replicates in the cells of the immune system, and primarily macrophages/monocytes and lymphocytes, and cause their destruction and immunosuppression (Gonda et al. 1987). In a study, it was observed that there was also decrease in CD4/CD8 ratio and an overall increase in lymphocyte, 2–6 weeks postinfection in calves inoculated with BIV, suggesting a possible immune dysfunction in BIV-infected calves (Zhang et al. 1997). The BIV replicates in fibroblast-like cells and is cytopathic in most, causing syncytia and cell death. In peripheral blood mononuclear cells (PBMCs) collected from naturally infected animals, BIV has been shown to infect and transcribe its genome in different subsets of cells, namely, CD3+, CD4+, CD8+, and γδ-T cells, B cells and monocytes (Whetstone et al. 1997; Wu et al. 2003).

17.10 Bovine Herpes Virus Infection

Bovine herpes virus 1 (BHV-1) is a causative agent of infectious bovine rhinotracheitis and causes broad immunosuppression in bovine, leading to decrease resistance to secondary bacterial and viral infections. The virus affects the functional properties of polymorphonuclear cells, macrophages, and lymphocytes (Tikoo et al. 1995). It also causes reduction in the number of CD4 and CD8 T lymphocytes. BHV-1 causes decreased mitogenic stimulation of PBMCs and expression of interleukin-2 receptor (Winkler et al. 1999). BHV-1 is also responsible for reduced expression of MHC class I molecules present on the surface of infected cells (Hariharan et al. 1993). The major histocompatibility complex (MHC) of cattle is known as bovine leukocyte antigen (BoLA). The BoLA is located on chromosome 23. The BoLA has been linked to variation in resistance to disease including bovine leukemia virus-induced lymphoma and mastitis (Table 17.2). Infection of monocytes and macrophages leads to impairment in the function of phagocytosis, antibody-dependent cell-mediated cytotoxicity (ADCC), and T-cell stimulation. The BHV-1 glycoprotein G (gG) is a chemokine binding protein that blocks chemokine binding, and this activity is responsible for partially mediating the effect of immunosuppression. The disease caused by BHV-1 is primarily associated with clinical syndromes such as rhinotracheitis, pustular vulvovaginitis, balanoposthitis, abortion, infertility, conjunctivitis, and encephalitis in bovine species (Nandi et al. 2009).

17.11 Hypersensitivity Reactions

Hypersensitivity reactions are immune responses that are exaggerated or inappropriate against an antigen or allergen. Under the Coombs and Gell classification of hypersensitivity, reactions are divided into four types. They all are different in terms of the manifestation of disease and pathological processes. Type I, type II, and type III hypersensitivity reactions are known as immediate hypersensitivity reactions because they occur within 24 h, and it is mediated by antibodies including IgE, IgM, and IgG, whereas type IV hypersensitivity reaction is known as delayed hypersensitivity, and it is T-cell mediated (Tomasiak-Łozowska et al. 2018).

Table 17.2 Major histocompatibility complex (MHC) alleles and disease susceptibility in cattle

Disease	Breed	Bovine MHC alleles	Effect
Enzootic bovine leukosis			
Seroconversion	Holstein	A14	Late
	Holstein	A15	Rapid
	Guernsey	A21	Late
	Guernsey	DA6.2 and A12	Rapid
Peripheral lymphocytes and B-cell numbers	Shorthorn	DA7	Resistance
	Shorthorn	DA12.3	Susceptibility
	Irish shorthorn	A6 and EU28R	Susceptibility
	Irish shorthorn	A8	Resistance
	Holstein	A12, A15, and DRB21C	Susceptibility
	Holstein	A14, A13, DRB22A, and DRB3 (ERmotif)	Resistance
Mastitis			
Clinical mastitis	Norwegian red	A2	Resistance
	Norwegian red	A16	Susceptibility
	Swedish red and white	DQ1A	Susceptibility
	Holstein	A11	Resistance
	Holstein	CA42	Susceptibility
Subclinical mastitis (cell count)	Icelandic	A19	Susceptibility
	Simmental (S) or S × red Holstein	A15	High
	Danish black pied	A11 and A30	Low
	Danish black pied	A21 and A26	High
California mastitis test	Holstein	A14	Low
Helminths			
Nematodes	Belmont red	A7 and CA36	Resistance
	Africander × Hereford	A9	Susceptibility
Protozoa			
Theileria parva	*Bos indicus*	Class I	Parasite entry
Ticks			
Boophilus microplus	Brahman × shorthorn	A6 and CA31	Susceptibility
Posterior spinal paresis	Holstein	A8	Susceptibility
Ketosis	Norwegian red	A2 and A13	Resistance
Retained placenta	Dutch Friesian	Compatibility	Susceptibility

17.12 Type I Hypersensitivity

Type I hypersensitivity reaction is also known as anaphylactic reaction. It is an immediate hypersensitivity reaction produced by the body in response to environmental proteins known as allergens, and it is mediated by IgE antibodies. Type I hypersensitivity reactions can be seen in bronchial asthma, allergic rhinitis, allergic dermatitis, food allergy, allergic conjunctivitis, and anaphylactic shock (Koike et al. 2018; Son et al. 2018).

Type I hypersensitivity reactions always occur in the individual previously sensitized to that allergen. The exposure of the individual with the allergen for the first time results in production of the immunoglobulin IgE, which binds to Fc receptors present on the surface of mast cells and basophils and, then on encountering with the same allergen, triggers cross-linking of mast cell cytophilic IgE, causing degranulation of mast cells and release of chemical mediators of inflammation that results into allergic reaction. There are two types of mediators: primary and secondary mediators that participate in this type of hypersensitivity reaction include histamine and lipid mediators such as platelet-activating factor (PAF), leukotriene C4 (LTC4), and prostaglandin D2 (PGD2) that cause a vascular leak, bronchoconstriction, inflammation, and hypermotility of intestine. Enzymes (e.g., tryptase causes tissue damage) and TNF cause inflammation. Eosinophils release cationic granule proteins, e.g., major basic protein (causes killing of host cells and parasites) and enzymes, e.g., eosinophil peroxidase, which participate in tissue remodeling (De et al. 2018).

17.13 Allergic Rhinitis

The allergic rhinitis, occurs as a result of inhalation of pollen or fungal spores and has been occasionally reported in cattle. Clinically, the affected cattle show nasal discharge, sneezing, lacrimation, nasal irritation, dyspnea, and nasal pruritus. In chronic cases, there may be formation of multiple small proliferative nodular-like growth in the nasal passage. Cytologic examination of the nasal discharge reveals increased concentration of eosinophils (Olchowy et al. 1995). Postmortem examination conducted in a herd of Jersey cattle affected with rhinitis shows nodules of 2 to 3 mm diameter on the mucosa of nasal conchae with an orange mucopurulent exudate (Raghuramula et al. 2012).

17.14 Acute Systemic Anaphylaxis

Acute systemic anaphylaxis or type I hypersensitivity reactions in cattle can result in atypical interstitial pneumonia as lungs are the major target organ, which is affected. Further, serotonin, kinin, and histamine are the major mediators of inflammation. Clinical signs are same as that produce an acute respiratory distress like dyspnea, hypertension due to constriction of pulmonary veins, and pulmonary edema. The concentration of histamine in plasma gets increased during anaphylaxis, whereas there is not as such increase in serotonin plasma concentration (Eyre et al. 1973). For example, anaphylactic reaction has been reported in cattle immediately after the administration intramuscular injection of penicillin-streptomycin with clinical signs including respiratory distress, urticaria, and lacrimation (Omidi 2009).

17.15 Milk Allergy

Milk allergy is an auto-allergic reaction in cattle wherein an immune response is elicited to its own alpha-casein protein of milk. The occurrence of milk allergy is highest in the high yielding breeds of cattle like Jersey and Guernsey, especially during the period of dry off or delay in milking. Retention of milk in the mammary gland for any reason can cause increased intramammary pressure, which allows subsequent leakage of alpha casein protein in the circulation and stimulation of immediate hypersensitivity through cytotropic IgE-mediated antibody. Generally, this protein does not get entry in the circulation, if the cow milked routinely that keep away increased intramammary pressure. Clinically, the condition is characterized by the presence of urticarial lesions in eyelids, lips, vulva, and skin. It may also lead to death when dyspnea is associated with pulmonary or laryngeal edema (Moroni et al. 2018).

17.16 Insect Bite Allergy

Infection of cattle with *Hypoderma bovis* (warble fly) may exhibit anaphylaxis as a result of rupture of pupal stage during its physical removal from the back of animal. The rupture of pupal stage results in release of coelom fluid in the sensitized animal, which may cause acute reaction and occasionally death of animal. Biting of certain insects like midges (*Culicoides* spp.) and black flies (*Simulium* spp.) may induce allergic dermatitis commonly known as Gulf coast itch, Queensland itch, or sweet itch. Further, infection of helminth's parasites such as *Fasciola hepatica* can induce IgE production, which is responsible for allergy and anaphylactic reaction (Chauhan and Joshi 2012).

17.17 Type II Hypersensitivity

Type II hypersensitivity is an antibody-dependent process, mediated by IgM or IgG targeting membrane-associated antigens. A sensitization phase leads to production of antibodies that recognize substances or metabolites that accumulate in cellular membrane structures. In the effector phase, antibodies-coated target cells, i.e., opsonization, lead to the destruction of cell through three mechanisms: (1) phagocytosis, (2) complement-mediated lysis, and (3) antibody-dependent cell cytotoxicity (ADCC). In first, IgG or IgM antibody target-coated cells bind via fc receptors present on the cells such as macrophages and neutrophils and mediate phagocytosis. Second, IgG or IgM antibodies mediate the killing of cells by binding with the cell surface antigen that leads to the activation of complement system via classical pathway. Activation of complement system causes generation of membrane attack complex (MAC), responsible for formation of pores in the cellular membrane of cells resulting in cytolysis. In third, i.e., antibody-dependent cell cytotoxicity, IgG antibodies bind with FcγRIII receptor present in the surface of NK cells and macrophages, mediating release of granular enzymes and perforin that results in cell death through apoptosis (David and Beenhouwer 2018).

17.18 Hemolytic Disease of Newborn Calf

Hemolytic disease of the newborn calf is an acute hemolytic anemia in which iso-immune blood group antibodies of dam cause destruction of the red blood cells of the fetus or newborn animal (Dimmock and Bell 1970). The occurrence of this disease is uncommon, but it may be encountered as a result of immunization of dam against babesiosis or anaplasmosis. Although, these vaccines provide immunity in the vaccinated animals, there is also production of antibodies against the blood group antigens present in the vaccine. These vaccines are prepared from the blood of animals affected with babesia or anaplasma, and contain the antigens against blood components also. Further, there will be production of iso-antibodies, when mating of such vaccinated dam is done with the bull carrying the same blood group antigen, due to reexposure with the same blood antigen. This ultimately leads to the transfer of iso-antibodies against the red cell antigen to the newborn calf through colostrum, resulting in hemolytic disease (Chauhan and Joshi 2012).

Normally, such calves are born healthy, but following ingestion of the colostrum and subsequently absorption of antibodies through intestines, they start exhibiting clinical signs of the disease such as acute hemolytic anemia, respiratory difficulty, and severe hemoglobinuria. The probability of hemolytic disease in newborn calves depends upon the frequency of vaccinations of dam, amount of colostrums ingested, and the time interval between the previous vaccination and calving (Dimmock 1973). Autopsy and histological findings reveal that mortality in acute cases occurred due to widespread intravascular coagulation consequently leading to deposition of fibrin in pulmonary capillaries and severe pulmonary edema. Detection of antibodies on red blood cells can be done by antiglobulin test.

17.19 Type III Hypersensitivity

Type III hypersensitivity reactions occur when soluble antibodies bind to antigen to form immune complexes in the body tissues, which are able to fix complement and produce acute inflammatory responses (Janeway et al. 2001). Normally, the immune complexes are formed in our body and are taken care by the various cellular mechanisms physiologically capable of removing foreign antigen from the system.

In some cases, formation of immune complexes gets enhanced when antigen is in excess of antibody, which escape phagocytosis gets deposited in tissues of various organs. Hence, the deposition of immune complexes can occur in any parts of the body (Powell et al. 2013). The common site for deposition of immune complexes includes: glomerular membrane results in glomerulonephritis, synovial membrane of joints causes arthritis, walls of blood vessels cause vasculitis, and lungs result in pneumonitis. Mainly deposition of intermediate-sized immune complexes occurs as they remain in circulation for longer period and are trapped in small capillaries and renal glomeruli leading to the inflammatory process, whereas small-sized immune complexes are not get trapped in blood vessels/capillaries, and large size immune complexes are insoluble and are quickly removed by the phagocytic cells from the circulation. Hence, the size of immune complexes plays important role in tissue deposition of immune complexes.

The binding of antigen with antibody causes the activation of classical complement pathway that leads to the generation of C3a and C5a anaphylatoxins. These anaphylatoxins have chemotactic properties for neutrophils and also stimulate the degranulation of basophils and mast cells that result in the release of vasoactive amines like histamine. These chemical mediators of inflammation act on blood vessels and cause increased vascular permeability, which facilitates the deposition of immune complexes on the wall of blood vessel and also attract phagocytic cells. The Fc region of antibody in immune complex also interacts with Fc receptors of platelets and gets bind to the Fc receptors on platelets leading to their aggregation, and platelets cause microthrombus formation on basement membrane, which further facilitate an increased vascular permeability through the action of vasoactive amines. The phagocytic cells present at the site of immune complex deposition may attempt to phagocytose the complexes deposited on basement membrane and are unable to do so because of their trapping in tissues. Thus, these phagocytic cells release lytic enzymes at the site of immune complex deposition leading to further tissue damage. Examples of type III hypersensitivity include serum sickness, Arthus reaction, and immune complex-mediated glomerulonephritis.

17.20 Serum Sickness

Serum sickness is the systemic immune complex phenomenon that has been observed due to the injection of foreign proteins or serum for prophylactic treatment of patient. The passively administered protein is recognized as foreign antigen by the host immune system, leading to the production of antibodies against them, which combines with foreign protein or serum, and there will be the formation of immune complexes. These circulating immune complexes get deposited in tissues and initiate a complement cascade, leading to inflammatory conditions like glomerulonephritis, arthritis, and vasculitis (Saczonek et al. 2018). For example, in diphtheria patient when anti-diphtheria horse serum is given, which is mistaken as foreign protein by the host immune system and the body, it initiates an immune responses against horse serum leading to serum sickness.

17.21 Arthus Reaction

The Arthus reaction is a local immune complex deposition phenomenon seen at local site in and around the wall of small blood vessels that will result in vasculitis. Generally, Arthus reaction is observed within 24 h of administration of antigen and is confined to the injection site (Gershwin 2017). The administration of antigen through subcutaneous or intradermal route into the humans and animals containing preformed antibody to that antigen, circulating antibodies will recognize the antigen and get bind to it that results in the activation of complement system. Activation of complement system induces release of chemotactic factors, C3a and C5a, which cause degranulation of mast cells and neutrophil chemotaxis (Krakowka 1989). It is characterized by severe pain, edema, swelling, and hemorrhage at the site of injection, which depend on the administered dose of foreign antigens. The amount of antibody present in blood is directly related with the severity of Arthus reaction in the skin (Culbertson and Kent 1935).

17.22 Immune Complex-Mediated Glomerulonephritis

Immune complex-mediated glomerulonephritis results due to the deposition of antigen-antibody complexes that are formed in the circulation in the capillary walls of glomeruli. Deposition of immune complexes causes activation of classical complement pathway, inflammation, neutrophil influx, and degranulation of mast cells that result in tissue destruction. In cattle, immune complex-mediated glomerulonephritis is thought to be associated with bovine viral diarrhea. It is reported that clinically healthy cattle persistently infected with the virus of bovine viral diarrhea, when examined for viral antigen and lesions by direct immunofluorescence against basement membrane of renal glomeruli, showed irregularly thick basement membrane with abundant deposition of eosinophils and mesangial cells in the glomeruli of kidneys (Cutlip and Coria 1980).

17.23 Type IV Hypersensitivity

Type IV hypersensitivity is also known as delayed-type hypersensitivity reactions. It is mediated by antigen-specific effector T cells rather than antibodies as in other types of hypersensitivity reactions. They are distinguished from other hypersensitivity reactions as they generally occur 1 to 3 days after exposure to the antigen. On exposure of body with the antigen, it is taken up, processed, and presented by antigen-presenting cells like macrophages or dendritic cells to T helper cells. The type 1 helper effector cells that recognize the specific antigen get activated to release chemokines, which cause the recruitment of macrophages to the site and hence release cytokines that mediate tissue injury. The IFN-γ causes activation of macrophages and enhances release chemical mediators of inflammation, whereas TNF-α and TNF-β activate endothelial cells and enhance vascular permeability and local tissue injury. The prototypical type IV hypersensitivity reaction is the tuberculin test, but similar reactions can occur after contact with sensitizing antigens (e.g., poison ivy and certain metals) and lead to epidermal reactions characterized by erythema, cellular infiltration, and vesicles (Salmon 2012).

17.24 Tuberculin Reaction

Tuberculin reaction is one of the important examples of the type IV hypersensitivity reaction. It is one of the standard methods to diagnose the tuberculosis in animals affected with bovine tuberculosis, which is mainly caused by the bacteria *Mycobacterium bovis* (Figs. 17.1 and 17.2). Tuberculosis is one of the main zoonotic diseases of cattle and buffalo, which results in considerable number of mortalities in these animals. Tuberculin was first time developed by Koch in 1890, and from then, various refinements are done to increase the sensitivity and specificity of the test (Good et al. 2018).

Normally, healthy animals, when injected with tuberculin purified protein derivative (PPD), do not show any reaction. In contrast, injection of tuberculin PPD into the skin of the animals already sensitized with mycobacterial antigens, it produces delayed-type hypersensitivity reaction associated with the influx of sensitized T lymphocytes and monocytes into the site of inoculation (Waters et al. 2000). Tuberculin testing is usually performed on the skin of middle neck and caudal, but the skin of neck is more sensitive as compared to the skin of caudal. Before

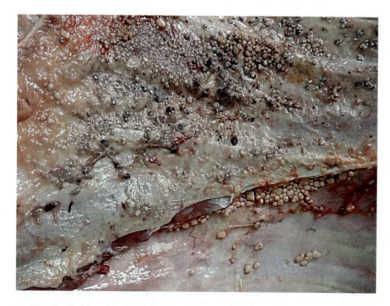

Fig. 17.1 Bovine tuberculosis (*Mycobacterium bovis*): Serosal surfaces of thorax and abdomen showed numerous pearly tubercle nodules

17.25 Johnin Reaction

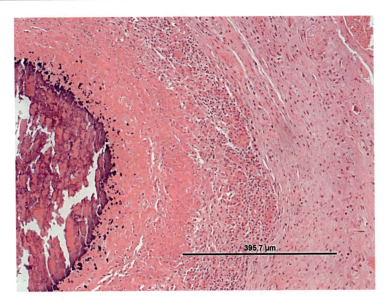

Fig. 17.2 Bovine tuberculosis (*Mycobacterium bovis*): Tuberculin reaction (type IV hypersensitivity)—central area of caseous necrosis with calcification (blue color), surrounded by epithelioid cells, Langhans giant cells, lymphocytes, and plasma cells with a fibrous capsule. H & E ×100

performing the test, testing site should be properly cleaned and shaved under the aseptic condition, and thickness of the skin should also be measured with the help of Vernier caliper. Then the tuberculin PPD should be injected intradermally with the help of tuberculin syringe. The dose of the tuberculin PPD should not be less than 2000 IU, and the correct injection is confirmed by the pea-like swelling at the site of injection. The animal is said to be positive only when thickness of the skinfold increases to double than the normal. Further, the injection site is examined for a reaction 72 h postinoculation with clinical signs of inflammation including redness, hot, pain, and edema (Table 17.3).

17.25 Johnin Reaction

A delayed-type hypersensitivity response is produced in animals after the intradermal injection of Johnin purified protein derivative (Johnin PPD) an extract of the bacteria *Mycobacterium avium* var. *paratuberculosis*. Johnin testing is done for the detection of paratuberculosis (Johne's disease), which is a chronic intestinal disease of ruminants, caused by *Mycobacterium avium* subspecies *paratuberculosis* (Maroudam et al. 2015). A positive test results in an increased thickness of skin (greater than 3 mm) at the site of injection within 72 h of intradermal injection of Johnin PPD. There is also a chance of significant cross-reactions due to the exposure of other environmental mycobacteria, such as *M. avium* species and *M. bovis*, or with

Table 17.3 Advantages and disadvantages of different tuberculin tests used in cattle

Tuberculin test	Application	Advantages	Disadvantages
Single intradermal (SID) test	Routine testing	Simple	Prone to false-positive results and poor sensitivity
Comparative intradermal tuberculin test (CIDT)	When avian tuberculosis or Johne's disease is prevalent	More specific than SID	More complex than SID
Short thermal tuberculin test	Use in postpartum animals and in infected animals	High efficiency	Time-consuming and risk for anaphylaxis
Stormont tuberculin test	Use in postpartum animals and in advanced cases	Very sensitive and accurate	Three visits are required and may sensitize an animal

vaccination for JD, resulting in a lack of specificity and a poor correlation with the infection status of the animal (Collins 1996). A nonspecific response can be clarified in cattle by the use of the comparative cervical skin test, because a stronger reaction will be given to the *M. avium* (PPD-A) injection site than to *M. bovis* (PPD-B) (Manning and Collins 2001).

17.26 Allergic Contact Dermatitis

Allergic contact dermatitis is also known as contact hypersensitivity. It is caused by the overreaction of immune system to a substance or chemical. It is a delayed-type hypersensitivity reaction, mediated by hapten-specific T cells (Saint-Mezard et al. 2004). Certain substances are responsible for causing contact dermatitis after single or multiple exposures of non-protein chemicals, i.e., haptens, that induce skin inflammation through the activation of innate skin immunity and cause irritant contact dermatitis or through activation of both innate and acquired specific immunity results into allergic contact dermatitis. It is observed that some dairy cattle have developed severe dermatitis that was suspected to have been caused by calcium cyanamide, as it is added to the material spread on the floor of the cattle shed to prevent environmental mastitis (Onda et al. 2008). Addition of calcium cyanamide to a mixture of manure and sawdust is a very effective method of reducing the levels of *Escherichia coli* (Minato et al. 2001).

17.27 Autoimmunity

Autoimmunity is the immune reaction of body against the self-antigen that elicits the prospect of "horror autotoxicus," a term coined by Paul Ehrlich to outline the perceived outrageous consequences of this condition (Kono and Theofilopoulos 2017). In other words, it is a state which results from a breakdown or failure of normal mechanism of body responsible for maintaining self-tolerance in B cells, T cells, or both, which allows immune response against its own cells and tissues. The illness that results due to immune reaction against the self is known as autoimmune diseases. Vitiligo is the autoimmune disease that has been reported in buffalo.

17.28 Vitiligo

Vitiligo is an acquired cutaneous disorder characterized by progressive loss of melanocytes and patchy depigmentation of the affected skin (Alikhan et al. 2011). It has been reported in brown- and dark-skinned buffaloes (Cockrill 1981). Etiology is not clear, but environmental, immunological, genetic, and neurological factors are assumed to play an important role; however, the exact pathogenesis remains unclear. Due to the reduction in tyrosinase activity, there is decreased conversion of tyrosine to melanin resulting in abnormal hair pigmentation (Mude and SyaamaSundar 2009). Affected animals show depigmented lesions at the site of face, muzzle, limbs, ventral, and dorsal surfaces of the body (Singh et al. 2016). Serum biochemical study of animals affected with vitiligo reveals low blood copper levels as compared to the normal. The copper forms an integral part of tyrosinase, which is involved in the conversion of tyrosine to melanin (Lerner and Fitzpatrick 1950). The deficiency of copper is very common in livestock (Kachhawaha 2003). In areas deficient in copper, there is low blood levels of copper intake from natural forages, and color coat of such animals is also affected (Radostits et al. 2000).

17.29 Conclusion

The immunopathological disorders include diseases of immune system, generally caused by an overactive immune response known as hypersensitivity reactions, an inappropriate reaction to self, i.e., autoimmunity or ineffective immune responses and immunodeficiency. Diseases associated with the defects of immune system directly or indirectly induce immunosuppression that provokes the chances of secondary infections or illness. There are different immunopathological disorders, which account for substantial morbidity and mortality in bovine species. Mortality is mainly seen in association with the secondary infections. The diagnosis of diseases related with immunologic origin always remains a major issue, but attentive collaboration of clinician and pathologist plays an important role to overcome this problem.

References

Alikhan A, Felsten LM, Daly M, Petronic-Rosic V (2011) Vitiligo: a comprehensive overview part I. introduction, epidemiology, quality of life, diagnosis, differential diagnosis, associations, histopathology, etiology, and work-up. J Am Acad Dermatol 65(3):473–491

Bhatia SS, Patil SS, Sood R (2013) Bovine immunodeficiency virus: a lentiviral infection. Indian J Virol 24(3):332–341

Bolin SR, McClurkin AW, Coria MF (1985) Effects of bovine viral diarrhoea virus cattle. Am J Vet Res 46:884–886

Bonilla FA, Oettgen HC (2010) Adaptive immunity. J Allergy Clin Immunol 125(2):33–40

Brewoo JN, Haase CJ, Sharp P, Schultz RD (2007) Leukocyte profile of cattle persistently infected with bovine viral diarrhea virus. Vet Immunol Immunopathol 115(3–4):369–374

Chase CCL (2013) The impact of BVDV infection on adaptive immunity. Biologicals 41:52–60

Chauhan RS, Joshi A (2012) Immunology for beginners. Kapish Prakashan, Gurgaon

Chinen J, Shearer WT (2010) Secondary immunodeficiencies, including HIV infection. J Allergy Clin Immunol 125(2):195–203

Cockrill WR (1981) The water buffalo: a review. Br Vet J 137(1):8–16

Collins MT (1996) Diagnosis of paratuberculosis. Vet Clin North Am Food Anim Pract 12:357–371

Culbertson JT, Kent JF (1935) The relationship of circulating antibody to the local inflammatory reaction to antigen (the Arthus phenomenon). J Immunol 29(1):29–39

Cutlip RC, AW MC, Coria MF (1980) Lesions in clinically healthy cattle persistently infected with the virus of bovine viral diarrhea—glomerulonephritis and encephalitis. Am J Vet Res 41(12): 1938–1941

David O, Beenhouwer MD (2018) Molecular basis of diseases of immunity. In: Molecular pathology, molecular basis of human disease, 2nd edn. Academic press, London, pp 329–345

De A, Rajagopalan M, Sarda A, Das S, Biswas P (2018) Drug reaction with eosinophilia and systemic symptoms. An update and review of recent literature. Indian J Dermatol 63(1):30–40

Dimmock CK (1973) Blood group antibody production in cattle by a vaccine against *Babesia argentina*. Res Vet Sci 15(3):305–309

Dimmock CK, Bell K (1970) Hemolytic disease of the newborn in calves. Aust Vet J 46(2):44–47

Eyre P, Lewis AJ, Wells PW (1973) Acute systemic anaphylaxis in the calf. Br J Pharmacol 47(3): 504–516

Falkenberg SM, Dassanayake R, Walz P, Neil J, Ridapath J (2018) Association between bovine viral diarrhea virus load in subsets of peripheral blood mononuclear cells (PBMC) in persistently infected animals and health outcome. J Immunol 200(1):25

Gamlen T, Richards KH, Mankouri J, Hudson L, McCauley J, Harris M, Macdonald A (2010) Expression of the NS3 protease of cytopathogenic bovine viral diarrhea virus results in the induction of apoptosis but does not block activation of the beta interferon promoter. J Gen Virol 91:133–144

Gershwin LJ (2017) Adverse reactions to vaccination: from anaphylaxis to autoimmunity. Vet Clin North Am Small Anim Pract 48(2):279–290

Gonda MA, Braun MJ, Carter SG, Kost TA, Bess JW Jr, Arthur LO, VanDerMaaten MJ (1987) Characterization and molecular cloning of a bovine lentivirus related to human immunodeficiency virus. Nature 330:388–391

Good M, Bakker D, Duignan A, Collins DM (2018) The history of *in vivo* tuberculin testing in bovine tuberculosis, a one health issue. Front Vet Sci 5:59

Hariharan MJ, Nataraj C, Sriikumaran S (1993) Down regulation of murine MHC class I expression by bovine herpes virus 1. Viral Immunol 6:273–284

Howard CJ (1990) Immunological responses to bovine virus diarrhoea virus infections. Rev Sci Tech 9:95–103

Janeway CAJ, Travers P, Walport M (2001) Hypersensitivity diseases. In: Immunobiology: the immune system in health and diseases, 5th edn. Garland science, New York, NY

Justiz V (2018) Immediate hypersensitivity reactions. In: StatPearls, vol 1, pp 1–123

Kachhawaha S (2003) Copper deficiency in Buffalo calves. Intas Polivet 4(2):238–239

Khodakaram-Tafti A, Farjanikish GH (2017) Persistent bovine viral diarrhea virus (BVDV) infection in cattle herds. Iran J Vet Res 18(3):154–163

Koike Y, Sato S, Yanagida N, Asaumi T, Ogura K, Ohtani K, Imai T, Ebisawa M (2018) Predictors of persistent milk allergy in children: a retrospective cohort study. Int Arch Allergy Immunol 175(3):177–180

Kono DH, Theofilopoulos AN (2017) Autoimmunity, 10th edn. Kelley and Firestein's textbook of rheumatology

Krakowka S (1989) Immunopathogenesis of arterial diseases in animals and man, vol 17. Department of Veterinary Pathology, College of Veterinary Medicine, the Ohio State University, Columbus, OH, p 1

Lambot M, Douart A, Joris E, Letesson JJ, Pastoret PP (1997) Characterization of the immune response of cattle against non-cytopathic and cytopathic biotypes of bovine viral diarrhoea virus. J Gen Virol 78:1041–1047

Lanyon SR, Hill FI, Reichel MP, Brownlie J (2014) Bovine viral diarrhoea: pathogenesis and diagnosis. Vet J 199:201–209

Lerner AB, Fitzpatrick TB (1950) Biochemistry of melanin. Physiol Rev 30(1):91–126

Manning EJB, Collins MT (2001) Mycobacterium avium subsp. paratuberculosis: pathogen, pathogenesis and diagnosis. Rev Sci Tech 20(1):133–150

Maroudam V, Mohana Subramanian B, Praveen Kumar P, Dhinakar RG (2015) Paratuberculosis: diagnostic methods and their constraints. J Vet Sci Tech 6:259

Maurer K, Krey T, Moennig V, Thiel HJ, Rumenapf T (2004) CD46 is a cellular receptor for bovine viral diarrhoea virus. J Virol 78:1792–1799

Meyling A, Houe H, Jensen AM (1990) Epidemiology of bovine virus diarrhoea virus. Rev Sci Tech 9:75–93

Minato K, Tamura T, Maeta Y (2001) The effect of sterilisation on *Escherichia coli* in cattle manure by adding nitrolime. Bulletin of the Hokkaido Animal Research Center, vol 24, p 21–22

Moroni P, Nydam DV, Ospina PA, Scillieri-Smith JC, Virkler PD, Watters RD, Welcome FL, Zurakowski MJ, Ducharme NG, Yeager AE (2018) Rebhon's diseases of dairy cattle, 3rd edn. Elsevier, Amsterdam, pp 389–465

Mude S, SyaamaSundar N (2009) Vitiligo in buffaloes. Vet World 2(7):282

Murphy KM, Travers P, Walport M (2007) Janeway's immunobiology, 7th edn. Garland science, New York, NY, London

Nagahata H (2004) Bovine leukocyte adhesion deficiency (BLAD). J Vet Med Sci 66(12):1475–1482

Nandi S, Kumar M, Manohar M, Chauhan RS (2009) Bovine herpes virus infections in cattle. Anim Health Res Rev 10(1):85–98

Notarangelo LD (2010) Primary immunodeficiencies. J Allergy Clin Immunol 125:182–194

Olchowy TW, Gershwin LJ, Dean DF (1995) Allergic rhinitis in a herd of cattle. J Am Vet Med Assoc 207(9):1211–1214

Omidi A (2009) Anaphylactic reaction in a cow due to parenteral administration of penicillin-streptomycin. Can Vet J 50(7):741–744

Onda K, Yagisawa T, Matsui T, Tanaka H, Yako J, Une Y, Wada Y (2008) Contact dermatitis in dairy cattle caused by calcium cyanamide. Vet Rec 163(14):418–422

Pac M, Bernatowska E (2016) Comprehensive activities to increase recognition of primary immunodeficiency and access to immunoglobulin replacement therapy in Poland. Eur J Pediatr 175(8):1099–1105

Padgett GA, Leader RW, Gorham JR, Omarry CC (1964) The familial occurrence of the chediak-higashi syndrome in mink and cattle. Genetics 49(3):505

Pedrera M, Gómez-Villamandos JC, Risalde MA, Molina V, Sanchez-Cordon PJ (2012) Characterisation of apoptosis pathways (intrinsic and extrinsic) in lymphoid tissues of calves inoculated with non-cytopathic bovine viral diarrhoea virus genotype. J Comp Pathol 146:30–39

Potgieter LN (1995) Immunology of bovine viral diarrhoea virus. Vet Clin North Am Food Anim Pract 11:501–520

Powell C, Thompson L, Murtaugh RJ (2013) Type III hypersensitivity reaction with immune complex deposition in 2 critically ill dogs administered human serum albumin. J Vet Emerg Crit Care 1:1–7

Radostits OM, Gay CC, Blood DC, Hinchcliff KW (2000) Textbook of the diseases of cattle, sheep, pigs, goats and horses, 9th edn, pp 1487–1499

Raghuramula N, Madhavannair K, Kalpna S (2012) Rhinitis associated with allergic nasal granuloma in Jersey cattle. Vet Rec 171(19):468–471

Raje N, Dinakar C (2015) Overview of immunodeficiency disorders. Immunol Allergy Clin North Am 35(4):599–623

Reimann KA, Letvin NL (1993) Immunodeficiency: an overview. In: Jones TC, Mohr U, Hunt RD (eds) Nonhuman primates I. Monographs on pathology of laboratory animals. Springer, Berlin, Heidelberg

Rouse BT, Horohov DW (1986) Immunosuppression in viral infections. Rev Infect Dis 8:850–873

Saczonek AO, Wygonowska E, Budkiewicz M, Waldemar P (2018) Serum sickness disease in a patient with alopecia areata and meniere disease after PRP procedure. Dermatol Ther 32:e12798

Saint-Mezard P, Rosieres A, Krasteva M, Berard F, Dubois B, Kaiserlian D, Nicolas JF (2004) Allergic contact dermatitis. Eur J Dermatol 14(5):284–295

Salmon JE (2012) Mechanism of tissue mediated tissue injury. In: Goldman's cecil medicine, vol 1, 24th edn. Elsevier, Amsterdam, pp 226–230

Sell S (1978) Immunopathology. Am J Pathol 3:215–275

Shiraishi M, Ogawah H, Ikeda M, Kawashima S, Ito K (2002) Platelet dysfunction in Chediak-Higashi syndrome-affected cattle. J Vet Med Sci 64(9):751–760

Shuster DE, Kehrli ME, Ackermann MR, Gilbert RO (1992) Identification and prevalence of a genetic defect that causes leukocyte adhesion deficiency in Holstein cattle. Proc Natl Acad Sci 89:9225–9229

Singh VP, Motiani RK, Singh A, Malik G, Aggarwal R, Pratap K, Mohan R (2016) Water Buffalo (Bubalus bubalis) as a spontaneous animal model of vitiligo. Pigment Cell Melanoma Res 29(4):465–469

Smith DA, Germolec DR (1999) Introduction to immunology and autoimmunity. Environ Health Perspect 107(5):661–665

Son JH, Park SY, Cho YS, Chung BY, Kim HO, Park CW (2018) Immediate hypersensitivity reactions induced by triamcinolone in a patient with atopic dermatitis. J Korean Med Sci 33(12):87

Tikoo SK, Campos M, Babiuk LA (1995) Bovine herpesvirus 1(BHV-1): biology, pathogenesis and control. Adv Virus Res 45:191–223

Tomasiak-Łozowska MM, Klimek M, Lis A, Moniuszko M, Bodzenta-Łukaszyk A (2018) Markers of anaphylaxis—a systematic review. Adv Med Sci 63(2):265–277

Turvey SE, Broide DH (2010) Innate immunity. J Allergy Clin Immunol 125(2):24–32

Umemura T, Katsuta O, Goryo M, Hayashi T, Itakura C (1983) Pathological findings in young Japanese black cattle. J Vet Med Sci 45:241–246

Waters WR, Palmer MV, Pesch BA, Olsen SC, Wannemuehler MJ, Whipple DL (2000) Lymphocyte subset proliferative responses of Mycobacterium bovis-infected cattle to purified protein derivative. Vet Immunol Immunopathol 77(3–4):257–273

Whetstone CA, Suarez DL, Miller JM, Pesch BA, Harp JA (1997) Bovine lentivirus induces early transient B-cell proliferation in experimentally inoculated cattle and appears to be pantropic. J Virol 71:640–644

Winkler MTC, Doster A, Jones C (1999) Bovine herpesvirus 1 can infect CD4+ T lymphocytes and induce programmed cell death during acute infection of cattle. J Virol 73:8657–8668

Wu D, Murakami K, Morooka A, Jin H, Inoshima Y, Sentsui H (2003) *In vivo* transcription of bovine leukemia virus and bovine immunodeficiency-like virus. Virus Res 97:81–87

Zhang S, Wood C, Xue W, Krunkenberg SM, Minocha HC (1997) Immune suppression in calves with bovine immunodeficiency virus. Clin Diagn Lab Immunol 4:232–235

Immunopathological Disorders in Sheep, Goat, Wild Animals, and Laboratory Animals

18

Key Points

1. Acute systemic anaphylaxis is the type I hypersensitivity, which is an emergency condition mediated by IgE that leads to an acute and life-threatening respiratory failure.
2. In sheep, major mediators of acute systemic anaphylaxis are histamine and later on leukotrienes.
3. Serotonin is the main chemical mediator of acute systemic anaphylaxis in case of rodents.
4. Allergic rhinitis in sheep is mainly caused by the *Oestrus ovis* larva in frontal sinus.
5. Autoimmune hemolytic anemia is reported in mice and rabbits, and antibodies are formed against erythrocytic antigen due to molecular changes in self-antigen.
6. Orf or contagious ecthyma caused by DNA parapox virus in small ruminants causes autoimmune disorder by giving rise to autoantibodies against basement membrane of epithelium.
7. Orf causes proliferative skin lesions on the lips, around the mouth, nostrils, and eyelids.
8. Johne's disease in small ruminants causes autoimmune disorder by giving rise to autoantibodies against HSP65 of MAP because of molecular mimicry with the various host proteins.
9. Knut is the autoimmune disorder reported in polar bear with high concentrations of autoantibodies in cerebrospinal fluid against the NR1 subunit of N-methyl-D-aspartate (NMDA) receptor.
10. Bluetongue, Border disease, and Jaagsiekte cause secondary immunodeficiencies in sheep.
11. Mouse mammary tumor virus and Murine leukemia virus cause secondary immunodeficiencies in murine.

18.1 Introduction

The immune system protects us against various infectious agents, toxic, and allergic substances (Chaplin 2010). It contains two interrelated responses, i.e., innate immune response and acquired immune response. These components of the immune system in coordination with each other give protection against any harmful agents. Immunopathological disorder arises when there is defect in immune system. The word immunopathology is derived from two words which are immunity and pathology. Immunity is the resistance of the body against any extraneous etiological factor due to interaction of chemical, humoral, and cellular reaction in the body. Pathology is the study of the anatomical, chemical, and physiological alterations from normal as a result of disease in animals. Immune system in our body is there to protect us from various diseases and help in maintaining the normal life, but in some cases rather than providing protection to the animals, immune response may prove fatal to animals. It shows that the protective immune response can also cause tissue damage (Sell 1978). Immunopathology includes the disorders of immune system, which are characterized by hypersensitivity, immunodeficiency, and autoimmunity. An overactive immune response is known as hypersensitivity reaction, an inappropriate reaction to self-antigen known as autoimmune reaction, and ineffective immune responses also known as immunodeficiency.

Hypersensitivity reaction is an exaggerated or elevated immune response against any antigen and is categorized into four types, namely, type I, immediate or IgE mediated; type II, cytotoxic; type III, immune complex mediated; and type IV, delayed-type hypersensitivity (Uzzaman and Cho 2012). The first three hypersensitivity reactions are the antibody mediated, while type IV is T-cell-mediated hypersensitivity. Immunodeficiency occurs due to failure or absence of essentials of the immune system such as complement system, lymphocytes, and phagocytes. Autoimmunity is defined as an immune response of the body against self-antigen or body's own tissues. Reactivity against self-antigen can arise either by triggering the receptors directly by autoantigen or through cross-reaction between foreign and self-antigens (Agmon-Levin and Shoenfeld 2010). In sheep and goat, wild, and laboratory animals, there are several immunopathological disorders that may prove fatal to animals including acute systemic anaphylaxis, allergic rhinitis, blood transfusion reactions, hemolytic diseases, immune-complex-mediated glomerulonephritis, transient hypogammaglobulinemia, bluetongue disease, mouse mammary tumor virus infection, simian immunodeficiency virus infection, murine leukemia virus infection, pemphigus foliaceus, autoimmune hemolytic anemia, autoimmune encephalitis etc. Cytokines play major role in the modulation of immune responses resulting in development of several immunopathological disorders (Table 18.1).

Table 18.1 List of important immunomodulatory cytokines

Interferons (IFN)	Colony-stimulating factors (CSF)	Pro-inflammatory cytokines	Anti-inflammatory cytokines
Type I (IFN-α/IFN-β)	IL-3/multi-CSF	IL-1	IL-4
Type II (IFN-γ)	Macrophage-CSF (M-CSF)	IL-6	IL-10
	Granulocyte-CSF (G-CSF)	IL-12	TGF-β
	Granulocyte-macrophage-CSF (GM-CSF)	TNF-α	

18.2 Hypersensitivity Reactions in Sheep, Goat, Wild Animals, and Laboratory Animals

Hypersensitivity reactions (HR) are immune responses that are exaggerated or inappropriate against an antigen or allergen. These are further categorized into type I, immediate or IgE mediated; type II, cytotoxic; type III, immune complex mediated; and type IV, delayed-type hypersensitivity (Tomasiak-Łozowska et al. 2018). First three types are the antibody-mediated hypersensitivity, but type IV hypersensitivity is cell mediated.

18.3 Type I Hypersensitivity

The anaphylactic reactions arise in response to environmental proteins, and allergens such as pollens or dust, vaccine, insect, food, mold, etc. are mediated by cytotropic IgE antibodies that are produced by the immune system. These antibodies (IgE) with the help of Fc receptor bind to mast cells and basophils. Now, IgE-bound mast cells and basophils are referred as sensitized. On subsequent exposure to the same antigen, there is a cross-linking between IgE antibodies, which results into release of chemical mediators of inflammation such as histamine and serotonin from degranulation of mast cells and basophils that cause inflammatory reactions. Type 1 hypersensitivity is an immediate immune reaction to an antigen (Sicherer and Leung 2009). These reactions can be seen in bronchial asthma, allergic rhinitis, allergic dermatitis, food allergy, allergic conjunctivitis, and anaphylactic shock in animals.

18.4 Acute Systemic Anaphylaxis

Acute systemic anaphylaxis is an emergency condition that leads to an acute and life-threatening respiratory failure. It is an IgE-mediated process. In sheep, the major mediators of acute systemic anaphylaxis are histamine and later on leukotrienes. Pulmonary signs are more prominent as major organ affected is the lungs. Clinically characterized by bronchospasm, laryngeal edema, constriction of blood vessels, shock, dyspnea, and increased pulmonary hypertension (Wang et al. 2019). Serotonin is the main chemical mediator of acute systemic anaphylaxis in case of rodents.

18.5 Allergic Rhinitis

Allergic rhinitis is an atopic reaction, mediated by IgE antibody, where mast cells immediately release histamine in large amount (Shamji et al. 2019). In sheep, it is mainly due to the *Oestrus ovis* larva in frontal sinus, but in other animals, it occurs due to the irritant like pollen grains, infection, drugs, etc. Allergic rhinitis is characterized by rhinorrhea, nasal obstruction, excessive lacrimation, and watery nasal discharge. In laboratory animals, conjunctivitis is also seen.

18.6 Type II Hypersensitivity

Antibody binding to the cell surface antigen, mediated by destruction of the cells, is the basic mechanism in type II hypersensitivity reactions (Rajan 2003). There are three ways by which antibody can cause the destruction of cells. First, antibody binds to the foreign erythrocytic antigen and acts as opsonin, and antibody-coated red cells are phagocytosed by the phagocytic cells with Fc and C3b receptors (Rajan 2003). Second, the combination of antibody and the red cell antigen activates the complement system and generates membrane attack complex, hence formation of pores into the foreign red cells. Third, antibody-dependent cell cytotoxicity (ADCC) mechanism plays a major role (Gell and Coombs 1963). Various cells such as macrophages, monocytes, NK cells, neutrophils, and basophils express receptors for antibody Fc region. These cells bind to the target cells through Fc receptors and initiate lysis of antibody-coated target cells by release of lytic components, tumor necrosis factor, perforins, etc. (Clynes and Ravetch 1995). Experimental studies in mice revealed that CD32a antibodies induced thrombocytopenia and type II hypersensitivity reactions in Fc fragment of IgG receptor IIa (FCGR2A) (Meyer et al. 2015). Extracellular microorganisms (*Staphylococci* and *Streptococci*) are capable of inducing type II antibodies to surface antigens of microorganisms and lead to C5a release and chemotaxis of polymorphonuclear leukocytes (PMNs) to site of infection. Certain drug reactions and vasculitides such as polyarteritis nodosa, sometimes agonist antibody to thyroid stimulating, and antagonist antibody to acetylcholine receptors, which mediate type II reactions (Gell and Coombs 1963).

18.7 Blood Groups

18.7.1 Sheep

By isoimmunization, five different agglutinins are produced in response to the antigens A, B, C, E, and G, and five isohemolysins independent from these agglutinins correspond to antigens D, H, I, J, and K. The A antigen is similar to R antigen (Rasmusen 1961). Blood group B of sheep is also complex and is reported to have more than 50 alleles. The blood group system of sheep somewhat resembles to those of cattle.

18.7.2 Goat

Ten antigens are detected by the use of isoimmune sera produced in sheep. The factor E, detected by agglutination, and factor J are detected by hemolysis. Also, the factor G is recognized by agglutination, and factor K is by hemolysis. The antigens A, B, C, D, H, and I are found in sheep and are not detected in goats. Some of the goats possess the antigens L, M, Q, and P, detected by hemolysis, and the factor O, detected by agglutination, or the antigen N, detected by both techniques. Hemolysis test is used for identification of erythrocyte antigen.

18.8 Blood Transfusion Reaction

As naturally occurring antibodies to the most of the erythrocyte antigen are absent in animals, first transfusion does not cause any discomfort or clinical reaction (Hale 1995). Hence, crossmatching or blood typing before first transfusion is not required. However, if the donor erythrocyte antigen is not identical to that of the recipient, it does stimulate antibody formation. The second time blood transfusion from the same animal or other animals with the identical antigen would induce type II reaction, which is mediated by circulating isoantibodies that are usually IgG type. There is a rapid agglutination of erythrocytes with intra- and extravascular erythrocyte destruction and hemolysis (Dhaliwal et al. 2004). The severity of transfusion reactions depends upon immunogenicity of the blood group antigen involved. The animal may suffer from generalized anaphylactic shock, hemoglobinemia, and disseminated intravascular coagulation (Swisher 1954). Incompatible blood transfusion involving minor antigen has a longer course (4–14 days) and causes progressive anemia and icterus. Direct antiglobulin test can be used for the diagnosis (Hohenhaus 2004). Crossmatching using donor's red blood cells and recipient serum will result in positive slide agglutination test.

18.9 Hemolytic Diseases

Hemolytic syndrome occurs after exposure to the certain chemicals and drugs in man and animals, with the appearance of erythrocyte inclusion bodies, i.e., Heinz-Ehrlich bodies (Webster 1949; Fertman and Fertman 1955). Various mechanisms impart association between infection and hemolysis (Berkowitz 1991). Further, autoantibody induction (e.g., *M. pneumoniae*), glucose-6-phosphate dehydrogenase (G6PD) deficiency (Beutler 1994), and antimicrobial drugs (e.g., penicillin) are capable to induce hemolytic syndrome. A deficiency of G6PD accounts for the hemolytic complications results due to primaquine and related compounds (Beutler 1959). An immunological mechanism induced by Fuadin has been described in hemolytic anemia (Arris 1956). In addition, certain infectious agents like Babesia, tick-borne protozoa, and *Bartonella bacilliformis* (a Gram-negative bacillus transmitted by the sandfly) cause extravascular hemolysis by direct erythrocytic invasion or alteration of red cell membrane (Dhaliwal et al. 2004) and make them immunologically foreign. *Trypanosoma rhodesiense* induces ADCC mediated through an alternative complement pathway (Flemmings and Diggs 1978), which is based on the assessment of extent of ADCC, measured by inhibition of incorporation of [3H] leucine as an indicator of metabolic integrity of trypanosome, antibody-mediated cytotoxicity, and also the immune hemolysis (Diggs et al. 1976).

Hemolytic disease is reported in hybrid fetus of sheep and goat. A hybrid fetus of sheep and goat dies due to hemolytic anemia, when antibodies to their own red blood cells cross the placenta from the maternal circulation (Alexander et al. 1967).

18.10 Type III Hypersensitivity

Type III hypersensitivity are inflammatory responses induced by classic complement activation, due to extracellular antibody (IgM and IgG) and antigen complexes. These responses are triggered by soluble immune complexes that deposit in various tissues, including the kidneys, joints, and small vessels of the blood. Activated complement system causes inflammation and changes in vascular permeability through the release of chemotactic agents that attract neutrophils to tissues, where the immune complexes are deposited and cause tissue damage as seen in vasculitis and glomerulonephritis. Irrelevant of the antigenic specificity of the antibodies, the site of type III hypersensitivity reactions depends entirely on where immune complexes get deposited (Birdsall 2015).

18.11 Sheep

Glomerulonephritis is the inflammatory condition, which is mediated by the deposition of antigen-antibody (IgG and IgM) complexes in glomerulus of the kidney. By attracting the circulating inflammatory cells or activating resident glomerular cells to release cytokines, vasoactive substances, and activators of coagulation immune complexes can damage glomerular structures of the kidney. However, the classical mediator of immune-complex-mediated glomerulonephritis is the complement system, typically C5b-9 membrane attack complex formation. The C5b-9 attacks membranes of glomerular cells, leading to cell activation that causes injury to glomerular cells by converting normal cells into resident inflammatory cells (Nangaku and Couser 2005). Immune-complex-mediated glomerulonephritis is also seen in case of ovine campylobacteriosis and lindane toxicity in sheep (Chauhan and Joshi 2012).

18.12 Rabbit

Multiple daily intravenous injections of bovine serum albumin (BSA) to the laboratory rabbits lead to the production of immune complexes, resulting in immune-complex-mediated glomerulonephritis and gastrointestinal lesions. Granular deposits of BSA, C_3, and rabbit IgG are also found in the gastrointestinal tract of approximately 50% of these rabbits. The immune complexes deposited in the GIT are mainly seen in the vessel walls, between the smooth muscle cells, near to the intestinal glands and the surface epithelium that induce injury to the gastrointestinal tract (Accinni et al. 1978).

18.13 Type IV Hypersensitivity

The type IV hypersensitivity reaction is a delayed hypersensitivity reaction, as typically it takes 48–72 h to develop. It is mainly mediated by subclasses of T cells mainly the Th_1 and Tc cells. The most classical example of the delayed-type hypersensitivity (DTH) reaction is tuberculin testing, i.e., immunologic response to intracellular microorganism particularly *Mycobacterium* (Fig. 18.1). The DTH results from interaction between the allergen, macrophages, and T cells. The antigens are processed by antigen-presenting cells (APC) such as macrophages, Langerhans cells, and dendritic cells and presented to helper T cells having MHC class II molecules. These cells are specifically called as sensitized T cells or T delayed-type hypersensitivity cells. Sensitized T helper cells release cytokines that induce a local inflammatory response in a sensitized individual. Delayed-type hypersensitivity can also occur against various fungi, parasites, virus, chemical agents, and allograft. The magnitude of the DTH can be determined in animals by measuring the thickness of the skin along with inflammatory signs, which is local but can also be systemic such as T-cell division and cytokine synthesis (Barailler et al. 2019; Pelzer et al. 2018). In guinea pigs, flea allergy dermatitis or flea bite hypersensitivity reactions are reported (Fig. 18.2).

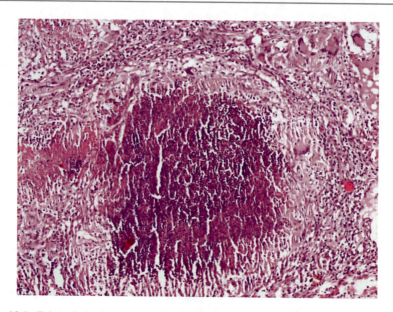

Fig. 18.1 Tuberculosis in goat (*Mycobacterium bovis*): Tuberculin reaction (type IV hypersensitivity)—central area of caseous necrosis with calcification (blue color), surrounded by epithelioid cells, Langhans giant cells, lymphocytes, and plasma cells with a fibrous capsule. H & E ×100

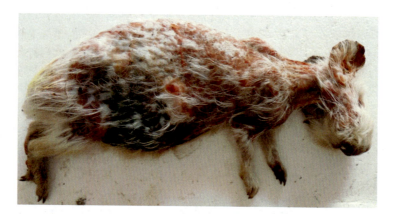

Fig. 18.2 Flea allergy dermatitis/flea bite hypersensitivity reaction in guinea pig: Guinea pig showed cutaneous lesions, dermatitis, pruritis, excoriation, alopecia, and eosinophilic lesions

18.14 Immunodeficiency in Sheep, Goat, Wild Animals, and Laboratory Animals

Immunodeficiency occurs due to failure or absence of essentials of the immune system such as complement system, lymphocytes, and phagocytes. These immunodeficiencies can be either primary also known as congenital or secondary which is also known as acquired (Pac and Bernatowska 2016).

18.15 Primary Immunodeficiency/Congenital Immunodeficiency

It is present in animals since their birth, and the defect in immunity is genetically determined (Notarangelo 2010). The congenital immunodeficiency is very rare in animals and has been reported due to defect in basic cellular components at the time of development. Various types of congenital immunodeficiencies are B-cell deficiencies, selective immunoglobulin deficiencies, T-cell immunodeficiencies, T-cell and B-cell deficiencies, complement deficiencies, and phagocyte deficiencies. The B and T lymphocytes are known as immune cells. The B cells differentiate into plasma cells that produce large amounts of immunoglobulins or antibodies. These antibodies fight against extracellular microorganisms. The T cells transform into helper T cells and cytotoxic or suppressor T cells. Helper T cells stimulate the production of antibodies. Hence in T-cell deficiencies, production of antibodies may be compromised up to an extent. T cells attack intracellular microorganisms such as fungi, viruses, and also neoplastic cells.

18.16 Severe Combined Immunodeficiency Disease (SCID)

The SCID is incompatible with life and more commonly affects young male. The SCID-affected young ones usually die within the first 2 years of life. The early stem cells failed to differentiate T and B lymphocytes. In more than 50% of cases, it is caused by a gene defect on the X chromosome. The gamma chain of the interleukin-2 (IL-2) receptor is encoded by a defective gene. This chain forms a molecular part of the receptors for IL-2, IL-4, IL-7, IL-11, IL-15, and IL-21. However, in few cases, severe combined immunodeficiency disorder is caused by defective genes that encode for nucleoside phosphorylase or adenosine deaminase that causes ribonucleotide reductase inhibition, which results into a defect in the DNA synthesis and cell replication. An autosomal recessive form of SCID occurred due to mutation in the genes encoding *RAG1* or *RAG2*. Clinically, the disease is manifested by a variety of opportunistic infections (Chinn and Shearer 2015).

18.17 Transient Hypogammaglobulinemia in Lamb

Transient hypogammaglobulinemia is mainly due to the defect in B lymphocytes. Hence, there is absence of any classes or subclasses of immunoglobulins. It occurs in neonates at 4–6 months of age. The maternal antibodies or immunoglobulins are catabolized slowly, which result into low level of immunoglobulins in the neonatal blood. During the period of transient hypogammaglobulinemia, neonates become immunocompromised and susceptible to various opportunistic pathogens (Chauhan and Joshi 2012).

18.18 Secondary Immunodeficiency/Acquired Immunodeficiency

Secondary immunodeficiencies are more common than primary immunodeficiencies. It may be acquired by the animal due to suppression of immune system by drugs, infections, deficiency of nutrition, neoplasm, environmental pollution, and trauma or surgery. Drugs including steroids (Ocon et al. 2017) affect the functions of immune cells, i.e., T and B lymphocytes. Viral infections can cause immunosuppression. For example, simian immunodeficiency virus affects mainly CD4+ T cells and downregulates the cellular immune responses. Malnutrition leads to secondary deficiency; for example, protein-energy malnutrition damages the cell-mediated immunity and phagocytosis; the ingestion of microorganisms is not affected; but the ability of phagocytic cells to destroy the intracellular organisms is hindered. Neoplastic diseases cause immunosuppression as they express Fas ligand that binds to Fas receptor of T cells and send signals for cell death and also by release of transforming growth factor beta (TGF beta), which itself is a potent immunosuppressor. Nutritional deficiency occurs may be due to burns, cancer, multiple trauma, chronic renal disease, and chronic infections. Zinc and iron deficiencies also affect immunity. Vitamin supplementation (B6 and B12), copper, and selenium play important role in normal functioning of the immune system (Rehman et al. 2017). Affected patients are relatively immunocompromised due to nonspecific cell activation that results into anergic immune responses, additionally increasing levels of cortisol induced by stress leading to inactivated immune state (Tschoeke and Ertel 2007). Due to rapid advancement, our environment is introduced with a large number of synthetic environmental pollutants such as pesticides, heavy metals, etc. leading to deleterious effect on immune system.

18.19 Bluetongue Disease

Bluetongue (BT) is caused by an arbovirus, which leads to acute disease in small ruminants. It is a vector-borne disease; *Culicoides* a biting midges act as a vector for transmission from one susceptible host to another (Legisa et al. 2013). The BTV induces immunosuppression in natural host sheep by hindering B-cell division in germinal centers, infects, and disrupts follicular dendritic cells, which leads to delayed production of high affinity and virus-neutralizing antibodies (Melzi et al. 2016). Further, the humoral immune response against second antigen is also hampered in BT disease. Thus, an arbovirus induces an acute immunosuppression by invading the host antiviral responses. Clinical manifestations are erosions of oral mucosa, erosions in/around nostrils, salivation, fever, edema of face and lips, apathy, lameness, conjunctivitis, coronitis, dysphagia, coronitis, muscle necrosis, and stiffness in limbs (Maan et al. 2012; Jenckel et al. 2015). Clinical signs may differ among hosts, however much more severe in sheep and some species of deer (Elbers et al. 2008).

18.20 Border Disease

Border disease (BD) is caused by border disease virus (BDV), which is a *Pestivirus* genus of family *Flaviviridae*. It is a congenital viral disease of sheep and goats. The BD is closely related to bovine virus diarrhea virus (BVDV) and classical swine fever virus. The BD is clinically characterized by abnormal body conformation and excessive hairy birth coat, the disease is known as "hairy-shaker disease" or "fuzzy" lambs (Nettleton et al. 1998). The BDV depresses the function of T helper cells and T cytotoxic cells, which leads to immunodeficiency in lambs. Further, there is a marked reduction in the circulating lymphocytes, which expressing the MHC class I antigen was also observed (Burrells et al. 1989).

18.21 Jaagsiekte Disease

Ovine pulmonary adenocarcinoma (OPA) is a contagious viral disease of adult sheep, which is caused by Jaagsiekte sheep retrovirus (JSRV). It is associated with a high rate of morbidity and mortality in the sheep; hence, there is a massive loss to the economy in the affected areas (Gomes et al. 2017; Jörger et al. 2017). The main clinical manifestation of the disease is tumor lesions in the lung. The JSRV is a carcinogenic retrovirus, which affects the epithelial cells of the lungs that result into the presence of a high number of neoplastic growths in the affected lungs (Martineau et al. 2011; Fan et al. 2003). The glandular transformation of the lung tissues and emphysema was seen on microscopic examination. The affected adult sheep shows respiratory signs such as dyspnea, nasal discharge, coughing, polypnea, and excessive fluid accumulation in the lungs (Salvatori et al. 2004; Caporale et al. 2005). The JSRV virus causes immunosuppression as it embedded its viral DNA into the host DNA (Spencer et al. 2003).

18.22 Feline Leukemia Virus

Feline leukemia virus (FeLV) is a pathogenic infectious disease of non-domestic feline species such as jaguars, bobcats, the most notably endangered puma subspecies, the Florida panther (*Puma concolor coryi*), and critically endangered Iberian lynx (Sleeman et al. 2001; Luaces et al. 2008; Filoni et al. 2012; Silva et al. 2016). The FeLV is also responsible for high mortality rate in domestic cats (Willett and Hosie 2013). The subgroup FeLV-A causes most of the infections, which is horizontally transmissible and replication competent (Jarrett and Russell 1978; Willett and Hosie 2013). Other FeLV subgroups are B, C, D, E, and T, which emerge after mutation or through recombination (Chiu et al. 2018). The FeLV results into neoplastic condition, immunosuppression, and hematopoietic disorders, mainly due to FeLV subgroups (Mullins et al. 1989; Hartmann 2012).

18.23 Mouse Mammary Tumor Virus

Mouse mammary tumor virus is a type B retrovirus that induces mammary neoplasia and, more rarely, T-cell lymphoma by insertional mutagenesis or through activation of proto-oncogenes (Salmons and Ginzburg 1987). In their 3' long terminal repeat (LTR), both endogenous and exogenous mouse mammary tumor viruses encode a superantigen (Sag), which is responsible for its tissue tropism especially toward the mammary tissue (Choi et al. 1991).

18.24 Feline Immunodeficiency Virus

The feline immunodeficiency virus (FIV) infects a broad range of cell types, likewise $CD4^+$ and $CD8^+$ T lymphocytes, B lymphocytes, and macrophages. That results into an eventual development of immunodeficiency in infected cats by the progressive loss of $CD4^+$ T cells (Pedersen et al. 1987; Brown et al. 1991; English et al. 1993).

18.24.1 Simian Immunodeficiency Virus Infection

Simian immunodeficiency virus infection is naturally occurring in several nonhuman primates such as world rhesus macaque, black mangabey, chimpanzee, and baboon. There are at least 40 different African monkey species that retain their own species-specific to SIV (Sharp and Hahn 2011). The virus encodes for genes, namely, tat, rev, nef, vif, and vpr. The Nef protein downregulated the expression of cellular receptor like CD4. Simian immunodeficiency virus infects mainly $CD4^+$ T lymphocytes, monocytes, and macrophages. In acute infection, there is marked initial decline in the gut $CD4^+$ T lymphocytes and a temporary reduction in peripheral blood $CD4^+$ T lymphocytes (Rout and Kaur 2014). Simian immunodeficiency virus will cause progressive lymphoid depletion in primary and secondary lymphoid organs. Inguinal rash and lymphadenopathy may develop after several weeks of infection.

18.24.2 Murine Leukemia Virus

The murine gammaretroviruses mainly affect laboratory animals such as rats, mice, and guinea pigs. This gammaretrovirus has both exogenous and endogenous forms with complex biology. Endogenous viruses induce reintegration during cell division, which leads to random distribution of copies throughout the genome of mouse and develops neoplasm rapidly. The exogenous strains of murine leukemia virus-inducing tumors with long latency period and typically are slowly transforming viruses. These virus strains promote characteristic of the disease which includes T-cell lymphoma, erythroleukemia, immunosuppression, and neurological disorders.

18.25 Autoimmunity

Autoimmunity is defined as an immune response of the body against self-antigen or body's own tissues. Reactivity against self-antigen can arise either by triggering the receptors directly by autoantigen or through cross-reaction between foreign and self-antigens (Agmon-Levin and Shoenfeld 2010).

18.26 Pemphigus Foliaceus

In this autoimmune disease, autoantibodies are formed against desmoglein-1 protein, which are components of desmosomes and form adhesion between epidermal cells. Pemphigus is a severe blistering disease that predominantly affects the skin and mucous membranes (Justiz Vaillant and Zito 2019). Clinically, characteristic lesions include pustules, crusts, ulceration, and alopecia resulting from destruction of adhesions between keratinocytes by autoantibodies (Olivry et al. 2006).

18.27 Autoimmune Hemolytic Anemia (AIHA)

It is reported in laboratory animals such as mice and rabbits. Here, the antibodies are formed against erythrocytic antigen due to molecular changes in self-antigen. The clinical signs are manifested by anemia, icterus, lethargy, and exercise intolerance. The autoimmune hemolytic anemia can be either IgG mediated known as warm AIHA or IgM mediated known as cold AIHA. Jaundice is the primary clinical sign in both. The laboratory diagnosis is done by a positive Coombs test, which recognizes the immunoglobulins and C3 on erythrocytes (Li et al. 2019).

18.28 Orf-Induced Autoimmunity

The orf disease is caused by DNA parapox virus. Orf is also known as contagious ecthyma (CE), a severe exanthematic dermatitis that mainly affects domestic and wild small ruminants (Peralta et al. 2015). Here the autoantibodies are formed against basement membrane of epithelium, and the typical clinical signs are proliferative skin lesions on the lips, around the mouth, nostrils, and eyelids. Orf is clinically characterized by the appearance of papules, vesicles, pustules, and rapidly growing scabs, which are primarily confined to the lips and muzzle of the affected animals (Cargnelutti et al. 2011).

18.29 Johne's Disease

Johne's disease is caused by infectious *Mycobacterium avium* subspecies *paratuberculosis* (MAP), which is an enteric inflammatory disease in small ruminants. Through heat shock proteins, MAP may trigger autoimmune antibodies. Mainly the HSP65 of MAP shows molecular mimicry with the various host proteins, so antibodies are produced against these HSPs. They also act upon the protein of host and stimulate autoantibodies and associated autoimmune disorders in small ruminants (Dow 2012).

18.30 Autoimmune Disease in a Polar Bear

An autoimmune disease is reported in a polar bear named "knut." It was found that high concentrations of specific autoantibodies against the NR1 subunit of N-methyl-D-aspartate (NMDA) receptor are present in Knut's cerebrospinal fluid (Dalmau et al. 2008). The pathological analyses exposed that polar bear suffered from encephalitis, which caused the seizures (Szentiks et al. 2014).

18.31 Conclusion

Immune system in our body protects us from various infectious agents and help in maintaining the normal life. Several immunopathological disorders are reported in sheep, goat, wild animals, and laboratory animals that arise from full or partial impairment of the immune system. Occurrence of acquired immunopathological disorders over the congenital is much higher. Simply, the destruction of host tissue may occur if there is a defective immune response, hyperresponsiveness, or response to self-antigen due to dysfunctional regulatory mechanisms. The process starts and continues through a series of definable steps that lead to a pathologic outcome. So, emphasis on awareness, investigation, and earlier diagnosis results into less morbidity and mortality due to immunopathological disorders.

References

Accinni BJR, Albini B, Ossi E, O'Connell DW, Pawlowski IB, Andres GA (1978) Deposition of circulating antigen-antibody complexes in the gastrointestinal tract of rabbits with chronic serum sickness. Am J Dig Dis 23(12):1098–1106

Agmon-Levin N, Shoenfeld Y (2010) Geoepidemiology of autoimmune rheumatic diseases. Nat Rev Rheumatol 6:468–476

Alexander G, William D, Bailey L (1967) Natural immunization in pregnant goats against red blood cells of their sheep and goat hybrid fetuses. Aust J Biol Sci 20:1217–1226

Arris JW (1956) Studies on the mechanism of a drug induced hemolytic anemia. J Lab Clin Med 47: 760

Barailler H, Milpied B, Chauvel A, Claraz P, Taïeb A, Seneschal J, Darrigade AS (2019) Delayed hypersensitivity skin reaction to hydroxychloroquine: successful short desensitization. J Allergy Clin Immunol 7(1):307–308

Berkowitz FE (1991) Hemolysis and infection: categories and mechanisms of their interrelationship. Rev Infect Dis 13:1151–1162

Beutler E (1959) The hemolytic effect of primaquine and related compounds-a review. Blood 14: 103

Beutler E (1994) G6PD deficiency. Blood 84:3613–3636

Birdsall HH (2015) Adaptive immunity. In: Mandell, douglas, and bennett's principles and practice of infectious diseases, 8th edn

Brown WC, Bissey L, Logan KS, Pedersen NC, Elder JH, Collisson EW (1991) Feline immunodeficiency virus infects both $CD4^+$ and $CD8^+$ T lymphocytes. J Virol 65:3359–3364

Burrells C, Nettleton PF, Reid HW, Miller HR, Hopkins J, McConnell I, Gorrell MD, Brandon MR (1989) Lymphocyte subpopulations in the blood of sheep persistently infected with border disease virus. Clin Exp Immunol 76(3):446–451

Caporale M, Centorame P, Giovannini A, Sacchini F, Di Ventura M, De Las HM, Palmarini M (2005) Infection of lung epithelial cells and induction of pulmonary adenocarcinoma is not the most common outcome of naturally occurring JSRV infection during the commercial lifespan of sheep. Virology 3389(1):144–153

Cargnelutti JF, Masuda EK, Martins M, Diel DG, Rock DL, Weiblen R, Flores EF (2011) Virological and clinico-pathological features of orf virus infection in experimentally infected rabbits and mice. Microb Pathog 50:56–62

Chaplin D (2010) Overview of immune response. J Allergy Clin Immunol 125(2):3–23

Chauhan RS, Joshi A (2012) Immunology for Beginners. Kapish Prakashan, Gurgaon

Chinn IK, Shearer WT (2015) Severe combined immunodeficiency disorders. Immunol Allergy Clin North Am 35(4):671–694

Chiu ES, Hoover EA, VandeWoude S (2018) A retrospective examination of feline leukemia subgroup characterization: viral interference assays to deep sequencing. Viruses 10:E29

Choi Y, Kappler JW, Marrack P (1991) A superantigen encoded in the open reading frame of the 3' long terminal repeat of the mouse mammary tumor virus. Nature 350:203–207

Clynes R, Ravetch JV (1995) Cytotoxic antibodies trigger inflammation through fc receptors. Immunity 3(1):21–26

Dalmau J, Gleichman AJ, Hughes EG, Rossi JE, Peng X, Lai M, Dessain SK, Rosenfeld MR, Balice-Gordon R, Lynch DR (2008) Anti-NMDA-receptor encephalitis: case series and analysis of the effects of antibodies. Lancet Neurol 7(12):1091–1098

Dhaliwal G, Patricia A, Cornett LM, Tierney JR (2004) Hemolytic anemia. Am Fam Physician 69: 11

Diggs C, Flemmings B, Dillon J, Snodgrass R, Campbell G, Esser K (1976) Immune serum-mediated cytotoxicity against Trypanosoma rhodesiense. J Immunol 116:1005–1009

Dow CT (2012) M. Paratuberculosis heat shock protein 65 and human diseases: bridging infection and autoimmunity. Autoimmune Dis 2012:1–6

Elbers AR, Backx A, Mintiens K, Gerbier G, Staubach C, Hendrickx G, van der Spek A (2008) Field observations during the bluetongue serotype 8 epidemic in 2006: II. Morbidity and mortality rate, case fatality and clinical recovery in sheep and cattle in The Netherlands. Prev Vet Med 87:31–40

English RV, Johnson CM, Gebhard DH, Tompkins MB (1993) In vivo lymphocyte tropism of feline immunodeficiency virus. J Virol 67:5175–5186

Fan H, Palmarini M, DeMartini JC (2003) Transformation and oncogenesis by Jaagsiekte sheep retrovirus. Curr Top Microbiol Immunol 275:139–177

Fertman MH, Fertman MB (1955) Toxic anemias and heinz bodies. Medicine 34:131

Filoni C, Catão-Dias JL, Cattori V, Willi B, Meli ML, Corrêa SH, Marques MC, Adania CH, Silva JC, Marvulo MF, Ferreira Neto JS, Durigon EL, de Carvalho VM, Coutinho SD, Lutz H, Hofmann-Lehmann R (2012) Surveillance using serological and molecular methods for the detection of infectious agents in captive Brazilian neotropic and exotic felids. J Vet Diagn Invest 24:166–173

Flemmings B, Diggs C (1978) Antibody-dependent cytotoxicity against Trypanosoma rhodesiense mediated through an alternative complement. Infect Immun 19(3):928–933

Gell PGH, Coombs RRA (1963) The classification of allergic reactions underlying disease. In: Clinical aspects of immunology. Blackwell Scientific Publication, Oxford, pp 217–237

Gomes M, Archer F, Girard N, Gineys B, Dolmazon C, Erny A, Mornex J, Leroux C (2017) Blocked expression of key genes of the angiogenic pathway in JSRV-induced pulmonary adenocarcinomas. Vet Res 48(1):76

Hale AS (1995) Canine blood groups and their importance in veterinary transfusion medicine. Vet Clin North Am Small Anim Pract 25:6

Hartmann K (2012) Clinical aspects of feline retroviruses: a review. Viruses 4:2684–2710

Hohenhaus AE (2004) Importance of blood groups and blood group antibodies in companion animals. Transfus Med Rev 18:117–126

Jarrett O, Russell PH (1978) Differential growth and transmission in cats of feline leukaemia viruses of subgroups A and B. Int J Cancer 21:466–472

Jenckel M, Bréard E, Schulz C, Sailleau C, Viarouge C, Hoffmann B, Höper D, Beer M, Zientara S (2015) Complete coding genome sequence of putative novel bluetongue virus serotype 27. Genome Announc 3:00016–00015

Jörger A, Acevedo C, Busley D, Ganter M, Schmiedl A, Humann-Ziehank E (2017) Stereological and biophysical characteristics of the ovine surfactant system and its changes caused by ovine pulmonary adenocarcinoma. Res Vet Sci 114:332–340

Justiz Vaillant AA, Zito PM (2019) Immediate hypersensitivity reactions. In: Stat Pearls, Treasure Island

Legisa D, Gonzalez F, De Stefano G, Pereda A, Santos MD (2013) Phylogenetic analysis of bluetongue virus serotype 4 field isolates from Argentina. J Gen Virol 94:652–662

Li TX, Sun FT, Ji BJ (2019) Correlation of IgG subclass with blood cell parameters in patients with autoimmune hemolytic anemia. J Exp Hematol/Chin Ass Pathophysiol 27(1):197–201

Luaces I, Doménech A, García-Montijano M, Collado VM, Sánchez C, Tejerizo JG, Galka M, Fernández P, Gómez-Lucía E (2008) Detection of feline leukemia virus in the endangered Iberian lynx (Lynx pardinus). J Vet Diagn Invest 20:381–385

Maan NS, Maan S, Belaganahalli MN, Ostlund EN, Johnson DJ, Nomikou K, Mertens PP (2012) Identification and differentiation of the twenty six bluetongue virus serotypes by RT–PCR amplification of the serotype-specific genome segment 2. PloS One 7:32601

Martineau HM, Cousens C, Imlach S, Dagleish MP, Griffiths DJ (2011) Jaagsiekte sheep retrovirus infects multiple cell types in the ovine lung. J Virol 85(7):3341–3355

Melzi E, Caporale M, Rocchi M, Martín V, Gamino V, di Provvido A, Marruchella G, Entrican G, Sevilla N, Palmarini M (2016) Follicular dendritic cell disruption as a novel mechanism of virus-induced immunosuppression. Proc Natl Acad Sci U S A 113(41):E6238–E6247

Meyer T, Davila M, Desai H, Carrillo LR, Brodie M, Amaya MR, Francis JL, Amirkhosravi A (2015) CD32a antibodies induce thrombocytopenia and type II hypersensitivity reactions in FCGR2A mice. Blood 126:19

Mullins JI, Hoover EA, Overbaugh J, Quackenbush SL, Donahue PR, Poss ML (1989) FeLV-F AIDS-induced immunodeficiency syndrome in cats. Vet Immunol Immunopathol 21:25–37

Nangaku M, Couser WG (2005) Mechanisms of immune-deposit formation and the mediation of immune renal injury. Clin Exp Nephrol 9(3):183–191

Nettleton PF, Gilray JA, Russo P, Dlissi E (1998) Border disease of sheep and goats. Vet Res 29(3–4):327–340

Notarangelo LD (2010) Primary immunodeficiencies. J Allergy Clin Immunol 125:S182–S194

Ocon AJ, Bhatt BD, Miller C, Peredo RA (2017) Safe usage of anakinra and dexamethasone to treat refractory hemophagocytic lymphohistiocytosis secondary to acute disseminated histoplasmosis in a patient with HIV/AIDS. BMJ Case Rep 2017:bcr2017221264

Olivry T, Lavoy A, Dunston SM, Brown RS, Lennon EM, Warren SJ, Prisayan P, Müller EJ, Suter MM, Dean GA (2006) Desmoglein-1 is a minor autoantigen in dogs with pemphigus foliaceus. Vet Immunol Immunopathol 110(3-4):245–255

Pac M, Bernatowska E (2016) Comprehensive activities to increase recognition of primary immunodeficiency and access to immunoglobulin replacement therapy in Poland. Eur J Pediatr 175(8):1099–1105

Pedersen NC, Ho EW, Brown ML, Yamamoto JK (1987) Isolation of a T-lymphotropic virus from domestic cats with an immunodeficiency-like syndrome. Science 235:790–793

Pelzer PT, Mutayoba B, Cobelens FGJ (2018) BCG vaccination protects against infection with mycobacterium tuberculosis ascertained by tuberculin skin testing. J Infect 77(4):335–340

Peralta A, Robles C, Martínez A, Alvarez L, Valera A, Calamante G, König GA (2015) Identification and molecular characterization of Orf virus in Argentina. Virus Genes 50(3):381–388

Rajan TV (2003) The Gell–Coombs classification of hypersensitivity reactions: a re-interpretation. Trends Immunol 24:7

Rasmusen BA (1961) Blood group in sheep. Ann N Y Acad Sci 97(1):306

Rehman AM, Woodd SL, Heimburger DC, Koethe JR, Friis H, PrayGod G, Kasonka L, Kelly P, Filteau S (2017) Changes in serum phosphate and potassium and their effects on mortality in malnourished African HIV-infected adults starting antiretroviral therapy and given vitamins and minerals in lipid-based nutritional supplements: secondary analysis from the nutritional support for African adults starting antiretroviral therapy (NUSTART). Br J Nutr 117(6):814–821

Rout N, Kaur A (2014) Cellular immune responses in natural and non-natural hosts of simian immunodeficiency virus infection. In: Natural hosts of SIV, pp 197–210

Salmons B, Ginzburg WH (1987) Current perspectives in the biology of mouse mammary tumor virus. Virus Res 8:81–102

Salvatori D, González L, Dewar P, Cousens C, de las Heras M, Dalziel RG, Sharp JM (2004) Successful induction of ovine pulmonary adenocarcinoma in lambs of different ages and detection of viraemia during the preclinical period. J Gen Virol 85:3319–3324

Sell S (1978) Immunopathology. Am J Pathol 3:215–275

Shamji MH, Thomsen I, Layhadi J, Kappen J, Holtappels G, Sahiner U, Switzer A, Durham SR, Pabst O, Bachert C (2019) Broad IgG repertoire in chronic rhinosinusitis with nasal polyps regulates pro-inflammatory IgE responses. J Allergy Clin Immunol 143(6):2086–2094.e2

Sharp PM, Hahn BH (2011) Origins of HIV and the AIDS pandemic. Cold Spring Harb Perspect Med 1(1):a006841

Sicherer SH, Leung DY (2009) Advances in allergic skin disease, anaphylaxis and hypersensitivity reactions to foods, drugs, and insects. J Allergy Clin Immunol 123:319–327

Silva CP, Onuma SS, de Aguiar DM, Dutra V, Nakazato L (2016) Molecular detection of feline leukemia virus in free-ranging jaguars (*Panthera onca*) in the pantanal region of mato grosso, Brazil. Braz J Infect Dis 20:316–317

Sleeman JM, KeaneJM J JS, Brown RJ, Woude SV (2001) Feline leukemia virus in a captive bobcat. J Wildl Dis 37:194–200

Spencer TE, Mura M, Gray CA, Griebel PJ, Palmarini M (2003) Receptor usage and fetal expression of ovine endogenous beta retroviruses: implications for coevolution of endogenous and exogenous retroviruses. J Virol 77(1):749–753

Swisher SN (1954) Studies of the mechanisms of erythrocyte destruction initiated by antibodies. Trans Assoc Am Physicians 17:124

Szentiks CA, Tsangaras K, Abendroth B, Scheuch M, Stenglein MD, Wohlsein P, Heeger F, Höveler R, Chen W, Sun W, Damiani A, Nikolin V, Gruber AD, Grobbel M, Kalthoff D, Höper D, Czirják GÁ, Derisi J, Mazzoni CJ, Schüle A, Aue A, East ML, Hofer H, Beer M, Osterrieder N, Greenwood AD (2014) Polar bear encephalitis: establishment of a comprehensive next-generation pathogen analysis pipeline for captive and free-living wildlife. J Comp Pathol 150(4):474–488

Tomasiak-Łozowska MM, Klimek M, Lis A, Moniuszko M, Bodzenta-Łukaszyk A (2018) Markers of anaphylaxis—a systematic review. Adv Med Sci 63(2):265–277

Tschoeke SK, Ertel W (2007) Immunoparalysis after multiple trauma. Injury 38(12):1346–1357

Uzzaman A, Cho SH (2012) Classification of hypersensitivity reactions. Allergy Asthma Proc 1:96–99

Wang KY, Friedman DF, DaVeiga SP (2019) Immediate hypersensitivity reaction to human serum albumin in a child undergoing plasmapheresis. Transfusion 2019(9999):1–3

Webster SJ (1949) Heinz body phenomenon in erythrocytes-a review. Blood 4:479

Willett BJ, Hosie MJ (2013) Feline leukaemia virus: half a century since its discovery. Vet J 195:16–23

Immunopathological Disorders in Swine and Equine

19

Key Points

1. In horses, major mediators of acute anaphylaxis are histamine and serotonin, which mainly affect lungs and intestine.
2. In pigs, major mediator of anaphylaxis is histamine, which mainly affects the lungs, but, in few cases, intestine may also involve.
3. Recurrent airway obstruction or heaves or chronic obstructive pulmonary disease is an asthma-like condition in mature horses following stabling and exposure to dusty hay and straw infected with fungus like *Aspergillus fumigatus*, *Faenia rectivirgula*, and *Thermoactinomyces vulgaris* allergen.
4. Hemolytic anemia of newborn foals and piglets is a type II hypersensitivity which occurs because of immune-mediated destruction of the neonate's RBCs by antibodies acquired from the dam in colostrum.
5. Diagnosis of the antibodies attacking the RBCs in case of alloimmune hemolytic anemia is done in direct Coomb or antiglobulin test.
6. African swine fever virus causes type III hypersensitivity in pigs, and the immune complex deposition consists of the ASFV antigen, IgG, and C3.
7. M antigen of *Streptococcus equi* causes purpura hemorrhagica (type III hypersensitivity), which is an acute, noncontagious, necrotizing vasculitis characterized by petechial or ecchymotic hemorrhage of the mucosa and subcutaneous tissue.
8. Equine agammaglobulinemia and Fell pony immunodeficiency syndrome are common primary immunodeficiency disorders in equine.
9. Equine agammaglobulinemia is a primary immunodeficiency which occurs due to defect in B cells and x-linked chromosome, mainly in male horses.
10. Severe combined immunodeficiency syndrome (SCID) is a primary immunodeficiency disorder of foals and piglets which occurs due to autosomal recessive gene defect in which young ones failed to produce both B and T lymphocytes whereas normal activity of the NK cells.

11. Equine recurrent uveitis is also known as moon blindness, iridiocyclitis, and periodic ophthalmia.
12. Equine recurrent uveitis is one of the common causes of vision loss in horses throughout the world, and autoantibodies are produced against the *Leptospira interrogans*, which cross-react with the retinoid-binding protein.
13. Equine polyneuritis is an autoimmune disorder of the horses characterized by sacral and coccygeal nerve paralysis. Affected horses have circulating antibodies against peripheral myelin protein, i.e., P2.

19.1 Introduction

The immune system has evolved to protect the living body from the infections, which are themselves evolving. The disorders of the immune system cause immunopathological diseases. Study of the diseases caused by the immune reaction is known as immunopathology. The word immunopathology is made up of two words having different meaning. First is immunity, i.e., the resistance of the body added by the interaction of the chemical, humoral, and cellular reaction in the body against the extraneous etiological factors, which is responsible for the occurrence of the diseases. The second word is the pathology, which is the study of the anatomical, chemical, and physiological alteration from the normal as a result of disease in animals. Immunopathology is mainly characterized by the three responses in the body. These are increased response to an antigen, also known as hypersensitivity; decrease response to an antigen, also known as immunodeficiency; and response to self-antigen, i.e., autoimmunity (Marshall et al. 2018).

19.2 Hypersensitivity

Hypersensitivity is the exaggerated or accelerated immune response to an antigen or allergen. These hypersensitivity reactions are classified by Coomb and Gell (1963) into two types. These are immediate hypersensitivity reactions and delayed-type reactions. Immediate-type hypersensitivity reaction includes type I hypersensitivity, i.e., anaphylaxis or allergy; type II hypersensitivity, i.e., cytotoxic; and type III hypersensitivity, i.e., immune complex mediated. Delayed-type hypersensitivity reaction includes only one type of hypersensitivity, i.e., type IV hypersensitivity also known as T-cell-mediated hypersensitivity (Uzzaman and Cho 2012).

19.3 Type I Hypersensitivity

Dr. Von Pirquet, an Austrian scientist and pediatrician, in 1906 noted that some of his patients overreacted to the things such as dust, pollen, or certain food ingredients, which are not harmful as such. So, he coined the term allergy for such overreaction from ancient Greek words allos meaning others or different and ergon meaning work or reaction (Shulman 2017). Type I hypersensitivity reactions are an acute inflammatory reaction which occurs as a result of release of biologically active substances from active mast cells and basophils, when cytotropic IgE antibody bounds to these cells. So, the main components of type I hypersensitivity are mast cells, basophils, and IgE antibodies (Stone et al. 2010). Mast cells are round to oval or stellate cells having round bean-shaped nucleus and darkly stained granules in cytoplasm (Gupta and Ghosh 1963). It is suggested that it originates from bone marrow but not precisely known. Life span of mast cells is very long, i.e., from several weeks to months. There are two types of mast cells, connective tissue mast cells having diameter 19–20 μm and mucosal mast cells having diameter 9–10 μm. Basophils are small round cells having diameter of 12–15 μm with bi- or trilobed nucleus and cytoplasm having intense reddish violet granules. Basophils originate from bone marrow and live up to 6 h in blood and few days in tissue. The IgE antibody is heat labile having molecular weight of 190,000 Da and originates from plasma cells located beneath the body surface. In 1921, Prausnitz and Kustner found a factor in serum of allergic subject and named it reaginic factor. In 1966, Dr. Kimishige Ishizaka found that these reaginic factors are allergic-specific immunoglobulin proteins, now called IgE (Platts-Mills et al. 2016). These IgE antibodies have half-life of 2–3 days in serum and few weeks when they bound to antibodies.

19.4 Pathogenesis of Type I Hypersensitivity

The entry of an antigen or allergen (example: pollen, dust, or food) in the body for the first time, it is presented and processed by antigen-presenting cells like dendritic cells and macrophages to the Th_2 cells and activate them. These activated Th_2 cells release the cytokines IL-4 and IL-5, which induce the activation of B cells and their conversion to plasma cells that release the IgE antibodies. These IgE antibodies bind to the mast cells or basophils through their Fc receptors. On reexposure to same antigen, there is cross-linking of two molecules of IgE antibodies binding on the mast cells or basophil by the antigen (Zhou 2012). This cross-linking is necessary for the degranulation of the mast cells and basophils and release of mediators of the type I hypersensitivity, which are responsible for the clinical manifestations (Knol 2006). There are two types of mediators released by mast cells and basophils. First are the primary mediators, which are preformed or already formed in these cells and release after the degranulation signals. These mediators include histamine, which increases vascular permeability, smooth muscle contraction, itching, and glandular secretion. Serotonin induces smooth muscle contraction and vasospasm. Proteases increase the bronchial mucus secretion and lead to degradation of blood basement membrane. Neutrophil chemotactic factor (NCF) and eosinophil chemotactic factor (ECF) result in neutrophil chemotaxis and eosinophil chemotaxis, respectively. Second mediators are secondary mediators, which are formed and release only after the degranulation signals. These mediators include platelet-activating factor (PAF), i.e., platelet aggregation and degranulation factor; leukotriene B is responsible for neutrophil and eosinophil chemotaxis; leukotriene C, D, and bradykinin are responsible for smooth muscle contraction and increase vascular permeability; and cytokines like IL–1 and TNF–α are responsible for systemic anaphylaxis and increased expression of cell adhesion, and IL-4 and IL–13, which again increases the IgE production.

19.5 Clinical Manifestation of Type I Hypersensitivity

- Acute Anaphylaxis
  In horse, major mediators of acute anaphylaxis are histamine and serotonin, which mainly affect lungs and the intestine. Clinical signs of acute anaphylaxis include bronchial or bronchiolar constriction leading to coughing, dyspnea, and eventually apnea. Severe diarrhea may also be observed. During PM examination, severe pulmonary emphysema and peribronchial edema are constant features. Edematous hemorrhagic colitis may also be observed (Eyer and Lewis 1973).
  In pigs, major mediator of anaphylaxis is histamine, which mainly affects the lungs, but, in few cases, intestine may also involve (Turnquist et al. 1993). Major clinical signs include pulmonary hypertension leading to dyspnea and death. Postmortem examination reveals severe pulmonary emphysema and peribronchial edema. Edematous hemorrhagic enteritis is also observed in some pigs, but in others, no gross intestinal lesions are observed.
- Specific allergic conditions
  - Food Allergy
    Entry of some of the specific food ingredients in the body act as allergen, and within a few seconds, clinical symptoms are observed. In horses, it is not so common. In case food allergy is observed in any horse, it mainly occurs due to soybean, peanut, alfalfa, etc. (Marsella 2013). Reported signs include recurrent urticarial, pruritic skin disease and anal pruritus. In swine, it mainly occurs due to soy meal, fish meal, peanut, and egg (Rupa et al. 2009). Reported sign includes skin pruritus.
  - Insect Bite Allergy
    This mainly occurs due to biting insects like *Culicoides*, *Simulium*, and *Stomoxys*. Saliva of these insects acts as allergen. Lesions are mainly found on face, mane, withers, rump, and tail. The disease is characterized by the urticaria, pruritus (Fig. 19.1) and secondary lesion of alopecia and crusting (Warger 2015).
- Recurrent Airway Obstruction or Heaves
  It is asthma-like condition in mature horses following stabling and exposure to dusty hay and straw. It is also known as chronic obstructive pulmonary disease. Fungus like *Aspergillus fumigatus*, *Faenia rectivirgula*, and *Thermoactinomyces vulgaris* (Seguin et al. 2012) are present in the hay or straw which act as allergen. The disease is mainly characterized by infiltration of neutrophils in airways (McGorum et al. 1993), excessive mucous production, coughing, and reduced dynamic lung compliance, i.e., reduced ability of lungs to scratch, which leads to increased pulmonary resistance and pulmonary arterial hypertension. Clinical

19.5 Clinical Manifestation of Type I Hypersensitivity

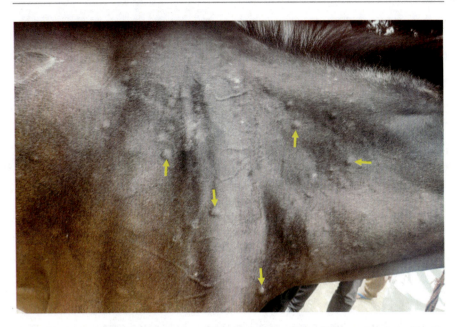

Fig. 19.1 Insect bite allergy due to type I hypersensitivity. Urticarial (arrow) and pruritic skin lesions due to biting insects like *Culicoides*, *Simulium*, and *Stomoxys* on face, mane, withers, rump, and tail

findings include coughing, intermittent bilateral mucopurulent to serous nasal discharge, and increased respiration (24–36/min). Excessive mucus production is considered to be the hallmark of the disease. It is studied that mucus cell number is increased due to the enhanced expression of EqMUC5AC gene (Gerber et al. 2003) and delayed apoptosis of the mucus cells (Bartner et al. 2006). Further, there is increased expression of the eCLCA1 gene due to goblet cell metaplasia and hyperplasia (Range et al. 2007). Normal horses have two phases of the expiration, but heaves-affected horses lack second phase of respiration (Cook and Rossdale 1963). Long-standing case of difficulty in breathing has heave line due to hypertrophy of abdominal oblique muscles (Leguillete 2003). Abnormal lung sounds (wheezing and cracking) and tracheal sounds (moist sound) are also ausculted during physical examination. During PM examination, one can observe that tissue damages are centered to airways and are less than 2 mm diameter. Lungs are pale, voluminous, and do not collapse. Histopathological examination shows alveolar emphysema, chronic bronchitis, diffuse epithelium, goblet cell hyperplasia, and cellular infiltration by mast cells, plasma cells, and lymphocytes. It was also observed that during chronic disease condition, the level of IFN–γ and IL–8 level increased to 2.5- and 3-fold times than normal, respectively (Ainsworth et al. 2003).

19.5.1 Diagnosis

Diagnosis is done by intradermal skin testing/wheal and flare reaction, passive cutaneous anaphylaxis test, radioimmunosorbent assay, and enzyme-linked immunosorbent assay (ELISA). In intradermal skin testing, suspected allergen is injected intradermally or scratched superficially. In positive cases, allergens degranulate the activated mast cells by cross-linking the two IgE antibodies molecules binding to the mast cells. Release of vasoactive amines by the mast cells results in the swelling (wheal) and erythema (flare) at the site of injection within few minutes. It reaches to its maximum intensity in 30 min and then decreases with time (Carr and Saltoun 2012). Passive cutaneous anaphylaxis test is used to detect the IgE antibodies. From affected animal, various dilutions of the serum are taken and injected into the skin of the normal animals. After 24–48 h, antigen is inoculated intravenously. In positive cases, acute inflammatory reaction develops at the site of injection of serum. With the help of ELISA, we can detect both antigen and allergen, and in radioallergosorbent test (RAST), we can detect IgE antibody in serum (Hamilton and Adkinson Jr. 2003).

19.6 Type II Hypersensitivity and Its Pathogenesis

It is also known as cytotoxic-type hypersensitivity reaction. In this reaction, antibody binds to the antigen and causes the destruction of the antigen. Antibodies produced cytotoxic reaction which occurs by three methods. First is by antibody-dependent cell cytotoxicity (ADCC). In ADCC, when antigen entered in the body, it is presented and processed by the antigen-presenting cells and produce antigen-specific antibody, which binds with that particular antigen. Cytotoxic cells bind with complex of antibody and antigen through Fc-binding receptors and promote the killing of the cells. Second is the complement-mediated cell destruction. Antigen-antibody complex leads to the induction of the complement reaction, which ends with the formation of the membrane attacking complex. It forms the pore in the cells thus promote the killing of the cells. Third is the antibody-mediated cell dysfunction. Here, antibodies bind to the receptors present in the body, and then the autoantibodies are produced against the fc receptor of the antibody and hence cause the destruction of the receptors (Viel et al. 2018).

19.7 Clinical Manifestation of Type II Hypersensitivity Reaction

- Alloimmune Hemolytic Anemia
  Hemolytic anemia of newborn horse and piglets occurs because of immune-mediated destruction of the neonate's red blood cells by antibodies acquired from the dam in colostrum (Seino 2010). The disease occurs naturally in foals and iatrogenic in piglets. In foals, the disease is initiated when fetal red blood cells expressed antigen derived from the stallion, whose blood group is differed from

19.7 Clinical Manifestation of Type II Hypersensitivity Reaction

Table 19.1 Major known blood groups in horses

Blood groups	Naturally occurring alloantibodies	Special considerations
EAA group	Minute amounts	Aa most important in neonatal isoerythrolysis
EAC group	Anti-ca in horses that are C-negative	–
EAQ group	Minute amounts	Qa most important in neonatal isoerythrolysis

the blood group from dam. In horses, there are 32 blood group antigens present, and most of antibodies are directed against Aa or Qa antigen (Table 19.1). The fetal antigen enters the dam blood during the last trimester of pregnancy and parturition due to transplacental hemorrhages, and dam isoantibodies are produced against those fetal antibodies (Kahn et al. 1991). The first pregnancy is without any adverse effects in foals, but on subsequent pregnancy with same stallion, hemolytic anemia occurs in newborn foal. The main occurrence of neonatal isoerythrolysis in pigs was manmade and related to repeated vaccination against hog cholera using the pooled blood, inactivated by addition of crystal violet of affected pigs (Goodwin et al. 1956). This vaccine contains erythrocytic antigen, and vaccination leads to the isoantibodies production against those antigens. If the piglet contains same erythrocytic antigen as the pig from whose blood, vaccine is prepared, and isoantibodies produced leads to hemolytic anemia in piglets. In swine, there are 15 blood group antigens recognized. Of these, A blood group is most important. In horses, the disease occurs in three forms. Peracute cases occur within 8–36 h of birth. Collapse of the foal is first indication. Severe hemoglobinuria is observed. Acute cases occur 2–4 days after birth. Jaundice is marked with moderate hemoglobinuria. Subacute cases occur 4–5 days after birth. In this case, jaundice is marked, but hemoglobinuria is absent. Observation during PM examination in foal shows swollen and friable liver. Spleen is greatly enlarged and is almost black. Piglet shows sign of jaundice at 24 h and weakness in 48 h. Most pigs dye by the fifth day. In per acute cases, piglets die within 12 h with acute anemia and no sign of jaundice and hemoglobinuria. In piglets, blood-stained peritoneal fluid and enlarged spleen are observed during PM (Radostits et al. 2006).

- Drug-Induced Type II Hypersensitivity
  Drugs like penicillin, quinine, and phenacetin are adsorbed on the surfaces of the RBC. These drugs act as antigen, and antibodies are produced against these drugs and bind to these drugs. This also leads to antibody-mediated RBC destruction by macrophage (Garratty 2009). Drugs like cephalosporin modify the RBC membrane, which leads to the adsorption of the nonspecific proteins on the surface of RBCs against which antibodies are produced, which cause destruction of the RBCs (Arndt and Garratty 2005).

19.7.1 Diagnosis

Diagnosis of type II hypersensitivity is done by Coomb test. The detection of the antibodies attacking the RBCs is done in direct Coomb test. It is also known as antiglobulin test. In this test, blood from affected animal is taken, and erythrocytes are washed. Then the anti-immunoglobulin reagent specific to that animal is added to the washed erythrocyte. In positive case, reagent binds with the antibodies attached on the surface of the RBCs, and agglutination of the RBC will occur, which is visible through naked eyes (Matthews and Newton 2010). Indirect Coomb testing is less frequently used in the animals. Indirect Coomb test is used to detect the antibodies present in the serum of the patients against the donor RBC during the transfusion reaction (Wardrop 2005).

19.8 Type III Hypersensitivity and Its Pathogenesis

The reaction of antibody and antigen in the body forms immune complexes. The deposition of the immune complex is depending on the size of these complexes. Generally, large-sized immune complexes get phagocytized, and small-sized immune complexes remain in the blood and do not get trapped in blood vessels. So, the main culprit of the type III hypersensitivity reaction is medium-sized immune complexes (Chauhan and Joshi 2012). These immune complexes get deposited in the endothelium in the blood vessels and cause changes where they get deposited. Deposited immune complexes activate the complement system and lead to the release of the complement C3a and C5a. These complements are potent anaphylotoxic and chemotactic factor for the neutrophil. They act on mast cells and basophils and lead to their degranulation, which releases the vasoactive amines. Vasoactive amines increase the permeability of the local blood vessels (Theofilopoulos and Dixon 1980a, b). The C3a opsonizes the immune complex, and neutrophils try to kill these opsonized immune complexes by lytic enzymes. As the immune complexes are attached to blood vessels, they do not get lysed, but released lytic enzymes damage the endothelium and also lead to further activation of the complement and formation of membrane-attacking complex, which again causes damage to the endothelium. Platelet aggregation can also be induced by the complements and results into formation of microthrombi (Tizard 2004). The type of lesions produced by the immune complex also depends on the site of deposition, for example, these immune complexes are deposited in the vessel wall of glomeruli results in glomerulonephritis.

19.8.1 Clinical Manifestation of Type III Hypersensitivity Reaction

- Serum Sickness
  Disease is caused by the formation of immune complexes, where antigen is soluble and exogenous. The immune complexes are formed in the circulation

and deposited in the organs like glomeruli, synovial membrane, lymph node, and skin. Immune complex formation leads to inflammation at the site of deposition. The deposition of immune complexes in the synovial membrane results in arthritis, if deposited in glomeruli cause glomerulonephritis, if deposited in lymph node cause lymphadenitis, and in skin it causes purpura. Clinical signs include fever, skin eruptions or purpura, lymphadenopathy, arthralgia, and polysynovitis. Albuminuria/proteinuria (glomerulonephritis) leads to acute renal failure (Kniker and Cochrane 1968). In horses, the circulating immune complexes are formed in recurrent airway obstruction (RAO) due to the immune response against endogenous and exogenous antigens (Niedźwiedź et al. 2014). In pigs, The immune complex deposition occurs in African swine fever disease in pigs, and this immune complexes consists of the African swine fever antigen, IgG, and C3 (Slauson and Vizcaino 1981)

- Purpura Hemorrhagica

It is an acute, noncontagious, aseptic necrotizing vasculitis, characterized by edema and petechial or ecchymotic hemorrhage of the mucosa and subcutaneous tissue (Wiender et al. 2006). The M antigen of *Streptococcus equi* helps in the formation of immune complexes. Immune complexes get deposited in the walls of capillaries with subsequent vasculitis and extravasation of blood and plasma (Akhurst and Valberg 2018). It is a sequel to vaccination against *Streptococcus equi* and infection of equine influenza virus, equine arteritis virus, equine herpesvirus type 1, *Streptococcus zooepidemicus*, *Rhodococcus equi*, or *Corynebacterium pseudotuberculosis* or by other antigens (Pusterla et al. 2003). Clinical findings include swelling of the head, limbs, and body; on mucosal surfaces, petechial hemorrhages are present; and skin of the limbs may slough. Fever, lethargy, and reluctance to move are also observed (Boyle 2016). During postmortem examination, one can observed that vasculitis also affects other organ systems, including the gastrointestinal tract and lungs.

19.8.2 Diagnosis

Type III hypersensitivity can be tentatively diagnosed by history and clinical signs. Tissue immune complexes can be detected by the immunofluorescence and other standard techniques, whereas immune complex in the fluid is diagnosed only when antigen is known (Theofilopoulos and Dixon 1980a, b).

19.9 Type IV Hypersensitivity and Its Pathogenesis

Type IV hypersensitivity is a delayed-type hypersensitivity reaction, which mainly involved cell-mediated immunity. There are two phases of the delayed-type hypersensitivity. First is the sensitizing phase, and the other is the effector phase. Sensitizing phase starts with the entry of antigen. When the antigen first time entered in the blood, they were presented and processed by antigen-presenting cells, which induce the Th₁ cell-mediated response and, in some cases, CD8⁺ T cells. It also generates the T memory cells, which respond to the specific antigens entering the body by any route (Stohlman 1991). Effector phase starts with the reexposure of the same antigen. These antigens were presented by Langerhans cells to memory T cells leading to generation of T effector cells. These effector Th₁ cells secrete a variety of cytokines that recruit and activate the macrophages and other inflammatory cells and lead to tissue damage, while T cytotoxic cells induce direct toxicity (Tizard 2004).

19.9.1 Clinical Manifestation of Type IV Hypersensitivity Reaction

- Allergic Contact Dermatitis
  Allergic contact dermatitis is also referred to as contact hypersensitivity. It is a cutaneous delayed-type hypersensitivity reaction produced by exposure of the external skin surface to nonirritant compounds, such as dyes and electrophilic metals. Constant use of these nonirritating compounds activates the effector Th₁ cells and leads to the release of various cytokines. Infiltration of the macrophages and other cells is promoted by these cytokines like IFN-γ, TNF-β, and IL-2 (Xu et al. 2000). Clinical findings include hyperemia, vesiculation, alopecia, and erythema. Allergic contact dermatitis causes intense pruritic lesions lead to self-inflicted injuries like excoriation and ulceration. In horses, it is characterized by the epidermal intracellular edema and lymphocytic inflammation with neutrophil infiltration (Felippe 2016).

19.9.2 Diagnosis

Diagnosis of type IV hypersensitivity reaction is mainly done by skin testing. Skin testing in this case is also known as patch testing. Patch testing is of two types, i.e., open and close patch testing. In open patch testing, the antigen is applied externally, and the region is covered with gauge. In close patch testing, antigen is injected intradermally. In positive case, there is swelling at the site of injection after 72 h along with signs of inflammation like redness, hot, swelling, and pain (Lazzarini et al. 2013).

19.10 Immunodeficiency Diseases

Immunodeficiency diseases are the rare disorders of the immune system, in which the immune system fails to protect the animals from pathogens, and thus the animal becomes susceptible to many infections and cancers. Immunodeficiency disorders are categorized into two types, i.e., primary immunodeficiency and secondary immunodeficiency. Primary immunodeficiency is congenital and mainly is caused by one or more than one defects in the immune system like deficiency of B lymphocytes, T lymphocytes, phagocytes, and complementary system (Raje and

Dinakar 2015). Secondary immunodeficiency diseases are those diseases which are acquired by the animal during its lifetime.

19.11 Primary Immunodeficiency Diseases

- Equine Agammaglobulinemia
  It is a primary immunodeficiency which occurs due to B-cell defect. Defect mainly occurs in male horses, so it is thought that it occurs due to defect in x-linked chromosome (Perryman 2000). The disease is characterized by normal count of T cells, the absence of B cell, which results into complete absence of all classes and subclasses of immunoglobulins. There is the absence of lymphoid follicle and germinal center in the spleen and lymph nodes (McGuire et al. 1976). Main defect arises in the maturation process of the precursor cells (Smith 2014). These foals survive up to 1–1.5 years, and there is recurrence of bacterial infections several times due to agammaglobulinemia. Diagnosis is mainly done by ELISA or immunoglobulin and lymphocyte testing (Smith 2014).
- Fell Pony Immunodeficiency Syndrome
  The disease is mainly found in dell and fell pony breed's foal. It is an autosomal recessive disease caused by mutation in the sodium/myo-inositol cotransporter gene (SLC5A3) on chromosome 26 leading to P446L substitution in the protein causing erythropoiesis failures and immune system compromisation (Fox-Clipsham et al. 2011). The disease mainly occurs in foals at the age of 4–12 weeks. The disease is characterized by the anemia, weakness, weight loss, and peripheral ganglionopathy. There is the absence of germinal center in lymphoid organs with lymphoid hypoplasia. The B-cell numbers in blood are less than the normal B-cell numbers (Scholes et al. 1998). With decline of antibodies in colostrum, there are increased chances of death of foal. In affected foals, in comparison to normal horses, there is no difference in the number of the $CD4^+$ and $CD8^+$ T cells, but due to secondary bacterial infections, there is increased expression of the CD11a/18 (Bell et al. 2001). The disease is diagnosed by the serum globulin testing and lymphoid testing.
- Severe Combined Immunodeficiency Syndrome
  It is an autosomal recessive gene defect in which young ones failed to produce both B and T lymphocytes, whereas normal activity of the NK cells in SCID affected foals (Lunn et al. 1995) and piglets (Powell et al. 2017). The animal becomes weak, there is reduction in its weight, and the animal becomes susceptible to many infections. The disease is mainly characterized by the lymphopenia and agammaglobulinemia. On necropsy, observable findings are complete absence of thymus and atrophy of other lymphoid organs (Powell et al. 2017). The SCID affection in foals, there is defect in the gene that encodes for the enzyme DNA-dependent protein kinase that helps in rejoining of the cut DNA segments, and the animal containing two copies of SCID gene only manifests the disease (Bernoco and Bailey 1998). It is shown that in horses, both V(D)J recombination and DNA-dependent protein kinase (DNA–PK) activity are

affected by SCID mutated gene (Wiler et al. 1995). In pigs, naturally SCID occurs due to the two mutations in the Artemis (DCLRE1C) gene, whereas X-linked SCID gene also artificially induced in pigs by interleukin-2 receptor gamma chain gene (IL2RG) and RAG1 and/or RAG2 genes disruption (Rajao et al. 2017). Disease is diagnosed by the decreased number of lymphocytes in blood, by histopathology where one can find the hypoplasia of the lymphoid organs. SCID genes can also be detected by the PCR.

19.11.1 Secondary Immunodeficiency Diseases

The secondary immunodeficiency diseases are the acquired immunodeficiency diseases, which mainly occur due to the drugs, diseases, deficiency of the nutrition, neoplasm, and environmental pollution (Chinen and Shearer 2010). The exposure of the animals with xenografts, due to their toxic nature, they cause immunosuppression. Drugs like corticosteroids affect both T helper cell function and antibody production. Corticosteroids impaired the maturation process of the dendritic cells and T lymphocytes and also inhibits IL-2, IL-3, IL-4, and IL-6 and hence inhibits the activation of the T cells (Youssef et al. 2016). Cyclosporine A, a fungal metabolite, depresses the cell-mediated immune responses by inhibiting the T lymphocyte activation due to inactivation of the calcineurin (Tedesco and Haragsim 2011). Aspirin used for the treatment of the rheumatoid arthritis reduced the platelet aggregation, decreased phagocytic activity of the neutrophils by inhibiting their extravasation, inhibit monocyte/macrophages tissue recruitment, and adhesion of the T cells to the endothelium (Hussain et al. 2011). Infection is caused by the equine herpes virus-1 associated with the nonspecific T-cell function suppression and clinically characterized by the leucopenia, neutropenia, and lymphopenia. The T lymphocytes are susceptible to the virus and help in the transfer of the virus (Poelaert et al. 2019).

In pigs, postweaning multisystemic wasting syndrome (PMWS) caused by porcine circovirus type 2 (Ghebremariam and Gruys 2005) leads to secondary immunosuppression by the depletion of the lymphocytes in the follicular and interfollicular areas along with infiltration of the macrophages in the lymphoid tissues (Segales et al. 2004). Trauma and surgery may also lead to the reduction in cell-mediated immunity by increasing the T helper 2 cell expressions which also decrease IL-12 expression (Marik and Flemmer 2012). Corticosteroids and prostaglandins released during surgery or trauma may also lead to immunosuppression. The use of various synthetic chemicals like pesticides, heavy metals, etc. affects the immune responses greatly. The residues found in animal food reach to the various tissues and produce the deleterious effects on the tissues. Pesticides like organochlorine compounds, organophosphates (OP), and synthetic pyrethroids reduce the humoral as well as the cell-mediated immune responses in animals. Some of them decrease the cytotoxic effects of the NK cells like OP compounds; some suppresses the expression of the MHC class I and hinder the maturation process of the dendritic cells like herbicides (Mokarizadeh et al. 2015). Heavy metals like lead and mercury also affect both humoral and cell-mediated immune responses. Mycotoxins present in food produce adverse effects on lymphoid organs leading to immunosuppression. Due to mycotoxins, there is decreased activity of both T and B lymphocytes, suppression of the antibody production, and impaired function of the macrophages and neutrophils (Oswald et al. 2005).

19.12 Autoimmune Disorders

Autoimmune diseases occur when the self molecules are attacked by the immune system. This occurs due to breakdown of an immunologic tolerance to autoreactive immune cells (Smith and Germolec 1999). Predisposing factors for the autoimmune diseases are associated with the genetic, infectious, and environmental factors. Mechanism for induction of the autoimmune diseases includes release of hidden antigens, antigens generated by molecular change, molecular mimicry, failure of regulatory control, and polyclonal lymphocyte activation (Chauhan and Joshi 2012). All these mechanisms are related with defect in immunological tolerance.

19.13 Clinical Manifestation of the Autoimmune Disorders

- Equine Polyneuritis
  This is the uncommon disease of the horses characterized by sacral and coccygeal nerve paralysis. Sometimes facial and trigeminal nerves are also affected. Affected horses have circulating antibodies against peripheral myelin protein, i.e., P2 (Kadlubowski and Ingram 1981). First clinical sign observed is hyperesthesia, which later followed by the paralysis (Hahn 2006). Affected parts include the tail, rectum, and bladder; sometimes facial paralysis is also observed. Affected animals have a history of poor tail tone, incontinence of the feces, and urine followed by complete paralysis of the perineal region leading to the retention of feces, cystitis, and scalding of limb with urine (Hahn 2008). During histopathological examination, it is observed that granulomatous inflammation develops in the region of extradural nerve roots due to the infiltration of the lymphocytes and macrophages (Galen et al. 2008) leading to pelvic limb paresis, ataxia, and sometimes atrophy of the focal gluteal muscle (Hahn 2008). ELISA is used to diagnose the antibodies against the myelin basic protein P2 (Ellison et al. 2015a). In a study, it is shown that about 45% of horses affected with equine protozoal myeloencephalitis are seropositive for the myelin protein P2 otherwise normal horses seronegative for the same protein (Ellison et al. 2015b).
- Equine Recurrent Uveitis
  It is one of the very common causes of vision loss in horses throughout the world and also known as moon blindness, iridiocyclitis, and periodic ophthalmia (Gilger and Deeg 2011). Autoantibodies are produced against the interphotoreceptor retinoid-binding protein and the S-protein with subsequent inter- and intramolecular spreading to both antigen-derived epitopes (Deeg et al. 2006). The antibodies

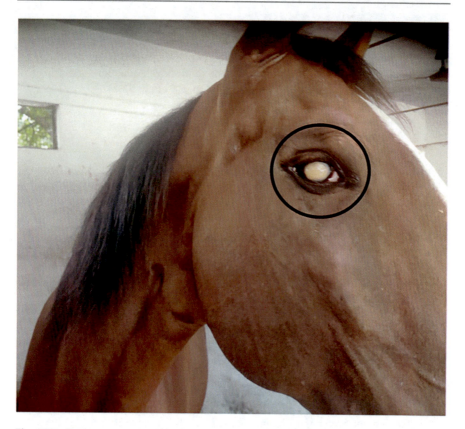

Fig. 19.2 Equine recurrent uveitis due to autoimmunity. Cataract, synechiae, lens dislocation, glaucoma, and phthisis bulbi, which progress to vision loss due to antibodies produced against *Leptospira interrogans* that cross react with the retinoid-binding protein

produced against *Leptospira interrogans* cross-reacts with the retinoid-binding protein and thus causes recurrence of disease. It was found that early antibodies and T lymphocytes response produced against the *Leptospira interrogans* lipoprotein Lru A and Lru B localized in inner membrane of the eye of horse lead to desequestration of the interphotoreceptor retinoid-binding protein (IRBP) and other antigens (Verma et al. 2005). There are two forms of the equine recurrent uveitis. Classical form is the most common form and characterized by the inflammation, which progresses to chronic end-stage uveitis after a period of quiescence. It is characterized by cataract, synechiae, and phthisis bulbi, which progress to vision loss (Fig. 19.2). Each attack gets progressively more severe and gradually spreads to involve other eye tissues until complete blindness results (Curling 2011). Insidious form is less severe in which low-grade inflammation does not resolve completely and progress to chronic clinical signs of equine recurrent uveitis (Gilger and Michau 2004).

- The Pemphigus Complex
It is the autoimmune disease of the skin and characterizes in three types. First is the pemphigus vulgaris, where autoantibody is formed against protein desmosomal cadherin called desmoglein-3 (Eming et al. 2019). Desmoglein-3 (DSG3) is a keratinocyte adhesion protein (Mao et al. 2017), so autoantibodies against DSG3 lead to loss of cell to adhesion in basal and suprabasal layers of deeper epidermis (Amagai et al. 1996). Clinical lesions in horse include initial blistering in the oral mucosa followed by spreading to all over the skin. Microscopic lesions include the separation of skin epithelial cells (Ramineni et al. 2015). Second is the pemphigus foliaceus, where autoantibody is formed against protein called desmoglein-1. The DSMG1 is a desmosomal protein which, through its adhesive function, maintains the structure of the epidermis (Hammers and Stanely 2013). Primary lesions often begin in head and extremities and secondary lesions to other areas. Lesions include exudates filled with vesicles, bullae, and pustules, which dry to form crust, scaling, and epidermal collarettes with extensive edema in legs and abdomen (Zabel et al. 2005). Third is bullous pemphigoid, where autoantibodies are produced against the type XVII collagen, which leads to the formation of the subepidermal vesicles (Karsten et al. 2018). In both equine and pigs, the IgG autoantibodies target the NC16A ectodomain of the collagen XVII, i.e., BP180 and BPAG2. Physical lesions in horses include multiple erythematous, ulcerated, crusty, and itchy lesions at head, medial thigh, and ventral thoracic region (Fontes et al. 2016). In pigs, lesion includes erythematous and pruritic patches that evolve into turgid, isolated, or clustered vesicles, which are rich in intact and degranulated eosinophils (Olivry et al. 2000).
- Systemic Lupus Erythematous
Systemic lupus erythematous is a debilitating, and often fatal autoimmune disease involves multiple organ system. Autoantibody production is poorly understood, but two hypotheses can be considered, i.e., impaired central or peripheral B-cell tolerance and increased circulating autoreactive B cells (Han et al. 2015). Autoantibodies thus produced cause tissue damage in host through type I hypersensitivity, type II hypersensitivity, and type III hypersensitivity. A filly shows the cutaneous lesions, which include lymphedema of the distal limbs, panniculitis, mucocutaneous ulceration, alopecia, and scaling (Geor et al. 1990). Systemic lupus erythematosus (SLE) is also observed in leptin transgenic pig showing symptoms like anemia, leucopenia, and thrombocytopenia as well as kidney and liver impairment (Chen et al. 2018). Diagnosis can be made by antinuclear antibody test, LE cell test, and lupus band test. The antinuclear antibody production is the hallmark of the systemic lupus erythematous, where the autoantibodies are produced against many different nuclear structures, including nucleic acids, ribonucleoproteins, and chromatin. Demonstration of the antinuclear antibodies is first done by immunofluorescent antinuclear antibody test; in positive cases, further test like CLIF, ELISA, and blotting test should be done for confirmation (Kumar et al. 2009). The demonstration of the lupus cell in bone marrow is also diagnostic. The lupus cells are the cells, which phagocytize the antibody and antinuclear antigen complex. Further, when skin lesions are

produced in SLE, the immunoglobulin deposited in the dermoepidermal junction and demonstrated as a linear band at the basement membrane zone. This band is known as lupus band. This lupus band demonstrated by the immunofluorescence or immunohistochemistry test can be diagnostic for the SLE (Reich et al. 2011).

19.14 Conclusion

Immunopathological disorders are highly lethal and most negligible disorders in the animals. There are only few cases reported in all over the world and almost negligible from India. The main problem is the lack of knowledge of the immunopathological disorders among the veterinarians. As the infectious diseases occur in large number and are easy to diagnose, it leads to narrowing of the thinking process toward only to infectious diseases and leads to the negligence of the immunopathological disorders. Further, researches should be done in the field of immunopathology in animals as it not only helps to understand the disease in animals but also in humans as animals can be the model for the human diseases. Further, the role of harmful chemicals like pesticides, herbicides, drugs, etc. in acquired immunopathological disorders should be studied further and should be considered while using them.

References

Ainsworth DM, Grunig G, Matychak MB, Young J, Wagner B, Erb HN, Antczak (2003) Recurrent airway obstruction (RAO) in horses is characterized by IFN-γ and IL- 18 production in Bronchioalveolar lavage. Vet Immunol Immunopathol 96(1–2):83–91

Akhurst SAD, Valberg SJ (2018) Immune—mediated muscle disease of the horse. Vet Pathol 55(1):68–75

Amagai M, Koch PJ, Nishikawa T, Stanley JR (1996) Pemphigus vulgaris antigen (Desmoglein 3) is localized in the lower epidermis, the site of blister formation in patients. J Investig Dermatol 106:351–355

Arndt PA, Garratty G (2005) The changing Spectrum of the drug induced immune hemolytic anemia. Semin Hematol 42(3):137–144

Bartner LR, Robinson NE, Kiupel M, Tesfaigzi Y (2006) Persistent mucus accumulation: a consequence of delayed bronchial mucous cell apoptosis in RAO-affected horses? Am J Physiol Lung Cell Mol Physiol 291(4):L602–L609

Bell SC, Savidge C, Taylor P, Knottenbelt DC, Carter SD (2001) An immunodeficiency in fell ponies: a preliminary study into cellular responses. Equine Vet J 33(7):687–692

Bernoco D, Bailey E (1998) Frequency of the SCID gene among Arabian horses in the USA. Anim Genet 29:41–49

Boyle AG (2016) Strangles and its complications. Equine Vet Educ 29:149–157

Carr TF, Saltoun CA (2012) Skin testing in allergy. Allergy Asthma Proc 33(1):6–8

Chauhan RS, Joshi A (2012) Hypersensitivity. In: Immunology for beginners. Kapish Prakashan Publication, Guragaon

Chen J, Zeng W, Pan W, Peng C, Zhang J, Su J, Long W, Zhao H, Zuo X, Xie X, Wu J, Nie L, Zhao HY, Wei HJ, Chen X (2018) Symptoms of systemic lupus erythematosus are diagnosed in leptin transgenic pigs. PLoS Biol 16(8):e2005354

Chinen J, Shearer WT (2010) Secondary immunodeficiency, including HIV infection. J Allergy Clin Immunol 125(2):S195–S203

Cook WR, Rossdale PD (1963) The syndrome of 'broken wind' in the horse. Proc R Soc Med 56: 972–977

Curling A (2011) Equine recurrent uveitis: classification, etiology and pathogenesis. Compend Contin Educ Vet 33(6):E1–E4

Deeg CA, Amann B, Raith AJ, Kasper B (2006) Inter- and intramolecular epitope spreading in equine recurrent uveitis. Investig Opthalmol Vis Sci 47(2):652–656

Ellison SP, Kennedy TJ, Li A (2015a) Neuritogenic peptides derived from equine myelin P2 basic protein detect circulating antibodies in ataxic horses. Int J Appl Res Vet Med 13(3):175–181

Ellison SP, Kennedy TJ, Li A (2015b) Serum antibodies against a reactive site of equine myelin protein 2 linked to polyneuritis Equi found in horses diagnosed with EPM. Int J Appl Res Vet Med 13(3):164–170

Eming R, Hennerici T, Backlund J, Feliciani C, Visconti KC, Willenborg S, Wohde J, Holmdahl R, Sønderstrup G, Hertl M (2019) Pathogenic IgG antibodies against Desmoglein 3 in pemphigus vulgaris are regulated by HLA-DRB1*04:02- restricted T cells. J Immunol 193:4391–4399

Eyer P, Lewis AJ (1973) Acute systemic anaphylaxis in the horse. Br J Pharmacol 48:426–437

Felippe MJ (2016) Equine clinical immunology. John Wiley & Sons, Hoboken, NJ

Fontes TN, Farias SS, Machado GAC, Mascarenhas MB, Silva AL, Brandao EB, Nogueira VA, Peixoto TC (2016) Equine bullous pemphigoid—case report. Braz J Vet Med 38(1):55–59

Fox-Clipsham LY, Carter SD, Goodhead I, Hall N, Knottenbelt DC, May PDF, Ollier WE, Swinburne JE (2011) Identification of a mutation associated with fatal foal immunodeficiency syndrome in the fell and dales pony. PLoS Genet 7(7):e1002133, 1–8

Galen GV, Cassart D, Sandersen C, Delguste C, Nollet H, Amory H, Ductatelle R (2008) The composition of the inflammatory infiltrate in three cases of polyneuritis Equi. Equine Vet J 40(2):185–182

Garratty G (2009) Drug induced immune hemolytic anemia. Hematol Am Soc Hematol Educ Program 2009:73–79

Geor RJ, Clark EG, Haines DM, Napier PG (1990) Systemic lupus erythematosus in filly. J Am Vet Med Assoc 197(11):1489–1492

Gerber V, Robinson NE, Venta RJ, Rawson J, Jefcoat AM, Hotchkiss JA (2003) Mucin genes in horse airways: MUC5AC, but not MUC2, may play a role in recurrent airway obstruction. Equine Vet J 35(3):252–257

Ghebremariam MK, Gruys E (2005) Postweaning multisystemic wasting syndrome (PMWS) in pigs with particular emphasis on the causative agent, the mode of transmission, the diagnostic tools and the control measures. A review. Vet Q 27(3):105–116

Gilger BC, Deeg C (2011) Equine recurrent uveitis. In: Gilger BC (ed) Equine ophthalmology, 2nd edn. Elsevier Saunders Publication Maryland Heights, St. Louis, MI, pp 317–349

Gilger BC, Michau TM (2004) Equine recurrent uveitis: new methods of management. Vet Clin Equine Pract 20:417–427

Goodwin RFW, Hayward BHG, Heard DH, Roberts GF (1956) Hemolytic disease of the newborn piglet. J Hyg 54(2):153–171

Gupta PCS, Ghosh S (1963) Tissue mast cell. Nature 197:506–507

Hahn CN (2006) Miscellaneous disorders of the equine nervous system: Horner's syndrome and Polyneuritis Equi. Clin Tech Equine Pract 5:43–48

Hahn CN (2008) Polyneuritis equi: the role of T-lymphocytes and importance of differential clinical signs. Equine Vet J 40(2):100

Hamilton RG, Adkinson NF Jr (2003) Clinical laboratory assessment of Ig E—dependent hypersensitivity. J Allergy Clin Immunol 111(2):687–701

Hammers CM, Stanely JR (2013) Desmoglein-1, differentiation, and disease. J Clin Invest 123(4): 1419–1422

Han S, Zhuang H, Shumyak S, Yang L, Reeves WH (2015) Mechanisms of autoantibody production in systemic lupus erythematosus. Front Immunol 6:228

Hussain M, Javeed A, Ashraf M, Yong Z, Mukhtar MM, Rehman MU (2011) Aspirin and immune system. Int Immunopharmacol 12(2012):10–20

Kadlubowski M, Ingram PL (1981) Circulating antibodies to the neuritogenic myelin protein P2 in neuritis of the cauda equine of the horse. Nature 293:299

Kahn W, Vaala W, Palmer J (1991) Neonatal Isoerythrolysis in newborn foals. Tierarztl Prax 19(5): 521–529

Karsten CM, Beckmann T, Holtsche MM, Tillmann J, Tofern S, Schulze FS, Heppe EN, Ludwig RJ, Zillikens D, König IR, Köhl J, Schmidt E (2018) Tissue destruction in bullous pemphigoid can be complement independent and may be mitigated by C5aR2. Front Immunol 9(488):1–12

Kniker WT, Cochrane CG (1968) The localization of circulating immune complexes in experimental serum sickness—the role of vasoactive amines and hydrodynamic forces. J Exp Med 127: 119–139

Knol EF (2006) Requirement of effective Ig E cross-linking on mat cells and basophils. Mol Nutr Food Res 50(7):620–624

Kumar Y, Bhatia A, Minz RW (2009) Antinuclear antibodies and their detection methods in diagnosis of connective tissue diseases: a journey revisited. Diagn Pathol 4:1–10

Lazzarini R, Duarte I, Ferreira AL (2013) Patch test. An Bras Dermatol 88(6):879–888

Leguillete R (2003) Recurrent airway obstruction—heaves. Vet Clin N Am Equine Pract 19(1): 63–86

Lunn DP, McClure JT, Schobert CS, Holmes MA (1995) Abnormal patterns of equine leucocyte differentiation antigen expression in severe combined immunodeficiency foals suggests the phenotype of normal equine natural killer cell. Immunology 84:495–499

Mao X, Cho MJT, Ellebrecht CT, Mukherjee EM, Payne AS (2017) Stat3 regulates desmoglein 3 transcription in epithelial keratinocytes. J Clin Investig 2(9):e92253

Marik PE, Flemmer M (2012) The immune response to surgery and trauma: implications for treatment. J Trauma Acute Care Surg 73(4):801–808

Marsella R (2013) Equine allergy therapy update on the treatment of environmental, insect bite hypersensitivity, and food allergies. Vet Clin North Am Equine Pract 29:551–557

Marshall JS, Warrington R, Watson W, Kim HL (2018) An introduction to immunology and immunopathology. Allergy Asthma Clin Immunol 14(2):49

Matthews J, Newton S (2010) The Coombs test. Clin J Oncol Nurs 14(2):143–145

McGorum BC, Dixon PM, Halliwell RE (1993) Responses of horses affected with chronic obstructive pulmonary disease to inhalation challenges with mould antigens. Equine Vet J 25: 261–267

McGuire TC, Banks KL, Evans DR, Poppie MJ (1976) Agammaglobulinemia in a horse with evidence of functional T lymphocyte. Am J Vet Res 37(1):41–46

Mokarizadeh A, Faryabi MR, Rezvanfar MA, Abdollahi M (2015) A comprehensive review of pesticides and the immune dysregulation: mechanisms, evidence and consequences. Toxicol Mech Methods 25(4):258–278

Niedźwiedź A, Jaworski Z, Kubiak K (2014) Circulating immune complexes and markers of systemic inflammation in RAO-affected horses. Pol J Vet Sci 17(4):697–670

Olivry T, Mirsky ML, Singleton W, Dunston SM, Boeeillo AK, Xu L, Traczyk T, Rosolia DL, Chan LS (2000) A spontaneous arising porcine model of bullous pemphigoid. Arch Dermatol Res 292(1):37–45

Oswald IP, Marin DE, Bouhet S, Pinton P, Taranu I, Accensi F (2005) Immunotoxicological risk of mycotoxins for domestic animals. Food Addit Contam 22(4):354–360

Perryman LE (2000) Primary Immunodeficiencies of horses. Vet Clin North Am Equine Pract 16(1):105–116

Platts-Mills TAE, Heymann PW, Commins S, Woodfolk JA (2016) The discovery of IgE 50 years on. Ann Allergy Asthma Immunol 116(3):179–182

Poelaert KCK, Cleemput JV, Laval K, Favoreel HW, Couck L, Broeck WV, Azab W, Nauwynck HJ (2019) Equine herpes virus 1 bridles T lymphocytes to reach its target organs. J Virol 93: e02098–e03018

Powell EJ, Cunnick JE, Tuggle CK (2017) SCID pigs: an emerging large animal NK model. J Rare Dis Res Treat 2(3):1–6

Pusterla N, Watson JL, Affolter VK, Magdesian KG, Wilson WD, Carlson GP (2003) Purpura haemorrhagica in 53 horses. Vet Rec 153:118–121

Radostits O, Gay C, Hinchcliff K, Constable P (2006) Veterinary medicine—a textbook of the disease of cattle, horses, sheep, pigs and goat, 10th edn. Saunders publication, Philadelphia, PA

Rajao DS, Loving LC, Waide EH, Gauger PC, Dekkers JCM, Tuggle CK, Vincent AL (2017) Pigs with severe combined immunodeficiency (SCID) are impaired in controlling influenza a virus infection. J Innate Immun 9(2):193–202

Raje N, Dinakar C (2015) Overview of immunodeficiency disorders. Immunol Allergy Clin North Am 35(4):599–623

Ramineni HB, Yerraguntla M, Pulimila S, Kukkapalli NB, Suryadevara V (2015) Pemphigus vulgaris: a rare case report. Int J Res Med Sci 3(6):1543–1544

Range F, Mundhenk L, Gruber AD (2007) A soluble secreted glycoprotein (eCLCA1) is overexpressed due to goblet cell hyperplasia and metaplasia in horses with recurrent airway obstruction. Vet Pathol 44(6):901–911

Reich A, Marcinow K, Birula RB (2011) The lupus band test in systemic lupus erythematosus patients. Ther Clin Risk Manag 7:27–32

Rupa P, Schmied J, Wilkie BN (2009) Porcine allergy and Ig E. Vet Immunol Immunopathol 132(1):41–45

Scholes SFE, Holliman A, May PDF, Holmes MA (1998) A syndrome of anaemia, immunodeficiency and peripheral ganglionopathy in fell pony foals. Vet Rec 142:128–134

Segales J, Domingo M, Chianini F, Majo N, Dominguez J, Darwich L, Mateu E (2004) Immunosuppression in postweaning multisystemic wasting syndrome affected pigs. Vet Microbiol 98:151–158

Seguin V, Garon D, Lavenant LS, Lanier C, Bouchart V, Gallard Y, Blanchet B, Diquelou S, Personent E, Ourry A (2012) How to improve the hygienic quality of forages for horses feeding. J Sci Food Agric 92:975–986

Seino KK (2010) Immune mediated anemia in ruminants and horses. In: Weiss DJ, Wardrop KJ, Schalm OW (eds) Schlam's veterinary hematology, 6th edn. Wiley-Blackwell, Hoboken, NJ

Shulman ST (2017) Clemon von Pirquet: a remarkable life and carrier. J Pediatr Infect Dis Soc 6(4):376–379

Slauson DO, Vizcaino JMS (1981) Leukocyte-dependent platelet vasoactive amine release and immune complex deposition in African swine fever. Vet Pathol 18:813–826

Smith BP (2014) Immunologic disorders. In: Large animal internal medicine, 5th edn. Elsevier Mosby Publication, St. Louis, MI

Smith DA, Germolec DR (1999) Introduction to immunology and autoimmunity. Environ Health Perspect 107(5):661–665

Stohlman SA (1991) Accessory cells control induction of CD4+ T cells with specific effector function. Res Immunol 142:50

Stone KD, Prussin C, Metcalfe DD (2010) IgE, mast cells, basophils, and eosinophils. J Allergy Clin Immunol 125(2):S73–S80

Tedesco D, Haragsim L (2011) Cyclosporine: a review. J Transplant 2012:1–7

Theofilopoulos AN, Dixon FJ (1980a) Detection of immune complexes: techniques and implications. Hosp Pract 15(5):107–121

Theofilopoulos AN, Dixon FJ (1980b) Immune complexes in human diseases. Am J Pathol 100(2):532–569

Tizard IR (2004) Veterinary immunology an introduction. Saunders Publication, Philadelphia, PA

Turnquist SE, Bouchard G, Fischer JR (1993) Naturally occurring systemic anaphylactic and anaphylactoid reactions in four groups of pigs injected with commercially available bacterins. J Vet Diagn Invest 5:103–105

Uzzaman A, Cho SH (2012) Classification of hypersensitivity reactions. Allergy Asthma Proc 13(1):96–94

Verma A, Artiushin S, Matsunaga J, Haake DA, Timoney JF (2005) LruA and LruB, novel lipoproteins of pathogenic Leptospira interrogans associated with equine recurrent uveitis. Infect Immun 73(11):7259–7266

Viel S, Pescarmona R, Belot A, Nosbaum A, Lombard C, Walzer T, Berard F (2018) A case of type 2 hypersensitivity to Rasburicase diagnosed with a natural killer cell activation assay. Front Immunol 9:110

Wardrop KJ (2005) The Coomb's test in veterinary medicine: past, present, future. Vet Clin Pathol 34(4):325–334

Warger B (2015) Immunoglobulin E and allergy. Equine Vet J 48(1):13–14

Wiender EB, Couetil LL, Levy M, Sojka JE (2006) Purpura haemorrhagica. Compendium equine edition, p 82–93

Wiler R, Leber R, Moore BB, VanDyk LF, Perryman LE, Meek K (1995) Equine severe combined immunodeficiency: a defect in V(D)J recombination and DNA-dependent protein kinase activity. Proc Natl Acad Sci U S A 92:11485–11489

Xu H, Bjarnason B, andElmets CA. (2000) Sensitization versus elicitation in allergic contact dermatitis: potential differences at cellular and molecular level. Am J Contact Dermat 11(4):228–234

Youssef J, Novosad SA, Winthrop KL (2016) Infection risk and safety of corticosteroid use. Rheum Dis Clin North Am 42(1):157–176

Zabel S, Mueller RS, Fieseler KV, Bettenay SV, Littlewood JD, Wagner R (2005) Review of 15 cases of pemphigus Foliaceus in horses and a survey of the literature. Vet Rec 157:505–509

Zhou C (2012) Mechanism of type I hypersensitivity. In: Multidisciplinary approaches to allergies. Advanced topics in science and technology in China. Springer, Berlin, Heidelberg

Immunopathological Disorders of Pet Animals

20

Key Points

1. Canine atopic dermatitis is a type 1 hypersensitivity reaction that occurs mainly due to inhalation of allergens, namely, molds, weed, and pollen grains associated with IgE antibodies in genetically predisposed individuals.
2. Flea allergy dermatitis is a type 1 hypersensitivity reaction and common skin disease in dogs and cats.
3. Lupus means horrible facial rashes and autoantibodies directed against RBCs, platelets, leucocytes, and nuclear antigen during type 3 hypersensitivity.
4. Lethal acrodermatitis is a primary immunodeficiency condition of adult bull terrier dogs which occurs due to T-cell defect and reduced serum IgE levels.
5. Lethal acrodermatitis affected dogs frequently suffer from skin infections like candidiasis.
6. Canine parvovirus and canine distemper virus cause secondary immunodeficiency.
7. Myasthenia gravis is a disorder of neuromuscular function in young dogs characterized by skeletal muscle weakness and fatigue.
8. Myasthenia gravis is mainly diagnosed by tensilon test.
9. Systemic lupus erythematosus, rheumatoid arthritis, autoimmune thyroiditis, and myasthenia gravis were the reported autoimmune disorders of pets.

20.1 Introduction

During the process of evolution, nature has provided a defense mechanism in the body of all living creatures that protect them from physical, chemical, and biological harmful effects. Immunopathology is the study of disease conditions resulting from immune reaction. Immunopathological disorders mainly include the hypersensitivity, autoimmune, and immunodeficiency disorders. In hypersensitivity disorders, type 1 hypersensitivity is the immediate immune reaction to an antigen (Sicherer and Leung 2009). In type 1 hypersensitivity, mast cell degranulation can lead to the release of inflammatory mediators including histamine, proteoglycans, serine proteases, and leukotrienes (Yamasaki and Saito 2005). Type 2 hypersensitivity also known as cytotoxic hypersensitivity is rare reaction that is typically caused by IgG and IgM antibodies (Brostoff et al. 1991). In type 3 hypersensitivity, there is formation of antigen-antibody complexes, which gets deposited in various tissues and joints leading to various kinds of disease conditions. Type 4 hypersensitivity is called delayed type because it takes more than 24 h to develop (Brostoff et al. 1991). There is allergic contact dermatitis, which mainly affects the pets and human beings. Hypersensitivity reactions are common, yet they are not often considered in treatment regimens because of lack of knowledge. Untreated hypersensitivities can contribute to a myriad of conditions including autoimmune diseases (Valenta et al. 2009). In case of pet animals, glomerulonephritis and systemic lupus erythematosus are the major autoimmune diseases. Immunodeficiency disorders are seen in pet animals due to defects in congenital inertness of the immune system. Many common diseases like canine parvovirus and canine distemper also cause immunodeficiency, which is also a very big concern nowadays.

20.2 Immunopathology

Immunopathology is the study of diseases or conditions resulting to immune reaction, or it is the study of the role of the immunological processes in the production of disease, its diagnosis, and treatment.

20.3 Types of Hypersensitivity

Type 1 hypersensitivity is an immediate reaction toward an antigen. When an antigen (allergen) comes in contact with the body, IgE antibody is produced. These IgE antibodies form a cross-linkage between each other and bind to fc receptors present on mast cells and produce primary and secondary mediators.

20.4 Disease Related to Type 1 Hypersensitivity

20.4.1 Anaphylactic Shock

Anaphylaxis is a severe life-threatening reaction. It is a serious allergic reaction that is rapid in onset and may cause death (Sampson et al. 2006). In case of the cattle, lungs are the major shock organ, and serotonin, kinin, and leukotrienes play an important role in anaphylaxis, while in case of sheep, histamine plays major role in anaphylaxis. In case of dogs, anaphylaxis reactions are severely marked. In case of the dogs, some antihistaminic drugs are also given as preventive medication in anaphylaxis.

20.4.2 Urticaria and Angioedema

The urticaria and angioedema manifest as a cutaneous hypersensitivity reaction to immunogenic stimuli. Urticaria is characterized by the development of wheals or angioedema or may be both (Zuberbier et al. 2014). Main etiology includes the drugs, vaccines, bacterins, food or food additives, stinging or biting insects, and plants.

20.4.3 Canine Atopic Dermatitis

Canine atopy is a hypersensitivity reaction to inhaled or cutaneously absorbed environmental antigens (allergens) in genetically predisposed individuals. Main etiology is the molds, weed, and pollen grains (Table 20.1). It is mainly associated with IgE antibodies with the environmental antigens (Halliwell 2006).

20.4.4 Flea Allergy Dermatitis (Flea Bite Hypersensitivity)

Flea allergy dermatitis is a common skin disease in dogs and cats sensitized to flea bites. The allergic feline patients will show four characteristic patterns of cutaneous signs indicative of pruritus and inflammation in head and neck with excoriation, self-induced alopecia, miliary dermatitis, and eosinophilic lesions (Hobi et al. 2011). Flea allergy dermatitis is the most frequently diagnosed hypersensitivity in cats (Miller et al. 2013).

Table 20.1 Comparison of the atopic dermatitis and allergic contact dermatitis

Features	Atopic dermatitis	Allergic contact dermatitis
Hypersensitivity	Type I hypersensitivity	Type IV hypersensitivity
Major allergens	Foods, pollens, fleas, inhaled allergens	Reactive chemicals and dyes in contact with skin
Clinical signs	Hyperemia, urticaria, and pruritus	Hyperemia, vesiculation, alopecia, and erythema
Distribution	Face, nose, eyes, feet, and perineum	Hairless areas, usually ventral abdomen, and feet
Pathology	Eosinophilic infiltration and edema	Mononuclear cell infiltration and vesiculation
Diagnosis	Intradermal testing and immediate response	Delayed response on patch testing
Treatment	Steroids, antihistamines, and hyposensitization	Steroids

20.5 Type 2 Hypersensitivity

When an allergen comes in contact with the body, the antibody binds to the cell surface antigen which causes destruction of cells. Type 2 hypersensitivities are also known as cytotoxic hypersensitivities. It is a rare reaction that is typically caused by IgG and IgM antibodies (Brostoff et al. 1991). Type 2 response may occur when the target antigen is part of the surface of a specific host cell or tissue. Type 2 hypersensitivities can be associated with autoimmune diseases, drug reactions, and transplantations (Brostoff et al. 1991). Biochemically, type 2 reactions occur, when IgG and IgM antibodies bind to host cells and tissues to form complexes that activate the complement pathway, which eliminates the host cells (Kornbrust et al. 1989; Brostoff et al. 1991). During type 2 hypersensitivities, mediators of acute inflammation, such as B cells, antibodies, and cytokines, are generated to induce cell lysis and death.

20.6 Disease Related to Type 2 Hypersensitivity

20.6.1 Incompatible Blood Transfusion

Generally, incompatible blood transfusion is reported in dog, cat, horse, pig, and goat. The naturally occurring isoantibodies to most of the erythrocyte antigens are absent in animal, so the first transfusion does not cause any discomfort, if donor erythrocyte antigen is not identical to recipient and it stimulates the antibodies production, the antibodies activate the complement cascade and causes hemolysis of donor erythrocytes (Tables 20.2 and 20.3).

20.7 Type 3 Hypersensitivity

Type 3 hypersensitivities are also mediated by IgG and IgM antibodies. Unlike a type 2 response, type 3 hypersensitivity is associated with responses to soluble antigens that are not combined with host tissues but with antibodies in the blood, which can then lead to inflammatory responses (Brostoff et al. 1991). As the number of antigen-antibody complexes increase, they can deposit in joints and various tissues such as kidneys, skin, and eyes leading to an inflammatory response, wherever they precipitate (Ellsworth et al. 2008). Research has suggested that type 3 reactions may contribute to certain systemic diseases such as systemic lupus erythematosus (SLE), serum sickness, and farmer lung (Coico and Sunshine 2009).

20.7 Type 3 Hypersensitivity

Table 20.2 Major known blood groups in dogs

Blood groups	Genetics	Naturally occurring alloantibodies	Special considerations
Dog erythrocyte antigen (DEA) 1.1	Codominant	None	Most important blood group during transfusions because it causes acute hemolytic reaction
DEA 1.2	RBC positive or negative for each 1.1 and 1.2	–	–
DEA 3	DEA 3 (dominant) and null	In some DEA-3 negative dogs, but results in delayed RBC survival	Rare; 23% of greyhounds are DEA 3–positive
DEA 4	DEA 4 (dominant) and null	None	~98% of dogs in the United States are DEA 4–positive
DEA 5	DEA 5 (dominant) and null	In some DEA-5 negative dogs, but results in delayed RBC survival	10% of dogs; as many as 30% of greyhounds are DEA 5-positive
DEA 7	DEA 7 (dominant) and null	None	99% of dogs in the United States are DEA 6–positive
Dalmatian (dal) blood type	–	None	100% of the general dog population; absent from Dalmatians

Table 20.3 Major known blood groups in cats

Blood groups	Genetics	Inheritance	Naturally occurring alloantibodies	Special considerations
A	AA, AA^{ab} or ab	A is dominant over B; A allele in cats is dominant to b and a^{ab}	Some may have low anti-B titer	Approximately 90% of cats are A positive
B	Bb or bb	B is recessive to A	All have high anti-A titer	Agglutinins and hemolysins resulting in severe transfusion reaction
AB	a^{ab}b or a^{ab}a^{ab}	Determined by a third allele *aab* that is recessive to *A* and dominant over *b*	Most have no alloantibodies	Rare
Mik	–	Some type A cats are Mik-negative, but most are Mik-positive	Mik-negative cats might have alloantibodies to Mik	Most type A cats are Mik-positive. Newly recognized group in domestic shorthair cats

20.8 Disease Related to Type 3 Hypersensitivity

20.8.1 Serum Sickness

In serum sickness, circulating immune complexes are deposited in tissues that initiate the inflammatory processes leading to glomerulonephritis and arthritis. This condition is also observed in case of serum therapy. In case of diphtheria, anti-diphtheria horse serum is given in man, which is recognized as foreign protein, and elicits an immune response detrimental to the host.

20.8.2 Arthus Reaction

It is observed in animals following administration of repeated injection of antigen until an appreciable amount of precipitating IgG antibody appears, and then on subsequent subcutaneous or intradermal injection of antigen, marked edema and hemorrhage is produced at the site of injection. There is intravascular clumping of platelets leading to occlusion of blood vessels and necrosis.

20.8.3 Glomerulonephritis

Glomerulonephritis is a kidney condition that involves damage or inflammation to the glomeruli. It may be caused by streptococcal, bacterial, viral, and parasitic antigens. The severity of a glomerulus disease usually reflected in terms of proteinuria (Lees et al. 2005). The primary glomerulus disease in dogs has more severe outcome, if urine protein to creatinine ratio exceeds 2.0 (Jacob et al. 2005). Generally, glomerulonephritis is seen in the middle-aged dogs, and there is formation of immune complexes in this disease, and these are deposited in glomerulus that led to the increased production of glomerulus cell lining the epithelium and then leucocyte infiltrate the glomerulus leads to thickening of glomerulus filtration membrane. This causes loss of glomerulus filtration membrane, which leads to decreased glomerulus filtration membrane. Main clinical signs are the increase in protein level in urine which leads to hypoproteinemia, ascites, edema, and hypercholesterolemia.

20.8.4 Type 4 Hypersensitivity

Type 4 hypersensitivity is also known as delayed-type hypersensitivity. Type 4 hypersensitivity response depends upon the T-cell interaction, which recruits other cells to the site of exposure (Brostoff et al. 1991). Two primary methods exist to verify type 4 hypersensitivity which are delayed skin testing and lymphocyte transformation test (Primeau and Adkinson 2001). Delayed skin testing is similar to an immediate-type skin test; however, the reaction is typically read after 24 or 72 h rather than 15 min after application of the antigens (Li 2002). Still, skin testing can pose the risk of developing adverse systemic reactions and appropriate training, and care must therefore be practiced to ensure the safety of patients (Reid et al. 1993). In addition, research has shown that skin testing may be unreliable for some antigens, such as food allergens (Sampson and Albergo 1984). Due to the limitations of skin testing (Rietschel 1996), alternative methods are currently being tested for the detection of type 4 hypersensitivities including the lymphocyte transformation test (Pichler and Tilch 2004).

20.9 Disease Related to Type 4 Hypersensitivity

20.9.1 Allergic Contact Dermatitis

Allergic contact dermatitis is the most common disease of skin with a great socio-economic importance (Uter et al. 1998). It is characterized by redness, papule, and vesicles followed by dryness of skin (Krasteva 1999). Several chemical and substances cause the allergic contact dermatitis like formaldehyde, carpet dyes, hair dyes, and various cosmetics (Fig. 20.1). Most of these substances are small molecules that can form complex with skin protein when applied on the skin; these complexes are internalized by antigen-presenting cells and processed. Further, along with MHC class 2 molecules presented to the T cells and intraepithelial vesicles are formed as a killing of antigen-presenting cells containing the chemical protein complex by the activated T cells. There is mild erythema, and red patches are seen in the animal body (Table 20.1).

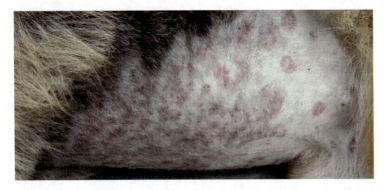

Fig. 20.1 Allergic contact dermatitis in dog due to chemical exposure: skin showed redness, erythema or red patches, papule, and dryness in the ventral abdomen

20.10 Autoimmune Diseases

Autoimmune diseases are the diseases that arise from the overactive immune response of the body against substances and tissue normally present in the body. Autoimmune diseases are pathological conditions identified by abnormal immune responses and characterized by autoantibodies and T-cell response to self-molecule by immune response reactivity (Invernizzi and Gershwin 2009).

20.11 Autoimmune Diseases of the Pet Animals

20.11.1 Systemic Lupus Erythematosus

The term lupus means the horrible facial rashes present in this disease, which mainly are two types of autoantibodies present in this disease tissue-specific autoantibodies and non-specific autoantibodies, and tissue-specific autoantibodies are formed against the red blood cells, platelets, and leucocytes, while nonspecific autoantibodies are directed against the nuclear antigen these autoantibodies are formed due to structure change in self-antigen at molecular level, exposer of sequestered antigen to the host immune response. This disease happens through the activation of various sensors of the innate immune response and can contribute to the initiation of the disease (Kontaki and Boumpas 2010). Factors which are important in the initiation of autoimmune response in systemic lupus erythematosus increase production of autoantigen during handling and presentation of lupus flares (Kontaki and Boumpas 2010). Diagnosis of systemic lupus erythematosus is done by lupus band test.

20.11.2 Rheumatoid Arthritis

Rheumatoid arthritis is characterized by deposition of immune complexes within the synovial tissue, and this disease is commonly seen in small and toy breed of dog. The cause of rheumatoid arthritis is unknown, although autoimmunity plays pivotal role in both chronicity and progression, and rheumatoid arthritis is considered a systemic autoimmune disease. In rheumatoid arthritis, autoantibodies are formed against altered immunoglobulins, and these antibodies are called rheumatoid factors. These autoantibodies are formed due to steric configurational changes in the IgG molecules, and these antibodies are deposited in the synovium and activate the complement. The presence of leukotrienes and platelet-activating factors causes infiltration of large number of neutrophils in the synovial fluid; the protease releases from the neutrophils cause degradation of articular cartilage. There is formation of pannus in rheumatoid arthritis, which consists of proliferating synoviocytes infiltrated with lymphocytes, plasma cells, and neutrophils. Diagnosis of this disease is done by mucin clot test.

20.11.3 Autoimmune Thyroiditis

This disease is caused by the reaction of immune system against the thyroid gland. Autoantibodies are formed in this disease against the thyroglobulin and thyrotropin receptors. Several mechanisms have been proposed that implicate iodine itself or the iodination of thyroglobulin as the cause of autoimmune thyroiditis, which have been reviewed (Wang and Baker 2011). The first model of experimental autoimmune thyroiditis was in rabbits induced by extract of thyroid with complete freund's adjuvant (Rose and Witebsky 1956). The main clinical signs of this disease include hypothyroidism; animal is dull and depressed; and animal is lethargic. Diagnosis of this disease is done by characteristic lymphocytic infiltration in thyroid biopsy.

20.11.4 Myasthenia Gravis

Myasthenia gravis is the disorder of neuromuscular function. This disease is characterized by skeletal muscle weakness and fatigue. This condition is generally seen in young dogs. In this disease, antibodies are formed against acetylcholine receptors, and the autoantibodies cross bind with the acetylcholine receptors, which prevent activation of adenylate cyclase and normal contraction. Binding of autoantibodies to acetylcholine receptors also blocks the access of acetylcholine to its receptors, and this inhibits the physiologic effect of acetylcholine. Myasthenia gravis is mainly diagnosed by tensilon test.

20.12 Immunodeficiency

The alterations that decrease the effectiveness or destroy the capabilities of the system to respond to various antigens are collectively designated as immunodeficiency. The immunodeficiency is of two types, namely, primary and secondary immunodeficiency. Primary immunodeficiency is congenital in nature and may be due to the defect in gene or chromosome. Secondary immunodeficiencies are the acquired due to the drugs, deficiency of nutrition, neoplasm, or environmental pollution. More than 300 genetically defined single-gene inborn errors of immunity are now recognized as a cause of primary immunodeficiency (Bousfiha et al. 2015). In primary immunodeficiency, there is immunoglobulin replacement and judicious use of prophylactic antibiotics, which can prevent the significant end-organ damage and improve long-term outcome and quality of life in many patients (Piguet et al. 2008).

20.13 Disorder Related to Primary Immunodeficiency

20.13.1 Severe Combined Immunodeficiency Syndrome (SCID)

This defect is due to inherited gene defect and an autosomal recessive gene causing abnormal purine metabolism. In SCID syndrome, stem cells are absent and unable to differentiate into T and B lymphocytes; there is hypoplasia of thymus, spleen, and lymph nodes were seen. Gene therapy has been shown to be effective in patient with adenosine deaminase deficiency and with X-linked SCID leading to survival. It is anticipated that gene therapy will be considered as a therapeutic option for a growing number of primary immunodeficiency in the coming years (Aiuti et al. 2009).

20.13.2 Lethal Acrodermatitis

This defect is due to T-cell defect, characterized by hypoplasia of T-dependent lymphoid tissues. Generally, this defect is seen in adult dogs. In bull terriers, related phenotypes termed as lethal acrodermatitis have been reported in scientific literature as early as 1986 (Jezyk et al. 1986). Lethal acrodermatitis in dogs is immunodeficient with a reduction in serum IgE level and frequently suffers from skin infections like candidiasis (McEwan et al. 2003).

20.13.3 Chediak-Higashi Syndrome

Chediak-Higashi syndrome is a rare autosomal recessive multisystem disorder. It is characterized by defect in granule morphogenesis with giant lysosome in leucocyte and other cells (Hoffman 2005). This syndrome is generally seen in Persian cats, characterized by dilution of hair pigmentation, ocular abnormality, and increased susceptibility to diseases. This disorder further culminates into lymphoproliferative syndrome progressing into pancytopenia (Hoffman 2005). In this disorder, the giant granules are seen in neutrophils. The diagnostic hallmark of Chediak-Higashi syndrome is the presence of giant violet to purple granules in leucocytes (Suresh and Nazia 1994).

20.14 Disorder Related to Secondary Immunodeficiency

20.14.1 Canine Parvovirus Infection

Canine parvovirus is the common intestinal pathogen of pups. This disease is characterized by rapid clinical signs, in which death can occur after few days of onset of clinical signs (Carman and Povey 1985; Parrish 1995). Myocarditis is seen after infection in neonatal puppies, where clinical signs are seen after few days of infections (Meunier et al. 1984; Sime et al. 2015). Canine parvovirus causes destruction of immunocyte, which leads to depletion of lymphoid tissues and cause immunodeficiency. The evolution of the virus raises the question about the efficacy of the vaccines, so understanding is very much required in case of this virus (Truyen 2006).

20.14.2 Canine Distemper

Canine distemper is a most common disease of dogs, canids, mustelids, procyonids, and viverrids (Appel and Gillespie 1972). The Canine distemper virus belongs to the family *Paramyxoviridae* and the genus *Morbillivirus*. It is a single-stranded RNA virus that is reported to cause a systemic disease globally (Deem et al. 2000). Canine distemper virus causes immunosuppression by activation of T suppresser cells. The virus causes high morbidity and mortality in a broad range of immune naïve host including some non-human primates and carnivores (Beineke et al. 2015; Martinez Gutierrez and Ruiz 2016).

20.14.3 Drug Therapy Defects

Aspirin drug used in therapy of rheumatoid arthritis causes immunosuppression, which leads to reduction in the platelet aggregation, phagocytic activity of neutrophils, and the lymphocytic function.

References

Aiuti A, Cattaneo F, Galimberti S, Benningh Off U, Cassani B, Callegaro L (2009) Gene therapy for immunodeficiency due to adenosine deaminase deficiency. N Engl J Med 360:447–458

Appel M, Gillespie JE (1972) Canine distemper monograph. In: Gard S, Hallauer C, Meyer KF (eds) Handbook of virus research. Springer Verlag, New York, NY, pp 34–63

Beineke A, Baumga Èrtner W, Wohlsein P (2015) Cross species transmission of canine distemper virus an update. J One Health 1:49–59

Bousfiha A, Jeddane L, Al-Herz W, Ailal F, Casanova J-L, Chatila T (2015) The 2015 IUIS phenotypic classification for primary immunodeficiency. J Clin Immunol 35:38–727

Brostoff J, Scadding GK, Male D, Roitt IM (1991) Introduction to immune responses. In: Clinical Immunology. Gower Medical Publishing, New York, NY

Carman PS, Povey RC (1985) Pathogenesis of canine parvovirus-2 in dogs hematology, serology and virus recovery. J Res Vet Sci 38:134–140

Coico R, Sunshine G (2009) Types II and type III hypersensitivity. In: Immunology a short course. John Wiley and Sons, Hoboken, NJ

Deem SL, Spelman LH, Yates R, Montali RJ (2000) Canine distemper in terrestrial carnivores a review. J Zoo Wildl Med 31:441–451

Ellsworth JL, Maurer M, Harder B, Hamacher N, Lantry M, Lewis KB (2008) Targeting immune complex mediated hypersensitivity with recombinant soluble human FcgammaRIA (CD64A). J Immunol 180:580–589

Halliwell R (2006) Revised nomenclature for veterinary allergy. J Vet Immunol Immunopathol 114:8–207

Hobi S, Linek M, Marignac G, Olivry T, Beco L, Nett C, Fontaine J, Roosje P, Bergvall K, Belova S (2011) Clinical characteristics and causes of pruritus in cats: a multicenter study on feline hypersensitivity-associated dermatoses. J Vet Dermatol 22:406–413

Hoffman R (2005) Defects in structure and function of lysosomes. In: Hoffman R, Edward J, Harvey J (eds) Hoffmans haematology basic principles and practice, chapter 46, 4th edn. Elsevier, Philadelphia, PA, pp 607–629

Invernizzi P, Gershwin ME (2009) The genetics of human autoimmune disease. J Autoimmun 33: 303–308

Jacob F, Polzin DJ, Osborne CA (2005) Evaluation of the association between initial proteinuria and morbidity rate or death in dogs with naturally occurring chronic renal failure. J Am Vet Med Assoc 226:393–400

Jezyk PF, Haskins ME, MacKay-Smith WE, Patterson DF (1986) Lethal acrodermatitis in bull terriers. J Am Vet Med Assoc 188:833–839

Kontaki E, Boumpas DT (2010) Innate immunity in systemic lupus erythematosus: sensing endogenous nucleic acids. J Autoimmun 35:318–321

Kornbrust D, Eydelloth R, Garratty G (1989) Investigations of the potential for five beta lactam antibiotics to elicit type II hypersensitivity reactions in rats and monkeys. J Fundam Appl Toxicol 12:558–566

Krasteva M (1999) Contact dermatitis II. Clinical aspects and diagnosis. Eur J Dermatol 9:144–159

Lees GE, Brown SA, Elliott J (2005) Assessment and management of proteinuria in dogs and cats: 2004 ACVIM forum consensus statement (small animal). J Vet Intern Med 19:377–385

Li JT (2002) Allergy testing. Am Fam Physician 66:621–624

Martinez Gutierrez M, Ruiz SJ (2016) Diversity of susceptible hosts in canine distemper virus infection a systematic review and data synthesis. BMC Vet Res 12:78

McEwan NA, Huang HP, Mellor DJ (2003) Immunoglobulin levels in bull terriers suffering from lethal acrodermatitis. Vet Immunol Immunopathol 96:235–238

Meunier PC, Cooper BJ, Appel MJ, Slauson DO (1984) Experimental viral myocarditis parvoviral infection of neonatal pups. J Vet Pathol 21:509–515

Miller WH, Griffin CE, Campbell KL (2013) Hypersensitivity disorders. In: Muller and kirks small animal dermatology, 7th edn. Elsevier, St. Louis, MI, pp 363–431

Parrish CR (1995) Pathogenesis of feline panleukopenia virus and canine parvovirus. Baillieres Clin Haematol 8:57–71

Pichler WJ, Tilch J (2004) The lymphocyte transformation test in the diagnosis of drug hypersensitivity. J Allergy 59:809–820

Piguet D, Tosi C, Luthi JM, Andresen I, Juge O, Redimune R (2008) NF liquid, a ready to use, high concentration intravenous immunoglobulin therapy preparation is safe and typically well tolerated in the routine clinical management of a broad range of conditions. Clin Exp Immunol 152:9–45

Primeau MN, Adkinson NF Jr (2001) Recent advances in the diagnosis of drug allergy. Curr Opin Allergy Clin Immunol 1:337–341

Reid MJ, Lockey RF, Turkeltaub PC, Platts Mills TA (1993) Survey of fatalities from skin testing and immunotherapy. J Allergy Clin Immunol 92:6–15

Rietschel RL (1996) Reproducibility of patch test results. Lancet 347:1202

Rose NR, Witebsky E (1956) Studies on organ specificity changes in the thyroid glands of rabbits following active immunization with rabbit thyroid extracts. J Immunol 76:417–427

Sampson HA, Albergo R (1984) Comparison of results of skin tests, RAST, and double-blind placebo controlled food challenges in children with atopic dermatitis. J Allergy Clin Immunol 74:26–33

Sampson HA, Munoz Furlong A, Campbell RL, Adkinson NF Jr, Bock SA, Branum A (2006) Second symposium on the definition and management of anaphylaxis summary report second National Institute of allergy and infectious disease, food allergy and anaphylaxis network symposium. J Allergy Clin Immunol 117:7–391

Sicherer SH, Leung DY (2009) Advances in allergic skin disease, anaphylaxis, and hypersensitivity reactions to foods, drugs, and insects. J Allergy Clin Immunol 123:319–327

Sime TA, Powell LL, Schildt JC, Olson EJ (2015) Parvoviral myocarditis in a 5 week old dachshund. J Vet Emerg Crit Care 25:765–769

Suresh M, Nazia B (1994) Chediak Hegashi syndrome a rare case report. Indian J Pediatr 31:8–1115

Truyen U (2006) Evolution of canine parvovirus a need for new vaccines. Vet Microbiol 117:9–13

Uter W, Schnuch A, Geier J, Frosch PJ (1998) Epidemiology of contact dermatitis. The information network of departments of dermatology (IVDK) in Germany. Eur J Dermatol 8:36–40

Valenta R, Mittermann I, Werfel T, Garn H, Renz H (2009) Linking allergy to autoimmune disease. J Trends Immunol 30:109–116

Wang S, Baker JR (2011) Immuno pathogenesis of thyroiditis. Edition Eisenbarth GS

Yamasaki S, Saito T (2005) Regulation of mast cell activation through FcepsilonRI. J Chem Immunol Allergy 87:22–31

Zuberbier T, Aberer W, Asero R, Bindslev Jensen C, Brzoza Z, Canonica GW, Church M, Ensina L, Giménez Arnau A, Godse K (2014) The EAACI/GA2LEN EDF/WAO guideline for the definition, classification, diagnosis, and management of urticaria, the 2013 revision and update. J Allergy 69:868–887

Techniques in Immunopathology 21

Key Points

1. Macrophage function test is performed to assess their ability to phagocytose the particulate material or bactericidal activity.
2. Type IV hypersensitivity reaction is applied in the diagnosis of some chronic diseases like tuberculosis, paratuberculosis (Johne's disease), and glanders.
3. Cells involved in type IV hypersensitivity reaction are T lymphocytes, macrophages, regulatory B lymphocyte, and basophils.
4. Enzyme-linked immunosorbent assay (ELISA) is a widely applicable and accepted test for determination of antibody titers in serum (Fig. 21.10).
5. Dot-immunobinding assay (DIA) is used as an alternative test for ELISA, and the basic principle of DIA and ELISA is same.
6. Agglutination test is a simple procedure that can be done when the antigen of interest is particulate (e.g., RBCs, bacteria) or when soluble antigen is coated onto particles such as tiny latex beads.
7. Particulate antigen reacts with antibodies in optimum proportions, and the epitopes of antigen bind and cross-link with the antibodies to form an agglutination or clumping.
8. IgM antibodies are more efficient to cause agglutination than IgG antibodies.
9. Immunoperoxidase techniques are used for the demonstration of antigen in tissues, type of lymphoid cells (T or B cells), and specific antibody-producing cells.
10. Immunoperoxidase technique requires peroxidase-labeled antibody to react with antigen present in tissues, which are detected by developing a color using chromogenic substrate 3,3′-diaminobenzidine (DAB).
11. Peroxidase antiperoxidase (PAP) technique involves three reagents, i.e., primary antibody, secondary antibody, and peroxidase antiperoxidase complex.
12. Avidin-biotin technique is considered one of the most sensitive techniques. The principle of this technique lies on the ability of egg white glycoprotein "avidin" to bind with four molecules of vitamin "biotin."

13. Cell-mediated immune response is estimated by lymphocyte blastogenesis assay, macrophage function test, and DTH reaction.

21.1 Collection of Blood and Serum

The blood is collected from animals and man through puncture of vein using syringe and needle. In some laboratory animals and poultry, however, it is collected directly from the heart. The sites of blood collection in different animal species are as under:

1. Cattle and buffalo	Jugular vein
2. Horse, camel, sheep, and goat	Jugular vein
3. Pig	Anterior vena cava, ear vein
4. Dog	Cephalic vein, recurrent tarsal vein
5. Rabbit	Heart
6. Mice	Heart, inner canthus
7. Poultry	Wing vein, heart
8. Man	Cephalic vein

The blood is collected for total leucocyte count (TLC), differential leucocyte count (DLC), macrophage blastogenesis assay and lymphocyte stimulation test, and for serum to carry out various serological tests. About 0.5 to 1.0 mL of blood collected in vials containing ethylenediaminetetraacetic acid (EDTA) is sufficient for TLC and DLC. Collect the blood under aseptic conditions preferably by using disposable syringe and needle. After collection of blood, the needle should be removed, and blood is transferred gently in vials containing anticoagulant. Mix the contents gently by rotating the vial in between palms. Vigorous shaking should be avoided in order to prevent the hemolysis.

The blood for macrophage functions and lymphocyte blastogenesis assay (LBA) is collected in separate sterile vials containing heparin as anticoagulant. Five milliliters of blood is sufficient for which take two to three drops of 1% heparin in syringe and rinse it before collection of blood. This amount is sufficient and will prevent the clotting. After collection, transfer about 2.0 mL of blood in vial meant for macrophage function test and 3.0 mL of blood in vial for LBA.

For serum, the blood is collected in sterile tubes without any anticoagulant. In order to obtain clear serum, the test tubes should be rinsed with sterile normal saline solution before collection of blood. As about 1.0–2.0 mL of serum is required for various serological tests, 4–5 mL of blood is collected in the test tube and kept in slanting position without any disturbance. The serum can be separated after 6–8 h of its collection. If there is any turbidity, the tube should be centrifuged to get clear serum. The serum can be stored at $-20\ °C$ until its further use in laboratory without any preservative for short period. If it is to be stored more than a month, then one drop of 0.01% merthiolate or sodium azide should be added in order to check the contamination (Chauhan 1995, 1998a).

21.2 Leucocyte Count

21.2.1 Total Leucocyte Count (TLC)

- Clean the Neubauer's chamber/hemocytometer. Put the coverslip on the area demarcated for counting.
- Suck fresh/anticoagulant mixed blood in white blood cell (WBC) diluting pipette up to 0.5 mark, and fill the pipette with WBC diluting fluid up to 11 mark.
- Hold the pipette in horizontal position, and remove rubber tube. Mix the contents by rotating the pipette in between palms.
- Discard first few drops from pipette, and then place a drop near the edge of coverslip to fill the space between coverslip and chamber.
- Keep counting the chamber after 1–2 min for settling of the cells.
- Count the cells under low power in four large/primary corner squares of the ruled area (Fig. 21.1).
- Cells on top of square and left side are included in count.
- Calculate WBC per µL of blood by multiplying 50 to the total number of cells counted in four large squares. It can be converted into per mL and per lit by further multiplying by 10^3 and 10^6, respectively.

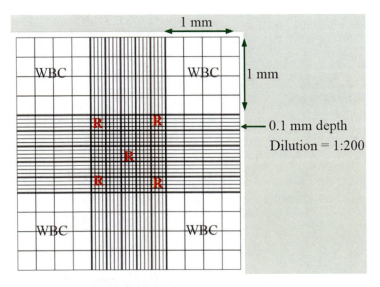

Fig. 21.1 Neubauer chamber (W = Counting area for leucocytes; R = Counting area for erythrocytes)

21.2.2 Differential Leucocyte Count (DLC)

- Prepare a thin blood smear on clean grease-free glass slide. Place a drop of blood on one end of slide, and spread as smear with the help of another slide using its edge at 45° angle (Fig. 21.2).
- Dry the smear in air, and mark the identification number in the thick portion of smear.
- Fix the smear in methanol for at least 5 min, and dry in air.
- Stain the smear with Giemsa stain diluted to 1:10 in PBS for 30 min or with Leishman's stain without fixing the smear.
- Wash the slide, dry in air, and examine under oil immersion microscope. Count at least 200 cells by battlement/zigzag method. Cells counted are neutrophils (Figs. 21.3a, 21.4), monocytes (Figs. 21.3b, 21.5), lymphocytes (Figs. 21.3c, 21.6), basophils (Fig. 21.3d), and eosinophils (Fig. 21.3e). Cell count is presented in percent (%).

21.2.3 Absolute Lymphocyte Count (ALC)

The absolute lymphocyte count is calculated from the data of DLC and TLC through the following formula:

$$\text{ALC}\,(10^3/\mu L) = \frac{\%\text{Lymphocyte} \times \text{TLC}\,(10^3/\mu L)}{100}$$

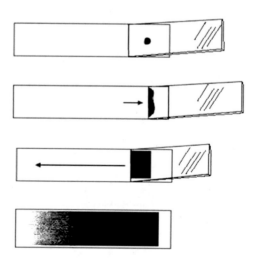

Fig. 21.2 Blood smear preparation for differential leucocyte count

21.2 Leucocyte Count

Fig. 21.3 Leucocytes. (**a**) neutrophil, (**b**) monocyte, (**b**) lymphocyte, (**d**) basophil, and (**e**) eosinophil

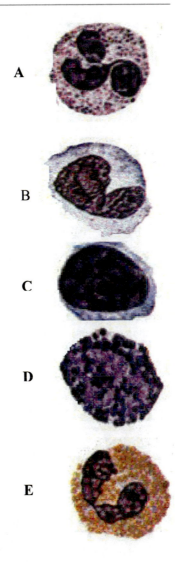

21.2.4 Absolute Neutrophil Count (ANC)

The absolute neutrophil count is calculated by using the neutrophil percentage of differential leucocyte count and total leucocyte count as follows:

$$\text{ANC}\left(10^3/\mu L\right) = \frac{\%\text{Neutrophils} \times \text{TLC}\left(10^3/\mu L\right)}{100}$$

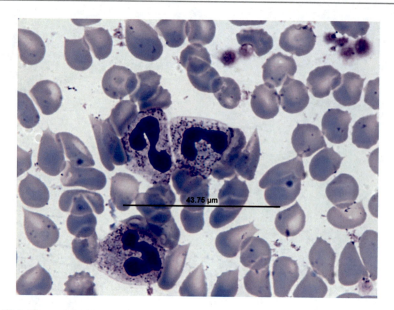

Fig. 21.4 Neutrophil of human in a blood smear. Polymorphonuclear (PMN) leukocyte with 3–5 nuclear lobes and fine granules within the cytoplasm

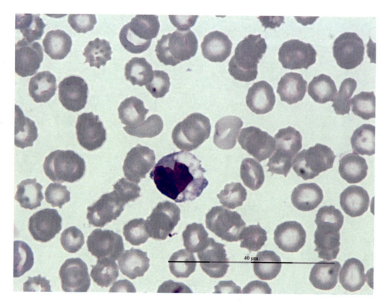

Fig. 21.5 Monocyte of dog in a blood smear. Largest mononuclear leukocyte has large eccentrically placed kidney bean-shaped nucleus with abundant vacuolated cytoplasm

21.3 Collection of Lymphoid Cells

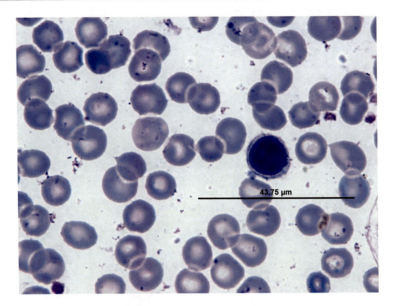

Fig. 21.6 Lymphocyte of human in a blood smear. Mononuclear leukocyte is small in size but bigger than RBCs. Lymphocytes have a regular, spherical nucleus and high nuclear:cytoplasmic ratio with scanty pale blue rim of cytoplasm

21.3 Collection of Lymphoid Cells

Lymphocytes/mononuclear cells are collected from blood, lymph nodes, mucosa-associated lymphoid tissue (MALT), respiratory-associated lymphoid tissue (RALT) and spleen for lymphocyte blastogenesis assay (LBA), enumeration of T- and B-cell population, subsets of T-cell population, and for their microscopic evaluation.

21.3.1 Blood

- Collect 3 mL of blood in sterilized vials containing heparin as anticoagulant under strict hygienic conditions.
- Mix 3 mL of RPMI-1640 medium in the blood.
- Take 3 mL of Histopapue-1077 in a centrifuge tube, and overlay the blood-RPMI mixture on histopaque carefully.
- Centrifuge it at 400 × g for 30 min at room temperature. Carefully aspirate the opaque layer with sterilized Pasteur pipette in a sterilized centrifuge tube (Fig. 21.7).
- Add RPMI-1640, and wash the cells for two times. Finally resuspend the cells in RPMI-1640 medium in desired concentration.

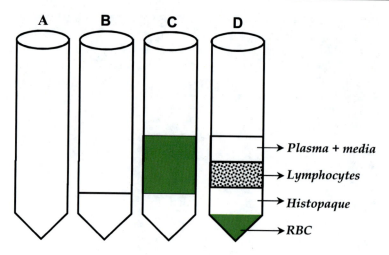

Fig. 21.7 Diagram showing separation of lymphocytes in histopaque. (**a**) Test tube, (**b**) histopaque, (**c**) blood over histopaque, and (**d**) separated lymphocytes

21.3.2 Prescapular Lymph Node

- Locate the prescapular lymph node under the anterior portion of scapula at slightly above the point of shoulder.
- Aspirate the lymphoid cells by puncturing with biopsy needle and syringe under strict aseptic conditions (Fig. 21.8).
- Collect the lymphoid cells in RPMI-1640, and filter through muslin cloth. Wash three times as described earlier.

21.3.3 Mesenteric Lymph Nodes

- Mesenteric lymph nodes are collected under general anesthesia or just after the death at necropsy and wash with sterile phosphate-buffered saline (PBS).
- Small pieces are cut in RPMI-1640 medium, and cell suspension is prepared.
- The cell suspension is filtered through muslin cloth or steel sieve and washed three times with RPMI-1640 medium as described earlier.
- Make desired concentration of cells in RPMI-1640 medium.

21.3.4 Mucosa-Associated Lymphoid Tissue (MALT)

- The lymphocyte and other mononuclear cells are collected from gut-associated lymphoid tissue (GALT) including Peyer's patches and respiratory-associated lymphoid tissue (RALT).

21.3 Collection of Lymphoid Cells

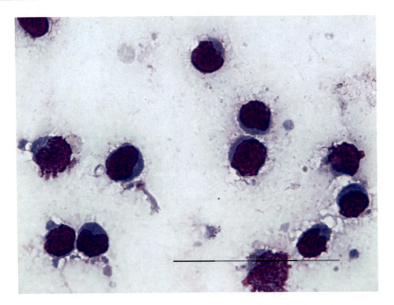

Fig. 21.8 Lymphocytes of dog in an aspirate from prescapular lymph node. Lymphocytes have a regular, spherical nucleus and high nuclear:cytoplasmic ratio with scanty, pale blue, agranular rim of cytoplasm

21.3.4.1 Peyer's Patches/Intestinal Lymphocytes

- Remove terminal ileum under general anesthesia or just after death.
- Wash in sterile PBS pH 7.2, cut longitudinally, and spread it in a petri dish.
- Remove the mucosal layer by scarping gently. Superficial scrapings of mucosa should be discarded.
- Deeper scrapings to the level of muscularis mucosae should be collected in RPMI-1640 medium and centrifuged at 900 × g for 10 min.
- The large mucoid pellets should be washed three times with RPMI-1640 medium.
- Filter the cells through muslin cloth, centrifuge at 400 × g, and make the desired concentration of cells.

21.3.5 Respiratory-Associated Lymphoid Tissue (RALT)

- Bronchi-associated lymphoid tissue (BALT) is collected just after the death of animal.
- Bronchial or mediastinal lymph nodes particularly at the bifurcation of trachea are collected.
- Collect the lymphoid cells as described in mesenteric lymph nodes.

21.3.6 Spleen

- Lymphoid cells from spleen are collected either through biopsy or after the death of animal.
- Since the spleen is the largest lymphoid organ, it can be located at the medial surface of the dorsal curvature of rumen below the diaphragm in cattle, buffaloes, sheep, and goats.
- Normally, the spleen is not palpable. But in case of enlargement of spleen, it can be palpated.
- From mice, poultry, and calves, splenic lymphoid tissue is collected just after death.
- Washing and separation of lymphocytes can be done as described for mesenteric lymph nodes.

21.4 Lymphocyte Blastogenesis Assay

- As described earlier, the lymphocytes are collected and resuspended in small amount of RPMI-1640 medium.
- The viability of the cells is tested by using 0.5% trypan blue dye exclusion test. In this, live lymphocytes do not take any stain, while dead cells are stained black. Finally, the live cell count is adjusted to 1×10^7 cells per mL in RPMI-1640 medium.
- For lymphocyte cultures, 96 well flat bottom culture plates are taken. Triplicate wells of cultures are prepared using 100 µL cell suspensions in each well. A set of three wells is kept as control, and 50 µL RPMI-1640 medium is further added. Second set of three wells is added with 50 µL medium containing concanavalin A (Con-A) or phytohemagglutinin-M (PHA-M) (5 µg/mL). A third set of triplicate wells is added with 50 µL of lipopolysaccharides (LPS) (5 µg/mL) in medium RPMI-1640.
- The plate is then sealed with cello tape and incubated for 68 h at 37 °C in incubator with 5% CO_2 tension.
- After incubation, 50 µL of 3-(4,5-dimethylthiazol-2-yl)-2,5-diphenyltetrazolium bromide (MTT) (4.0 mg/mL) is added to all wells, and plate is again sealed and incubated for another 4 h at 37 °C in CO_2 incubator.
- Thereafter, the liquid contents of the wells are discarded, and 100 µL of acid isopropanol [0.04 N hydrochloric acid (HCl) in isopropanol] is added in each well.
- The isopropanol is mixed by micropipette using separate tips of each set of wells.
- The absorbance of each well is determined in spectrophotometer at wavelength of 570 nanometer (nm).
- The optical density (OD) of triplicate wells is averaged, and the mean OD of mitogen-stimulated cultures is obtained by subtracting the mean OD of control wells from mean OD of wells with mitogen and presented as delta OD.

- The delta OD of Con-A/PHA-M is plotted on graph for the calculation of stimulation index of T-lymphocyte/T-lymphocyte blastogenesis assay.
- The delta OD of mitogen LPS is plotted on separate graph for calculating the index stimulation of B-lymphocyte blastogenesis (Schultz and Adams 1978; Chauhan and Singh 1992a).

21.5 Macrophage Function Test

Macrophage functions are determined to assess their ability to phagocytose the particulate material or bactericidal activity. For the purpose, peripheral blood macrophages and polymorphonuclear cells or peritoneal macrophages are collected.

- For peripheral blood phagocytic cells, collect 5.0 mL of blood in heparin vials, and add equal amount of RPMI-1640 medium. Take 5.0 mL of Histopapue-1119 in a conical centrifuge tube, and overlay blood-media mixture on Histopaque-1119 slowly.
- Centrifuge the tube at 400 × g for 10–15 min, and collect the upper opaque layer, which contains mostly phagocytic cells including polymorphonuclear and mononuclear cells.
- The peritoneal macrophages are collected by injecting mineral oil intraperitoneally 2–3 days before the start of experiment. The animal/poultry is sacrificed, or under anesthesia, peritoneal cavity is opened to collect the peritoneal fluid. One can also collect the peritoneal fluid from mouse or small animal similarly.
- The phagocytic cells in peritoneal fluid are centrifuged to remove debris and are washed three times with RPMI-1640 medium.
- The live and dead cell count is performed by using trypan blue dye exclusion method as described earlier.
- Adjust the desired concentration of phagocytic cells to perform nitroblue tetrazolium (NBT) reduction assay or bactericidal activity of the cells (Schultz and Adams 1978; Chauhan and Singh 1992a).

21.5.1 Nitroblue Tetrazolium Test

- The phagocytic cells are incubated in a tube containing:
  - 0.3 mL of 0.2% NBT in PBS
  - 0.2 mL of cell suspension (1×10^7/mL)
  - 0.1 mL of activated plasma (1 mL of plasma +15 μL of endotoxins incubated at 37 °C for 30 min)
- Tubes are incubated in water bath at 37 °C for 30 min.
- Stop the reaction by adding cold PBS.
- Centrifuge the cell suspension at 500 × g for 5 min, and discard the supernatant.
- Resuspend the cells in 0.5 mL of PBS. Put a drop of cell suspension on clean dry glass slide and make smear. Dry in air and fix in methanol for 2 min.

- Counter stain the cells with safranin (0.5%) for 2 min. Dry and mount in dibutyl phthalate polystyrene xylene (DPX) mountant.
- NBT-positive cells are counted in percent.
- Cells which contain black/blue granules of NBT dye in the cytoplasm are called as NBT-positive cells (Fig. 21.12).

21.5.2 Bactericidal Activity

- Take a culture tube and add.
  - 3.0 mL of macrophage cell suspension (1×10^7/mL)
  - 1.0 mL of *Staphylococcus aureus* or *E. coli* (2×10^7/mL)
  - 0.4 mL of normal animal serum
- Incubate it at 37 °C for 30 min in shaker.
- Stop the reaction by adding cold PBS/Hank's balanced salt solution (HBSS).
- Centrifuge the cell suspension at $400 \times g$ for 2–3 min, and discard supernatant.
- Wash the sediment for at least three times with HBSS, and finally resuspend the cells in 4.0 mL of HBSS.
- Incubate the cell suspension for 2 h at 37 °C.
- Collect 0.1 mL of cell suspension at the time of start of incubation (0 h).
- Collect 0.1 mL of cell suspension at 1 h and 2 h incubation.
- Add 1 mL of distilled water, and disrupt the cells by vigorous pipetting.
- Prepare tenfold dilutions in test tube.
- Take 0.1 mL from each dilution, and plate it on nutrient agar or tryptose soya agar plates. Incubate the plates over night at 37 °C.
- The discrete colonies are counted, and the count of bacteria per mL is calculated. Compare the bacterial counts at 0, 1 h, and 2 h.
- Normally at 1 h, the phagocytic cells kill the 50–70% organisms after phagocytosis; but as the capacity of the macrophages reduces, the bacterial count is not much affected.

21.6 Delayed-Type Hypersensitivity (DTH) Reaction

Application of an allergen (antigen) intradermally into a previously sensitized animal results in hot and painful swelling at the site after 48–72 h of injection. Microscopic examination of such skin sections reveales the presence of heavy infiltration of mononuclear cells comprising mostly of lymphocytes. These are the manifestation of type IV hypersensitivity reaction and are applied in the diagnosis of some chronic diseases like tuberculosis, paratuberculosis (Johne's disease), and glanders. The cells involved in this reaction are T lymphocytes, macrophages, regulatory B lymphocyte, and basophils (Schultz and Adams 1978; Chauhan and Singh 1992a; Tizard 1996).

21.6.1 Allergens

(a) Tuberculin purified protein derivative (PPD) for diagnosis of tuberculosis
(b) Johnin PPD for diagnosis of Johne's disease
(c) Mallein PPD for diagnosis of disease
(d) Chemicals:
  - Dinitrochlorobenzene (DNCB)
  - Dinitroflurobenzene (DNFB)

These are used for the assessment of cell-mediated immunity in experimental animals through DTH reaction.

21.6.2 Tuberculin Test

- In bovines, tuberculin is injected in the skin of neck.
- In poultry, the tuberculin is injected in wattles. 0.1 mL of tuberculin/PPD is injected intradermally using tuberculin syringe.
- Prior to tuberculin injection, skin should be cleaned and shaved with razor. The thickness of skin fold is measured using vernier caliper.
- The reaction is read after 72 h of injection. Positive reaction is characterized by hot, red, and painful swelling with an increase in double the normal skin thickness (Figs. 21.9, 21.10).

21.6.3 Johnin Test

- Johnin test is also done like that of tuberculin test.
- Instead of tuberculin/PPD, for Johnin test, either Johnin or PPD is used. 0.1 mL of Johnin is injected in clean and shaved skin of neck using tuberculin syringe. After

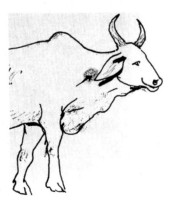

Fig. 21.9 Diagram showing of tuberculin reaction

48–72 h of injection of Johnin, the thickness of skin fold is measured using vernier caliper and is compared with normal thickness of skin. Two times increase in the thickness of skin is considered positive for Johne's disease in animals (Fig. 21.11).

21.6.4 Mallein Test

- Just like tuberculin, mallein is derived from the causative agent of glanders, i.e. *Pseudomonas mellei*.
- For the test, inject 0.2 mL of mallein intradermopalpebrally (IDP) in the skin of lower eyelid using tuberculin syringe.
- The test is read after 48 h, and a positive reaction is characterized by edema of eyelid, blepharospasm, and severe purulent conjunctivitis with ocular discharges (Fig. 21.12).

21.6.5 DNCB-/DNFB-Induced DTH Reaction

- The skin of the area to be tested is cleaned and shaved with the help of a razor.
- About 1 cm^2 area of skin is marked with marker pen for the test.
- 0.25 mL of DNCB or DNFB (10 mg/mL) is injected in the marked area intradermally.

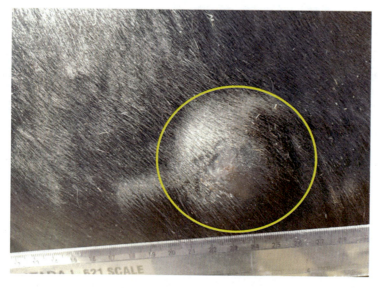

Fig. 21.10 Diagram showing tuberculin reaction in cattle due to delayed-type hypersensitivity (DTH) reaction

21.6 Delayed-Type Hypersensitivity (DTH) Reaction

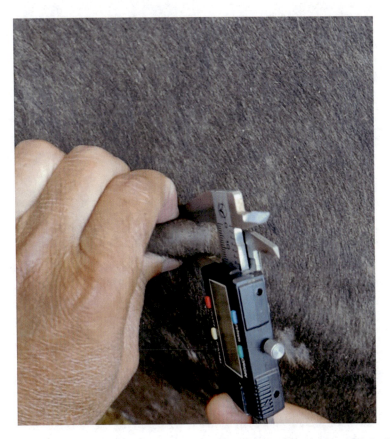

Fig. 21.11 Diagram showing Johnin reaction in cattle due to delayed-type hypersensitivity (DTH) reaction

Fig. 21.12 Photograph showing mallein reaction

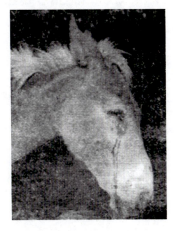

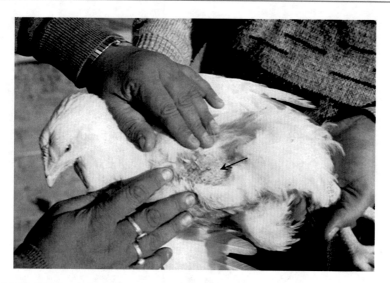

Fig. 21.13 Diagram showing separation of lymphocytes in histopaque. (**A**) Test tube, (**B**) histopaque, (**C**) blood over histopaque, and (**D**) separated lymphocytes

- The vehicle for the DNCB/DNFB is used as such on another side/part of skin to serve as control.
- After 2 weeks of sensitization, 0.25 mL of DNCB or DNFB (1 mg/mL) is again injected intradermally on the same area of skin.
- Vehicle is applied similarly on control side of skin so as to compare the results.
- Measure the thickness of skin with the help of vernier caliper at 0, 12, 24, 36, 48, and 60 h of post challenge. Examine the challenged area for erythema, induration, ulceration, and scab formation (Figs. 21.13, 21.14 and 21.15).
- Compare the skin thickness of DNCB/DNFB applied area with that of control area of skin (Tizard 1996).

21.7 Gamma Globulins in Serum

- Take 5.7 mL of ammonium sulfate-sodium chloride (19.5% and 2.03%, respectively) in a centrifuge tube, and overlay 0.3 mL of clear serum on it.
- Mix gently and keep the mixture on ice bath for 15 min and centrifuge at $1250 \times g$ for 10 min.
- Dissolve the precipitate in 0.2 mL of normal saline solution, and repeat the process of precipitation.
- Finally dissolve all precipitates in 2.0 mL of normal saline solution, and add 5.0 mL of biuret reagent. Keep the mixture for 10 min at room temperature.
- Read the optical density at 555 nm using a spectrophotometer against the controls of normal saline (Schultz and Adams 1978; Chauhan and Singh 1992a).

21.7 Gamma Globulins in Serum

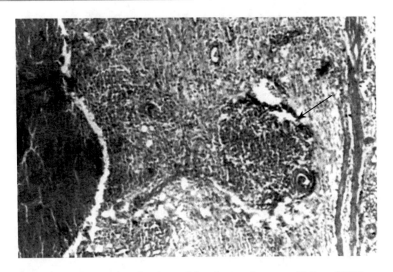

Fig. 21.14 Photomicrograph showing delayed-type hypersensitivity (DTH) reaction-lymphofollicular lesions

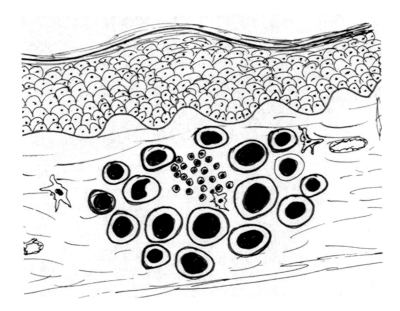

Fig. 21.15 Diagram showing microscopic picture of delayed-type hypersensitivity (DTH) reaction

21.8 Measurement of Antibody Titer

Various primary binding tests and secondary binding tests are used to measure the amount of antibody levels within a patient's blood (Table 21.1). The amount and diversity of antibodies correlate to the strength of the body's immune response. The antibody titer can be measured for a number of diseases (Worthington 1982).

21.8.1 Enzyme-Linked Immunosorbent Assay (ELISA)

- Enzyme-linked immunosorbent assay (ELISA) is a widely applicable and accepted test for determination of antibody titer in serum (Fig. 21.10).
- For detection of antibodies in serum, take a polystyrene 96 well round bottom/flat bottom microtiter plate, and coat the wells with 100 µL of antigen diluted in coating buffer. Keep the plate at 4 °C overnight after covering it with aluminum foil or in polythene (Figs. 21.16a and 21.17).
- Wash the plate three times (5 min each) with washing solution, and tap the plate after each washing against any soft paper/towel to get rid of any unadsorbed material in the well.
- To block the unsaturated sites of polystyrene wells, 5% skimmed milk or 2% BSA or 1% gelatin in washing solution is used. Add 100 µL of blocking solution in each well, and keep it for at least 1 h at 37 °C.
- Wash and tap the polystyrene plate three times (5 min each) as described earlier.
- Apply 100 µL of appropriately diluted serum in duplicate wells, and keep the plate at 37 °C for 2 h (Figs. 21.16b and 21.17).
- Wash and tap the polystyrene plate three times (5 min each) as described earlier.

Table 21.1 Minimum detectable levels of antibody protein by various immunological tests

Tests	Protein (µg/mL)
Primary binding tests	
Enzyme-linked immunosorbent assay (ELISA)	0.0005
Competitive radioimmunoassay	0.00005
Secondary binding tests	
Gel precipitation	30
Ring precipitation	18
Antitoxin neutralization	0.06
Bacterial agglutination	0.05
Complement fixation test	0.05
Passive hemagglutination	0.01
Hemagglutination inhibition	0.005
Virus neutralization	0.00005
Bactericidal activity	0.00005
In vivo test	
Passive cutaneous anaphylaxis	0.02

21.8 Measurement of Antibody Titer

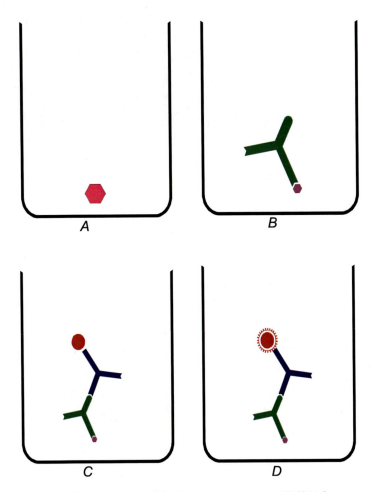

Fig. 21.16 Diagram showing enzyme-linked immunosorbent assay (ELISA) for measurement of antibody titer

- Add 100 μL of appropriately diluted antispecies IgG peroxidase conjugate in each well, and incubate the plate for 1 h at 37 °C (Figs. 21.16c, d and 21.17).

Note

1. If antibody titer is to be determined in cattle, conjugate should be antibovine IgG peroxidase conjugate.

Fig. 21.17 Diagram showing enzyme-linked immunosorbent assay (ELISA) for measurement of antibody titer against bluetongue virus

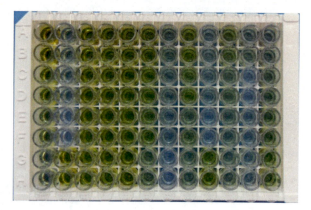

2. If antibody titer is to be determined in poultry, conjugate should be anti-chicken IgG-peroxidase conjugate.
3. If antibody titer is to be determined in mice, conjugate should be anti-mouse
- IgG-peroxidase conjugate.
  Wash and tap the plate three times (5 min each) as described earlier.
- Apply 100 µL of substrate o-phenylenediamine dihydrochloride (OPD) in each well, and note the time. Stop the reaction within 30 min by using 1 N sulfuric acid (100 µL per well) (Figs. 21.16 and 21.17).
- Read the absorbance on ELISA reader at 492 nm.
- Calculate ELISA values dividing the OD of test samples with that of negative controls.

$$\text{ELISA value} = \frac{\text{OD of test}}{\text{OD of negative control}}$$

It the ELISA value is more than 2, then it is considered significant diagnostic value.

Note:
For the measurement of various isotypes of immunoglobulins like IgA, IgM, IgG, etc., the procedure of ELISA will remain same as described above except the type of conjugate, which should be as follows:

For detection of the levels of IgA in serum, fluid, milk, or any other secretions, use anti species IgA-peroxidase conjugate. The titers of IgM are measured in serum by using anti-species IgM-peroxidase conjugate (Schultz and Adams 1978; Worthington 1982).

21.9 Dot Immunobinding Assay (DIA)

Dot immunobinding assay (DIA) is used as an alternative test for plate ELISA. The basic principle of DIA and ELISA is same. In DIA, in place of polystyrene plates, nitrocellulose strips are used. It involves the direct application of antigen on nitrocellulose bound to a plastic surface and detection of antigen-antibody complexes by development of colored dot using chromogenic substrate (Golden 1991; Chauhan and Singh 1992b; Chand and Chauhan 2001). The procedure to perform DIA for the determination of antibody titers is as follows (Fig. 21.18):

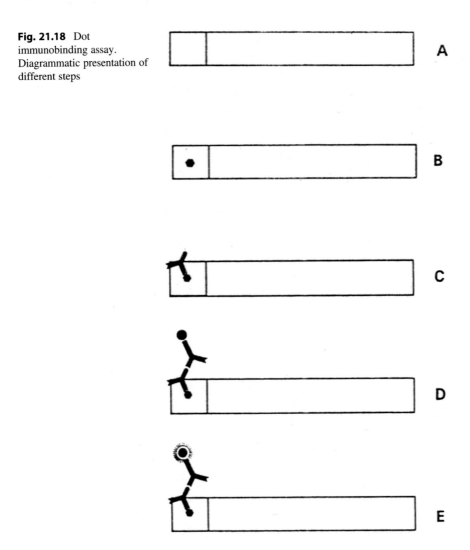

Fig. 21.18 Dot immunobinding assay. Diagrammatic presentation of different steps

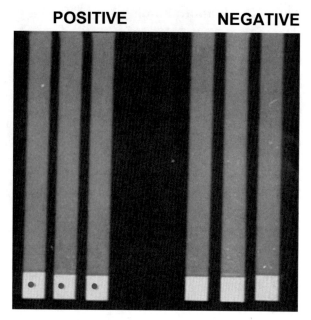

Fig. 21.19 Photograph showing dot immunobinding assay

- Take dipsticks and wash in PBS (pH 7.2) for 1–2 min and dry in air (Fig. 21.18a).
- Place a drop of antigen (1–2 µL) in the middle of the nitrocellulose bound to the plastic strips (Fig. 21.18b).
- Leave the dipsticks for few min at room temperature for drying, and then place the dipsticks in 5% skimmed milk or 2% BSA in PBS-Tween (pH 7.2) at 37 °C for 1 h for blocking unadsorbed sites.
- Wash the dipsticks in PBS-Tween, three times of 2–3 min each.
- Place the dipsticks in optimally diluted serum samples in PBS-Tween at 37 °C for 1 h (Fig. 21.18c).
- Wash the dipsticks in PBS-Tween three times of 2–3 min each.
- Place the dipsticks in optimally diluted anti-species IgG peroxidase conjugate for 30 min at 37 °C (Fig. 21.18d).
- Wash the dipsticks in PBS-Tween three times of 2–3 min each.
- Place the dipsticks in chromogenic substrate (diaminobenzidine tetra hydrochloride 0.5 mg/mL) containing 1 µL/mL of 30% H_2O_2. A positive reaction is characterized by development of a brown dot at the site of antigen deposition. Dot appears within a min, and reaction can be stopped by washing the dipsticks in running tap water (Figs. 21.18e and 21.19).
- The dipsticks are dried and can be stored in polythene bags for a longer period.

Note:
Use separate dipsticks for each dilution, if the antibody titer is measured.

Table 21.2 Role of specific immunoglobulin classes in serological assays

Property	IgG	IgM	IgA	Equine IgG3/IgG(T)
Agglutination	+	+++	+	−
Complement Activation	+	+++	−	−
Precipitation	+++	+	±	±
Neutralization	+	++	+	+
Time of appearance (days)	3–7	2–5	3–7	3–7
Time to peak titer (days)	7–21	5–14	7–21	7–21

- For measurement of isotype-specific antibody titers, use separate conjugates of separate conjugates of respective isotypes given as under:

  IgA---------- Anti-species IgA peroxidase conjugate
  IgM---------- Anti-species IgM peroxidase conjugate
  IgG---------- Anti-species IgG peroxidase conjugate

21.10 Agglutination Test

Agglutination is a simple procedure that can be done when the antigen of interest is particulate (e.g., RBCs, bacteria) or when soluble antigen is coated onto particles such as tiny latex beads. Because antibodies are bivalent, they can cross-link particulate antigens resulting in agglutination. Particulate antigen reacts with antibodies in optimum proportions, and the epitopes of antigen bind and cross-link with the antibodies to form an agglutination or clumping. The agglutination can be seen to the naked eyes or require light microscopic examination. Antibodies differ in their ability to cause agglutination. The IgM antibodies are more efficient to cause agglutination than IgG antibodies (Table 21.2). Addition of more antibodies in a suspension of antigenic particles results in inhibition of agglutination because each particle may be coated by antibodies. This inhibition of agglutination during high concentrations of antibody is called as prozone. The presence of non-agglutinating antibodies results in formation of prozone. These non-agglutinating antibodies are named as incomplete antibodies. The reason for their lack of agglutinating activity is location of epitopes deeper within the surface of the particle, and cross-linking cannot occur. Agglutination test is commonly employed in various immunodiagnostic procedures in veterinary field (Chauhan 1995; Tizard 1996; Chauhan 1998a).

21.11 Immunofluorescence Techniques

Immunofluorescence techniques (IFT) are used for the detection of antigen in cells/tissues/organs using either smears or sections. This is considered as one of the confirmatory tests in many infectious diseases of man and animals. For example,

IFT is being used as confirmatory test for diagnosis of rabies in animals and man. Using IFT, antigen can be demonstrated in tissue sections, biopsy materials, cells, exfoliated cells, impression smear, scrapped cells, etc. It is used to identify various subsets of T and B lymphocytes using monoclonal markers. Formalin-fixed tissue sections can also be used after digestion with proteolytic enzymes to get better results. This test is simple, rapid, and quite sensitive but requires a fluorescent microscope (Chauhan 1995; Tizard 1996; Chauhan 1998a). The following two procedures, direct and indirect, are routinely used in immunofluorescent tests.

21.11.1 Direct Method

- Prepare smear or tissue section or scrapped cells on a clean glass slide. Fix the smears in chilled acetone or methanol (Fig. 21.20a).
- Apply primary antibody directed against specific antigen (to be detected) and conjugated with fluorescein isothiocyanate (FITC) dye for 30 min at room temperature (Figs. 21.20b, c).
- Wash the slide in PBS (pH 7.2) for 2–3 min.
- Mount the slide in 50% buffered glycerol, and examine under fluorescent microscope (Fig. 21.20).

21.11.2 Indirect Method

- Prepare smear or tissue sections or scrapped cells on clean glass slide. Fix the smear in chilled acetone or methanol.
- Apply primary antibody on slide for 30 min at room temperature.
- Wash in PBS (pH 7.2) 3 times of 5 min each.
- Apply secondary antibody directed against species of primary antibody, e.g., if primary antibody raised in rabbit then secondary antibody should be anti-rabbit (IgG) conjugated with FITC dye for 30 min at 37 °C.
- Wash in PBS (pH 7.2) three times of 5 min each.
- Mount the slide in buffered glycerol and examine under fluorescent microscope (Figs. 21.21, 21.22, and 21.23).

21.12 Immunoperoxidase Techniques (IPT)

Immunoperoxidase techniques are used for the demonstration of antigen in tissues, type of lymphoid cells (T or B cells), and specific antibody-producing cells. The techniques are based on the principle of ELISA and IFT and require peroxidase-labeled antibody to react with antigen present in tissues, which are detected by developing a color using chromogenic substrate 3,3′-diaminobenzidine (DAB) tetrahydrochloride. The slides prepared by these techniques are permanent in nature and can be stored for years. The color developed is seen by using ordinary

21.12 Immunoperoxidase Techniques (IPT)

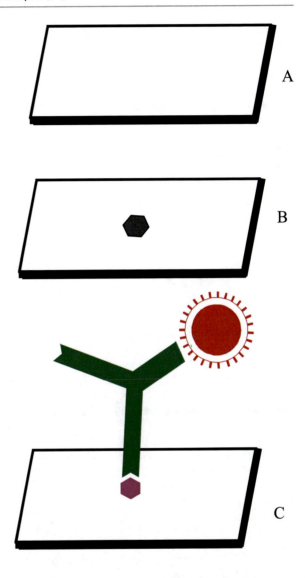

Fig. 21.20 Diagram showing direct immunofluorescence test

microscope and hence does not require any expensive equipment like fluorescent microscope. This technique is also useful in studying the role of dual infections using previous paraffin blocks (Wilchek and Bayer 1984; Chauhan et al. 1998).

The main disadvantage of immunoperoxidase technique is the presence of endogenous peroxidase in various cells like leucocytes, which may give false-positive results. To overcome this problem, before applying primary antibody, the endogenous peroxidase should be removed, and one should always keep control slides for comparative studies.

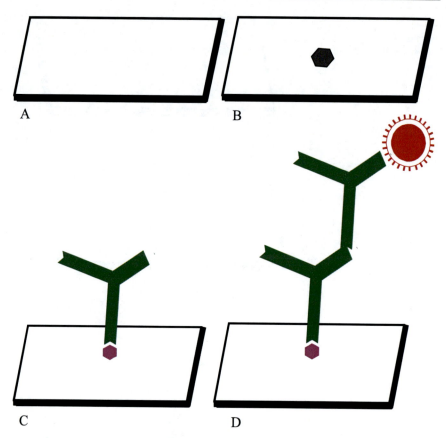

Fig. 21.21 Diagram showing indirect immunofluorescence test. (**a**) clean glass slide, (**b**) antigen on a smear or tissue section, (**c**) primary antibody binds with antigen, and (**d**) immunofluorescence

In this technique, tissues are preserved in formol saline or buffered formalin. However, to have a better contrast, formol sublimate fixative is used, which can be prepared by mixing 9 part saturated mercuric chloride and 1 part commercial formaldehyde. Tissues are fixed in formol sublimate for 24 h, and then fixative is replaced with 80% ethanol.

In addition to direct and indirect methods, several modifications of IPT have been described.

21.12.1 Antigen Detection

Paraffin-embedded tissue sections of 4–5 μ thickness are prepared from tissues as described elsewhere using standard histopathological procedures (Wilchek

21.12 Immunoperoxidase Techniques (IPT)

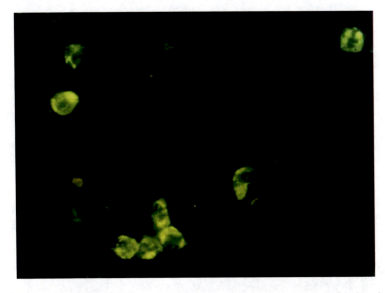

Fig. 21.22 Photomicrograph showing immunofluorescence for demonstration of antigen in cells

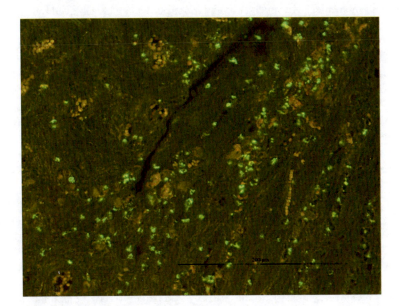

Fig. 21.23 Photomicrograph showing immunofluorescence for demonstration of bluetongue virus antigen in pregnant uterus

and Bayer 1984; Chauhan et al. 1998). The slides of tissue sections are dried in incubator or at room temperature and are processed as under:

- Slides are gently warmed on hot plate/spirit lamp and are placed in xylene-I for 10–15 min in order to remove the paraffin. Thereafter, the slides are placed in xylene-II for 10–15 min and xylene+ ethanol (1:1) for 10 min. Hydration of tissue sections is done in descending series of ethanol, viz., absolute ethanol-I, absolute ethanol-II, 95%, 90%, 80%, and 70% ethanol for 5 min in each dilution.
- Slides are finally taken in water for clearing, where extra wax and sections are removed with the help of muslin cloth and fingertip. The slides are then washed in clean tap water.
- If the tissues are fixed in formol sublimate, then remove the mercuric chloride deposits from tissues. For this purpose, the slides are kept in Gram's iodine for 5 min followed by immersion in 0.5% sodium thiosulfate solution of 5 min. The slides are washed in 0.2 M PBS (pH 7.2) for few min.
- The endogenous peroxidase is quenched by placing the slides in 0.01 M periodic acid solution for 10 min followed by in 0.003 M sodium borohydride solution for 30 min. The slides are washed in 0.2 M PBS (pH 7.2) 3 times of 5 min each.
- The major drawback of formalin fixation of tissues is the masking of tissue antigens due to formation of methylene cross-bridges between reactive sites on protein molecules. The reversal of antigen masking can be achieved by two most common procedures including enzymatic digestion (trypsin, proteinase K, pronase, ficin, and pepsin) or heat-based (0.01 M citrate buffer, pH 6.0; 1 mM EDTA, pH 8.0; and 20 mM Tris/0.65 mM EDTA/0.0005% Tween, pH 6.0 by microwave or autoclave) antigen retrieval method. The slides are washed in 0.2 M PBS (pH 7.2) three times of 5 min each.
- Cover the sections with blocking reagent (3% w/v bovine serum albumin in TBS) for 20 min to block the nonspecific binding sites. Remove excess blocking reagent, and do not wash at this stage.
- Now slides are ready for application of primary antibody directed against antigen. The primary antibody is applied in optimum dilutions for 24 h at 4 °C. The slides are then washed in 0.2 M PBS three times of 5 min each.
- The slides are now kept in optimally diluted secondary antibody conjugated with peroxidase for 2 h at room temperature. The secondary antibody should be directed against the species of primary antibody, i.e., if primary antibody is raised in rabbits, the secondary antibody should be anti-rabbit IgG-peroxidase conjugate. Thereafter, the slides are washed in 0.2 M PBS (pH 7.2) thrice for 5 min each.
- The slides are then kept in freshly prepared 0.05% diaminobenzidine tetrahydrochloride in PBS containing 0.01% hydrogen peroxide for 5 min and wash the slides in running tap water for 5 min to stop the reaction.
- Slides are dehydrated in ascending series of ethanol, i.e., 70%, 80%, 90%, 95%, and absolute ethanol for 5 min in each dilution. Thereafter, slides are kept in absolute ethanol + xylene mixture (1:1) for 5 min, xylene I and II for 10–15 min each for clearing.

21.12 Immunoperoxidase Techniques (IPT)

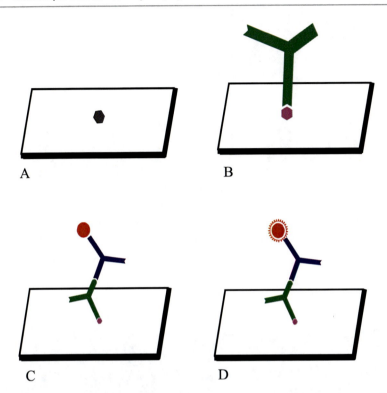

Fig. 21.24 Diagram showing indirect immunoperoxidase test. (**a**) antigen in a tissue section, (**b**) primary antibody binds with Ag, (**c**) secondary antibody binds with primary antibody and antigen complex, and (**d**) peroxidase reaction of substrate

- Finally, the slides are mounted with coverslip using DPX mountant and placed in incubator for 2–4 h for drying. The slides are examined under light microscope; the presence of antigen is characterized by brown- to red-colored cells under a light blue background. Compare the results with control slides for proper interpretation (Figs. 21.24, 21.25, and 21.26).

21.12.2 Enumeration of T and B Cells

- For enumeration of T and B cells, three sets of the slides having sections of lymphoid organs are used. In place of sections, the smears of peripheral blood lymphocytes or impression smears of lymph nodes/spleen can be used (Chauhan 1998b).
- The slides or tissue sections (4–5 μ thick) are dried in incubator or room temperature. The slides are slightly warmed at hot plate/sprit lamp and are placed in xylene I for 10–15 min. Thereafter, the slides are kept in xylene II for 10–15 min and in xylene + absolute ethanol (1:1) for 5 min.

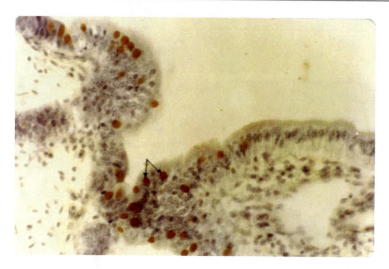

Fig. 21.25 Photomicrograph showing detection of antigen by immunoperoxidase technique

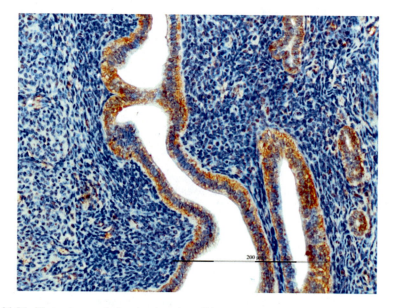

Fig. 21.26 Photomicrograph showing detection of bluetongue virus antigen in luminal epithelium, endometrial glands, and stromal cells of pregnant uterus by immunoperoxidase technique

- Hydration of tissue sections is done in descending series of ethanol, viz., absolute ethanol, 95%, 90%, 80%, and 70% ethanol. Thereafter, the slides are placed in water for cleaning of extra wax and sections. Clean the slides in running tap water.
- For removal of mercuric chloride deposits, slides are placed in Gram's iodine for 5 min followed by immersion in 0.5% sodium thiosulfate solution for 5 min; slides are washed in 0.2 M PBS (pH 7.2) 3 changes of 5 min each.
- In order to remove the endogenous peroxidase, the slides are kept in 0.01 M periodic acid solution for 10 min followed by 0.003 M sodium borohydride solution for 30 min. Finally, the slides are washed in 0.2 M PBS (pH 7.2) thrice for 5 min each.
- Now the monoclonal antibody derived against the T- and B-lymphocyte subsets is to be applied on each slide. For this, separate section/slide is to be used for each T- and B-lymphocyte subset and keep the slides at 4 °C for 24 h. Thereafter, wash the slides in 0.2 M PBS (pH 7.2) thrice for 5 min each.
- Apply secondary antibody, i.e., anti-mouse IgG peroxidase conjugate in appropriate dilution for 2 h at room temperature. Wash the slides with 0.2 M PBS (pH 7.2) thrice for 5 min each.
- The slides are now placed in substrate solution containing 0.05% DAB in PBS along with 0.01% hydrogen peroxide for 5 min and wash the slides in running tap water for 5 min to stop the reaction.
- Counterstain the slides in Harris hematoxylin for 5 min, differentiate in acid alcohol by just 1 dip, and bleach in ammonia water by dipping for 1–2 s. Wash the slides in running tap water.
- Dehydration is done in ascending series of ethanol, viz., 70%, 80%, 90%, 95%, and absolute ethanol for 5 min in each dilution, and then the slides are kept in absolute ethanol + xylene (1:1) solution for 5 min. Clearing is done in xylene I and II by placing the slides for 10–15 min.
- Slides are mounted in DPX using coverslips. Examine the slides for the presence of T- and B-lymphocyte subsets, and count the cell number in percent. Positive cells are characterized by their golden brown to red color, while others will take bluish color (Fig. 21.27).

21.13 Peroxidase Antiperoxidase (PAP) Techniques

The peroxidase antiperoxidase (PAP) technique has the same principle like indirect peroxidase method. However, it involves three reagents, i.e., primary antibody, secondary antibody, and peroxidase antiperoxidase complex. The PAP complex includes an enzyme known as horseradish peroxidase and its antibody. The primary antibody is specific to antigen, and secondary antibody is capable of binding with both primary antibody and PAP complex, because both are produced in same animal species. It is considered that PAP techniques are comparatively more sensitive than the direct and indirect immunoperoxidase techniques (Wilchek and Bayer

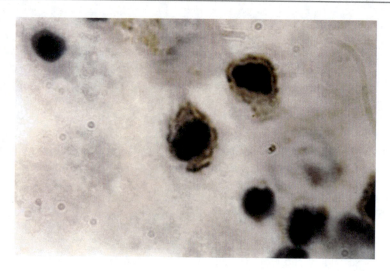

Fig. 21.27 Photomicrograph showing demonstration of T and B-cell subsets by immunoperoxidase technique

1984; Chauhan et al. 1998). However, it takes more time to complete. It has following steps:

- Tissue sections are cleaned in water after rehydration, and the slides are placed in Gram's iodine for 5 min followed by 5 min in sodium thiosulfate.
- Wash the slides in PBS at least for three times of 5 min each. In order to remove the endogenous peroxidase, place the slides in periodic acid for 10 min followed by in sodium borohydride for 30 min. Wash the slides in PBS three times for 5 min each.
- Apply primary antibody on tissue sections, and place them in a moist chamber at 4 °C in refrigerator overnight. Wash the slides in PBS three times for 5 min.
- Apply secondary antibody (antispecies of primary antibody) on tissue sections for 1 h at 37 °C. Wash the slides in PBS three times for 5 min each.
- Apply PAP complex for 30 min at 37 °C, and wash the slides in PBS 3 changes for 5 min each.
- Apply substrate DAB for 5 min, and wash the slides in running tap water.
- Stain with hematoxylin for 5 min, dip in acid alcohol, dip in ammonia water, and dehydrate in ascending series of ethanol, i.e., 70%, 80%, 90%, and absolute ethanol for 5 min in each.
- Clear in absolute ethanol + xylene for 5 min, xylene I and xylene II for 15 min each.
- Mount in DPX and examine under microscope.
- The presence of antigen is determined by golden brown red color against light blue background (Fig. 21.28).

21.14 Avidin-Biotin Complex Techniques

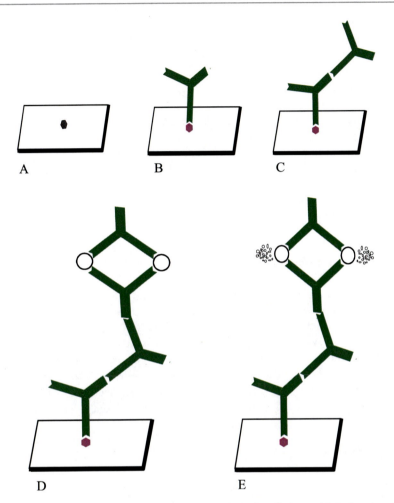

Fig. 21.28 Diagram showing peroxidase antiperoxidase (PAP) techniques. (**a**) Antigen in a tissue section or smear, (**b**) antibody binds with primary antibody + antigen. (**d**) PAP complex binds with (**c**) and (**e**). Peroxidase reaction of substrate on (**d**)

21.14 Avidin-Biotin Complex Techniques

The avidin-biotin techniques are considered one of the most sensitive techniques than any other immunoperoxidase method. The main basis of this technique lies on the ability of egg white glycoprotein "avidin" to bind with four molecules of vitamin "biotin." In avidin-biotin methods, the secondary antibody is labeled with biotin, which is detected by either avidin labeled with peroxidase or bridged avidin-biotin method or using an avidin-biotin complex. Because of high sensitivity, avidin-biotin techniques are useful, where the antigens are present in very meager amounts (Wilchek and Bayer 1984). Three methods of these techniques are described as under.

21.14.1 Enzyme-Labeled Avidin-Biotin Method

In this method, the secondary antibody is conjugated with biotin, and peroxidase is conjugated with avidin. After application of primary antibody, biotinylated antibody is applied for 1 h at 37 °C, and then slides are washed three times for 5 min each. Avidin conjugated with peroxidase is then applied for 1 h at 37 °C. After washing, substrate like DAB is applied for development of color, counterstain the slides with hematoxylin, dehydrate in ascending series of ethanol, clear in xylene, and mount in DPX (Fig. 21.29).

21.14.2 Bridged Avidin-Biotin Method

In this method, biotin is labeled with secondary antibody. The avidin is used as such, while biotin conjugated with peroxidase is used as detector. After application of primary antibody and washing, the secondary antibody labeled with biotin is applied for 1 h at 37 °C. Wash the slides three times in PBS for 5 min each. Then apply avidin 10 mg/mL in PBS for 5 min each. The biotin conjugated with peroxidase is applied for 1 h at 37 °C. Wash the slides in PBS three times for 5 min each. Apply substrate like DAB for 5 min, and then counterstain in hematoxylin. Dehydrate the slides in ascending series of ethanol, clear in xylene, and mount in DPX (Fig. 21.30).

21.14.3 Avidin-Biotin Complex Method

In this method, biotinylated secondary antibody is used with avidin-biotin complex conjugated with peroxidase. After application of primary antibody and secondary biotinylated antibody on section, the slides are washed in PBS three times for 5 min each. Apply avidin-biotin complex conjugated with peroxidase for 1 h at 37 °C. The avidin-biotin mixture contains 5 µg avidin and 2 µg biotin conjugated with peroxidase in 1 mL PBS. Slides are washed in PBS, and then substrate (chromogen DAB and H_2O_2) is applied on sections for 5 min. Slides are washed in running tap water to stop the reaction. The sections are counterstained in hematoxylin, dehydrate in ethanol, clear in xylene, and mount in DPX (Fig. 21.31).

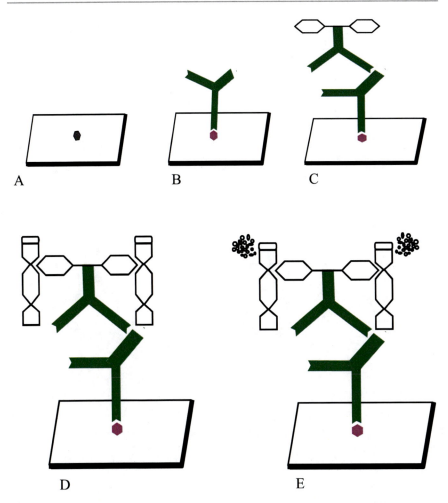

Fig. 21.29 Diagram showing enzyme labeled avidin-biotin techniques. (**a**) antigen in a smear or tissue section, (**b**) primary antibody binds with antigen, (**c**) secondary antibody labeled with biotin binds with (**b**), (**d**) avidin conjugated with peroxidase binds with (**c**), and (**e**) peroxidase reaction with substrate

21.15 Detection of Immune Complex

21.15.1 Kidneys

Immune complexes are formed as a result of antigen-antibody reaction in the body; normally, they are phagocytosed by macrophages and removed from the system. However, when immune complex formations accelerated, these complexes get deposited in the glomerulus and cause inflammation of kidneys leading to

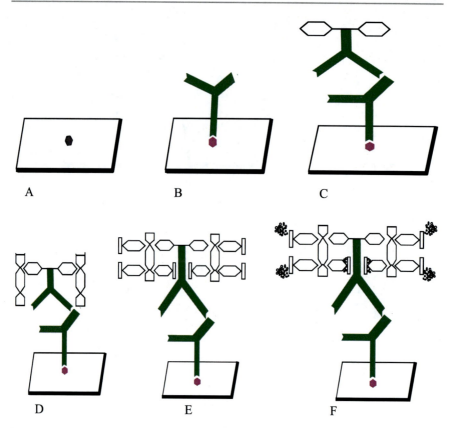

Fig. 21.30 Diagram showing bridged avidin-biotin techniques. (**a**) antigen in a smear or tissue section, (**b**) primary antibody binds with antigen, (**c**) secondary antibody conjugated with biotin binds with (**b**), (**d**) avidin binds with (**c**), (**e**) biotin conjugated with peroxidase binds with Avidin at (**d**) and (**f**) peroxidase reaction of substrate

glomerulonephritis. Thus, the demonstration of immune complexes in glomerulus is considered diagnostic for glomerulonephritis and type III hypersensitivity reaction, even if the exact cause remains unidentified. For the detection of immune complexes, IgM, IgG, IgA, or C3 are localized in glomeruli of formalin-fixed and paraffin-embedded kidney sections (Schultz and Adams 1978; Chauhan 1998a, 1998b).

The tissues from kidneys are collected in formol sublimate and, after 24 h of fixation, replaced with 80% ethanol. Sections of 4–5 μ are cut using routine histological procedures. For staining of immune complexes, the following procedure is followed:

- Take four sets of sections of kidney, slightly warm them on flame of spirit lamp or hot plate, and place in xylene I for 15 min. Slides are then transferred in xylene II for 10–15 min and finally in xylene + ethanol (1:1) mixture for 5 min. The slides

21.15 Detection of Immune Complex

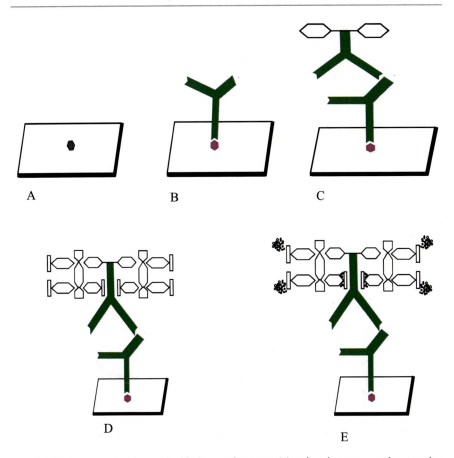

Fig. 21.31 Diagram showing avidin-biotin complex assay. (**a**) antigen in a smear or tissue section, (**b**) primary antibody binds with antigen, (**c**) secondary antibody labeled with biotin binds with (**b**), (**d**) avidin-biotin–peroxidase conjugate binds with (**c**), and (**e**) peroxidase reaction of substrate

are hydrated in ascending series of ethanol, 95%, 90%, 80%, and 70% ethanol, 5 min in each dilution.
- Slides are taken in running tap water and cleared in order to remove the extra wax and sections. Clean in fresh water.
- Place the slides in Gram's iodine for 5 min and then in sodium thiosulfate for 5 min. Thereafter, wash the slides in 0.2 M PBS (pH 7.2) thrice for 5 min each.
- Place the slides in periodic acid for 10 min and then in sodium thiosulfate for 5 min. Thereafter wash the slides in 0.2 M PBS (pH 7.2) thrice for 5 min each.
- Treat the slides with trypsin and calcium chloride solution for 1 h at 37 °C. Wash the slides in 0.2 M PBS (pH 7.2) thrice for 5 min each.
- Place anti-IgA peroxidase conjugate on slide I, anti IgG peroxidase conjugate on slide II, anti-IgM peroxidase conjugate on slide III, and anti-C3 peroxidase conjugate on slide IV for 2 h at room temp. Wash the slides in 0.2 M PBS thrice for 5 min each.

- Apply substrate 0.05% DAB and 0.01% hydrogen peroxide in PBS for 5 min, and thereafter wash the slides in running tap water to stop the reaction.
- Counterstain the slides in hematoxylin for 5 min and then given just one dip in acid alcohol for differentiation and one dip in ammonia water for bleaching. Thereafter, wash the slides in running tap water to stop the reaction.
- Dehydrate the slides in ascending series of ethanol, i.e., 70%, 80% 90%, 95%, and absolute ethanol for 5 min in each dilution. Slides are then placed in xylene + absolute ethanol (1:1) for 5 min. Clear the slides in xylene I for 15 min and then in xylene II for 15 min.
- Mount the slides with coverslip using DPX mountant. Examine the sections, and localize the immune complexes in the glomerulus, as it gives golden brown/red color (Figs. 21.32 and 21.33).

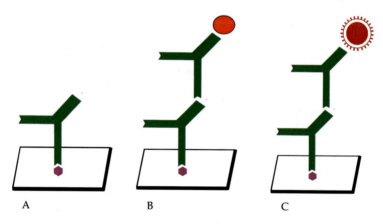

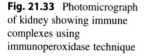

Fig. 21.32 Diagram showing immune complexes in kidneys. (**a**) antigen-antibody complex in a smear or tissue section, (**b**) secondary antibody peroxidase conjugated binds with Ag-Ab complex, and (**c**) peroxidase reaction with substrate

Fig. 21.33 Photomicrograph of kidney showing immune complexes using immunoperoxidase technique

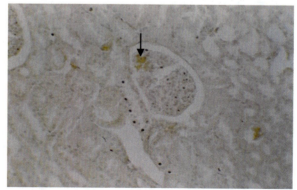

21.15.2 Serum

In serum, the immune complexes are detected by using ELISA, and the antigen-antibody complexes are first separated from the serum by using poly ethylene glycol-6000 (PEG-6000) using following procedure:

- Take 1 mL of serum, mix drop by drop 1 mL of 8% PEG-6000, and constantly stir the mixture. Leave it for 1 h at room temperature, and then centrifuge it at 1500 × g for 1 h at 4 °C. Discard the supernatant and suspend the pellet in 2 mL of 4% PEG-6000 and centrifuge again. Discard the supernatant, and finally dissolve the pellet in 0.5 mL of PBS (pH 7.2).
- Coat the polystyrene ELISA plates with antibodies against the agent for which immune complexes are detected. But these antibodies should be raised in any animal species other than that in which the immune complexes are detected. Keep the plate at 4 °C for overnight for coating. Thereafter, wash and tap the plate, with PBS-Tween three times of 5 min each.
- Apply the diluted precipitate of serum in PBS as prepared above. Dilutions can be made two-fold like 1:2, 1:4, 1:8, 1:16, 1:32, and so on. Keep the plate in incubator at 37 °C for 1 h. Thereafter, wash and tap plate with PBS-Tween for three times of 5 min each.
- Apply anti-species IgG peroxidase conjugate in proper dilution (anti-species in which immune complexes are detected). Place the plate in incubator at 37 °C for 1 h; thereafter, wash and tap the plate with PBS–Tween for three times of 5 min each.
- Apply substrate OPD for at least 30 min, and stop the reaction using 1 N H_2SO_4.
- Read the OD in spectrophotometer, and calculate the ELISA value. The ELISA value more than 2 is positive for the presence of immune complexes in serum (Fig. 21.34).

21.16 Microscopic Evaluation of Lymphoid Organs

21.16.1 Processing of Tissues

- The tissues from lymphoid organs, viz., lymph nodes (Fig. 21.35), spleen (Fig. 21.36), Peyer's patches, bursa, thymus, etc. are collected in 10% formol saline or 10% buffered formalin.
- Size of the tissue should not be more than 5 mm in length and/or width.
- Tissues should be cut with sharp object and should be directly collected in fixative.
- After 12–24 h of fixation, the tissue pieces are kept in capsules and are washed in running tap water at least for 12 h.
- The tissue blocks are dehydrated in ascending series of ethanol starting from 50% and then in 70%, 80%, 90%, 95%, absolute ethanol I, and absolute ethanol II for

Fig. 21.34 Diagram showing immune complexes in serum. (**a**) coating of capture antibody, (**b**) immune complexes in serum, (**c**) secondary antibody peroxidase conjugate binds with (**b**), and (**d**) peroxidase reaction with substrate

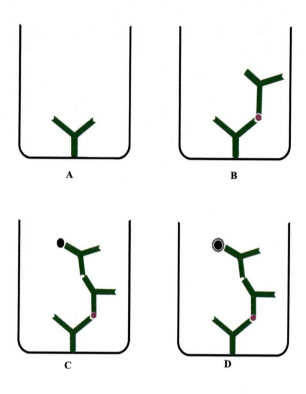

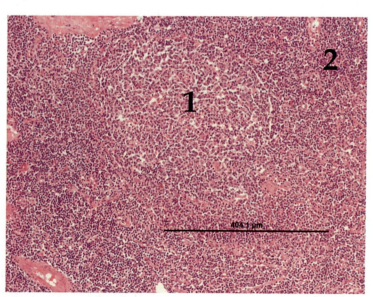

Fig. 21.35 Microscopic evaluation of lymph node in sheep. Histology of lymph node showed lymphoid follicle (1) in cortex (2). H&E ×100

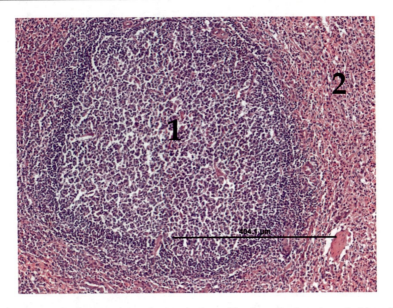

Fig. 21.36 Microscopic evaluation of spleen in sheep. Histology of spleen showed white pulp (1) in red pulp (2). H&E ×100

1 h in each. The tissues should be agitated either mechanically or in automatic tissue processor.
- The volume of ethanol should be at least 50 times more than the tissue placed for dehydration.
- After dehydration, clearing of tissues is done in xylene I and xylene II for 1 h each but before that tissues are placed in mixture of absolute ethanol + xylene (1:1) for 1 h.
- In place of xylene, benzene or toluene can also be used at least for 3 h as their action of clearing is slow.
- After clearing, the tissues are placed in paraffin wax at 60–62 °C. Here, tissues are required three changes in paraffin I, paraffin II, and paraffin III, 1 h in each. Paraffin wax should be melted, free from dust, or any other coarse particles.
- After 3 h impregnation of tissue blocks in paraffin wax, the blocks are formed in molds using molten wax. The tissues are placed in molds in such a way that desired surface should be downward on the base of mold. The mold is then filled with molten paraffin wax, and then the blocks are cooled at room temperature or in cold water.
- The blocks are removed from the molds and are trimmed in order to reduce the wax around the tissues by rubbing on hot plate or by using knife. Identification number is fixed on one side of the block by touching the block with the small paper kept on it, which bears the number, with hot forceps or knife.

- The blocks are fixed on block holders. This is done by touching the block with warm block holder and kept it in cold water.
- Trimming of the blocks is done on microtome at 10–15 µm in order to fully expose the tissue.
- The blocks are kept on ice before section cutting for at least 1–2 h. Sections of 4–5 µm are cut on microtome using sharp knife having no nicks.
- The ribbon of sections is placed in tissue floatation bath filled with water at about 60–65 °C temperature. After proper spread, the sections are taken on glass slide. The glass slides are coated with sticky material, which consists of egg white and glycerine in 1:1 (v/v) ratio.
- Generally, 4–5 slides are prepared from each block and kept in incubator for drying.

21.16.2 Staining

- For routine staining, hematoxylin and eosin stains are used in histopathological evaluation of any tissue.
- The slides are slightly warmed either on flame of spirit lamp or in incubator and place them in xylene for 10–15 min in order to remove the paraffin from the tissue sections and slide.
- The slides are then placed in another set of xylene for 10–15 min and in xylene + alcohol (50:50) mixture for 10 min.
- The slides are then placed in descending series of absolute ethanol, 95%, 90%, 80%, 70%, and 50% ethanol for 5 min in each dilution and finally into water.
- Clean the slides with fingertip by using muslin cloth, and leave only 1–2 good quality sections on each slide. Extra paraffin on slides should be removed and wash the slides in running tap water.
- Dip the slides in acid alcohol for few seconds for differentiation. Wash the slides in running tap water, and then dip in ammonia water for few seconds for bluing, and place in running tap water to remove ammonia.
- Place the slides in eosin stain for 2–5 min, and quickly proceed for dehydration in ascending series of ethanol, i.e., 70%, 80%, 90%, 95%, absolute ethanol I, and absolute ethanol II for 5 min in each dilution.
- Place the slides in absolute ethanol + xylene (50:50) for 5 min, and then clearing of the sections is done in xylene by placing the slides in xylene I and xylene II for at least 10–15 min in each. Clearing in xylene II can be extended for 1–2 h.
- The slides are mounted with coverslip using DPX mountant. For this, the coverslip of desired size and shape is kept on filter paper, and one to two drops of mountant is placed on coverslip. Take out the slides from xylene, and place on coverslip in such a way that the sections are touched with mountant, press gently, and lift the slide. Remove air bubble, if any, by pressing the coverslip with the forceps, and keep the slides in horizontal position in a tray for drying.
- After drying for 1–2 days at room temperature, clean the slides with muslin cloth and xylene to remove the spots of stain, paraffin, or mountant. Label the slides

with a piece of paper, and stick it on one corner of the slide using appropriate adhesive.
- Slides are examined under microscope for histopathological alterations on hematoxylin and eosin staining; nuclei of the cells take blue stain, while cytoplasm takes pink or red color.

21.17 Evaluation of Xenobiotics

Rapid advancement in human civilization has brought a large number of synthetic chemicals in our environment. These include pesticides, heavy metals, gases, etc. which are widely used in agriculture and animal husbandry and are distributed throughout the world as environmental pollutants. Majority of these compounds are beneficial when used for specific purpose, handled properly, and applied judiciously. However, many of them become contaminated of the environment either by improper application or due to their persistence in the ecosystem in soil, water, plant, and animal tissue (Chauhan 1998b).

Immune system is considered to be a more sensitive indicator of toxicity assays especially for environmental contaminants and pollutants, which may have residual effect in the ecosystem. Thus, immunotoxicology has become one of the widely accepted and well-recognized research areas of public health concern, which deals with undesirable effects produced by the compound/xenobiotics as a result of interaction of immune system. These harmful effects are required to be studied in every biological and chemical endeavor especially in domestic animals, birds, and man.

This dose of a particular chemical, i.e., insecticide, weedicide, herbicide, rodenticide, fungicide, and heavy metals like lead, mercury, cadmium, nickel, copper, etc., is given to experimental animals, and the immune status of the animals is assessed in comparison to untreated controls at least for 2–3 months at an interval of weekly or 10 days using the following parameters:

21.17.1 Humoral Immune Response

Humoral immune response is measured by using the following parameters:

21.17.1.1 Estimation of Serum Globulins
For estimation of serum globulins, one has to estimate the total protein content and serum albumin and calculate the serum globulins quantity by subtracting the serum albumin values from total protein values. The clinical chemistry reagent kits are available for the estimation of serum proteins and for serum albumin.

21.17.1.2 Serum Gamma Globulins
For the estimation of gamma globulins in serum, take 5.7 mL of ammonium sulfate-sodium chloride solution (19.5% ammonium sulfate, 2.03% sodium chloride;

pH 6.4) in a test tube, and overlay 0.3 mL of clear serum on it. Mix the contents by gently inverting the tube at least 6 times, and place it on ice bath for 15 min. Centrifuge the contents at 3000 rpm for 10–15 min, and discard the supernatant. Repeat the process twice, and finally dissolve the contents in 2.0 mL of normal saline solution (NSS). Add 5.0 mL of biuret reagent, and keep it for 10 min at room temp. Make a blank with 2.0 mL of NSS and 5 mL of biuret reagent in test tube and mark as "B." Make a standard by placing 2.0 mL of 0.15% BSA, and add 5.0 mL of biuret reagent in the tube and mark as "S." Read the absorbance against blank at 555 nm, and calculate serum gamma globulin by using the following equation:

$$\text{Serum gamma globulin (Gram/100 mL)} = \frac{\text{OD of test}}{\text{OD of standard}}$$

21.17.1.3 Estimation of Specific Antibody Titer

The specific antibody titer is measured by using ELISA or dot immunobinding assay (DIA) as described earlier.

21.17.1.4 Enumeration of B Lymphocytes

B-Lymphocyte Blastogenesis Assay

This is carried out in sterilized culture plates using peripheral blood lymphocytes (PBLs) or splenic lymphocytes and mitogen lipopolysaccharide. The test procedure is similar to that of LBA described earlier utilizing MTT dye.

Immunoperoxidase Method

This technique has also been described earlier. The cells-producing antibodies are specific for antigen and are counted in tissue sections of lymph nodes, spleen, intestine, etc. using immunoperoxidase techniques. In this various isotypes (IgG, IgA, and IgM), producing cells could also be enumerated.

21.17.2 Cell-Mediated Immune Response

In order to assess the effect of xenobiotics on cell-mediated immune response, the following procedures are used:

21.17.2.1 Lymphocyte Blastogenesis Assay (LBA)

Using peripheral blood lymphocytes or from splenic lymphocytes, this test is performed in 96 well culture plate using the mitogens Con-A or PHA as described earlier.

21.17.2.2 Macrophage Function Test

This has also been described earlier in detail and can be carried out on peripheral blood leucocytes or peritoneal macrophages.

21.17.2.3 DTH Reaction

This has also been described earlier in detail and can be carried out using tuberculin or chemical allergen.

The evaluation of any xenobiotics can be made by utilizing the data from the abovementioned assays. However, the results so obtained are compared with that of the parallel untreated control. Any significant effect on immune system based on the above parameters is highlighted, and the xenobiotics on such instances are evaluated as immunosuppressive, immunostimulant, or immunounresponsive.

References

Chand P, Chauhan RS (2001) Dot Immunobinding assay (theory & practice). SIIP, Pantnagar
Chauhan RS (1995) Textbook of veterinary clinical and laboratory diagnosis. Jay Pee Brothers Medical Publishers, New Delhi
Chauhan RS (1998a) Laboratory manual of immunopathology. G.B. Pant University, Pantnagar
Chauhan RS (1998b) Diagnostic techniques in immunotoxicity. In: Advances in veterinary toxicology, pp 41–48
Chauhan RS, Singh NP (1992a) Cell mediated immune response in rotavirus infected calves. Leucocytes migration inhibition assay. J Comp Pathol 107:115–118
Chauhan RS, Singh NP (1992b) Rapid diagnosis of rotavirus infection in calves by dot immunobinding assay. Vet Rec 130:381
Chauhan RS, Singh GK, Seema G (1998) Immunohistochemistry: principle and applications. Introduction SIIP, pp 11–27
Golden CA (1991) Overview of the state of the art of immunoassay screening tests. J Am Vet Med Assoc 198:827–830
Schultz RD, Adams LS (1978) Immunologic methods for detection of humoral and cellular immunity. Vet Clin North Am 8:721–753
Tizard IR (1996) Veterinary immunology- an introduction, 5th edn. W.B. Sanders, Singapore
Wilchek M, Bayer EA (1984) The avidin-biotin complex in immunology. Immunol Today 5:39–43
Worthington RW (1982) Serology as an aid to diagnosis: uses abuses. N Z Vet J 30:93–97

Molecular Biology Techniques of Pivotal Importance in Veterinary Diagnostics

22

Key Points

1. Polymerase chain reaction (PCR) is a molecular biology technique used to produce hundreds to millions of copies of a specific DNA segment by amplifying the extremely small number of DNA segments.
2. PCR is carried out in a machine known as thermal cycler, which performs the process of repetitive heating and cooling.
3. Primers are single-stranded RNA or DNA sequences that range in length from 20 to 30 nucleotides.
4. Bacteria *Thermus aquaticus* can tolerate temperatures as high as 80 °C, which is the source of the enzyme Taq DNA polymerase.
5. Taq DNA polymerase is used to create a new strand of DNA during PCR.
6. Denaturation is the process of separation of hydrogen bonds between the bases in the two strands of template DNA using high temperature.
7. Annealing allows the primers to hydrogen link to a specific place on the single-stranded template DNA.
8. Microarray is a multiplex chip with 2D array and matching of DNA samples with known identity and unknown DNA samples or probes is done based on base pairing rules.
9. The purpose of lateral flow assay is to determine if a target analyte is present or absent in a sample (matrix) without the need of complex or expensive equipment.
10. Lateral flow assay works by chromatographic principle and immunological recognition system.
11. Complement fixation test (CFT) is a widely used immunological test for the diagnosis of microbial infections and rheumatic diseases by detecting the serum antibodies that are unique to a certain disease.
12. High-performance liquid chromatography (HPLC) is a greatly enhanced version of column chromatography and analytical chemistry method for separating, identifying, and quantifying the individual components in a mixture.

© The Author(s), under exclusive license to Springer Nature Singapore Pte Ltd. 2024
R. S. Chauhan et al., *Essentials of Veterinary Immunology and Immunopathology*,
https://doi.org/10.1007/978-981-99-2718-0_22

13. Confocal microscopy is an optical imaging technique that uses point lighting and a spatial pinhole to eliminate out-of-focus light in specimens that are thicker than the focal plane.
14. Confocal microscopy improves the optical resolution, contrast of a micrograph, and most specialized fluorescence imaging technique.
15. Confocal microscopy makes it possible to create three-dimensional structures from the photos that are collected.
16. A specialized form of flow cytometry is called as fluorescence-activated cell sorting (FACS), and fluorescent dyes are used to mark live or dead cells and sort the cells into different groups.

22.1 Polymerase Chain Reaction (PCR)

The polymerase chain reaction (PCR) is a molecular biology technique used in the laboratory to produce hundreds to millions of copies of a specific DNA segment by amplifying the extremely small number of tiny genes or DNA segments. The PCR was invented in 1983 by Kary Mullis, an American scientist. The PCR is most commonly used instrument in biological and medical research facilities.

22.1.1 Principle

The PCR uses the same principle as DNA polymerase, which starts from a double-stranded region and synthesizes a complementary strand of DNA in the 5′ to 3′ direction using a single-stranded template. In PCR, two primers are used, each complementary to an opposing strand of the DNA that has been denatured. The primers are organised in such a way that each primer extension reaction guides DNA synthesis toward the other. Forward and reverse primers control the synthesis of a DNA strand, which can then be primed by a forward primer. This results in the synthesis of the area of DNA bordered by the two primers from scratch. Because the deoxynucleotides and primers are abundant, the synthesis procedure is repeated by heating the freshly synthesized DNA to split the strands and cooling to allow the primers to anneal to their complementary sequences. The PCR is carried out in a machine known as thermal cycler, which performs the process of repetitive heating and cooling.

22.1.2 Ingredients

The PCR requires five main ingredients:

1. Deoxynucleotides to provide nucleosides and energy for DNA synthesis
2. DNA polymerase II

3. Forward and reverse primers (short stretches of DNA that initiate the PCR reaction)
4. DNA template to be duplicated
5. Magnesium-containing buffer to achieve proper reaction conditions

22.1.3 Primers

Primers are single-stranded RNA or DNA sequences that range in length from 20 to 30 nucleotides. The primers are intended to be complementary in a sequence to small regions of DNA on each end of the sequence to be replicated. The primers are the starting site for DNA synthesis. Only once the primer has bound can the polymerase enzyme bind and begin to form the new complementary strand of DNA from the loose DNA bases. Normally, this stage takes between 10 and 30 s.

22.2 Taq DNA Polymerase

The Taq DNA polymerase is an enzyme derived from the bacteria *Thermus aquaticus*, which lives in hot springs and can survive temperatures exceeding 80 °C. This bacterial DNA polymerase is particularly stable at high temperatures, which means it can survive the heat required to break the DNA strands apart during the denaturing stage of PCR. The ideal temperature for the enzyme Taq polymerase to form the complementary strand is 72 °C. DNA polymerase initially binds to the primer before adding the DNA bases one by one to the single strand in the 5' to 3' direction.

22.2.1 Three Stages in PCR

There are three major steps or stages in PCR: denaturation, annealing, and extension stages.

22.2.1.1 Denaturation Stage
During denaturation, a heat-induced separation of a double-stranded DNA template into two single stranded template occurs. During this stage, the mixture containing template DNA and other components were heated to 94-98 °C. The hydrogen bonds between the bases in the two strands of template DNA are destroyed by the high temperature, causing the two strands to separate. Two single DNA strands are formed as a result, and these will act as template for the formation of more new DNA strands. To ensure that all the DNA strands have completely split, it is critical that the temperature remains at this level for an extended length of time. This process normally takes between 30 s to 1 min.

22.2.1.2 Annealing Stage

The DNA primers can bind to the template DNA during annealing when the temperature is lowered. The reaction condition is cooled to 48–65 °C during the annealing step. This allows the primers to hydrogen link to a specific location on the single-stranded template DNA (the temperature varies depending on the melting temperature of the primers). This process normally takes between 30 s to 1 min.

22.2.1.3 Extension Stage

During extension, the temperature is raised, and the Taq polymerase enzyme is used to create a new strand of DNA. This is the final stage, and the temperature is raised to 72 °C to allow a unique Taq DNA polymerase enzyme that adds DNA bases to create new DNA. A new DNA strand and a double-stranded DNA molecule formation are the end results. The length of the DNA sequence being amplified determines how long this step takes, although it usually takes around 1 min to copy 1000 DNA bases.

All three stages of PCR are repeated around 20–40 times to make more number of copies of the DNA sequences. The new DNA fragments are synthesized during PCR also serve as a template to which the DNA polymerase enzyme can bind and begin DNA copies formation. As a result, in a very short duration of time, an enormous numbers of copies of the given DNA segment are created. With certain high-speed machines, a whole PCR reaction can be completed in a few hours, if not less than an hour. After PCR, the amount and size of the DNA fragments generated may be determined using an electrophoresis technique (Fig. 22.1).

22.2.2 Applications of PCR

The PCR tests are quick, sensitive, and precise. PCR is a valuable technique in many fields of biotechnology, molecular biology, and medicine. Because PCR primers target specific DNA, it may create specific DNA fragments or genes from materials

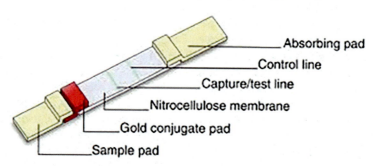

Fig. 22.1 PCR detection of amplified product (257 bp) of p72 or B646L gene of African swine fever virus (ASFV) using the OIE recommended primer sets PPA-1(F) and PPA-2(R). Lane M: 100 bp DNA ladder; L1—Positive control; L2 to L10—ASFV suspected samples; L11—Negative sample; L12—Negative control

containing many distinct genomes, such as soil, water, and blood. The PCR has become a key component of various infectious agents and disease diagnostic procedures. PCR is also utilized in forensic sciences, where it is used as part of DNA fingerprinting technique in criminal cases.

22.3 Microarray

Microarray is used to analyze the expression of several genes in a single reaction rapidly and efficiently. In the microarray, the mRNA molecule is hybridized to the DNA template from which it is originated. An array is an orderly arrangement of tens of thousands of either probes, reporters, DNA, cDNA, oligonucleotides, and spotted samples are immobilized on a solid support or surface such as microscope glass slides or silicon chips or nylon membrane or Illumina. The quantity of mRNA bound to each site on the microarray provides the information on the level of expression of the different genes in the cell. The concept of microarray was first introduced by Tse Wen Chang in 1983.

22.3.1 Principle

The microarray is a multiplex chip with 2D array and matching of DNA samples with known identity and unknown DNA samples or probes that are done based on base pairing rules. Microarray technique is originated from Southern blotting technology, in which DNA fragments are attached to a substrate and then probed with a known DNA sequences. The principle of microarray technique is the hybridization between two DNA strands by formation of hydrogen bonds between complementary nucleotide base pairs, which occurs when complementary nucleic acid sequences bind with each other to produce hybridization between two DNA strands. A nucleotide sequence with more numbers of complementary base pairs has tighter non-covalent bonds between the two strands. After washing off non-specific binding sequences, only strongly paired strands will remain hybridized. Target sequences that are labeled with fluorescent, silver, or chemiluminescence bind to a probe sequences to produce a signal that is influenced by the hybridization conditions such as temperature and washing after hybridization.

22.3.2 Types of Microarrays

The DNA microarray or DNA chip such as complementary DNA (cDNA), oligonucleotide, bacterial artificial chromosome (BAC), and single nucleotide polymorphism (SNP) microarrays have become the most sophisticated and widely used technique. The MMChips are used to monitor the microRNA populations. Protein-protein interactions are studied or optimized using protein and peptide microarrays. Other microarrays are tissue microarray, cellular or transfection microarray, chemical compound microarray, antibody microarray, carbohydrate or glycoarray, phenotype microarray, and reverse phase protein microarray.

22.3.3 DNA Microarray

The DNA microarray is a collection of microscopic DNA spots attached to a solid surface. DNA microarray is used to genotype a multiple regions of a genome and to quantify the expression levels of large numbers of genes simultaneously. Each DNA spot contains picomoles (10−12) of a specific DNA sequences. These spots contain short sequences of a gene or other DNA elements that are used to hybridize a cRNA (also called anti-sense RNA) or cDNA sample. Probe-sample hybridization is usually quantified by detection of fluorophore-labeled targets to determine the relative abundance of nucleic acid sequences in the sample.

22.3.4 Applications of Microarrays

Microarrays can be used for forensic analysis, genotyping or targeted resequencing, measuring predisposition to disease, identifying the drug candidates, evaluating the germline mutations in individuals or somatic mutations in cancers, assessing the loss of heterozygosity, genetic linkage analysis, to detect single-nucleotide polymorphisms (SNPs) among alleles within or between populations, and to measure the changes in gene expression profiling.

22.4 Lateral Flow (Immuno) Assay

22.4.1 Principle

Lateral flow (immuno) assay (LFA) is also known as immunochromatography technique, strip test, or sol particle immunoassay (SPIA). Lateral flow assays are simple devices and used to detect the presence or absence of an antigen or antibody or target analyte in the sample (matrix) without the need for any specialized and sophisticated equipment. The liquid sample or its extract containing the analyte of interest are moved along a strip of polymeric material thereby passing various zones, where molecules have been attached that exert more or less specific interactions with the analyte. The LFA works by chromatographic principle and immunological recognition system.

22.4.2 Parts of LFA Device

The surface layer of a standard LFA format carries the sample from the sample application pad through the conjugate release pad, along the strip across the detection zone, and up to the absorbent pad. Because the membrane is usually thin and fragile, it is attached with a nylon or plastic basic layer to allow handling and cutting easier. The strips are housed in a plastic holder and the reading window and sample application window are only exposed outside. Currently used membrane strips are made from nitrocellulose, nylon, polyethersulfone, polyethylene, and fused silica. Typically, cross-linked silica or cellulose is used to make the sample application pad. The conjugate release pad is made up of cross-linked silica, and it has close contact with the strip material and the sample application pad. The conjugate release pad is labelled with the analyte or recognition element, which are dried and after adding the fluid sample, material in the conjugate release pad will interact with the sample fluid during its flow. The antigen-antibody interactions can be initiated and will continue during the chromatographic processes.

Labels are made of coloured or fluorescent nanoparticles with sizes of 15–800 nm, allowing an unobstructed flow of sample through the membrane. Labels are often made of colloidal gold or latex; less often made of selenium, carbon, or liposomes. To facilitate optical detection, latex nanoparticles are colored. For visualization of liposomes colored fluorescent or bioluminescent dyes can be incorporated.

The strip is sprayed with a minimum of two lines: a test line and a control line. The sample analyte can provide the required visible reaction at the test line, together with the reporter. The response at the control line verifies that the liquid is flowing through the strip properly. In order to perform the multianalyte testing or semiquantitative evaluation of the response, more test lines can be applied. The capillary force of the strip material causes the liquid to travel, but to keep a continous flow, an absorbent pad is attached at the distal side of the strip (Fig. 22.2). This absorbent pad will wick the liquid to the end of the strip, thus maintaining the flow. Lateral flow immunoassay (LFIA) is the term used for the tests that exclusively uses the antibodies as recognition elements. Nucleic acid lateral flow immunoassay

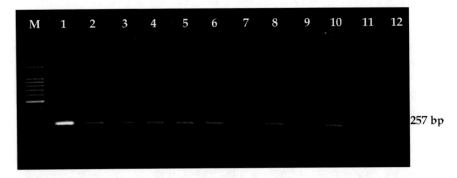

Fig. 22.2 PCR detection of amplified product (257 bp) of p72 or B646L gene of African swine fever virus (ASFV) using the OIE recommended primer sets PPA-1(F) and PPA-2(R). Lane M: 100 bp DNA ladder; L1 – Positive control; L2 to L10 – ASFV suspected samples; L11 - Negative sample; L12 - Negative control

(NALFIA) is a method that combines antigen-antibody interaction with specific tagged double-stranded amplicon detection following PCR. Nucleic acid lateral flow assay (NALF) is a method that allows for the specific nucleic acid hybridization of amplicons using immobilized complementary probes.

22.4.2.1 Membrane Material

The most often used membrane for strip material is made of nitrocellulose. Other polymeric materials are nylon, polyethersulfone, polyethylene, and fused silica. Polyethersulfone substance was used in the NALF format. Desired features for the selection of strip material are the capillary forces of the carrier material, improved capillary flow time, ease of binding, and immobilization of the proteins required for sequential selection, reaction, and detection. Various pore size diameters ranging from 0.05 to 12 µm are available for nitrocellulose membrane. The pore size and the material are important for the transport of the label. The nitrocellulose material should be stored at ambient temperature and humidity, because at low humidity, handling of the material can be difficult due to accumulation of static electricity. Larger pore size may widen the test line and the sensitivity of the test may be reduced, because faint lines of positivity can be missed.

22.4.3 Material of the Sample Pad

The sample pad should possess the property of even distribution of the sample to the conjugate pad. The sample pad should be impregnated with proteins, detergents, viscosity enhancers, and buffer salts to enhance the flow rate of the sample, to increase the sample viscosity and reaction time at the conjugate pad, and to chemically modify the sample for binding at the test line. The selection of material for the sample pad is depending on the aim of the test and the properties of the sample.

22.4.3.1 Material of the Absorbent Pad

The primary function of the absorbent pad is to wick the fluid through the membrane. When an appropriate absorbent pad is utilized, the sample volume can be increased, resulting in an increased sensitivity. Most often cellulose filters are used as a absorbent pad.

22.4.3.2 Material and Size of the Label

Nowadays, colloidal gold and colored latex particles are used most often as material of the label. Carbon and selenium are used as colored nanoparticles. Chemiluminescent and fluorescent nanoparticles are used less often. An important requirement for the nanoparticle labels is their colloidal stability in solution and this can be achieved by coating the binding proteins on the surface of the nanoparticles. It was observed that employing larger particles improved the sensitivity of the test but utilizing the particles larger than 40 nm lowered the stability of the colloid. However, it was reported that gold nanoparticles of 80 nm size, provided the optimum results.

22.4.3.3 Recognition Element

The sensitivity of the LFIA is largely depends on the affinity of the specific primary antibodies. When secondary anti-species antibodies are labelled, the primary antibodies can be titrated for checking concentration for optimal response.

22.4.3.4 Position of the Test Line

The performance of the assay depends on the location of the test line in the strip. When the test line is placed farther downstream from the sample application side of the strip, there is more contact time available. Optimum results are obtained, when the speed of movement of the sample fluid decreases with distance.

22.4.4 Optimization

The first step in the development of LFA diagnostic assay is usually the optimization of the concentration of the recognition element and the label. The second step during LFA development is standardizing the optimal position of the test line. The selection of the strip material, label, and detection method are often depends on the personal choice of the researcher.

22.4.5 Diagnostic Applications

The LFA is frequently employed to detect the pregnancy, function or failure of internal organs (such as heart attack, renal failure, or diabetes), infection or contamination with specific pathogens, including biowarfare agents, presence of toxic substances in food, feed, or the environment, and drug misuse.

22.4.6 Advantages of LFA

The results of LFA are usually obtained within 10–20 min, and it showed high sensitivity, selectivity, and ease of use. Further, it gives qualitative or semiquantitative results. It requires small sample volume and usually designed for individual tests.

22.5 Complement Fixation Test

Complement fixation test (CFT) is an immunological test, which can be used to detect the antibodies in the serum that are specific to certain disease. The CFT is widely used for the diagnosis of microbial infections and rheumatic diseases. However, the usage of CFT in clinical diagnostic laboratories has decreased as a result of the development of alternative serological techniques like ELISA and nucleic acid-based detection techniques like PCR. A group of serum proteins are known as the complement system, which reacts with antigen-antibody complexes. If this reaction takes place on a cell surface, it will cause transmembrane pores to form, which can cause the destruction of the cells.

22.5.1 Principle

The principle of CFT is based on the ability of the antibodies in the test serum to bind to their respective antigens results in formation of complement-activating antigen-antibody immune complexes. The antigen and antibodies are incubated in the presence of guinea pig serum, which acts as a source of complement. The indicator system in CFT is antibody coated sheep RBCs (sRBCs). When specific antigen and antibody are present in the test system, they utilize the complement; hence, the complement is not available to lyse the added antibody-coated sheep RBCs. When antigen or antibody is lacking specificity in the test system, the complement is available to lyse the sensitized sRBCs, because the complement is not fixed. The test can be performed in small test tubes (Wasserman's tubes), haemagglutination plates, or microtitration plates.

22.5.2 Procedure

The following steps are followed while performing the CFT:

1. Serum should be isolated from the infected and convalescent animal blood.
2. It is necessary to destroy the complement proteins present in the infected and convalescent animal serum and replace them with a predetermined quantity of standardized complement proteins. The serum should be heated at 56 °C for 30 min to destroy the complement proteins without destroying the antibodies. Compared to antibodies, complement proteins are much more vulnerable to destruction by heat.
3. The serum is also added with a known quantity of standard complement proteins. Guinea pig serum is a rich source of complement, hence it is routinely used to obtain the complement proteins.
4. The antigen of interest should be added to the serum.
5. Hemolysin: Rabbit antiserum against sheep erythrocytes can be prepared, inactivated at 56 °C for 30 min, and a hemolytic titer of 2 units per 0.5 mL is determined.
6. The sRBCs have been pre-bound to anti-sRBC antibodies are added to the serum.

22.5.3 Interpretation of Results

1. During a positive reaction, antibodies against the antigen of interest present in the infected and convalescent animal serum binds to the antigen and forms antigen-

antibody complexes. The binding of the complement to an antigen-antibody complexes, results in depletion of complement, and is not available to interact with sensitized RBCs. Hence, sensitized RBCs remain unlysed and settle to the bottom of the wells to form a button.
2. During a negative reaction, antibodies against the antigen of interest are absent in the sample, hence the complement will not be depleted. Further, the complement remains free to interact with the sRBC-Ab complexes, causing them to lyse the sRBCs results in formation of red or pink solution.

22.5.4 Detection of Antigen

Most frequently, the CFT is used for the detection of antibodies. For the detection of antigen, infected and convalescent animal serum should be supplemented with specific antibody to induce the formation of antigen-antibody complexes, complement and indicator sRBC.

22.5.5 Quantitative Testing

The test can be performed for quantitative purpose by making serial dilutions of infected and convalescent animal serum and determining the highest dilution factor that can show a positive CF test. This titer is correlated with the dilution factor.

22.5.6 Applications of CFT

The CFT has been used for the determination of antimicrobial antibodies or antigen in infected and convalescent animal sera and direct measurement of complement activity using antibody-sensitized RBCs. The CFT is well-known simple protocol, easy to perform, reliable, inexpensive, and ideal for screening purposes. However, it requires long time to obtain the results and the laborious protocol. This test is used for diagnosis of certain diseases, including African horse sickness, brucellosis (confirmatory test for international trade), anaplasmosis (standard test for detection of carrier animals), babesiosis, eperythrozoonosis, epizootic hemorrhagic disease, bluetongue, contagious bovine pleuropneumonia (CBPP), glanders, sporadic bovine encephalomyelitis, enzootic abortion in ewes, Q-fever, Yersiniosis, Melioidosis etc.

22.6 High-Performance Liquid Chromatography (HPLC)

22.6.1 Principle

High-performance liquid chromatography is also referred to as high-pressure liquid chromatography (HPLC) and is a powerful tool in analysis of samples. The HPLC is basically a greatly improved version of column chromatography. The HPLC is an analytical chemistry method for separating, identifying, and quantifying the individual components in a sample containing mixture of components. It depends on the pumps to pass a pressurized (up to 400 atmospheres) liquid solvent containing the sample mixture through a column filled wit a solid adsorbent material more quickly. Each component in the sample interacts slightly differently with the adsorbent material, causing various flow rates for the different components and leading to the separation of the components as they flow out the column.

Further, it allows a smaller tiny particle size for the column packing material, which provides a significantly greater surface area for interactions between the stationary phase and the molecules passing through it. This allows a better separation of the components of the mixture. The HPLC is extremely sensitive and highly automated technique.

22.6.2 Types of HPLC

Different types of HPLC techniques are aqueous normal-phase chromatography, size-exclusion chromatography, ion-exchange chromatography, bioaffinity chromatography, displacement chromatography, normal-phase chromatography, partition chromatography, and reversed-phase chromatography (RPC).

22.6.2.1 Normal-Phase HPLC

The principle of normal-phase HPLC is same as that of thin layer chromatography or column chromatography. The normal-phase HPLC is not most commonly used method. The solvent is non-polar (hexane), and the column is filled with tiny silica particles. A typical column measures 150 to 250 mm in length and has an interior diameter of less than 4.6 mm. Polar compounds in the mixture being passed through the column will stick longer to the polar silica than the non-polar compounds. Therefore, the non-polar compounds pass through the column more quickly.

22.6.2.2 Reversed-Phase HPLC

Reversed-phase HPLC is the most widely employed HPLC method. The column size is same in this type, but the silica has been changed to make it non-polar by having lengthy hydrocarbon chains attached to its surface (either 8 or 18 carbon atoms). A polar solvent such as mixture of water and alcohol (methanol) is used. There is a strong attraction between the polar solvent and the polar molecules in the mixture being transported through the column. There is a weak interaction between

22.6 High-Performance Liquid Chromatography (HPLC)

the polar molecules in the solution and the hydrocarbon chains attached to the silica (the stationary phase). Therefore, polar molecules in the mixture can spend most of their time moving with the solvent.

Non-polar compounds in the mixture will tend to form attractions with the hydrocarbon groups because of van der Waals dispersion forces. Therefore, they spend less time in solution in the solvent and move slowly through the column. The polar molecules will travel through the column more quickly.

22.6.3 Procedure

22.6.3.1 Injection of the Sample
The sample is injected by complete automatically due to the involvement of pressures.

22.6.3.2 Retention Time
The time taken for a particular compound to travel through the column to the detector is known as retention time. This period of time is calculated from the time at which the sample is injected to the point at which the display shows a maximum peak for that compound. Retention time varies with different compounds. The retention period may vary for a particular compound depending on:

- Pressure applied (influences the flow rate of solvents)
- Nature of the stationary phase (depends on material made and particle size)
- Exact composition of the solvent
- Temperature of the column

22.6.3.3 The Detector
There are several ways of detecting when a compound has passed through the column. Ultraviolet absorption is a widely used and easy method for detection. Various organic compounds absorb UV light at different wavelengths. The amount of light absorbed may depend on the amount of particular compound that is passing through the beam at the time. Water absorbs at wavelength below 190 nm and methanol absorbs at wavelength below 205 nm. Methanol-water mixture solvent absorbs at wavelength greater than 205 nm.

22.6.3.4 Interpreting the Output from the Detector
The output will be recorded as a series of peaks and each peak representing a compound in the mixture passing through the detector and absorbing UV light. Careful monitoring of the column conditions and the retention time can help to identify the compounds present in the sample. The quantities of the compounds present in the sample can also be measured using the peaks. The area under the peak is proportional to the amount of compound in the sample, which has passed the detector, and this area can be calculated automatically by the computer linked to the display. The area under the peak would be less, but the retention time would remain

the same, if the solution contained a less concentration of the compound. If two different compounds present in the mixture of sample and the relative amounts of these substances were not possible to detect using the UV absorption method.

22.6.4 Applications of HPLC

The HPLC has been used in the field of medicine (for the detection of vitamin D levels in blood serum), vetero-legal (for the detection of performance-enhancing drugs in urine), research (for the separation of components of a complex biological sample or similar synthetic chemicals from each other), and manufacturing (during the production process of pharmaceutical and biological products).

22.7 Confocal Microscopy

Confocal microscopy is an optical imaging technique that uses point illumination and a spatial pinhole to eliminate the out-of-focus light in specimens that are thicker than the focal plane. Confocal microscopy improves the optical resolution and contrast of a micrograph. It enables the reconstruction of three-dimensional structures from the obtained images. Marvin Minsky invented the principle of confocal imaging in 1957 with the intention of overcoming some of the drawbacks of traditional wide-field fluorescence microscopes.

22.7.1 Principle

The confocal microscope employs point illumination and a pinhole in an optically conjugate plane in front of the detector to eliminate out-of-focus signal. The optical resolution of images, particularly in the sample depth direction, is significantly better than that of wide-field microscopes, because only fluorescence light is extremely close to the focal plane can be detected.

The confocal microscopy is a most specialized fluorescence imaging technique, and it relies on the same principles of traditional epifluorescence microscope does to form an image. Fluorescence is a two-stage process, where a fluorescent molecule or fluorophore absorbs photons from a particular wavelength of light, and this absorption event then triggers the fluorophore to emit photons of light at a longer wavelength than its absorption. In green fluorophore, the majority of the excitation is in the blue range from 470 to 490 nanometers (nm), and the emission is in the green, which ranges from 510 to 550 nm. When compared to a traditional fluorescence microscope, the confocal microscope provides increased contrast, sharpness, and resolution in the image and creates the three-dimensional data sets. Confocal microscopes utilize the lasers for excitation. Lasers are monochromatic and highly collimated light sources that provide tons of power and does not need a separate excitation filter.

22.7 Confocal Microscopy

The confocal microscopes use an adjustable aperture diaphragm called a pinhole to physically reject fluorescence emission from planes outside the primary focus plane of the objective. The larger pinhole diameter causes more focal planes that may contribute to the image, and smaller pinhole diameter results in fewer planes that may contribute to the image. The diameter of the pinhole is expressed in Airy units (AU) on a confocal microscope. In addition to the pinhole diameter, the numerical aperture of the objective lens has the largest influence on overall resolution. Numerical aperture is the ratio of diameter of lens to its focal length. Numerical aperture is the measure of its ability to gather light and to resolve fine specimen detail while working at a fixed object (or specimen) distance. Resolution is the ability to view closely adjacent structures as separate and distinct. The choice of objective lens will control the numerical aperture. The numerical aperture directly influences the resolution of the lens. Along with the numerical aperture, the wavelength of emission light by the fluorophore will play a role in the resolution of the instrument. The shorter wavelength of light may give the high resolution. Objectives are designed for imaging in high refractive index solutions such as glycerol or oil.

In confocal imaging, the photomultipliers (PMTs) are employed to produce relatively lengthy pulses, in the range of about 20 ns. Primarily, detectors are highly sensitive PMTs due to the light-rejecting nature of a confocal microscope. These are essentially single-spot cameras that maximize the light signals by amplifying the signals over a photoelectric device. Light intensity is the number of photons per unit time detected in a given picture element. The intensity is expressed as "counts per second" in the photon-counting mode.

The variables that affect the thickness of the optical section are:

- Pinhole diameter
- Numerical aperture of the lens
- Wavelength of emission light
- Refractive index of any immersion fluid required by the objective

22.7.2 Applications of Confocal Microscope

Nowadays, confocal microscopy is widely utilized in high-quality imaging and analysis technique in the field of biomedical sciences. It is used for locating the individual genes on the individual chromosomes using fluorescence PCR and hybridization. It is also used for live cell imaging and imaging inside a cell or tissue. Further, confocal microscopy is used for protein trafficking, in which, where a protein of interest is attached or located can be identified by using green fluorescent protein (GFP), or other fluorochromes to track intracellular protein movement. Using specific fluorescent dyes, confocal imaging is used to analyze the subcellular functions including pH gradients and membrane potentials. It is also used to measure the intracellular changes in the ion concentrations of substances like calcium, sodium, magnesium, zinc, and potassium. It is an extremely useful technique for capturing the images of a variety of biological specimens.

22.7.3 Advantages of Confocal Microscopy

The benefits of confocal microscope are decreased blurring of the image from light scattering, increased resolution, improved signal-to-noise ratio, clear examination of thick specimens, Z-axis scanning, perception of depth in Z-sectioned images, and magnification can be adjusted electronically. It is possible to capture very sharp three-dimensional images of the sample. Further, it eliminates out-of-focus noise by improving the resolution and considerably enhancing the sensitivity of the machine.

22.7.4 Cons of Confocal Microscope

The time required to capture the images from approximately 50 z optical slices is around 15 min, which makes the image acquisition procedure often quite time-consuming. Only a few laboratories have confocal microscope facilities because of the high purchasing and maintaining costs of the confocal microscope.

22.8 Fluorescence-Activated Cell Sorting (FACS)

A specialized type of flow cytometry is called as fluorescence-activated cell sorting (FACS). It is a technique for sorting (separating) a one biological cell type at a time from a heterogeneous mixture of biological cells into two or more containers based upon the specific light scattering and fluorescence properties of each cell (Parks et al. 1979; Tsien 1998). The FACS provides a fast, objective and quantitative recording of fluorescent signals from the individual cells as well as physical separation of cells of a specific interest. Based on their size and fluorescence color, the FACS can quickly separate the cells in a suspension. Mack Fulwyler invented the first cell sorter in 1965 utilizing the Coulter principle. Len Herzenberg modified it and came up with the term FACS (Herzenberg et al. 1976; Tsien 1998).

22.8.1 Principle

Fluorescent dyes are used to label the live or preserved cells. Individual cells are sorted based on their fluorescence markers. Frequently used for cell cycle studies and cell purification based on the cell surface protein expression. In multicellular organisms, all the cells have identical DNA, but their proteins differ greatly. As a result, it is feasible to separate and distinguish between cells that differ phenotypically from one other. Further, it is feasible to determine the number of cells that expressed particular protein of interest and how much of that protein expressed in those cells (Anderson et al. 1996; Bigos et al. 1999).

22.8.2 Mechanism of FACS

- FACS machine has following parts: one laser and two light detectors (one for forward scatter to measure a cell size and one for fluorescence).
- A cell suspension comprising target cells that have been fluorescently labeled is directed into a thin stream, so that the cells pass one after the other in a single file. The dye is labelled with an antigen-specific monoclonal antibody and binds with the antigen in the cells of interest.
- A nozzle produces a thin stream vibrates at 40,000 cycles per second, which divides the stream into 40,000 distinct droplets each second. These droplets may contain a cell.
- A laser beam is directed at the stream just before it breaks up into droplets.
- As each labeled cell passes through the beam and its resulting fluorescence is detected by a photocell.
- The laser light scattered by the cells is used to count the cells. The size of the cells can also be measured using this scattered light.
- The laser light excites the dye, which emits a color of light that is detected by the photomultiplier tube or light detector. A computer can determine which cells need to be isolated and collected by collecting the data from the scatter and fluorescence light.
- If the signals from the two detectors meet either of the criteria set for fluorescence and size, an electrical charge (positive or negative) is given to the stream.
- As they move between two charged metal plates, the droplets maintain their charge.
  - Positively-charged droplets are attracted by the negatively-charged plate and vice versa.
  - Uncharged droplets (those without cells or with cells that fails to meet the desired criteria of size and fluorescence) pass straight and directly into a third container and are then discarded.
- The end result is three tubes with pure subpopulations of cells. Each tube contains a known number of cells, and the level of fluorescence is also recorded for each cell.
- FACS device has a maximum sorting rate of 3,000,000 cells per minute (Herzenberg et al. 1976; Tsien 1998).

22.8.3 Procedure

- Stain the cells with fluorescent dye labeled with an antigen-specific monoclonal antibody under sterile conditions.
- Resuspend the cells in Hank's balanced salt solution (HBSS) or a serum-free medium containing antimicrobials, and keep the sample on ice.
- Samples must have a volume of more than 0.5 mL with a cell density of not less than 15×10^6/mL, and cells must be in a single-cell suspension.

- After trypsinization, adherent cells should be resuspended thoroughly, and cell clumps should be eliminated by passing cells through a cell-strainer with a 5 mM EDTA solution.
- Sometimes, large number of dead cells can cause clumping through the release of genomic DNA and this can be prevented by DNAse (10 U/ml).
- Cell culture medium is not the ideal buffer for sorting because pH indicators such as phenol red can cause emission interference and calcium in the medium can be precipitated by phosphates in buffers used in the sorting machine.
- A basic sorting buffer is cation-free PBS containing 1 mM EDTA, 25 mM hydroxyl ethyl piperazine ethane sulfonic acid (HEPES), pH 7.0, and 1% serum.
- The default nozzle used by the machine has a 100 μm opening.
- Control sample is needed for adjusting the machine settings and sort the cells (Herzenberg et al. 1976; Tsien 1998).

22.8.4 Quantifying the FACS Data

1. FACS data collected by the computer can be displayed in two different ways. It gives information about how many cells were sorted into each color? The number of cells with each degree of fluorescence is plotted on the Y-axis, while the intensity of the green or red fluorescence is plotted on the X-axis. This approach works best when all the cells are either green, red, or unlabeled, and no cells are labelled for both colors (Fig. 22.3).
2. The red fluorescence intensity is plotted on the Y-axis, while the green fluorescence intensity is plotted on the X-axis. The individual black dots represent individual cells in each quadrant. The top right quadrant contains no cells labeled with both red and green, and bottom left quadrant contains many unlabeled cells. The level of fluorescence was higher in the green cells than the red cells (Fig. 22.4). This way of graphing the data is particularly helpful if cells are present that have been labeled with both red and green (Fig. 22.5) (Herzenberg et al. 1976; Tsien 1998).

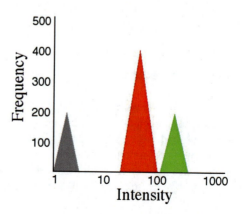

Fig. 22.3 Quantifying the FACS data